Pleural Diseases

Fourth Edition

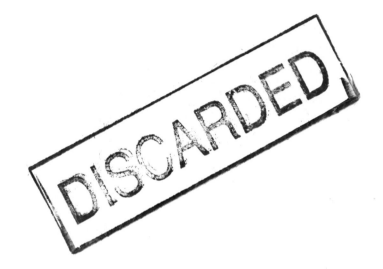

J74.33

DISCARDED

Pleural Diseases

Fourth Edition

Richard W. Light, M.D., F.C.C.P.

*Professor of Medicine, Pulmonary Division, Vanderbilt University;
Director of Pulmonary Disease Program, Department of Pulmonary
Medicine, Saint Thomas Hospital, Nashville, Tennessee*

LIPPINCOTT WILLIAMS & WILKINS
A **Wolters Kluwer** Company
Philadelphia • Baltimore • New York • London
Buenos Aires • Hong Kong • Sydney • Tokyo

A 020759

THE LIBRARY
POSTGRADUATE CENTRE
MAIDSTONE HOSPITAL

WF 700

0028469

Acquisitions Editor: Joyce-Rachel John
Developmental Editor: Kerry B. Barrett
Production Editor: John C. Vassiliou
Manufacturing Manager: Benjamin Rivera
Cover Designer: Mark Lerner
Compositor: The PRD Group
Printer: Edwards Brothers

© **2001 by LIPPINCOTT WILLIAMS & WILKINS**
530 Walnut Street
Philadelphia, PA 19106 USA
LWW.com

All rights reserved. This book is protected by copyright. No part of this book may be reproduced in any form or by any means, including photocopying, or utilized by any information storage and retrieval system without written permission from the copyright owner, except for brief quotations embodied in critical articles and reviews. Materials appearing in this book prepared by individuals as part of their official duties as U.S. government employees are not covered by the above-mentioned copyright.

Printed in the USA

Library of Congress Cataloging-in-Publication Data
Light, Richard W.
    Pleural diseases / Richard W. Light.—4th ed.
      p. ; cm.
    Includes bibliographical references and index.
    ISBN 0-7817-2777-4
    1. Pleura—Diseases.   I. Title.
    [DNLM: 1. Pleural Diseases. WF 700 L723p 2001]
  RC751 .L48   2001
  616.2′5—dc21   00-065522

Care has been taken to confirm the accuracy of the information presented and to describe generally accepted practices. However, the author and publisher are not responsible for errors or omissions or for any consequences from application of the information in this book and make no warranty, expressed or implied, with respect to the currency, completeness, or accuracy of the contents of the publication. Application of this information in a particular situation remains the professional responsibility of the practitioner.

The author and publisher have exerted every effort to ensure that drug selection and dosage set forth in this text are in accordance with current recommendations and practice at the time of publication. However, in view of ongoing research, changes in government regulations, and the constant flow of information relating to drug therapy and drug reactions, the reader is urged to check the package insert for each drug for any change in indications and dosage and for added warnings and precautions. This is particularly important when the recommended agent is a new or infrequently employed drug.

Some drugs and medical devices presented in this publication have Food and Drug Administration (FDA) clearance for limited use in restricted research settings. It is the responsibility of the health care provider to ascertain the FDA status of each drug or device planned for use in their clinical practice.

10 9 8 7 6 5 4 3 2 1

This book is dedicated to my many friends throughout the world who have collaborated with my study of pleural disease.

Contents

Preface

The first three editions of *Pleural Diseases* were well received. Since the third edition was published in 1995, there has been a rapid advancement of knowledge concerning pleural diseases. Accordingly, the publishers have requested that I prepare a fourth edition.

As I prepared the fourth edition, I was impressed with how much new information concerning pleural diseases has become known during the past 5 years. New references have been added for nearly every disease of the pleura discussed in this book. Highlights of changes include the following:

Two new chapters have been added to this edition. There is a chapter on pleural effusions due to diseases of the heart. Included in the chapter is new information about diagnosis, pleural fluid characteristics, and management of patients with pleural effusions after coronary artery bypass surgery. There is also a new chapter on pleural disease in obstetrics and gynecology. This chapter covers pleural effusions due to the ovarian hyperstimulation syndrome, fetal pleural effusions, postpartum pleural effusions, Meigs' syndrome, and pleural effusion due to endometriosis.

The recommended approach to the patient with an undiagnosed pleural effusion has been altered. The use of spiral CT scans in the evaluation of patients with pleural effusion to establish the diagnosis of pulmonary embolism or to demonstrate parenchymal or mediastinal abnormalities is now recommended. The diagnosis of tuberculous pleuritis is now established by demonstrating elevated levels of adenosine deaminase or gamma interferon in the pleural fluid. In centers where it is available, thoracoscopy has largely replaced needle biopsy of the pleura in evaluating patients with undiagnosed pleural effusions.

The therapy of malignant pleural effusion continues to evolve. In the previous edition, I recommended talc as the sclerosing agent of choice. However, since it is now clear that intrapleural talc induces acute respiratory distress syndrome in a small percentage of cases, talc is no longer recommended. Rather, doxycycline is recommended as the sclerosing agent of choice in conjunction with tube thoracostomy, while pleural abrasion is the recommended procedure when pleurodesis is attempted at the time of thoracoscopy. In addition, the feasibility of treating malignant pleural effusions on an outpatient basis with indwelling catheters is discussed.

Since the previous edition, I have altered my recommended approach to the management of parapneumonic effusions. It is now recommended that all patients initially undergo a therapeutic rather than a diagnostic thoracentesis. If the fluid never recurs, one need not worry about the pleural effusion. If the fluid cannot be removed, then the patient can be subjected either to a tube thoracostomy with the instillation of fibrinolytic agents or a thoracoscopy with the breakdown of loculations and the optimal placement of chest tubes. If these treatments are unsuccessful, the patient should be subjected to decortication. The definitive procedure for the treatment of the parapneumonic effusion should be performed within 10 days of the patient initially being seen.

Other new areas which are covered in this edition include spontaneous bacterial pleuritis which occurs in conjunction with cirrhosis and ascites and is analogous to spontaneous bacterial peritonitis, and the pleural effusions that occur as a complication of bone marrow transplantation, drowning, and rupture of a mediastinal cyst. The clinical manifestations, diagnosis, and treatment of two recently described primary malignancies of the pleura, namely, pyothorax associated lymphoma and body cavity lymphoma, are discussed. The pleural effusions which occur secondary to Rocky Mountain Spotted Fever and ehrlichiosis are also discussed.

It is my hope that this fourth edition will continue to provide a practical, updated reference for health care professionals who care for patients with pleural disease.

Richard W. Light, M.D.

Preface to the First Edition

Approximately one million patients develop a pleural effusion each year. Pleural effusions may occur with many different infections or as a complication of pulmonary disease. Additionally, pleural effusions frequently complicate malignant disease, heart disease, liver disease, gastrointestinal disease, kidney disease, and collagen vascular disease. Yet there are no recent books on pleural disease to guide the practicing physician in determining the origin of a pleural effusion or in managing a patient with pleural disease. Moreover, diseases of the pleura receive only superficial treatment in books on pulmonary disease or internal medicine.

This book is intended primarily as a reference book for physicians who take care of patients with pleural diseases. Recent advances in the knowledge of pleural disease make publication of this volume timely. In this one volume, the practicing physician will have a comprehensive discussion of all aspects of pleural disease.

The first three chapters discuss the anatomy, physiology, and radiology of the pleura. The next chapter describes the clinical manifestations of pleural disease and discusses in depth the various diagnostic tests that might be used to establish the etiology of a pleural effusion. In Chapter 5, I present my recommended approach to the patient with an undiagnosed pleural effusion. The following 13 chapters contain discussions of the various disease states that can be associated with a pleural effusion. For each disease, the pathophysiology, clinical manifestations, diagnosis, and management of pleural effusion are outlined. In Chapters 19 through 21, pneumothorax, hemothorax, and chylothorax are presented, respectively. Pleural thickening not associated with pleural fluid is covered in Chapter 22. The next two chapters are devoted to those procedures used most often in managing patients with pleural disease, namely, diagnostic and therapeutic thoracentesis, pleural biopsy, and tube thoracostomy. The final chapter includes a description of the various drainage systems used with chest tubes.

It is my hope that publication of this book will result in better and more cost-effective management of patients with pleural disease.

Richard W. Light, M.D.

Acknowledgments

Many individuals contributed to this book and I acknowledge the following: Dr. Michael Rodriguez and Dr. Phillip Moyers who sought new radiographs for this edition. Many hours were devoted by Drs. Barrett Conner, Y.C. (Gary) Lee, and K. Hassaan Mohamed and Mr. Jeffrey Rogers and Mr. Tommie Johnson to reviewing the book's content. My present administrative assistant, Ms. Ada Chako-Moore and my previous administrative assistant, Ms. Sheila Rupp, who spent hours gathering new references and proofreading the manuscript. My wife, Judi Light, who carefully read every chapter and constantly encouraged me to proceed with the book. And finally, I thank Joyce-Rachel John, Acquisitions Editor, and Kerry Barrett, Associate Developmental Editor, at Lippincott Williams & Wilkins for their constant support while the book was prepared.

Acknowledgments

Pleural Diseases

Fourth Edition

1

Anatomy of the Pleura

The pleura is the serous membrane that covers the lung parenchyma, the mediastinum, the diaphragm, and the rib cage. This structure is divided into the visceral pleura and the parietal pleura. The visceral pleura covers the lung parenchyma, not only at its points of contact with the chest wall, diaphragm, and mediastinum but also in the interlobar fissures. The parietal pleura lines the inside of the thoracic cavities. In accordance with the intrathoracic surfaces that it lines, it is subdivided into the costal, mediastinal, and diaphragmatic parietal pleura. The visceral and the parietal pleura meet at the lung root. At the pulmonary hilus, the mediastinal pleura is swept laterally onto the root of the lung. Posterior to the lung root, the pleura is carried downward as a thin double fold called the pulmonary ligament.

A film of fluid (pleural fluid) is normally present between the parietal and the visceral pleura. This thin layer of fluid acts as a lubricant and allows the visceral pleura covering the lung to slide along the parietal pleura lining the thoracic cavity during respiratory movements. The space, or potential space, between the two layers of pleura is designated as the pleural space. The mediastinum completely separates the right from the left pleural space in humans. As previously mentioned, only a thin layer of fluid is normally present in this space, so it is a potential rather than an actual space. Many diseases are associated with increased amounts of pleural fluid, however, and a large segment of this book is directed toward an understanding of these diseases.

EMBRYOLOGY OF THE PLEURA AND PLEURAL SPACE

The body cavity in the embryo, the coelomic cavity, is a U-shaped system with the thick bend cephalad. The cephalad portion becomes the pericardium and communicates bilaterally with the pleural canals, which, in turn, communicate with the peritoneal canals. With development, the coelomic cavity becomes divided into the pericardium, the pleural cavities, and the peritoneal cavity through the development of three sets of partitions: (a) the septum transversum, which serves as an early, partial diaphragm; (b) the pleuropericardial membranes, which divide the pericardial and pleural cavities; and (c) the pleuroperitoneal membranes, which unite with the septum transversum to complete the partition between each pleural cavity and the peritoneal cavity. This newly formed pleural cavity is fully lined by a mesothelial membrane, the pleura (1).

When the primordial bronchial buds first appear, they and the trachea lie in a median mass of mesenchyme, cranial and dorsal to the peritoneal cavity. This mass of mesenchymal tissue is the future mediastinum and separates the two pleural cavities. In humans, no communication normally exists between the two pleural cavities. As the growing primordial lung buds bulge into the right and left pleural cavities, they carry with them a covering of the lining mesothelium, which becomes the visceral pleura. As the separate lobes evolve, they retain their mesothelial covering. This covering becomes the visceral pleura in the fissures. The lining mesothelium of the pleural cavity becomes the parietal pleura (2).

HISTOLOGY OF THE PLEURA

The parietal pleura over the ribs and intercostal spaces is composed of loose, irregular connective tissue covered by a single layer of mesothelial cells. Within the pleura are blood vessels, mainly capillaries, and lymphatic lacunas. The lacunas are specialized initial lymphatics shaped like flat cisterns and are located over the intercostal spaces, at least in sheep (3). The mean thickness of the parietal pleura in sheep is 20 to 25 μm, whereas the distance from the microvessels to the pleural space is 10 to 12 μm. Deep to the parietal pleura is the endothoracic fascia. This continuous band of dense irregular connective tissue, composed mainly of collagen and elastin, covers the ribs and intercostal spaces and varies in thickness from 75 to 150 μm (3).

The anatomy of the visceral pleura differs markedly from that of the parietal pleura and also varies among species, primarily by its thickness. The dog, cat, and monkey have a thin visceral pleura, whereas humans, sheep, cows, pigs, and horses have a thick visceral pleura (4). The distinction between lungs with a thick or thin visceral pleura is important physiologically because the blood supply is dependent on the thickness of the pleura. In animals with a thick visceral pleura, the predominant source of blood is the systemic circulation; in those with a thin pleura, the predominant source of blood is the pulmonary circulation (4).

Histologically, a thick visceral pleura is composed of two layers: the mesothelium and connective tissue. Blood and lymph vessels and nerves are located in the connective tissue. Animals with a thick visceral pleura have a layer of dense connective tissue of varying thickness interposed between the mesothelium and the blood vessels (4). In sheep, the visceral pleura ranges in thickness from 25 to 83 μm (compared with 10 to 25 μm for the parietal pleura) and the distance from the microvessels to the pleural space ranges from 18 to 56 μm (compared with 10 to 12 μm for the parietal space) (3).

The connective tissue layer in the visceral pleura has two important functions: (a) It contributes to the elastic recoil of the lung, which is important in expelling air from the lung, and (b) it restricts the volume to which the lung can be inflated, thereby protecting the lung (5). In the visceral pleura, fibers of the elastic and collagenous systems are clearly interdependent elements. Collagenous fibers are interwoven in a pleated structure that closely resembles the osiers of a wicker basket, suggesting that collagen fibers allow the lung volume to increase up to a point of maximal stretching of the system (5). The pleural contribution to lung elastic recoil pressure originates from the elastic network, which returns to its resting position when inspiratory pressures are negligible (5).

Both the visceral and the parietal pleura are lined with a single layer of flat mesothelial cells. These mesothelial cells range in size from 6 to 12 μm in diameter (6). With scanning electron microscopy (7), the pleural surface is found to either be flattened or bumpy (Fig. 1.1). The bumpy areas include most of the visceral pleura and portions of the parietal pleura, including the subcostal regions and the pleural recesses. The bumpy areas appear to result from a lack of rigidity of the underlying structures (6).

Scanning electron microscopy also demonstrates that microvilli are present diffusely over the entire pleural surface (Fig. 1.1), but the distribution of the microvilli is irregular. The density of the microvilli ranges from less than a few to more than 600 per 100 square μm, with a mean of about 300 (1). The microvilli are most numerous on the inferior parts of the visceral pleura and the anterior and inferior mediastinum on the parietal pleura (1). At corresponding regions in the thoracic cavity, more microvilli are present on the visceral pleura than on the parietal pleura. The microvilli are approximately 0.1 μm in diameter, and their length varies from 0.5 to 3.0 μm (1).

The exact function of these numerous microvilli has yet to be defined. At one time it was believed that their presence increased the capacity of the visceral pleura to absorb pleural fluid. This is probably incorrect because recent observations have indicated that the visceral pleura plays a limited role in the absorption of pleural fluid. It is now thought that the most important function of the microvilli is to enmesh glycoproteins that are rich in hyaluronic acid, especially in the lower thorax, to lessen the friction between

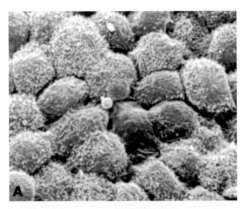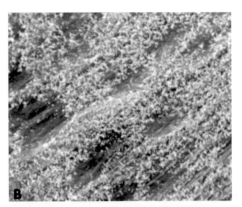

FIG. 1.1. Scanning electron microscopic studies of the pleura. **A:** Bumpy pleural surface with cellular borders irregularly depressed. Note that the number of microvilli present on each cell is variable. (Original magnification: 1,300×). **B:** Flattened pleural surface with indistinct cell boundaries and sparse microvilli. (Original magnification: 1250×). (From Wang NS. The regional difference of pleural mesothelial cells in rabbits. *Am Rev Respir Dis* 1974;110:623–633, with permission.)

the lung and the chest wall (7). Moreover, as mentioned earlier, a thin rim of fluid normally separates the visceral and parietal pleura. Impingement of the microvilli from one pleural surface into the opposing pleural surface could possibly help to maintain this thin rim of fluid (8), but this is controversial (9).

The mesothelial cells are active cells, and they are sensitive and responsive to various stimuli. In cell culture, mesothelial cells have been shown to produce type I, type II, and type IV collagens, elastin, fibronectin, and laminin, and to express intermediate filaments typical of both epithelial cells and fibroblasts (10). Mesothelial cells also express procoagulant activity due to a tissue factor that binds factor VII at the cell surface (11). Mesothelial cells have also been demonstrated to produce nitric oxide (12) and transforming growth factor β-1 (13).

The mesothelial layer is very fragile. At thoracotomy in patients without clinical pleural disease, focal denudation of mesothelial cells is common (14). When the normal layer of mesothelial cells lining the pleura is disrupted, the defect is repaired through mitosis and migration of the mesothelial cells (14, 15). When irritated, they retract but retain continuity with adjacent cells by projections called cellular bridges. Mesothelial cells frequently are dislodged from the pleural surfaces and thereby are free in the

pleural fluid. When free in the pleural space, the cells become round or oval (15). Their cytoplasm is rich in organelles. From this state, they may be transformed into macrophages capable of phagocytosis and erythrophagocytosis (15). Such transformed cells frequently have vacuoles in their cytoplasm. Not all the macrophages in pleural fluid evolve from mesothelial cells; some definitely evolve from peripheral blood mononuclear cells, and some may evolve from alveolar macrophages (16). An immunologic role for the macrophages derived from the mesothelial cells has been suggested (16).

PLEURAL FLUID

The major considerations in the understanding of pleural fluid are volume, thickness, cellular components, and physicochemical factors.

Volume

Normally, a small amount of pleural fluid is present in the pleural space. The mechanisms responsible for this small amount of residual fluid are discussed in Chapter 2. Although no reliable data on normal human pleural fluid are available, several studies have been conducted on the pleural fluid in normal animals. Miserocchi and Agostoni carefully measured the volume of pleural fluid in normal rabbits and dogs (17). They found that the rabbits' pleural spaces contained about 1.0 mL pleural fluid, whereas the dogs' pleural spaces contained about 2.4 mL pleural fluid. Sahn et al. (18) reported that there was 0.4 mL fluid in the rabbits' pleural spaces, but these researchers did not measure the fluid that adheres to the pleural surface and accounts for approximately 50% of the total pleural fluid (17).

Thickness

The small amount of residual pleural fluid appears to be distributed relatively evenly throughout the pleural space. Therefore, the pleural fluid behaves as a continuous system. Albertine and associates studied the thickness of pleural fluid in rabbits by four different methods (9). They found that the average arithmetic mean width of the pleural space was slightly more narrow near the top (18.5 μm) than at the bottom (20.3 μm). Pleural space width in the most dependent recesses, such as the costodiaphragmatic recess, reached 1 to 2 mm. They were unable to find any contacts between the visceral and parietal pleura. Because the microvilli of the mesothelial cells in the visceral and parietal pleural do not interdigitate, the frictional forces between the lungs and chest wall are low (9).

Cells

Normal pleural fluid, at least in rabbits and dogs, contains significant numbers of white blood cells and few red blood cells. Miserocchi and Agostoni reported that rabbit and dog pleural fluid contains about 2,450 and 2,200 white blood cells per mm^3, respectively (17). In the rabbit, 32% of the cells were mesothelial cells, whereas 61% were mononuclear cells and 7% were lymphocytes. In the dog, 70% of the cells were mesothelial cells, 28% were mononuclear cells, and 2% were lymphocytes. Sahn and colleagues also studied normal rabbit pleural fluid and reported a total white cell count of 1,500 per mm^3, with the differential count revealing 70% monocytes, 11% lymphocytes, 9% mesothelial cells, 7% macrophages, and 2% polymorphonuclear leukocytes (18). The variance in the differential count in these series may be related to the stains used and the definition of mesothelial cells and macrophages.

Physicochemical Factors

A small amount of protein is normally present in the pleural fluid. In rabbits, the protein concentration averages 1.33 g per dL, whereas in dogs, it averages 1.06 g per dL (17). The mean oncotic pressure in the pleural fluid is 4.8 cm H_2O in rabbits and 3.2 cm H_2O in dogs (17). Protein electrophoresis demonstrates that the electrophoretic pattern for pleural fluid is similar to that of the corresponding serum, except that low-molecular-weight proteins such as albumin are present in relatively greater quantities in the pleural fluid.

Interestingly, the ionic concentrations in pleural fluid differ significantly from those in serum. The pleural fluid bicarbonate concentration is increased by 20% to 25% relative to that of plasma, whereas the major cation (Na^+) is reduced by 3% to 5%, and the major anion (Cl^-) is reduced by 6% to 9%. The concentration of K^+ and glucose in the pleural fluid and plasma appears to be nearly identical (19). The gradient for bicarbonate persists when the animals are given a carbonic anhydrase inhibitor. When unilateral artificial pleural effusions of distilled water were produced in rats, electrolyte equilibrium between pleural fluid and venous plasma was reached in about 40 minutes, but the foregoing gradients persisted. The pleural fluid P_{CO_2} is about the same as the plasma P_{CO_2}. Accordingly, in view of the elevated pleural fluid bicarbonate, the pleural fluid is alkaline with respect to the plasma pH (19). These gradients for electrolytes suggest that an active process is involved in pleural fluid formation. The significance of such an active process remains to be defined.

BLOOD SUPPLY OF THE PLEURA

The parietal pleura receives its blood supply from the systemic capillaries. Small branches of the intercostal arteries supply the costal pleura, whereas the mediastinal pleura is supplied principally by the pericardiacophrenic artery. The diaphragmatic pleura is supplied by the superior phrenic and musculophrenic arteries. The venous drainage of the parietal pleura is primarily by the intercostal arteries, which empty into the inferior vena cava or the brachiocephalic trunk.

The blood supply to the visceral pleura is dependent on whether the animal has a thick or thin pleura. In general, the blood supply to the visceral pleura in animals with a thin pleura originates from the pulmonary circulation, whereas the blood supply in animals with a thick pleura originates from the systemic circulation via the bronchial arteries. Albertine and co-workers have demonstrated in sheep, an animal with a thick pleura, that the bronchial artery supplies the visceral pleura completely and exclusively (4). Because humans have a thick visceral pleura, the visceral pleura is probably also supplied by the bronchial artery, but there is still controversy (20) concerning this factor. The venous drainage of the visceral pleura is through the pulmonary veins.

PLEURAL LYMPHATICS

The lymphatic vessels of the costal pleura drain ventrally toward nodes along the internal thoracic artery and dorsally toward the internal intercostal lymph nodes near the heads of the ribs. The lymphatic vessels of the mediastinal pleura pass to the tracheobronchial and mediastinal nodes, whereas the lymphatic vessels of the diaphragmatic pleura pass to the parasternal, middle phrenic, and posterior mediastinal nodes.

The visceral pleura is abundantly endowed with lymphatic vessels. These lymphatics form a plexus of intercommunicating vessels that run over the surface of the lung toward the hilum and also penetrate the lung to join the bronchial lymph vessels by passing in the interlobular septa. Although lymph may flow in either direction, all lymph from the visceral pleura eventually reaches the lung root either by penetrating the lung or by flowing on the surface of the lung. Fluid from the pleural space does not enter the lymphatics in the visceral pleura in humans.

The lymphatic vessels in the parietal pleura are in communication with the pleural space by means of stomas that range in diameter from 2 to 6 μm (Fig. 1.2) (21). These stomas have a round or slitlike shape and are found mostly on the mediastinal pleura and on the intercostal surface, especially in the depressed areas just inferior to the ribs in the lower thorax. Few stomas are present in other portions of the parietal

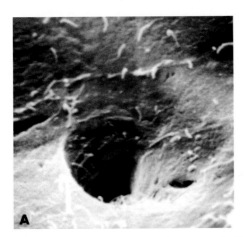
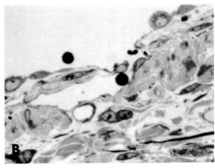

FIG. 1.2. Lymphatics of the parietal pleura. **A:** Scanning electron microscopic study of the parietal pleura in the rabbit demonstrating a lymphatic stoma. Microvilli and micropinocytic openings on the mesothelial surface are both much smaller than the stoma. (Original magnification: 6,500×.) **B:** Toluidine blue stain demonstrating a red blood cell at the stoma of a lacuna. (Original magnification: 1,000×.) (From Wang NS. The preformed stomas connecting the pleural cavity and the lymphatics in the parietal pleura. *Am Rev Respir Dis* 1975;111:12–20, with permission.)

pleura (3, 21). The distribution of stomas is similar to the distribution of particulate matter injected into the pleural space (see Chapter 2).

The lymphatic vessels in the parietal pleura have many branches. Some submesothelial branches have dilated lymphatic spaces called lacunas (Fig. 1.2B) (21). Stomas are found only over the lacunas. At the stoma, the mesothelial cells with their microvilli are in continuity with the endothelial cells of the lymphatic vessels. When red blood cells or carbon particles are injected into the pleural space, they collect around the stomas and in the lacunas and lymphatic vessels (Fig. 1.2B) (3, 21). Therefore, these stomas with their associated lacunas and lymphatic vessels are thought to be the main pathway for the elimination of particulate matter from the pleural space (3, 21).

The existence of such stomas has been difficult to demonstrate in humans. Gaudio et al. (6) were unable to demonstrate any such stomas in specimens from 30 patients undergoing thoracic surgical procedures. Peng and associates (14) were able to demonstrate stomas in only two of their nine human specimens. However, more recently Li was able to demonstrate human pleural stomata in the diaphragmatic pleura (22). The stomata were usually round or oval in shape and about 6.2 μm in diameter. The stomata were not present in the visceral pleura or the parietal pleura on the chest wall. The majority were quite deep, forming channels that seemed to connect the pleural cavity with the underlying lymphatic lacunae. Interestingly, in the golden hamster, there are many stomata but there are none in the diaphragmatic pleura (23).

No stomas are seen in the visceral pleura, and the lymphatic vessels of the visceral pleura are separated from the mesothelial cells by a layer of connective tissue. The lack of stomas in the visceral pleura explains the observation that particulate matter injected in the pleural space is removed through the parietal pleura (see Chapter 2).

Kampmeier's Foci

Kampmeier in 1928 described small milky spots in the dorsal and caudal portion of the medi-astinum in rats and humans (1). Microscopically, the foci are an aggregate of lymphocytes, histiocytes, plasma cells, and other mononuclear cells around central lymphatic or vascular vessels. It has been suggested that the black spots in patients with parietal anthracosis correspond to the Kampmeier foci and that the distribution of asbestos fibers in the pleura is also concentrated in these foci (24). It has been hypothesized that the high concentrations of asbestos in these foci leads to the development of pleural plaques and mesothelioma (24).

INNERVATION OF THE PLEURA

Sensory nerve endings are present in the costal and diaphragmatic parietal pleura. The intercostal nerves supply the costal pleura and the peripheral part of the diaphragmatic pleura. When either of these areas is stimulated, pain is referred to the adjacent chest wall. In contrast, the central portion of the diaphragm is innervated by the phrenic nerve, and stimulation of this pleura causes the pain to be perceived in the ipsilateral shoulder. The visceral pleura contains no pain fibers and may be manipulated without causing unpleasant sensation. Therefore, the presence of pleuritic chest pain indicates inflammation or irritation of the parietal pleura.

REFERENCES

1. Wang NS. Anatomy of the pleura. *Clin Chest Med* 1998;19:229–240.
2. Gray SW, Skandalakis JE. Development of the pleura. In: Chretien J, Bignon J, Hirsch A, eds. *The pleura in health and disease. Lung biology in health and disease.* Volume 30. New York: Marcel Dekker, 1985:319.
3. Albertine KH, Wiener-Kronish JP, Staub NC. The structure of the parietal pleura and its relationship to pleural liquid dynamics in sheep. *Anat Rec* 1984;208:401–409.
4. Albertine KH, Wiener-Kronish JP, Roos PJ, et al. Structure, blood supply, and lymphatic vessels of the sheep's visceral pleura. *Am J Anat* 1982;165:277–294.
5. Lemos M, Pozo RM, Montes GS, et al. Organization of collagen and elastic fibers studied in stretch preparations of whole mounts of human visceral pleura. *Anat Anz* 1997;179:447–452.
6. Gaudio E, Rendina EA, Pannarale L, et al. Surface morphology of the human pleura: a scanning electron microscopic study. *Chest* 1988;92:149–153.
7. Wang NS. The regional difference of pleural mesothelial cells in rabbits. *Am Rev Respir Dis* 1974;110:623–633.
8. Miserocchi G, Agostoni E. Pleural liquid and surface

pressures at various lung volumes. *Respir Physiol* 1980; 39:315–326.

9. Albertine KH, Wiener-Kronish JP, Bastacky J, et al. No evidence for mesothelial cell contact across the costal pleural space of sheep. *J Appl Physiol* 1991;70:123–143.

10. Antony VB, Sahn SA, Mossman B, et al. Pleural cell biology in health and disease. *Am Rev Respir Dis* 1992;145:1236–1239.

11. Idell S, Zwieb C, Kumar A, et al. Pathways of fibrin turnover of human pleural mesothelial cells in vitro. *Am J Respir Cell Mol Biol* 1992;7:414–426.

12. Owens MW, Milligan SA, Grisham MB. Nitric oxide synthesis by rat pleural mesothelial cells: induction by growth factors and lipopolysaccharide. *Exp Lung Res* 1995;21:731–742.

13. Gerwin BI, Lechner JF, Reddel RR, et al. Comparison of production of transforming growth factor-beta and platelet-derived growth factor by normal human mesothelial cells and mesothelioma cell lines. *Cancer Res* 1987;47:6180–6184.

14. Peng M-J, Wang NS, Vargas FS, et al. Subclinical surface alterations of human pleura. *Chest* 1994;106:351–353.

15. Efrati P, Nir E. Morphological and cytochemical investigation of human mesothelial cells from pleural and peritoneal effusions. A light and electron microscopy study. *Isr J Med Sci* 1976;12:662–673.

16. Bakalos D, Constantakis N, Tsicricas T. Distinction of mononuclear macrophages from mesothelial cells in pleural and peritoneal effusions. *Acta Cytol* 1974;18: 20–22.

17. Miserocchi G, Agostoni E. Contents of the pleural space. *J Appl Physiol* 1971;30:208–213.

18. Sahn SA, Willcox ML, Good JT Jr, et al. Characteristics of normal rabbit pleural fluid: physiologic and biochemical implications. *Lung* 1979;156:63–69.

19. Rolf LL, Travis DM. Pleural fluid-plasma bicarbonate gradients in oxygentoxic and normal rats. *Am J Physiol* 1973;224:857–861.

20. Bernaudin JF, Fleury J. Anatomy of the blood and lymphatic circulation of the pleural serosa. In: Chretien J, Bignon J, Hirsch A, eds. *The pleura in health and disease. Lung biology in health and disease.* Volume 30. New York: Marcel Dekker, 1985:101–124.

21. Wang NS. The preformed stomas connecting the pleural cavity and the lymphatics in the parietal pleura. *Am Rev Respir Dis* 1975;111:12–20.

22. Li J. Ultrastructural study on the pleural stomata in humans. *Funct Dev Morphol* 1993;3:277–280.

23. Shinohara H. Distribution of lymphatic stomata on the pleural surface of the thoracic cavity and the surface topography of the pleural mesothelium in the golden hamster. *Anat Rec* 1997;249:16–23.

24. Boutin C, Dumortier P, Rey F, et al. Black spots concentrate oncogenic asbestos fibers in the parietal pleura. Thoracoscopic and mineralogic study. *Am J Respir Crit Care Med* 1996;153:444–449.

2

Physiology of the Pleural Space

The pleural space is the coupling system between the lung and the chest wall, and, accordingly, it is a crucial feature of the breathing apparatus. The pressure within the pleural space (the pleural pressure) is important in cardiopulmonary physiology, because it is the pressure at the outer surface of the lung and the heart and the inner surface of the thoracic cavity. Because the lung, the heart, and the thoracic cavity are all distensible, and because the volume of a distensible object depends on the pressure difference between the inside and the outside of the object and its compliance, the pleural pressure plays an important role in determining the volume of these three important structures.

PLEURAL PRESSURE

If the thorax is opened to atmospheric pressure, the lungs decrease in volume because of their elastic recoil, while at the same time, the thorax enlarges. With the thorax open, the volume of the thoracic cavity is about 55% of the vital capacity, whereas the volume of the lung is below its residual volume. With the chest closed and the patient relaxed, the respiratory system is at its functional residual capacity (FRC), which is approximately 35% of the total lung capacity (1). Thus, at FRC, the opposing elastic forces of the chest wall and lung produce a negative pressure between the visceral and the parietal pleura, which is called the pleural pressure. This pressure surrounds the lung and is the primary determinant of the volume of the lung. The pleural pressure represents the balance between the outward pull of the thoracic cavity and the inward pull of the lung (1).

Pleural Liquid Pressure versus Pleural Surface Pressure

There has been a controversy for many years as to whether there are two pleural pressures or one (2). The two different pressures had been proposed to explain a discrepancy obtained when the pleural pressure was measured in two different ways. If the pressure was measured using fluid filled catheters, the vertical gradient obtained was approximately 1 cm H_2O per cm vertical height. This pressure was designated the pleural liquid pressure and was believed to represent the pressure that influenced the absorption of fluid. If the pressure was measured using surface balloons or suction cups, then a gradient of 0.5 cm H_2O per cm vertical height was obtained. This pressure was designated the pleural surface pressure and represented the balance between the outward pull of the thoracic cavity and the inward pull of the lung. It now appears that there is only one pressure and that the discrepancies in the pressures arose because of the distortion due to the catheters (3). It should be noted, however, that there is still a school of researchers who believe in the two different pressures (4, 5).

Measurement

The pleural pressure can be measured directly by inserting needles, trocars, catheters, or balloons into the pleural space. Direct measurement of the pleural pressure is not usually made because of the danger of producing a pneumothorax or of introducing infection into the pleural space. Rather, the pleural pressure is measured indirectly by a balloon positioned in the esophagus. Because the esophagus is a compliant structure situated between the two pleural spaces, esophageal pressure measurements provide a close approximation of the pleural pressure at the level of the balloon in the thorax (6). Estimation of pleural pressure by means of an esophageal balloon is not without difficulties (6). The volume of air within the balloon must be small, so that the balloon is not stretched and the esophageal walls are not displaced; otherwise, pleural pressure estimates are falsely elevated. Moreover, the balloon must be short and must be placed in the lower part of the esophagus. It has been demonstrated that reliable measurements of esophageal pressures can be made with micromanometers (7). The use of the micromanometer should circumvent some of the problems associated with esophageal balloons.

Gradients

Only one value for the pleural pressure is obtained when it is estimated by an esophageal catheter or balloon. It should be emphasized, however, that the pleural pressure is not uniform throughout the pleural space. A gradient in pleural pressure is seen between the superior and the inferior portions of the lung, with the pleural pressure being lowest or most negative in the superior portion and highest or least negative in the inferior portion (3). The main factors responsible for this pleural pressure gradient are probably gravity, mismatching of the shapes of the chest wall and lung, and the weight of the lungs and other intrathoracic structures (1).

The magnitude of the pleural pressure gradient appears to be approximately 0.50 cm H_2O per cm vertical distance (3). It should be noted that over the past 30 years, there have been many studies directed at measuring the pleural pressure gradient and the resulting values have ranged from 0.20 to 0.93 cm H_2O per cm vertical distance (3). The results have been largely dependent on the method used (3). It appears that the higher values were obtained with catheters that were large relative to the narrow pleural space and accordingly produced distortion of the pleura with subsequent alterations in the measured pressures (3).

In the upright position, the difference in the pleural pressure between the apex and the base of the lungs may be 12 cm or more. Because the alveolar pressure is constant throughout the lungs, the end result of the gradient in the pleural pressure is that different parts of the lungs have different distending pressures. The pressure–volume curve is thought to be the same for all regions of the lungs; therefore, the pleural pressure gradient causes the alveoli in the superior parts of the lung to be larger than those in the inferior parts of the lung. The pleural pressure gradients also account for the unevenness in the distribution of ventilation.

PLEURAL FLUID FORMATION

Fluid that enters the pleural space can originate in the pleural capillaries, the interstitial spaces of the lung, the intrathoracic lymphatics, the intrathoracic blood vessels, or the peritoneal cavity.

Pleural Capillaries

The movement of fluid between the pleural capillaries and the pleural space is believed to be governed by Starling's law of transcapillary exchange (8). When this law is applied to the pleura as indicated in Equation 2.1 below

$$\dot{Q}_f = Lp \cdot A[(P_{cap} - P_{pl}) - \sigma_d(\pi_{cap} - \pi_{pl})]$$

where Q_f is the liquid movement; L_p is the filtration coefficient per unit area or the hydraulic water conductivity of the membrane; A is the surface area of the membrane; P and π are the hydrostatic and oncotic pressures, respectively, of the capillary (cap) and pleural (pl) space; and σ_d is the solute reflection coefficient for protein, a measure of the membrane's ability to restrict the passage of large molecules (9). Widely varying values for σ_d have been reported. For example, the σ_d of the canine visceral pleura has been reported to exceed 0.80 (9), indicating a marked restriction in the movement of large molecules such as albumin. In contrast, the σ_d of the pig mediastinal pleura was reported to be between 0.02 and 0.05, indicating little restriction in the movement of large molecules (8).

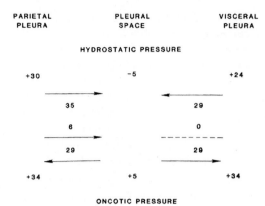

FIG. 2.1. Various pressures that normally influence the movement of fluid in and out of the pleural space in species with a thick visceral pleura, such as humans.

Estimates for the magnitude of the pressures affecting fluid movement from the capillaries to the pleural space in humans are shown in Fig. 2.1. When the parietal pleura is considered, a gradient for fluid formation is normally present. The hydrostatic pressure in the parietal pleura is approximately 30 cm H_2O, whereas the pleural pressure is about -5 cm H_2O. The net hydrostatic pressure is therefore $30 - (-5) = 35$ cm H_2O and favors the movement of fluid from the capillaries in the parietal pleura to the pleural space. Opposing this hydrostatic pressure gradient is the oncotic pressure gradient. The oncotic pressure in the plasma is approximately 34 cm H_2O. Normally, the small amount of pleural fluid contains a small amount of protein and has an oncotic pressure of about 5 cm H_2O (10), yielding a net oncotic pressure gradient of $34 - 5 = 29$ cm H_2O. Thus, the net gradient is $35 - 29 = 6$ cm H_2O, favoring the movement of fluid from the capillaries in the parietal pleura to the pleural space.

The net gradient for fluid movement across the visceral pleura in humans is probably close to zero, but this has not been demonstrated (Fig. 2.1). The pressure in the visceral pleural capillaries is approximately 6 cm H_2O less than that in the parietal pleural capillaries because the visceral pleural capillaries drain into the pulmonary veins. Because this is the only pressure that differs from those affecting fluid movement

across the parietal pleura and because the net gradient for the parietal pleura is 6 cm H_2O, it follows that the net gradient for fluid movement across the visceral pleura is approximately zero. It is also likely that the filtration coefficient (L_p) for the visceral pleura is substantially less than that for the parietal pleura because the capillaries in the visceral pleura are much farther from the pleural space than those in the parietal pleura (11).

The movement of pleural fluid is not the same across all the parietal pleura. Wang and Lai-Fook (12) used Evans blue–dyed albumin to study regional pleural filtration of prone anesthetized rabbits. They reported that there appeared to be more fluid formation across the parietal pleura over the ribs compared with the intercostal spaces. In contrast, pleural liquid absorption was primarily in the parietal pleura adjacent to the intercostal space rather than in the parietal pleura overlying the ribs. There was also more fluid formation over the caudal than over the cranial ribs (12). If the breathing frequency was increased, more fluid was formed (12).

The transpleural exchange of fluid is species dependent. Humans and sheep have a thick visceral pleura and its blood supply is from the bronchial artery rather than the pulmonary artery (13). However, many species, such as the rabbit and the dog, have a thin visceral pleura that receives its blood supply from the pulmonary circulation. In such a situation, as shown in Fig. 2.2, the net gradients favor pleural fluid formation across the parietal pleura and pleural fluid absorption through the visceral pleura.

Interstitial Origin

In recent years, it has been demonstrated that the origin of much of the fluid that enters the pleural space is the interstitial spaces of the lungs. Either high pressure or high permeability pulmonary edema can lead to the accumulation of pleural fluid. When sheep are volume overloaded to produce high-pressure pulmonary edema, approximately 25% of all the fluid that enters the interstitial spaces of the lungs is cleared from the lung via the pleural space (14). Within 2 hours of starting the volume overloading, the amount

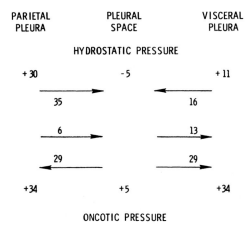

FIG. 2.2. Various pressures that normally influence the movement of fluid in and out of the pleural space in species with a thin STvisceral pleura, such as the dog. See text for explanation.

of fluid entering the pleural space increases, and within 3 hours, the protein concentration in the pleural fluid is the same as that in the interstitial spaces of the lungs (14). The amount of pleural fluid formed is directly related to the elevation in the wedge pressure. Increases in pleural fluid accumulation only occur after the development of pulmonary edema (15).

The pulmonary interstitial space is probably also the origin of the pleural fluid in patients with congestive heart failure. The likelihood of a pleural effusion increases as the severity of pulmonary edema increases (16). In addition, the presence of pleural effusions is more closely correlated with the pulmonary venous pressure than with the systemic venous pressure (16).

The amount of fluid that enters the pleural space is also increased when there is increased interstitial fluid due to high-permeability pulmonary edema. When increased-permeability edema was induced in sheep by the infusion of oleic acid, again, pleural fluid accumulated only after pulmonary edema developed (17). In this study, there was no morphologic evidence of pleural injury. When pulmonary edema is induced by xylazine (18) or hyperoxia (19) in rats, or by ethchlorvynol in sheep (20), the high-protein pleural fluid appears to originate in the interstitial spaces of the lungs. The pleural fluid associated with experimental *Pseudomonas* pneumonia in rabbits originates in the lung (21). It is likely that the origin of the pleural fluid with many conditions associated with lung injury, such as pulmonary embolization and lung transplantation, is also the interstitial spaces of the lung (2).

In experimental studies of hydrostatic and increased permeability edema, a pleural effusion develops when the extravascular lung water has reached a critical level for a certain amount of time (22). The necessary level of edema appears to be between 5 and 8 g of fluid per gram of dry lung whether the edema is secondary to hydrostatic edema, oleic acid lung injury, or alphanaphthyl thiourea lung injury (22). With increasing levels of interstitial fluid, it has been shown that the subpleural interstitial pressure increases (23). The barrier to movement of fluid across the visceral pleura appears to be weak, even though the visceral pleura is thick (24). Therefore, once the subpleural interstitial pressure increases, it follows that fluid will traverse the visceral pleura to the pleural space.

Peritoneal Cavity

Pleural fluid accumulation can occur if there is free fluid in the peritoneal cavity and if there are openings in the diaphragm. Under these conditions, the fluid will flow from the peritoneal space to the pleural space because the pressure in the pleural cavity is less than the pressure in the peritoneal cavity. The peritoneal cavity is the origin of the pleural fluid in hepatic hydrothorax, Meigs' syndrome, and peritoneal dialysis (25).

Thoracic Duct or Blood Vessel Disruption

If the thoracic duct is disrupted, lymph will accumulate in the pleural space, producing a chylothorax (see Chapter 23). The rate of fluid accumulation with chylothorax can be more than 1,000 mL per day. When the thoracic duct is lacerated in dogs, sizeable pleural effusions begin to develop almost immediately (26). In a like manner, when a large blood vessel in the thorax is disrupted owing to trauma or disease, blood can accumulate rapidly in the pleural space, producing hemothorax (see Chapter 22).

Origin of Pleural Fluid Normally

The rate of pleural formation in normal sheep is approximately 0.01 mL per kg per hour (27). It appears that in normal individuals, the origin of most pleural fluid is the capillaries in the parietal pleura (27). It certainly does not appear to be the interstitial spaces of the lung because the protein level in the interstitial spaces is normally about 4.5 g per dL, whereas the protein level in normal pleural fluid is only about 1 to 1.5 g per dL. From Fig. 2.1, it appears unlikely that it is the visceral pleura. Likewise, both a lymphatic origin and a peritoneal cavity origin appear unlikely. Supporting evidence for this thesis has been provided by Broaddus et al. (27). These workers measured the vascular pressures and the pleural fluid protein levels in sheep of different ages. They found that the systemic vascular pressures progressively increased with age, whereas the pleural fluid protein levels progressively decreased with age. They concluded that their findings supported their thesis because higher vascular pressures should produce pleural fluid with lower protein levels (27). Studies in rabbits with Evans blue–dyed albumin have demonstrated that most fluid originates in the parietal pleura over the ribs (12).

PLEURAL FLUID ABSORPTION

Lymphatic Clearance

From Fig. 2.1, one might have the impression that pleural fluid should continuously accumulate because the Starling equation favors fluid formation through the parietal pleura and there is no gradient for fluid absorption through the visceral pleura. Fluid clearance through the pleural lymphatics is thought to explain the lack of fluid accumulation normally. The pleural space is in communication with the lymphatic vessels in the parietal pleura by means of stomas in the parietal pleura. No such stomas are present in the visceral pleura. Proteins, cells, and all other particulate matter are removed from the pleural space by these lymphatics in the parietal pleura (28–31).

The amount of fluid that can be cleared through these lymphatics is substantial. Stewart found that the mean lymphatic flow from one pleural space in seven patients was 0.40 mL per kg

per h (32), whereas Leckie and Tothill found that the mean lymphatic flow was 0.22 mL per kg per h in seven patients with congestive heart failure (33). In both of these studies, marked variability was noted from one patient to another. If these results in patients with congestive heart failure are extrapolated to the normal person, a 60-kg individual should have a lymphatic drainage from each pleural space on the order of 20 mL per h or 500 mL per day.

Experimental work with sheep, a species with a thick visceral pleura similar to that of humans, suggests that most of the fluid that enters the pleural space in sheep is removed through the lymphatics. Broaddus et al. produced artificial hydrothoraces in awake sheep by injecting an autologous protein solution at a volume of 10 mL per kg, with a protein level of 1.0 g per dL (34). These investigators found that the hydrothorax was removed almost completely by the lymphatics in a linear fashion at a rate of 0.28 mL per kg per hour. The linearity suggests that the lymphatics operate at maximum capacity once the volume of the pleural liquid exceeds a certain threshold. Note that the capacity for lymphatic clearance is 28 times as high as the normal rate of pleural fluid formation.

In the foregoing experiments of Broaddus et al. (34), the fluid introduced into the pleural space had an oncotic pressure of about 5 cm H_2O, and from Fig. 2.1, one might speculate that if fluids with oncotic pressures other than 5 had been introduced, the equilibrium would have been altered such that fluid would enter the pleural space from the visceral pleura in animals with high oncotic pressures and would leave the pleural space through the visceral pleura in animals with low oncotic pressures. This does not appear to be the case. Aiba and associates produced artificial pleural effusions in dogs with protein levels ranging from 0.1 to 9.0 g per dL (35). Even when the induced pleural effusion had a protein level of 0.1 g per dL, there was no increase in the concentration of protein with time, indicating that the low oncotic pressure did not induce a rapid efflux of fluid out of the pleural space. When the protein concentration of the induced effusions was above 4 g per dL, the concentration of protein in the pleural fluid did gradually decrease with time, indicating a net transfer of protein-free fluid into the pleural space. The net amount of fluid entering the pleural space even with a protein level of 9.0 g per dL was only 0.22 mL per kg per hour, however. This degree of fluid flux is similar to the lymphatic clearance of 0.22 mL per kg per hour reported in the same studies. Additional evidence supporting a primary role for the pleural lymphatics in pleural fluid absorption comes from the studies of Shinto and Light (36). They performed serial thoracenteses on patients undergoing vigorous diuretic therapy for congestive heart failure and reported that the protein and lactate dehydrogenase (LDH) levels in the pleural fluid changed very little over a 24- to 72-hour period, even though the volume of the pleural fluid decreased rapidly. If the fluid had been removed via the capillaries in the visceral pleura, then the protein and LDH concentrations should have increased. These observations strongly suggest that most pleural fluid is removed through the lymphatics in the parietal pleura in species with a thick visceral pleura, such as humans.

Clearance through Capillaries in Visceral Pleura

Until the mid-1980s, it was thought that the primary route for the exit of fluid from the pleural space was through the capillaries in the visceral pleural (37). This conclusion was based primarily on experiments in animals with a thin pleura. It is easily seen from Fig. 2.2 that in animals with a thin pleura, there is a sizable gradient for the movement of fluid from the pleural space into the capillaries in the visceral pleura. In addition, fluid probably moves across a thin visceral pleura more easily than it moves across a thick pleural membrane. For the reasons cited earlier, however, it appears that in humans, almost all pleural fluid is removed via the lymphatics in the parietal pleura. Nevertheless, it should be noted that this view is not accepted by all (38).

The foregoing should not be interpreted as indicating that small molecules do not move across the pleural surfaces. Indeed, water and small-sized molecules exchange easily across both pleural surfaces (39). When hydrothoraces are induced in dogs, the clearance rate for para-aminohippurate (PAH) (molecular weight 216) is about 2 mL per kg per hour (35). When urea is injected

into patients with pleural effusions, its concentration decreases much more rapidly than does that of radiolabeled protein (40). Indeed, the urea clearance rate is several hundred milliliters per hour (40). Because urea and water have comparable molecular weights, one can assume that the rates of exchange for urea and water across the pleural membranes are similar. Therefore, several hundred milliliters of water probably traverse the pleural membranes each day, but the net movement is only a few milliliters because the osmolarity is nearly identical on each side of the membrane.

PATHOGENESIS OF PLEURAL EFFUSIONS

Pleural fluid accumulates when the rate of pleural fluid formation exceeds the rate of pleural fluid absorption. The main factors that lead to increased pleural fluid formation or decreased pleural fluid absorption are tabulated in Table 2.1. Normally, a small amount (0.01 mL per kg per hour) of fluid constantly enters the pleural space from the capillaries in the parietal pleura. Almost all of this fluid is removed by the lymphatics in

TABLE 2.1. *General causes of pleural effusions*

Increased pleural fluid formation
 Increased interstitial fluid in the lung
  Left ventricular failure, pneumonia and
   pulmonary embolus
 Increased intravascular pressure in pleura
  Right or left ventricular failure, superior
   vena caval syndrome
 Increased permeability of the capillaries
  in the pleura
  Pleural inflammation
  Increased levels of vascular endothelial
   growth factor (VEGF)
 Increased pleural fluid protein level
 Decreased pleural pressure
  Lung atelectasis or increased elastic recoil
   of the lung
 Increased fluid in peritoneal cavity
  Ascites or peritoneal dialysis
 Disruption of the thoracic duct
 Disruption of blood vessels in the thorax
Decreased pleural fluid absorption
 Obstruction of the lymphatics draining the
  parietal pleura
 Elevation of systemic vascular pressures
  Superior vena caval syndrome or right
   ventricular failure
 ?Disruption of the aquaporin system in the pleura

the parietal pleura, which have a capacity to remove at least 0.20 mL per kg per hour. Note that this provides a safety factor of nearly 20.

INCREASED PLEURAL FLUID FORMATION

Increased pleural fluid formation can occur when there is increased pulmonary interstitial fluid or when one of the terms in Starling's equation (Equation 2.1) is changed such that more fluid is formed.

Increased Interstitial Fluid

The most common cause of increased pleural fluid formation is increased interstitial fluid in the lung. As mentioned earlier, whenever the amount of edema in the lung exceeds 5 g per gram of lung dry weight, pleural fluid accumulates whether the edema is high protein or low protein (22). This appears to be the predominant mechanism for the formation of pleural effusions in patients with congestive heart failure, parapneumonic effusions, the acute respiratory distress syndrome, and lung transplantation.

Increased Hydrostatic Pressure Gradient

If there is an increase in the gradient between the intravascular pressure and the pleural pressure, there will be an increase in the rate of pleural fluid formation through Starling's equation (Equation 2.1). Increases in the intravascular pressure can occur with right ventricular failure, left ventricular failure, pericardial effusions, or the superior vena cava syndrome. The most common situation producing a decrease in the pleural pressure is bronchial obstruction leading to atelectasis of a lower lobe or a complete lung. A decrease in the pleural pressure also occurs when the visceral pleura becomes coated with a collagenous peel and the lung becomes trapped. In these instances, the pleural pressure can become very negative (below -50 cm H_2O) (41). Decreased pleural pressures can also contribute to pleural fluid accumulation with diseases in which the elastic recoil of the lung is increased.

Increased Capillary Permeability

It can also be seen from Equation 2.1 that increased permeability of the pleura can also lead to increased pleural fluid formation. In Equation 2.1, a generalized increase in the pleural permeability is reflected by an increase in L_p (hydraulic conductivity). It is thought that increased levels of vascular endothelial growth factor (VEGF) increase the permeability of the capillaries and may be at least partially responsible for the accumulation of pleural fluid in certain instances (42, 43). VEGF receptors have been demonstrated on mesothelial cells (43), and the levels of VEGF are higher in exudative effusions than in transudative pleural effusions (42, 43). Of course, if the pleural surfaces become inflamed, the permeability of the capillaries may be increased.

Decreased Oncotic Pressure Gradient

A decrease in the oncotic pressure gradient can also lead to increased pleural fluid formation through its influence on Starling's equation (Fig. 2.1). For example, if the protein level in the serum and pleural fluid are identical, then there should be gradients of 35 and 29 cm H_2O from the parietal and visceral pleura, respectively, (instead of the normal 6 and 0 cm H_2O) favoring pleural fluid formation. Increased pleural fluid protein levels occur with increased permeability pulmonary edema, hemothorax, and with conditions in which the permeability of the pleural capillaries is increased. This mechanism, however, is probably not too important because when sheep are given a pleural effusion with a protein level of 9.0 g per dL, the rate of fluid entry into the pleural space is only 0.22 mL per kg per hour (35). The rate of fluid formation is approximately equal to the capacity of the lymphatics for reabsorption. Moreover, hypoproteinemia is thought to be a very uncommon cause of pleural effusion (44).

Presence of Free Peritoneal Fluid or Disruption of the Thoracic Duct or an Intrathoracic Blood Vessel

If there is free fluid in the peritoneal cavity, it will lead to pleural fluid accumulation if there is a hole in the diaphragm (25). In like manner, chyle will accumulate in the pleural space if there is a disruption in the thoracic duct, and blood will accumulate in the pleural space if there is disruption of a blood vessel in the thorax.

Decreased Pleural Fluid Absorption

Obstruction of Lymphatics

The most common cause of a decrease in the pleural fluid absorption is obstruction of the lymphatics draining the parietal pleura. Normally, the lymphatic flow from the pleural space is about 0.01 mL per kg per hour or 15 mL per day, but the capacity of the lymphatics is about 0.20 mL per kg per hour or 300 mL per day. Lymphatic blockade is probably one of the major factors that contributes to the development of a malignant pleural effusion. Leckie and Tothill studied the lymphatic flow in eight patients with lung carcinoma and six patients with metastatic breast carcinoma, and found that the mean lymphatic flow was only 0.08 mL per kg per hour (33). Obviously, pleural effusions would not have developed in these patients unless excess fluid had also been entering the pleural space. Unless the lymphatic flow is markedly impaired, another factor must be present in addition to lymphatic disease to produce a pleural effusion given the excess reserve capacity of the lymphatics.

Elevation of Systemic Venous Pressures

Because the lymphatics drain into the systemic venous circulation, elevation of the pressures in the central veins decreases the lymphatic flow. Pleural effusions develop in sheep when the pressure in the superior vena cava is increased. Allen et al. (45) found that pleural fluid accumulated over a 24-hour period when the pressure in the superior vena cava exceeded 15 mm Hg. The amount of pleural fluid that accumulated increased exponentially as the pressure was increased. Comparable amounts of pleural fluid accumulated in both pleural spaces. A total of 500 mL of pleural fluid accumulated when the pressure was 27 to 28 mm Hg. These workers reported that the larger the pleural effusion, the higher the protein level. They concluded that the pleural effusions developed because of (a) lymph leakage out of the lymphatics that pass through the chest (these include the thoracic duct and the diaphragmatic and pulmonary lymphatics); or (b) obstruction of lung or chest wall lymphatics with subsequent leakage of interstitial fluid into the pleural space (45).

Disruption of the Aquaporin System

The aquaporins (AQPs) are a family of proteins that transport water across membranes (46). At least four different AQPs are in the lung. Although knockout mice lacking the aquaporins normally found in the lung do not have obvious problems with fluid exchange in the lungs, in other situations, the lack of an AQP has profound consequences. For example, deletion of AQP-1 in mice results in a severe defect in urinary-concentrating ability and the mice become profoundly dehydrated when deprived of water (46). It is unknown whether abnormalities in the AQP system affect the movement of fluid in and out of the pleural space (46). However, it has been shown that AQP-1 provides a major route for osmotically driven water transport across the peritoneal barrier in peritoneal dialysis (47).

WHY IS THERE NO AIR IN THE PLEURAL SPACE?

Because the pleural pressure is negative at functional residual capacity and throughout most of the respiratory cycle, why is there normally no air in the pleural space? Gases move in and out of the pleural space from the capillaries in the visceral and parietal pleura (48). The movement of each gas is dependent on its partial pressure in the pleural space, as compared with that in the capillary blood. The sum of all the partial pressures in the capillary blood averages 706 mm Hg ($P_{H_2O} = 47$, $P_{co_2} = 46$, $P_{n_2} = 573$, and $P_{o_2} = 40$ mm Hg). Therefore, a net movement of gas into the pleural space should occur only if the pleural pressure is below 706 mm Hg or below −54 mm Hg relative to atmospheric pressure. Because mean pleural pressures this low hardly ever occur, the pleural space normally remains gas free.

If air is discovered in the pleural space, it means that one of three things has occurred: (a) a communication exists or has recently existed between the alveoli and the pleural space; (b) a communication exists or has recently existed between the atmosphere and the pleural space; or (c) gas-producing organisms are present in the pleural space.

When air does enter the pleural space and thereby produces a pneumothorax, its rate of absorption depends on the difference between the sum of the partial pressures in the pleural space and in the capillary blood. The sum of the partial pressures in the pleural space is close to atmospheric pressure. Because the sum of the partial pressures in the capillary blood is most dependent on the P_{n_2}, this sum can be rapidly reduced by having the patient breathe supplemental oxygen, which reduces the P_{n_2} of the capillary blood without changing the other partial pressures substantially. In patients who have small pneumothoraces, administration of supplemental oxygen facilitates the reabsorption of the pneumothorax (49).

HOW IMPORTANT IS THE PLEURAL SPACE?

The pleural space serves as the coupling system between the lung and the chest wall. The thin rim of fluid that normally separates the parietal from the visceral pleura is thought to facilitate the movements of the lung within the thoracic cavity. Therefore, what are the consequences of obliterating the pleural space? Surprisingly, patients with obliterated pleural spaces appear to suffer no significant ill effects. Gaensler studied the pulmonary function of four patients before and 6 to 17 months after they had been subjected to pleurectomy (50). The mean vital capacity and maximal breathing capacity were virtually identical preoperatively and postoperatively. Moreover, the ventilation and oxygen uptake on the operated side, as compared with the intact side, were unchanged postoperatively.

Fleetham et al. (51) studied regional lung function in four men who had undergone thoracotomy

for pleurodesis 2 to 9 years previously. They found that in all subjects, boluses of xenon inhaled slowly at functional residual capacity were distributed more to the apex and less to the base of the lung on the operated side than on the intact side. These researchers believed, however, that these minor differences were probably not clinically significant.

Further evidence for the lack of importance of the pleural space is provided by studies of elephants. The pleural space of both Asian and African elephants has been found to be obliterated by connective tissue (37). Whether this observation reflects the normal condition is controversial. Nevertheless, that many of these large mammals function without a pleural space indicates the relative lack of importance of this structure for normal function. The potential pleural space plays a major role in many disease states, however.

The pleural space may be important in clearing fluid from the interstitium of the lung. When noncardiogenic pulmonary edema is produced in sheep through the intravenous injection of oleic acid, approximately 20% of the fluid that enters the interstitium of the lung is removed by the lymphatics in the parietal pleura after the fluid crosses the visceral pleura to the pleural space (17). The relevance of this observation to disease in humans is yet to be proved. The infrequency of unilateral pulmonary edema in patients with a previous pleurodesis makes one skeptical about the clinical significance of these findings.

PHYSIOLOGIC EFFECTS OF A PLEURAL EFFUSION

The presence of fluid in the pleural space affects three different systems, namely, the diaphragm, the lung, and the heart.

Effects on the Diaphragm

As fluid accumulates in a pleural space, the corresponding hemidiaphragm may be depressed by the weight and pressure even though the upper level of the effusion appears unchanged with respect to the rib cage or the mediastinal structures (52). Mulvey classified the changes in the diaphragm resulting from pleural fluid into three groups as seen on the plain film and fluoroscopy. In order of severity, this diaphragmatic classification included the domed normal-functioning hemidiaphragm, the flattened fixed hemidiaphragm, and the inverted hemidiaphragm with paradoxical excursions. The group with a domed normal-functioning diaphragm usually is relatively asymptomatic even though the pleural effusion may be large. The second group with the flattened fixed hemidiaphragm has a lung that is not ventilated normally and the diaphragm does not move. Mulvey noted that several patients with a fixed flattened hemidiaphragm improved symptomatically postthoracentesis even though the volume of aerated lung and the upper level of fluid appeared essentially unchanged. The third group, which has inversion of the diaphragm and paradoxical movement of the diaphragm on respiration, has the most severe dyspnea. Mulvey believes that inversion of the diaphragm occurs more commonly than is generally appreciated. The right diaphragm is much less likely to become inverted because of the liver (52).

Effects on the Lung

When fluid is present in the pleural space, one of two things must happen: (a) the lung must lose volume, or (b) the thoracic cavity must get larger. Therefore, it is not surprising that presence of fluid in the pleural space produces restrictive ventilatory dysfunction. When a saline solution is instilled into the pleural spaces of dogs, both the FRC and the total lung capacity (TLC) decrease with increasing amounts of saline added to the pleural space (53). When the volume of saline additions were 9%, 25%, and 45% of the control TLC, the decrease in FRC was about one third the amount of saline solution added. The other two thirds of the saline volume must therefore have increased the volume of the thoracic cavity. The enlargement of the thoracic cavity occurred predominantly because of downward displacement of the diaphragm. The decrease in the TLC was about 20% that of the added saline volume. Accordingly, there was no decrease in the inspi-

ratory capacity. Most of the volume decrease occurred in the lower lobe; the upper lobe retained its original volume. The esophageal pressure remained unchanged at both FRC and TLC.

In humans, the presence of a pleural effusion also produces restrictive ventilatory dysfunction. Our group obtained spirometry before and 24 hours after thoracentesis in 26 patients from whom a mean of 1,740 mL pleural fluid was withdrawn (54). In these patients, the mean vital capacity improved 410 ± 390 mL. Patients in this study with higher pleural pressures after the removal of 800 mL of pleural fluid and patients with a smaller decrease in the pleural pressure after the removal of 800 mL pleural fluid had greater improvements in the FVC after thoracentesis.

Wang and Tseng studied the pulmonary functions before and after thoracentesis in 21 patients with pleural effusion and an inverted diaphragm detected with ultrasound (55). They removed a mean of 1,610 mL of pleural fluid and reported that the mean FVC improved by 317 mL, the mean FEV_1 improved by 234 mL, and the mean $P(A - a)O_2$ improved from 40.3 to 31.9 mm Hg. The changes in pulmonary function were very similar to the changes that we observed in our series of patients who did not have known diaphragmatic inversion (54). It is interesting that the patients in Wang and Tseng's series were very dyspneic before the thoracentesis and the dyspnea was improved after the thoracentesis (55).

Estenne et al. (56) measured respiratory mechanics in nine patients before and 2 hours after removal of 600 to 2,750 mL (mean = 1,818 mL) of pleural fluid. Before the thoracentesis, the forced vital capacity (FVC) varied from 22% to 51% of predicted. After thoracentesis, the mean FVC and FRC increased only 300 and 460 mL, respectively.

Estenne et al. (56) attributed the relief of dyspnea following thoracentesis to a reduction in the size of the thoracic cage, which allows the inspiratory muscles to operate on a more advantageous portion of their length–tension curve. They found that, after thoracentesis, there was a shift in the inspiratory pleural pressure–volume curve such that the maximal pressures generated by the inspiratory muscles at a given lung volume were markedly more negative.

The maximal inspiratory pressure (MIP) at TLC was -16 cm H_2O before thoracentesis and improved to -25 cm H_2O after thoracentesis. The highest MIP went from -41 cm H_2O before thoracentesis to -52 cm H_2O after thoracentesis. Relieving the downward displacement of the diaphragm by the pleural fluid is probably the primary explanation for these observations.

The Pa_{O_2} is usually decreased and the alveolar—arterial O_2 gradient is usually increased in patients with pleural effusions. When bilateral pleural effusions are induced in pigs, there is a marked decrease in the Pa_{O_2} when the volume of the effusion exceeds 30 mL per kg (57). Agusti et al. (58) studied the oxygenation status of nine patients before and immediately after thoracentesis (693 $\pm$ 424 mL pleural fluid) with the multiple inert gas technique. They found that the mean $P(A - a)O_2$ difference was 29 mm Hg before thoracentesis and remained at 29 postthoracentesis (58). They showed that the intrapulmonary shunt is the main mechanism underlying arterial hypoxemia in patients with pleural effusion and that the shunt does not change significantly after thoracentesis (58). In an earlier study, the oxygenation status actually deteriorated after thoracentesis (59). In this study of 19 patients, the mean Pa_{O_2} fell from 70.4 mm Hg before thoracentesis to 61.2 mm Hg 20 minutes after the procedure and remained reduced to 64.4 mm Hg 2 hours after thoracentesis before returning to baseline 22 hours later. However, a recent study in patients with adult respiratory distress syndrome (ARDS), who were receiving mechanical ventilation, demonstrated that the removal of pleural fluid led to a significant improvement in the oxygenation status and the lung compliance (60).

Four separate studies have compared the oxygenation status of patients with pleural effusions when the patients were lying on their side (61–64). In all three studies, there was a small improvement in the mean oxygenation status when the patient was positioned with the lung without the effusion dependent. It was noted, however, in one study that patients with a severe reduction of their FVC had a lower Pa_{O_2} with the normal lung down, whereas patients with less severe reductions in their pulmonary function tests had a higher Pa_{O_2} with the normal lung down (63). In another study, eight of 30 patients (27%) had a higher Pa_{O_2} when the side without the effusion was dependent (64).

Effects on the Heart

It appears that the presence of a pleural effusion may compromise the cardiac function of some patients with large pleural effusions. It has been shown in dogs (65) that the induction of a large pleural effusion leads to right ventricular diastolic collapse and an associated decrease in cardiac output. In dogs with artificially induced bilateral pleural effusions, the occurrence of the right ventricular diastolic collapse occurs when the pleural pressure is about 4 mm Hg (65). Pleural pressures this high are frequently seen in patients with large pleural effusions (41). There have also been two reports of patients with large pleural effusions associated with compromised cardiac output (66, 67). In both cases, the cardiac output improved after therapeutic thoracentesis. In one of the cases, left ventricular diastolic collapse was documented (67). The frequency of cardiac compromise in patients with large pleural effusions remains to be determined. In one study in pigs, there was no decrease in the cardiac output when bilateral pleural effusions of 40 mL per kg were induced (57).

Many patients with pleural effusions complain of exercise intolerance; however, therapeutic thoracentesis does not appear to increase exercise tolerance in many patients. Over the past several years, we have performed symptom-limited maximal exercise tests on 25 patients before and 24 hours following a therapeutic thoracentesis, during which a mean of 1,700 mL pleural fluid was withdrawn (68, 69). Before the thoracentesis, the exercise tolerance of the patients was markedly limited, with a mean maximal workload of only 71 watts. However, after thoracentesis, the maximal workload tolerated increased to only 78 watts. Only 11 of the patients were able to achieve a higher workload after thoracentesis. There was no significant change in either the hypoxic or hypercapnic drives after thoracentesis. Most of the patients that we studied had malignant pleural effusions, and it appeared that general disability due to the underlying disease rather than compromised pulmonary function was responsible for the exercise limitation in many patients.

REFERENCES

1. Ward ME, Roussos C, Macklem PT. Respiratory mechanics. In: Murray JF, Nadel JA, eds. *Textbook of respiratory medicine.* Philadelphia: W.B. Saunders, 1994:90–138.
2. Broaddus VC, Light RW. Disorders of the pleura: general principles and diagnostic approach. In: Murray JF, Nadel JA, eds. *Textbook of respiratory medicine.* Philadelphia: W.B. Saunders, 2000:1995–2012.
3. Lai-Fook SJ, Rodarte JR. Pleural pressure distribution and its relationship to lung volume and interstitial pressure. *J Appl Physiol* 1991;70:967–978.
4. Agostoni E, D'Angelo E. Pleural liquid pressure. *J Appl Physiol* 1991;71:393–403.
5. Del Fabbro M. An improved technique for studying pleural fluid pressure and composition in rabbits. *Exp Physiol* 1998;83:435–448.
6. Milic-Emili J, Mead J, Turner JM, et al. Improved technique for estimating pleural pressure from esophageal balloons. *J Appl Physiol* 1964;19:207–211.
7. Hartford CG, Rogers GG, Turner MJ. Correctly selecting a liquid-filled nasogastric infant feeding catheter to measure intraesophageal pressure. *Pediatr Pulmonol* 1997;23:362–369.
8. Parameswaran S, Brown LV, Ibbott GS, et al. Hydraulic conductivity, Albumin reflection and diffusion coefficients of pig mediastinal pleura. *Microvasc Res* 1999;58:114–127.
9. Kinasewitz GT, Groome LJ, Marshall RP, et al. Role of pulmonary lymphatics and interstitium in visceral pleural fluid exchange. *J Appl Physiol* 1984;56:355–363.
10. Miserocchi G, Agostoni E. Contents of the pleural space. *J Appl Physiol* 1971;30:208–213.
11. Albertine KH, Wiener-Kronish JP, Staub NC. The structure of the parietal pleura and its relationship to pleural liquid dynamics in sheep. *Anat Rec* 1984;208:401–409.
12. Wang PM, Lai-Fook SJ. Regional pleural filtration and absorption measured by fluorescent tracers in rabbits. *Lung* 1999;177:289–309.
13. Albertine KH, Wiener-Kronish JP, Roos PJ, et al. Structure, blood supply, and lymphatic vessels of the sheep's visceral pleura. *Am J Anat* 1982;165:277–294.
14. Broaddus VC, Wiener-Kronish JP, Staub NC. Clearance of lung edema into the pleural space of volume-loaded anesthetized sheep. *J Appl Physiol* 1990;68:2623–2630.
15. Allen S, Gabel J, Drake R. Left atrial hypertension causes pleural effusion formation in unanesthetized sheep. *Am J Physiol* 1989;257(2 Pt 2):H690–H692.
16. Wiener-Kronish JP, Matthay MA, Callen PW, et al. Relationship of pleural effusions to pulmonary hemodynamics in patients with congestive heart failure. *Am Rev Respir Dis* 1985;132:1253–1256.
17. Wiener-Kronish JP, Broaddus VC, Albertine KH, et al. Relationship of pleural effusions to increased permeability pulmonary edema in anesthetized sheep. *J Clin Invest* 1988;82:1422–1429.
18. Amouzadeh HR, Sangiah S, Qualls CW Jr, et al.
Xylazine-induced pulmonary edema in rats. *Toxicol Appl Pharmacol* 1991;108:417–427.
19. Bernaudin JF, Theven D, Pinchon MC, et al. Protein transfer in hyperoxic induced pleural effusion in the rat. *Exp Lung Res* 1986;10:23–38.
20. Miller KS, Harley RA, Sahn SA. Pleural effusions associated with ethchlorvynol lung injury result from visceral pleural leak. *Am Rev Respir Dis* 1989;140:764–768.
21. Wiener-Kronish JP, Sakuma T, Kudoh I, et al. Alveolar epithelial injury and pleural empyema in acute *P. aeruginosa* pneumonia in anesthetized rabbits. *J Appl Physiol* 1993;75:1661–1669.
22. Wiener-Kronish JP, Broaddus VC. Interrelationship of pleural and pulmonary interstitial liquid. *Ann Rev Physiol* 1993;55:209–226.
23. Bhattacharya J, Gropper MA, Staub NC. Interstitial fluid pressure gradient measured by micropuncture in excised dog lung. *J Appl Physiol* 1984;56:271–277.
24. Payne DK, Kinasewitz GT, Gonzalez E. Comparative permeability of canine visceral and parietal pleura. *J Appl Physiol* 1988;65:2558–2564.
25. Kirschner PA. Porous diaphragm syndromes. *Chest Surg Clin N Am* 1998;8:449–472.
26. Hodges CC, Fossum TW, Evering W. Evaluation of thoracic duct healing after experimental laceration and transection. *Vet Surg* 1993;22:431–435.
27. Broaddus VC, Araya M, Carlton DP, et al. Developmental changes in pleural liquid protein concentration in sheep. *Am Rev Respir Dis* 1991;143:38–41.
28. Cooray GH. Defensive mechanisms in the mediastinum, with special reference to the mechanics of pleural absorption. *J Pathol Bacteriol* 1949;61:551–567.
29. Courtice FC, Simmonds WJ. Absorption of fluids from the pleural cavities of rabbits and cats. *J Physiol* 1949;109:117–130.
30. Burke H. The lymphatics which drain the potential space between the visceral and the parietal pleura. *Am Rev Tuberc Pulmon Dis* 1959;79:52–65.
31. Wang NS. The preformed stomas connecting the pleural cavity and the lymphatics in the parietal pleura. *Am Rev Respir Dis* 1975;111:12–20.
32. Stewart PB. The rate of formation and lymphatic removal of fluid in pleural effusions. *J Clin Invest* 1963;42:258–262.
33. Leckie WJH, Tothill P. Albumin turnover in pleural effusions. *Clin Sci* 1965;29:339–352.
34. Broaddus VC, Wiener-Kronish JP, Berthiauma Y, et al. Removal of pleural liquid and protein by lymphatics in awake sheep. *J Appl Physiol* 1988;64:384–390.
35. Aiba M, Inatomi K, Homma H. Lymphatic system or hydro-oncotic forces. Which is more significant in drainage of pleural fluid? *Jpn J Med* 1984;23:27–33.
36. Shinto RA, Light RW. The effects of diuresis upon the characteristics of pleural fluid in patients with congestive heart failure. *Am J Med* 1990;88:230–233.
37. Agostoni E. Mechanics of the pleural space. *Physiol Rev* 1972;52:57–128.
38. Agostoni E, Zocchi L. Starling forces and lymphatic drainage in pleural liquid and protein exchanges. *Respir Physiol* 1991;86:271–281.
39. Pistolesi M, Miniati M, Giuntini C. Pleural liquid and solute exchange. *Am Rev Respir Dis* 1989;140:825–847.
40. Nakamura T, Iwasaki Y, Tanaka Y, et al. Dynamics of pleural effusion estimated through urea clearance. *Jpn J Med* 1987;26:319–322.

41. Light RW, Jenkinson SG, Minh V, et al. Observations on pleural pressures as fluid is withdrawn during thoracentesis. *Am Rev Respir Dis* 1980;121:799–804.

42. Cheng C-S, Rodriguez RM, Perkett EA, et al. Vascular endothelial growth factor in pleural fluid. *Chest* 1999;115:760–765.

43. Thickett DR, Armstrong L, Millar AB. Vascular endothelial growth factor (VEGF) in inflammatory and malignant pleural effusions. *Thorax* 1999;54:707–710.

44. Eid AA, Keddissi JI, Kinasewitz GT. Hypoalbuminemia as a cause of pleural effusions. *Chest* 1999;115:1066–1069.

45. Allen SJ, Laine GA, Drake RE, et al. Superior vena caval pressure elevation causes pleural effusion formation in sheep. *Am J Physiol* 1988;255:H492–H495.

46. Verkman AS, Matthay MA, Song Y. Aquaporin water channels and lung physiology. *Am J Physiol Lung Cell Mol Physiol* 2000;278:L867–L879.

47. Yang B, Folkesson HG, Yang J, et al. Reduced osmotic water permeability of the peritoneal barrier in aquaporin-1 knockout mice. *Am J Physiol* 1999;276:C76–C81.

48. Magnussen H, Perry SF, Willmer H, et al. Transpleural diffusion of inert gases in excised lung lobes of the dog. *Respir Physiol* 1974;20:1–15.

49. Northfield TC. Oxygen therapy for spontaneous pneumothorax. *Br Med J* 1971;4:86–88.

50. Gaensler EA. Parietal pleurectomy for recurrent spontaneous pneumothorax. *Surg Gynecol Obstet* 1956;102:293–308.

51. Fleetham JA, Forkert L, Clarke H, et al. Regional lung function in the presence of pleural symphysis. *Am Rev Respir Dis* 1980;122:33–38.

52. Mulvey RB. The effect of pleural fluid on the diaphragm. *Radiology* 1965;84:1080–1086.

53. Krell WS, Rodarte JR. Effects of acute pleural effusion on respiratory system mechanics in dogs. *J Appl Physiol* 1985;59:1458–1463.

54. Light RW, Stansbury DW, Brown SE. The relationship between pleural pressures and changes in pulmonary function after therapeutic thoracentesis. *Am Rev Respir Dis* 1986;133:658–661.

55. Wang JS, Tseng CH. Changes in pulmonary mechanics and gas exchange after thoracentesis on patients with inversion of a hemidiaphragm secondary to large pleural effusion. *Chest* 1995;107:1610–1614.

56. Estenne M, Yernault J-C, De Troyer A. Mechanism of relief of dyspnea after thoracocentesis in patients with large pleural effusions. *Am J Med* 1983;74:813–819.

57. Nishida O, Arellano R, Cheng DC, et al. Gas exchange and hemodynamics in experimental pleural effusion. *Crit Care Med* 1999;27:583–587.

58. Agusti AG, Cardus J, Roca J, et al. Ventilation-perfusion mismatch in patients with pleural effusion: effects of thoracentesis. *Am J Respir Crit Care Med* 1997;156:1205–1209.

59. Brandstetter RD, Cohen RP. Hypoxemia after thoracentesis: a predictable and treatable condition. *JAMA* 1979;242:1060–1061.

60. Talmor M, Hydo L, Gershenwald JG, et al. Beneficial effects of chest tube drainage of pleural effusion in acute respiratory failure refractory to positive end-expiratory pressure ventilation. *Surgery* 1998;123:137–143.

61. Sonnenblick M, Melzer E, Rosin AJ. Body positional effect on gas exchange in unilateral pleural effusion. *Chest* 1983;83:784–786.

62. Neagley SR, Zwillich CW. The effect of positional changes on oxygenation in patients with pleural effusions. *Chest* 1985;88:714–717.

63. Chang SC, Shiao GM, Perng RP. Postural effect on gas exchange in patients with unilateral pleural effusions. *Chest* 1989;96:60–63.

64. Romero S, Martin C, Hernandez L, et al. Effect of body position on gas exchange in patients with unilateral pleural effusion: influence of effusion volume. *Respir Med* 1995;89:297–301.

65. Vaska K, Wann LS, Sagar K, et al. Pleural effusion as a cause of right ventricular diastolic collapse. *Circulation* 1992;86:609–617.

66. Negrus RA, Chachkes JS, Wrenn K. Tension hydrothorax and shock in a patient with a malignant pleural effusion. *Am J Emerg Med* 1990;8:205–207.

67. Kisanuki A, Shono H, Kiyonaga K, et al. Two-dimensional echocardiographic demonstration of left ventricular diastolic collapse due to compression by pleural effusion. *Am Heart J* 1991;122:1173–1175.

68. Shinto RA, Stansbury DW, Brown SE, et al. Does therapeutic thoracentesis improve the exercise capacity of patients with pleural effusion? *Am Rev Respir Dis* 1987;135:A244.

69. Shinto RA, Stansbury DW, Fischer CE, et al. The effect of thoracentesis on central respiratory drive in patients with large pleural effusions. *Am Rev Respir Dis* 1988;137:A112.

3

Radiographic Examinations

PLEURAL EFFUSIONS

Typical Arrangement of Free Pleural Fluid

Two main factors influence the distribution of free fluid in the pleural space. First, the pleural fluid accumulates in the most dependent part of the thoracic cavity because the lung is less dense than pleural fluid. In essence, the lung floats in the pleural fluid. Second, the lobes of the lung maintain their traditional shape at all stages of collapse owing to their elastic recoil (1). The shape of a lobe when it is partially or completely collapsed is a miniature replica of its shape when fully distended.

Bearing in mind that the distribution of fluid within the free pleural space obeys the law of gravity and that the lung maintains its shape when compressed, it is easy to predict the distribution of excess pleural fluid. The fluid first gravitates to the base of the hemithorax and comes to rest between the inferior surface of the lung and the diaphragm, particularly posteriorly, where the pleural sinus is the most inferior. As more fluid accumulates, the fluid spills out into the costophrenic sinuses posteriorly, laterally, and anteriorly. Additional fluid spreads upward in a mantle-like fashion around the convexity of the lung and gradually tapers as it assumes a higher position in the thorax.

Based on this pattern of fluid accumulation, the typical radiographic appearance of a pleural effusion of moderate size (1,000 mL) is as follows. In the posteroanterior projection (Fig. 3.1A), the lateral costophrenic angle is obliterated. The density of the fluid is high laterally and curves gently downward and medially with a smooth, meniscus-shaped upper border to terminate at the mediastinum. The layer of fluid is narrower at the mediastinal border than at the costal border; the reason for this difference is that the mediastinal surface of the lower lobe of the lung possesses less elastic recoil because it is fixed at the hilum and pulmonary ligament (1). In the lateral projection (Fig. 3.1B), the upper surface of the fluid density is semicircular, high anteriorly and posteriorly, and curving smoothly downward to its lowest point approximately midway between the sternum and the posterior chest wall.

Frequently, a "middle lobe step" is observed on the lateral radiograph (Fig. 3.1B). The explanation for the middle lobe step is that as pleural fluid accumulates, the first affected lobe is the lower lobe because it is the most dependent. Therefore, it starts to shrink and to float but maintains its shape. The middle lobe is unaffected and maintains its full volume. Accordingly, the result is a shrunken lower lobe with a middle lobe that retains its usual size. Radiographically, the fluid is mostly in the posterior part of the chest (Fig. 3.1B).

On the basis of the radiologic appearance, one might surmise that the height of the pleural fluid is greater laterally. The true upper limit of pleural fluid, however, is usually the same throughout the hemithorax (2). The meniscus shape is seen because the layer of fluid is of insufficient depth to cast a discernible shadow when viewed *en face* (Fig. 3.2).

Radiologic Signs

With the patient in the upright position, fluid first accumulates between the inferior surface of the lower lobe and the diaphragm. If the amount of

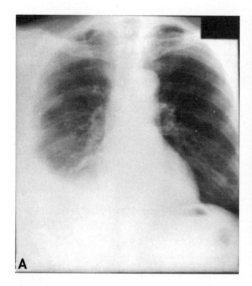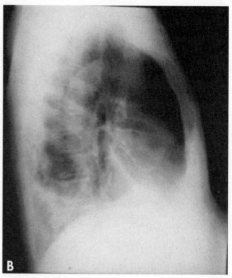

FIG. 3.1. Typical arrangement of free pleural fluid. **A:** Posteroanterior view revealing obliteration of the lateral costophrenic angle. Note that in this figure, a small amount of fluid appears in the lateral aspect of the minor fissure. **B:** Lateral view revealing obliteration of the diaphragmatic outline. Note that fluid is present in both major and minor fissures so that the right middle lobe is well outlined.

fluid is small (~75 mL), it may occupy only this position without spilling into the costophrenic sinuses. With this small amount of fluid, the normal configuration of the diaphragm is maintained, and the chest radiograph does not indicate that pleural fluid is present. When more fluid accumulates, it spills over into the posterior costophrenic angle and obliterates that sinus as viewed in the lateral projection (Fig. 3.1B). The normally sharp posterior costophrenic angle is obliterated by a shallow, homogeneous shadow whose upper surface is meniscus shaped. The pleural line up the posterior thoracic wall is also widened. Anytime the posterior costophrenic angle is obliterated or the posterior part of one or both diaphragms is obscured, the presence of pleural fluid is suggested, and further diagnostic efforts should be made. Moreover, if both posterior costophrenic angles are clear and sharp, the presence of clinically significant amounts of free pleural fluid can be nearly excluded.

Increasing amounts of fluid blunt the lateral costophrenic angle of the posteroanterior radiograph. Collins et al. (3) injected fluid into the pleural spaces of upright cadavers. They demonstrated that at least 175 mL pleural fluid had to be injected before the lateral costophrenic angle was blunted, and in some cases, more than 500 mL pleural fluid could be present without blunting the lateral costophrenic angle. As more fluid accumulates, the entire outline of the diaphragm on the affected side is lost, and the fluid extends upward around the anterior, lateral, and posterior thoracic walls. This fluid produces opacification of the lung base and the typical meniscus shape of the fluid, as demonstrated in Fig. 3.1.

Subpulmonic or Infrapulmonary Effusions

At times, for unknown reasons, substantial amounts of pleural fluid (over 1,000 mL) can be present and may remain in an infrapulmonary location without spilling into the costophrenic sulci or extending up the chest wall. Such pleural fluid accumulations are called subpulmonic or infrapulmonary pleural effusions (Fig. 3.3). Although the posterior costophrenic angle is usually blunted, at times it is perfectly clear (1).

The following radiologic characteristics are common to most cases of subpulmonic effusions (1), and the presence of one or more of these characteriistics should serve as an indication for

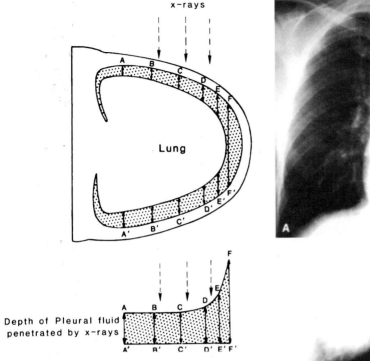

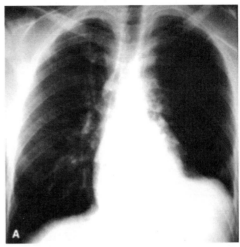

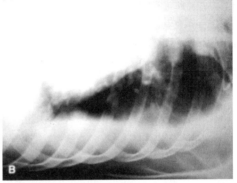

FIG. 3.2. Diagrammatic explanation for the meniscus shape of pleural fluid. The distance between the lung and the chest wall is the same around the entire lung. The depth of the fluid when viewed *en face* AA' to CC' is not sufficient to increase the radiodensity. More laterally at DD' to FF', however, the x-ray beam passes through more and more pleural fluid, so that an increase in density is radiologically evident.

FIG. 3.3. Subpulmonic pleural effusion. **A:** Posteroanterior chest radiograph showing apparent elevation of the left diaphragm with the apex of the apparent diaphragm more lateral than usual. **B:** Lateral decubitus film of this patient showing free pleural fluid. (Courtesy of Dr. Harry Sassoon.)

decubitus examinations to rule out the possibility of a subpulmonic pleural effusion: (a) apparent elevation of one or both diaphragms; (b) in the posteroanterior projection with subpulmonic effusions, the apex of the apparent diaphragm is more lateral than usual, near the junction of the middle third and the lateral third of the diaphragm, rather than at the center of the diaphragm; (c) the apparent diaphragm slopes much more sharply toward the lateral costophrenic angle (Fig. 3.4); (d) if the subpulmonic effusion is on the left side, the lower border of the lung is separated farther from the gastric air bubble than usual; normally, the top of the left diaphragm on the posteroanterior view is less than 2 cm above the stomach air bubble (4); a separation greater than 2 cm suggests a subpulmonic effusion, but of course, it can also be due to subdiaphragmatic fluid accumulation; if no gastric air bubble is present, the ingestion of a carbonated beverage by the patient will allow evaluation of this sign; (e) in the lateral projection, the major fissure often bows anteriorly where it meets the convex upper margin of the fluid; a small amount of fluid is usually apparent in the lower end of the major fissure at its junction with the infrapulmonary effusion; and (f) the lower lobe vessels may not be seen below the apparent diaphragmatic border.

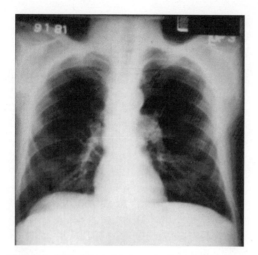

FIG. 3.4. Subpulmonic pleural effusion. Note that the right lateral costophrenic angle is clear, but the apex of the right diaphragm is more lateral than usual, and the apparent diaphragm slopes sharply toward the lateral costophrenic angle.

Diaphragmatic Inversion

At times, the weight of the fluid may cause the diaphragm to become inverted so that its normally convex superior border becomes concave. This inversion occurs much more commonly with effusions on the left, but it can occur with effusions on the right (5). Radiologically, the gastric air bubble is pushed inferiorly, and the superior border of the diaphragm is concave upward rather than convex. When viewed under fluoroscopy, such inverted diaphragms move paradoxically with respiration, rising on inspiration and descending on expiration (6). At times, patients with large left pleural effusions suddenly become dyspneic coincidentally with the development of inversion of the left diaphragm. In such instances, therapeutic thoracentesis is indicated (see Chapter 25). The removal of some of the pleural fluid restores the normal configuration to the diaphragm and rapidly relieves the patient's symptoms (6).

Supine Position

Until this time, I have only discussed the radiologic characteristics of pleural effusions with the patient in the upright position. Many chest radiographs, however, particularly those in acutely ill patients, are obtained with the patient in the supine position. When the patient is supine, pleural fluid gravitates to the posterior parts of the thoracic cavity. Because the pleural fluid is spread over a large area, considerable quantities must be present before any radiographic changes are seen.

The presence of free pleural fluid elicits several signs on the supine radiograph. These signs include blunting of the costophrenic angle, increased homogeneous density superimposed over the lung, loss of the hemidiaphragm silhouette, apical capping, elevation of the hemidiaphragm, decreased visibility of lower lobe vasculature, and accentuation of the minor fissure (7, 8). None of these signs are present in some patients with a small-to-moderate–sized pleural effusion. In one study (7), none of these radiologic signs were present in nine of 16 patients with small effusions (defined as measuring less than 1.5 cm on the decubitus radiograph) and in three of 13 patients with moderate effusions (defined as measuring 1.5 to 4.5 cm on the decubitus radiograph). In a second study, the supine chest radiograph suggested the presence of pleural fluid in 29 of 30 patients (97%) who had more than 300 mL pleural fluid (9). In this study, increased homogenous density, blunted costophrenic angle, and loss of diaphragm silhouette were the most accurate signs in diagnosing pleural effusion with an accuracy of about 80% (9). The increased homogeneous density in the majority of cases with pleural effusion was limited to the lower one or two thirds of the lung field or was more pronounced there (9).

The earliest sign is blunting of the costophrenic angle (7). Subsequently, increased density of the hemithorax, loss of the hemidiaphragm, and decreased visibility of the lower lobe vasculature occur. Apical capping does occur with pleural effusion, but it does not appear to be related to the size of the pleural effusion (7). Elevation of the hemidiaphragm and accentuation of the minor fissure are insensitive signs in that they occur in a minority of patients and they are not related to the size of the effusion (7).

Three characteristics serve to differentiate the increased density due to pleural fluid from that due to a parenchymal infiltrate. First, if the density is caused by pleural fluid, the vascular structures of the lung will be readily visible through the density in a properly exposed film. Any intrapulmonary process that produces a similar density, however, obliterates the vascular structure by the "silhouette effect." Second, if the density is due to pleural fluid, it is usually completely homogeneous. In contrast, infiltrates caused by intrapulmonary processes are usually less homogeneous. Third, air bronchograms are present only if the increased density is due to a parenchymal infiltrate.

Atypical Effusion

The typical arrangement of fluid in the pleural space depends on an underlying lung free of disease and therefore having uniform elastic recoil. If the lung underlying the effusion is diseased, the elastic recoil of the diseased portion is frequently different from that of the remainder of the lung, and fluid accumulates most where the elastic recoil is greatest. Therefore, an atypical collection of pleural fluid is an indication of underlying parenchymal as well as pleural disease. For example, if disease in a lower lobe increases its elastic recoil, fluid will collect posteromedially. Accordingly, in the posteroanterior projection, the opacity is higher on the mediastinal than on the axillary border, in contrast to the typical appearance in which the opacity is higher at the axillary border. Moreover, the upper surface curves downward and laterally toward the lateral costophrenic sulcus and thereby simulates atelectasis and consolidation of the middle and lower lobes. In the lateral projection, the upper border of the density roughly parallels the major fissure, beginning high in the thorax posteriorly and running downward and anteriorly to the anterior costophrenic sulcus. For the interested reader, Fleischner has detailed the radiographic appearance of atypical pleural fluid accumulation in disease affecting all the individual lobes (10).

Loculated Effusion

Pleural fluid may become encapsulated by adhesions anywhere between the parietal and the visceral pleura or in the interlobar fissures. Because the encapsulation is caused by adhesions between contiguous pleural surfaces, it occurs most frequently in association with conditions that cause intense pleural inflammation, such as empyema, hemothorax, or tuberculous pleuritis. Loculations occurring between the lung and the chest wall produce a characteristic radiographic picture. When viewed in profile (Fig. 3.5), the loculation is D-shaped, with the base of the D against the chest wall and the smooth convexity protruding inward toward the lung because of the compressibility of the lung parenchyma. If the loculation is in the lower part of the thoracic cavity, its lower border may not be visible. Loculation may be differentiated from parenchymal infiltrates by the absence of air bronchograms. A definitive diagnosis of loculated pleural effusion is best established by ultrasound (see the section of this chapter on ultrasound). Because multiple locules are common, the demonstration of one locule should serve as an indication to search for additional locules.

Loculation in the Fissures

The plane of the lung fissures is such that fluid encapsulated in the fissure is usually seen in profile in the lateral view. Fluid encapsulated in a fissure has a profile similar to a biconvex lens. Its margins are sharply defined and blend imperceptibly into interlobar fissures (Fig. 3.6). In some situations, the loculated effusion may simulate a mass on the posteroanterior radiograph. This situation is most frequently seen in patients with congestive heart failure, and because the fluid absorbs spontaneously when the congestive heart failure is treated, these fluid collections have been termed vanishing tumors or pseudotumors. The most common location of these "tumors" is in the right horizontal fissure (11). The distinctive configuration of the loculated interlobar effusion should establish the diagnosis. The disappearance of the apparent mass as the effusion resolves definitely establishes the diagnosis.

At times, it is difficult to differentiate encapsulated fluid in the lower half of a major fissure from atelectasis or combined atelectasis and consolidation of the right middle lobe. The following

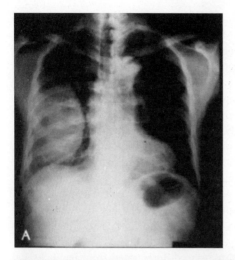

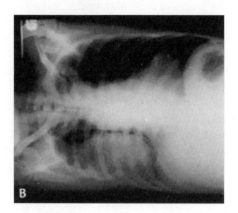

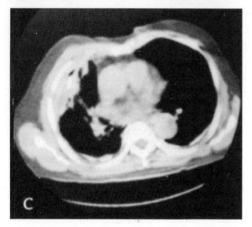

FIG. 3.5. Loculated pleural effusion. **A:** Posteroanterior radiograph demonstrating a D-shaped density, with base of the D against the right lateral chest wall. **B:** Right lateral decubitus radiograph demonstrating the absence of free pleural fluid in the same patient. **C:** CT scan demonstrating parenchymal involvement adjacent to loculated pleural effusion. This patient has an anaerobic infection of the lung and pleural space.

three points help make the distinction (1). First, if the minor fissure is visible as a separate shadow, the diagnosis of encapsulated fluid is certain. Second, encapsulated fluid does not usually obscure the border of the right side of the heart; in contrast, middle lobe atelectasis almost invariably does. Third, in the lateral projection, loculated effusions usually have a convex border on one or both sides. When the right middle lobe is diseased, the borders of the shadow are either straight or slightly concave.

RADIOLOGIC DOCUMENTATION

Most of the changes discussed in the previous sections are suggestive rather than diagnostic of the presence of pleural fluid. For example, blunting of the posterior or lateral costophrenic angles can be due to pleural effusion, but it can also be caused by pleural thickening or hyperinflation of the lung. Pleural effusion can obliterate one or both diaphragms on the lateral radiograph, but so can atelectasis or parenchymal infiltrates. Therefore, when the posteroanterior or the lateral chest radiograph suggests a pleural effusion, further radiographic studies are needed to document the presence of pleural fluid. If the pleural fluid is free, lateral decubitus radiographs are recommended. If the fluid is loculated, ultrasound examinations are preferred. The computed tomography (CT) scan is also useful in documenting both free and loculated pleural effusions.

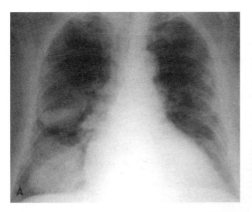 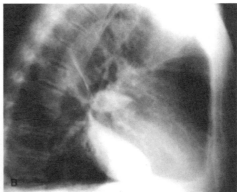

FIG. 3.6. Posteroanterior **(A)** and lateral **(B)** radiographs of a patient with congestive heart failure. **A:** Two masslike lesions are visible in the lower right lung field. **B:** The biconvex configuration of loculated fluid in both the major and the minor fissures is evident. With treatment of the patient's heart failure, the lung fields cleared, and the apparent masses disappeared. (Courtesy of Dr. Harry Sassoon.)

Lateral Decubitus Radiographs

The basis for the use of the lateral decubitus view is that free fluid gravitates to the most dependent part of the pleural space. The patient is placed in the lateral recumbent position, with the suspect side dependent. Sufficient radiolucent padding should be placed between the table top and the patient so an unobstructed tangential view of the dependent chest wall can be obtained. The x-ray film should be exposed with a high voltage to ensure that the interface between the fluid and the lung can be identified.

In the decubitus view, free pleural fluid is evidenced by a homogeneous density with a straight horizontal superior border between the dependent chest wall and the lower border of the lung (Fig. 3.7). This appearance is due to the lung floating in the fluid. By injecting fluid into the pleural space of cadavers, Moskowitz and colleagues have demonstrated that as little as 5 mL pleural fluid can be seen on properly exposed decubitus radiographs (12). Fluid is more easily demonstrated if the decubitus radiographs are obtained at full expiration rather than at full inspiration (13). The amount of free pleural fluid can be semiquantitated by measuring the distance between the inner border of the chest wall and the outer border of the lung (Fig. 3.7): the greater this distance, the more free pleural fluid. Empirically, I have found that when this distance is less than 10 mm, diagnostic thoracentesis is difficult because the amount of pleural fluid is small. Accordingly, I rarely attempt a diagnostic thoracentesis when the thickness of the pleural fluid on the decubitus radiograph is less than 10 mm.

Many patients suspected of having pleural effusions have apparent pleural thickening on the posteroanterior chest radiograph. When decubitus views are obtained in such patients, one must compare the distance between the lung and chest wall in the decubitus view to that in the posteroanterior view. If the distance between the lung and the chest wall is not at least 10 mm greater on the decubitus view, the patient does not have a significant amount of free pleural fluid.

In general, bilateral decubitus chest radiographs should be ordered. The film with the suspect side superior is informative because, in this view, the fluid gravitates toward the mediastinum. With the fluid shifted away from the chest wall and the lung, one can more readily assess the underlying lung for infiltrates or atelectasis (Fig. 3.7C). In addition, if the lateral costophrenic angle is blunted on the posteroanterior view and is clear on the decubitus view with the suspect side superior, one can be certain that the blunting is caused by free pleural fluid.

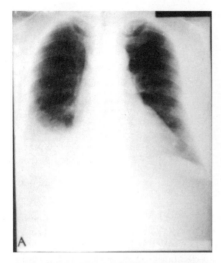

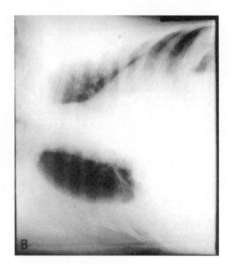

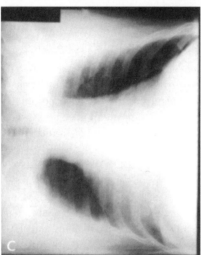

FIG. 3.7. A: Posteroanterior radiograph demonstrating blunting of the right costophrenic angle. **B:** Right lateral decubitus radiograph of the same patient demonstrating a large amount of free pleural fluid. **C:** Left lateral decubitus radiograph demonstrating that the lower right lung field is clear of parenchymal infiltrates.

Frequently, when decubitus radiographs are obtained, confusion exists as to which side is down. An arrow is usually seen on the x-ray film, but is the arrow pointing up or down in relation to the patient's position? Four radiologic characteristics allow the interpreter to ascertain the position of the patient when the radiograph was obtained. First, the dependent lung receives a greater percentage of the perfusion and therefore is more radiodense. Second, with the patient in the decubitus position, the abdominal pressure is greater on the dependent side; thus, the diaphragm on the dependent side is pushed higher in the thoracic cavity than the contralat-

eral diaphragm. Third, the radiolucent padding or examination table is often evident outside the thoracic cavity on the dependent side (Fig. 3.7). Fourth, if air–fluid levels are present in the stomach or the intestines, the air will always be on the superior side.

Semisupine Oblique Radiographs

Many patients are too ill or are in too much pain to tolerate decubitus chest radiographs. An alternate procedure that can be used to document free pleural fluid is to obtain oblique chest radiographs with the patient in the semisupine position. The patient assumes a position 45 to 65 degrees backward from the vertical plane. The individual's right side is lowered for separate views of both sides. Then the horizontal radiograph is centered to give a clear view of the dorsal half of the thorax. Films are obtained at full inspiration and full expiration. Pleural fluid is considered to be present when the thickness of the pleural shadow is greater on expiration than on inspiration. In one study, the semisupine oblique technique correctly demonstrated the presence of pleural fluid in 38 of 39 patients in whom fluid was demonstrated with decubitus radiographs. Moreover, in only five of 73 patients did the oblique semisupine films suggest fluid when none could be demonstrated by the decubitus technique (14).

Ultrasound

Ultrasound is very useful in the study of pleural disease (15). It can be used in several different situations, including the following: (a) identification of the appropriate location for an attempted thoracentesis, pleural biopsy, or chest tube placement; (b) identification of pleural fluid loculations; and (c) distinction of pleural fluid from pleural thickening (16). The advantages of ultrasound over CT are the ease and speed with which the examination can be performed, the availability of portable units that can be brought to the bedside of seriously ill patients, the lack of ionizing radiation, the relatively low cost, and the capacity to diagnose and distinguish an associated subphrenic process (16). With ultrasound, one can also assess the thickness of the parietal pleura and identify pleural nodules and focal pleural thickening (17). Last, with ultrasound, one can determine whether there is fusion of the visceral and parietal pleura. Given these advantages, there is no doubt that ultrasound has been underused in the assessment of pleural disease in the United States.

For simplicity, pleural fluid collections with ultrasound can be characterized as echo free (anechoic), complex septated if there are fibrin strands or septa floating inside the anechoic pleural effusions, complex nonseptated if heterogeneous echogenic material is inside the anechoic pleural effusion, and homogeneously echogenic if homogeneously echogenic spaces are present between the visceral and parietal pleura. In one recent series of 320 patients with pleural effusions, 172 (54%) were anechoic, 50 (16%) were complex nonseptated, 76 (24%) were complex septated, and 22 (7%) were homogeneously echogenic (17). Interestingly, all the patients who had complex-nonseptated, complex-septated, or homogeneously echogenic results had exudative pleural effusions. Patients who had anechoic effusions could have either transudative or exudative pleural effusions (17).

Sonographic examination of the pleura should be performed with plane or convex probes of 3.5, 5.0, 7.0, or even 10.0 MHz using the intercostal space as an acoustic window (18). The high-frequency transducer improves resolution in the near field so internal echoes in a solid lesion are easier to image, which helps the examiner distinguish solid lesions from cystic lesions. In addition, near-field reverberation artifacts, which might otherwise obscure fluid close to the skin, are reduced. Real-time scanning is preferred to conventional static scanning because it allows one to assess the changing configuration of pleural fluid with respiration, it is easier to use in the intercostal spaces, and it requires less time to scan large areas (16). The best distinguishing characteristic of a pleural fluid collection on ultrasound is that it changes its shape with respiration (19).

Ultrasound is accurate at identifying the presence of pleural fluid. In one recent study of 60 patients with congestive heart failure, CT scans demonstrated pleural effusions in 52 of the 60 (87%) (20). Ultrasound demonstrated pleural fluid in over 90% of the patients in whom the fluid was identified with CT (20). It has been suggested that color Doppler ultrasound is superior to real-time gray-scale ultrasound in the identification of pleural fluid (21). With the color Doppler ultrasound, pleural fluid is identified because it provides a color signal. In one report of 51 patients with minimal pleural effusions, color Doppler ultrasound correctly demonstrated color in 33 of 35 (94%) patients with pleural fluid but was negative in the 16 patients without pleural fluid. In contrast, real-time gray-scale ultrasound identified fluid in all 35 patients with fluid but also in five of 16 patients without fluid (21).

Another situation in which ultrasound is being used more and more is in the evaluation of the trauma patient (22, 23). Ma et al. reported that the ultrasound performed by emergency room physicians correctly identified 24 of 25 hemothoraces (96%) (22). In another study of 360 patients, 39 of 40 hemothoraces were detected by ultrasound, whereas 37 were detected by chest radiograph. The performance time for ultrasonography was significantly faster than that for chest radiography (1.3 versus 14.2 minutes) (23).

Ultrasonic techniques are useful in identifying the appropriate site for thoracentesis (16, 17, 24). The appropriate site can be identified both in patients with loculated pleural effusions and in those with small amounts of pleural fluid. In addition to identifying the site for aspiration, the appropriate depth for aspiration can also be ascertained, thereby increasing the safety of the procedure. It is important to perform the thoracentesis at the time the fluid is identified by ultrasound. When the skin is only marked at the time of the ultrasonic examination and the patient is sent back to the ward, the patient is frequently in a different position when the thoracentesis is attempted. In such instances, the relationship between the skin and the pleural fluid is altered, and the thoracentesis attempt may occur at the wrong location (24). Of course, the utility of the ultrasonic examination for pleural fluid depends upon the skill and the interest of the ultrasonographer. Performing the thoracentesis in the presence of the ultrasonographer will also improve the capabilities of the ultrasonographer by providing immediate feedback. At the present time at my hospital, most thoracenteses are performed by a radiologist with ultrasound guidance. The safety of this method is documented by the observation that of the 251 thoracenteses performed during a recent 6-month period, only 13 patients developed a pneumothorax and only one of these required a chest tube (25).

Computed Tomography

The availability of CT has markedly improved our ability to assess pleural abnormalities ra-diologically. Pleural abnormalities can be more readily detected and distinguished from lung parenchymal and extrapleural disease by CT than by standard radiographs because these anatomic compartments are distinct on the cross-sectional image with CT (26). Pleural collections or masses tend to conform to the pleural space. As with chest radiographs, the angle of the lesion with the chest wall may help identify whether the lesion is pleural or parenchymal. If the angle of the abnormality with the chest wall is acute, then the lesion probably has a parenchymal origin, whereas if the angle is obtuse, the lesion probably has a pleural origin. Sometimes, however, the CT findings are as ambiguous as the radiographs, particularly when there is atelectasis or pneumonia, or when a pleural collection forms acute angles with the chest wall.

Free-flowing pleural fluid produces a sickle-shaped opacity in the most dependent part of the thorax posteriorly (Fig. 3.8) (16). Loculated fluid collections are seen as lenticular opacities of fixed position. When free fluid lies in the posterior costophrenic recess adjacent to the diaphragm, it may be difficult to differentiate from ascites. Several CT features have been described that aid in the differentiation of pleural fluid from ascites. These are the displaced crus sign, the interface sign, the diaphragm sign, and the bare-area sign (16). With the displaced crus sign, the

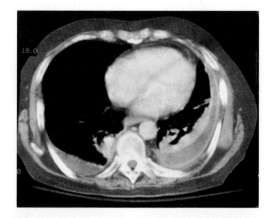

FIG. 3.8. CT scan with contrast demonstrating bilateral pleural effusions, the left larger than the right. Note how the parenchyma on the left is enhanced in comparison to the collection of pleural fluid.

displacement of the diaphragmatic crus away from the spine by the fluid indicates that the fluid is in the pleural space. In contrast, ascites lies lateral and anterior to the crus. With the interface sign, a sharp interface can be identified between the fluid and the liver or spleen, and this interface indicates that ascites is present. This line is much less distinct if pleural fluid is present. With the diaphragm sign, fluid that is outside the diaphragm is pleural fluid, whereas fluid that is inside the diaphragm is ascites. With the bare-area sign, restriction of ascites by the coronary ligaments from the bare area of the liver indicates that the patient has ascites.

CT is effective at demonstrating abnormalities in the lung parenchyma that are obscured on the conventional chest radiograph by the pleural disease. Chest CT is particularly useful in distinguishing empyema with air–fluid levels from lung abscess, as discussed subsequently. In patients with pleural effusions, CT can also identify pleural thickening, which suggests that the patient has an exudative effusion. In one study, 36 of 59 exudative effusions (61%) had associated pleural thickening, whereas only 1 of 27 transudates (4%) had associated pleural thickening (27). An added bonus with CT is the clear demonstration of bone pathology such as metastases or tuberculosis.

Chest CT is not indicated in all patients with suspected pleural disease. The density coefficients from CT are not specific enough to distinguish among parenchymal lesions, solid pleural masses, or pleural collections of serous fluid, blood, or pus (28). Ultrasonic examinations are preferred over CT when the primary question is whether pleural fluid is present.

CT examinations of the chest have also provided additional information concerning the effects of a pleural effusion on the underlying lung. Paling and Griffin reviewed the chest CT obtained in the supine position of 46 cases with a moderate or large pleural effusion (29). The volume of the underlying lung, particularly the lower lobe, was reduced in all patients, and there was atelectasis of the underlying lung in 44 of the 46 (96%) patients. In 19 patients, there was segmental collapse of the lower lobe. In seven patients, the atelectatic segment was so large as to produce an appearance initially suggestive of

complete collapse of the lower lobe. Recognition that the lower lobe was at least in part inflated depended on identification of the major fissure anterior to the airless lung, identification of lower lobe bronchi and vessels surrounded by aerated lung on more cephalad sections, and the presence of an identifiable inferior pulmonary vein in the normal location within aerated lung. In 25 of 46 patients, the lower lobe collapse involved all except the superior segment, which tended to remain aerated. Recognition of a major degree of volume loss in the lower lobe depended on identification of the bronchial anatomy serving the airless lung and on the loss of an identifiable inferior pulmonary vein, which was buried within the collapsed lung.

CT examinations of the chest have also been used to evaluate the major and minor fissures. In one report, 100 CT scans of patients with normal lungs were reviewed to determine the normal characteristics of the major fissures and the minor fissure. Each major fissure was imaged most often as a lucent band, less often as a line, and least often as a dense band. In contrast, the minor fissure was imaged as a lucent area, which was usually triangular with its apex at the hilar region (30).

Magnetic Resonance Imaging

Magnetic resonance imaging (MRI) has generated considerable interest as a safe and sensitive technique for imaging human pathologic conditions. The technique basically consists of inducing transitions between energy states by causing certain atoms to absorb and transfer energy. This is accomplished by directing a radio frequency pulse at a substance placed within a large magnetic field. Measures of the time required for the material to return to a baseline energy state (relaxation time) can be translated by a complex computer algorithm to a visual image. There are two time constants associated with relaxation, called T1 and T2. The T1 relaxation time characterizes a time constant with which the nuclei align in a given magnetic field. In contrast, T2 reflects the time constant for loss of phase coherence of excited spins (31, 32).

With MRI, the lungs are seen as regions of black signal intensity similar to the black appearance of the lungs on CT. When evaluating the soft tissues, however, several differences are noted. The subcutaneous fat on MRI has bright signal intensity, compared with the low signal intensity with CT. On MRI, the vascular structures including the aorta and main, left, and right pulmonary arteries are seen as regions of signal void (black) that is distinct from the surrounding mediastinal fat. With noncontrast CT, the vessels and masses have a similar attenuation. The bony structures on MRI may be seen as regions of bright signal intensity because of the fat within the marrow or low intensity for cortical bone (32).

Pleural effusions can be identified with MRI. A pleural fluid collection is visualized as an area of abnormally low signal intensity on T1-weighted images that increases in brightness on T2-weighted images. This characteristic is consistent with the relatively long T1 and T2 values of pleural fluid. With MRI, different types of pleural fluid collections such as transudative fluid, chylothorax, hemothorax, or pus may appear somewhat different, but their characteristics are not sufficiently distinct as to be diagnostic. A diagnostic thoracentesis is certainly more definitive and less expensive.

In summary, MRI of the chest at the present time is less satisfactory than ultrasound or CT in identifying the presence of a pleural effusion. For patients with mesothelioma, the CT and MRI provide comparable information in most instances. The MRI is superior to CT in revealing solitary foci of chest wall invasion and endothoracic fascia involvement, and also in showing diaphragmatic muscle invasion. However, these findings do not affect surgical treatment (33). At present, there are no definite clinical indications for MRI of the chest in the management of patients with pleural disease.

AIR–FLUID LEVELS IN THE PLEURAL SPACE

When both air and fluid are present in the pleural space, an air–fluid level is apparent on radiographs obtained in the erect position (Fig. 3.9). An air–fluid level is manifested as an absolutely straight line parallel to the bottom of the radiograph. Of course, if the radiograph is obtained with the patient supine, no air–fluid level will be present unless it is a cross-table lateral view. The presence of an air–fluid level in the pleural space indicates that air has gained entry into the pleural space. The differential diagnosis includes bronchopleural fistula from pulmonary infections, spontaneous pneumothorax

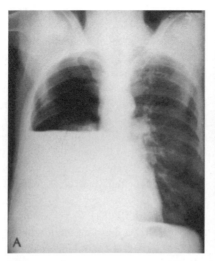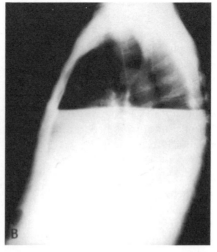

FIG. 3.9. Posteroanterior **(A)** and lateral **(B)** radiographs of a patient with a hydropneumothorax. Note that the air–fluid level extends throughout the length and width of the hemithorax. This hydropneumothorax followed an attempted thoracentesis in this patient with a massive right pleural effusion.

with pleural effusion, trauma (iatrogenic or non-iatrogenic), the presence of gas-forming organisms in the pleural space, and rupture of the esophagus into the pleural space. Air–fluid levels in the pleural space must be distinguished from air–fluid levels in dilated loops of bowel entering the thoracic cavity through a diaphragmatic hernia. Contrast media studies of the gastrointestinal tract are diagnostic in doubtful cases.

It is frequently difficult to distinguish a loculated pyopneumothorax with a bronchopleural fistula from a peripheral lung abscess. This differentiation is important because pyopneumothorax should be treated on an emergency basis with pleural drainage (see Chapter 9), whereas a lung abscess usually responds to antibiotics and postural drainage alone. Both ultrasound and CT are useful in distinguishing between these two conditions. With ultrasonic examination during hyperventilation, asymmetric motion of the proximal (chest wall–parietal pleura) and the distal (visceral pleura–lung) interface occurs when the process is in the pleural space. If the process is within the lung parenchyma, the proximal and distal interfaces (anterior and posterior walls of the cavity) move symmetrically (34).

Empyema with a bronchopleural fistula can also be distinguished from a lung abscess by chest CT (28). With CT scanning, a pyopneumothorax is characterized by unequal fluid levels on positional scanning that closely approximate the chest wall. The space characteristically has a smooth, regular margin that is sharply defined without side pockets. The appearance of the cavity often changes with variations in the patient's position. In contrast, a lung abscess is typically round with an irregular, thick wall and has an air–fluid level of equal length in all positions. When the patient's position is changed, the shapes of the cavity and of the mass do not change. Frequently, multiple side pockets are adjacent to the main cavity. An additional distinguishing feature is that the larger empyemas displace the adjacent lung and lung abscesses do not (28).

CT is not infallible in distinguishing empyemas from lung abscesses. Bressler et al. (35) reviewed the CT scans from 71 patients in whom the question was whether the individual had a lung abscess or empyema. In five of the 71 patients, the foregoing morphologic criteria were insufficient to make the distinction. The intravenous administration of a bolus of contrast medium in conjunction with CT was diagnostically useful. The demonstration of vessels within a lesion unequivocally identifies the lesion as parenchymal rather than pleural. Moreover, after administration of sufficient amounts of contrast material, pulmonary parenchyma is enhanced, whereas most pleural lesions show minimal or no enhancement (35).

Another condition that must be differentiated from empyema in a patient with air–fluid levels in the chest is fluid-filled bullae or lung cysts in which the CT findings may resemble those of empyema. On CT scan, the fluid-filled cavities have many characteristics of loculated pleural fluid collections including lenticular shape; air–fluid levels of different length on orthogonal views; uniform, smooth inner walls; and mass effect on the adjacent lung. Two features are useful in differentiating fluid-filled cysts from empyema: (a) cysts tend to be located in the upper lobes and the air–fluid levels are limited by fissures, and (b) one notes the absence of preexisting or coexisting large pleural effusion with fluid-filled cysts (36).

QUANTITATION OF THE AMOUNT OF PLEURAL FLUID

It is possible to estimate with some degree of reliability the amount of pleural fluid with either ultrasonography or lateral decubitus chest radiographs. Eibenberger et al. (37) studied 51 patients who had lateral decubitus chest radiographs and sonography while supine. The thickness of the fluid on the lateral decubitus radiograph and on sonography was measured just cranial to the base of the lung. Subsequent to these studies, the patients underwent therapeutic thoracentesis with removal of all of the pleural fluid. The relationship between the measurements and the amount of fluid withdrawn is shown in Fig. 3.10. It can be seen in Fig. 3.10 that the amount of fluid is more closely correlated with the ultrasonic measurement than with the lateral decubitus measurement. Note also that

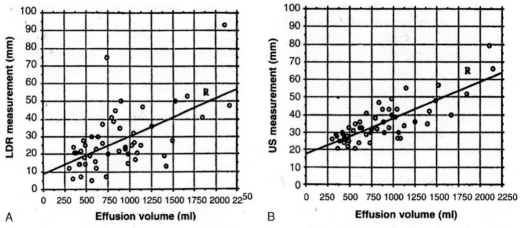

FIG. 3.10. Correlation of actual volume of pleural effusion with **(A)** thickness of fluid on the lateral decubitus radiograph and with **(B)** thickness of fluid on sonography. Values are from 51 patients before thoracentesis. The sonographic measurements were more closely correlated with the volume of the fluid (R = 0.80) than were the lateral decubitus measurements. (From Eibenberger KL, Dock WI, Ammann ME, et al. Quantification of pleural effusions: sonography versus radiography. *Radiology* 1994;191:681–684, with permission.)

on the lateral decubitus radiograph, a fluid thickness of 30 mm corresponds to a volume of 1,000 mL, whereas on the ultrasound measurement, a fluid thickness of 40 mm corresponds to a volume of 1,000 mL.

The amount of pleural fluid can also be semiquantitated from the posteroanterior and lateral chest radiographs (38). Blackmore et al. (38) have demonstrated that when there is more than 50 mL pleural fluid present, the pleural fluid becomes visible on the lateral radiograph as a meniscus posteriorly. When there is more than 200 mL fluid present, a meniscus can be identified in the lateral costophrenic angle of the posteroanterior radiograph. When there is more than 500 mL pleural fluid present, the meniscus obscures the entire hemidiaphragm.

Massive Effusion

When an entire hemithorax is opacified, one should first examine the position of the mediastinum because its position is influenced by the pleural pressures (Fig. 3.11). If the pleural pressure is lower on the side of the effusion, the mediastinum will be shifted toward the side of the effusion (Fig. 3.11A). Alternately, if the pleural

pressure is higher on the side of the effusion, the mediastinum will be shifted toward the contralateral side (Fig. 3.11B). Of course, if the mediastinum is invaded by tumor or other infiltrative processes, it will be fixed, and no shift will be evident on the posteroanterior radiograph.

When the patient's mediastinum is shifted toward the side of the effusion, the lung underlying the effusion is usually diseased. In such a case, overexpansion of the contralateral lung produces an enlarged retrosternal clear space on the lateral view. By far the most common cause of this radiographic picture is complete obstruction of the ipsilateral main stem bronchus by a neoplasm. Therefore, if the mediastinum is shifted toward the side of the effusion, the initial diagnostic procedure should be bronchoscopy to assess the patency of the bronchial tree. If an obstructing lesion is found, thoracentesis is not recommended because it is unnecessary diagnostically, and it carries an increased risk because of the negative pleural pressure, which can lead to a pneumothorax or reexpansion pulmonary edema. If no obstructing lesion is found, removal of large amounts (greater than 1,000 mL) of pleural fluid should only be attempted if pleural pressures are monitored (39).

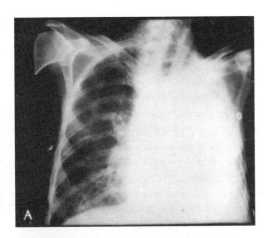

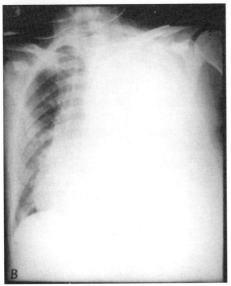

FIG. 3.11. A: Massive pleural effusion with marked shift of the trachea and mediastinum toward the side of the effusion. This patient had a bronchogenic carcinoma obstructing the left main bronchus. **B:** Massive pleural effusion with marked shift of the trachea and mediastinum away from the side of the effusion.

When the patient's mediastinum is shifted toward the contralateral side, an active process in the pleural space has led to the accumulation of pleural fluid. In such instances, not only is the ipsilateral lung completely nonfunctional, but the function of the contralateral lung is also compromised (Fig. 3.11B). A therapeutic thoracentesis (see Chapter 25) should be performed

immediately to attempt, at least, to restore the mediastinum to midline. The most common cause of massive pleural effusion with mediastinal shift is metastatic disease of the pleura (40), but tuberculosis, empyema, cirrhosis with hepatothorax, chylothorax, hemothorax, and congestive heart failure may also cause this picture. If the mediastinum is midline in a patient with a massive pleural effusion, the mediastinum is usually invaded by tumor. At times, most of the mediastinum is in the midline, but the tracheal air shadow is shifted. This picture is suggestive of bronchogenic carcinoma (41).

CT scan and ultrasound are both quite useful in evaluating patients with unilateral hemithorax opacification. Yu et al. (42) evaluated these two diagnostic modalities in 50 patients with unilateral hemithorax opacification. Either procedure can demonstrate whether the opacification is due to fluid, a tissue mass, or a combination. It is interesting that nine of the 50 patients in the above-mentioned series (18%) had no fluid in their pleural space. Both procedures are very effective in demonstrating pleural or parenchymal abnormalities, whereas only CT scan effectively demonstrates mediastinal involvement (42).

PLEURAL THICKENING

The pleura may become thickened over the convexity of the thorax and occasionally in the interlobar fissure.

Radiologic Signs

Normally, no line is visible between the inside of the chest wall and the outer border of the lung, but in response to inflammation of the pleura, the lung may become separated from the chest wall by a pleural line. After an episode of pleuritis, the thickness of the pleural line may be 1 to 10 mm. The pleural thickening that follows pleural inflammation results almost exclusively from fibrosis of the visceral pleural surface. The thickening may be either localized or generalized. If the pleural thickening is localized, it most commonly involves the inferior portions of the thoracic cavity because that is where the pleural fluid containing inflammatory mediators accumulates.

Frequently with localized pleural thickening, the costophrenic angles are partially or completely obliterated. In such instances, decubitus radiographs (see the foregoing section of this chapter on decubitus radiographs) are indicated to rule out free pleural fluid. The main significance of localized pleural thickening is as an index of previous pleural inflammation.

Following intense pleural inflammation, such as occurs with a massive hemothorax, pyothorax, or tuberculous pleuritis, generalized pleural thickening of an entire hemithorax may occur. This thickening is again due to the deposition of fibrous tissue on the visceral pleura. The thickness of the pleura may exceed 2 cm. Frequently, the inner aspect of this "peel" is calcified, providing an accurate measurement of the thickness of the peel. If the patient is symptomatic and if the underlying lung is functional, decortication (see Chapter 24) may provide symptomatic relief.

Apical Thickening

The pleura in the apex of the lungs sometimes becomes thickened. Although in the past, apical pleural thickening was usually attributed to tuberculosis (1), tuberculosis is not responsible for most cases at the present time. Renner et al. (43) studied the apical pleura at autopsy in 19 patients with radiologically visible pleural thickening and found no evidence of tuberculosis in any of the patients. However, the apical cap is commonly present in patients who have upper lobe fibrosis secondary to tuberculosis. The frequency of apical pleural thickening increases with age, and the authors suggested that the apical pleural thickening might be related to the healing of pulmonary disease in the presence of chronic ischemia (43). Apical pleural thickening is frequently bilateral but can be unilateral (43). Gross asymmetry should raise the suspicion of apical pulmonary carcinoma or Pancoast's tumor.

Asbestos-Induced Thickening

Pleural thickening can also result from asbestos exposure (see Chapter 24). In contrast to other types of pleural thickening, the parietal pleura rather than the visceral pleura is thickened following asbestos exposure. The pleural thickening can either be localized, in which case the thickenings are called pleural plaques, or generalized (44). An average of 30 years elapses between the first exposure to asbestos and the appearance of pleural plaques (44). The pleural thickening or plaques associated with asbestos exposure are usually bilateral, more prominent in the lower half of the thorax, and follow the rib contours (45). The pleural thickening due to asbestos exposure eventually becomes calcified. The calcification ranges from small linear or circular shadows, which are usually situated over the diaphragmatic domes, to complete encirclement of the lower portion of the lungs. CT of the chest is more sensitive than other radiologic procedures in identifying both pleural thickening and pleural calcification due to asbestos exposure (46).

In obese patients, subcostal fat may mimic pleural thickening. Typically, it appears as a symmetric, smooth, soft tissue density that parallels the chest wall and is of greatest thickness over the apices. In problem cases, subcostal fat can be distinguished from either diffuse thickening or localized plaques with CT. On CT, subcostal fat can be identified as low-density tissue internal to the ribs and external to the parietal pleura (16).

PNEUMOTHORAX

The radiographic signs of a pneumothorax are influenced by two factors (1). First, air in the pleural space accumulates in the highest part of the thoracic cavity because air is less dense than the lung. Second, the lobes of the lung maintain their traditional shape at all stages of collapse. Note that these are the same factors that influence pleural fluid accumulation. The only difference is that with pneumothorax, air rises to the apex of the hemithorax and causes early collapse of the upper lobes of the lung, whereas with pleural effusion, the pleural fluid falls to the bottom of the hemithorax and collapses the lower lobes.

The pleural pressure is normally negative, because of the balance between the inward pull of the lung and the outward pull of the chest wall. If air is introduced into the pleural space, the lung becomes smaller, the thoracic cavity enlarges, and the pleural pressure increases. If 1,000 mL of air enters the pleural space, the lung decreases in volume by about 600 mL, whereas the thoracic cavity will increase in volume by about 400 mL (Fig. 21.1). The ipsilateral pleural pressure becomes less negative, and because the contralateral pleural pressure remains unchanged, the mediastinum will shift toward the contralateral side. The ipsilateral diaphragm is also lowered on account of the increased pleural pressure and resultant decreased transdiaphragmatic pressure. An enlarged hemithorax, a depressed diaphragm, and a shifted mediastinum do not mean that a tension pneumothorax is present.

Radiologic Signs

A definitive radiologic diagnosis of pneumothorax can be made only when a visceral pleural line can be identified (Fig. 3.12). The visceral pleural line is evident as a faint but sharply defined line separating the lung parenchyma from the remainder of the thoracic cavity, which is clear and devoid of lung markings. Although one might suppose that the partially collapsed lung would have increased density radiologically, it does not for the following reasons. First, blood flow through the partially collapsed lung, which contributes substantially to the density radiologically, decreases proportionally to the degree of collapse. Second, the thorax is a cylinder, and with a pneumothorax, the presence of air both anterior and posterior to the partially collapsed lung decreases the overall density of the lung. The radiologic density of the lung does not increase until the lung loses approximately 90% of its volume. Complete atelectasis of a lung due to pneumothorax is characterized ipsilaterally by an enlarged hemithorax, a depressed diaphragm, a shift of the mediastinum to the contralateral side, and a fist-sized mass of increased density at the lower part of the hilum representing the collapsed lung (Fig. 3.13).

The diagnosis of pneumothorax is usually easily established by demonstrating the visceral pleural line on the posteroanterior radiograph. With small pneumothoraces, however, the visceral pleural line may not be visible on the routine radiographs. In such cases, one of the following two procedures can establish the diagnosis: (a) radiographs can be obtained in the upright position in full expiration; the rationale is that, although the volume of gas in the pleural space is constant, with full expiration, the lung volume

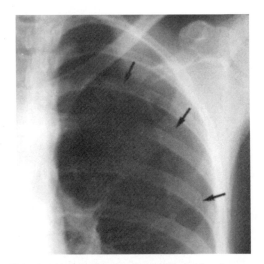

FIG. 3.12. Posteroanterior radiograph of a patient with a pneumothorax on the left side. Note the obvious pleural line (*arrows*) separating the lung from the air in the pleural space. The density of the radiograph inside and outside the pleural line is similar. Note also that a bleb (*upper arrow*) is present along the surface of the apical pleural line. This bleb was probably responsible for the pneumothorax. (Courtesy of Dr. Harry Sassoon.)

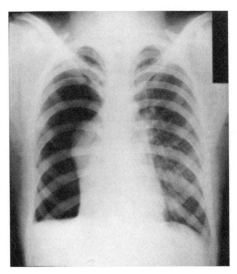

FIG. 3.13. Posteroanterior radiograph of a patient with a pneumothorax and complete atelectasis of the right lung.

is reduced, and therefore, the percentage of the hemithorax occupied by air increases, making identification of the visceral pleural line much easier; and (b) radiographs can be obtained in the lateral decubitus position, with the side of the suspected pneumothorax superior; the free air in the pleural space rises, increasing the distance between the lung and the chest wall; additionally, fewer conflicting shadows are seen over the lateral chest wall than at the apex. It appears that the decubitus position is the most sensitive for detecting a pneumothorax. Carr et al. (47) obtained conventional chest radiographs and CT scans on cadavers in which varying amounts of intrapleural air had been introduced. They found that the lateral decubitus film was most sensitive (88%) for the diagnosis of pneumothorax, followed by the erect (59%) and supine (37%) views. These researchers reported that the pneumothorax was always detected in the lateral decubitus position when there was more than 40 mL of intrapleural air. In addition, they found that a CT scan was no more sensitive than the decubitus views (47).

Pneumothoraces are more difficult to recognize on lateral projections than on posteroanterior projections. In one series, the pneumothorax could not be identified on the lateral projection in 13 of 122 patients (11%) (48). When the pneumothorax is identifiable, the displaced pleural line is more frequently anteriorly or posteriorly and is less commonly at the lung apex. In 10% of the patients, an air–fluid level was the only recognizable finding of a pneumothorax on the lateral projection (48).

Skin folds may superficially mimic a pleural line and possibly lead to a misdiagnosis of pneumothorax. A skin fold results in an abnormal edge with a sharp black–white interface laterally, with gradual fading of the density from white to black medially (Fig. 3.14). In contrast, there is no such fading medial to the line with pneumothorax. In addition, lung markings are seen peripheral to the edge of the skin fold, in contrast to absence of lung markings peripheral to the line of a pneumothorax (49).

It is much more difficult to establish the diagnosis of pneumothorax on a supine radiograph. In a review of 88 critically ill patients with 112 cases of pneumothorax, 30% of the cases were

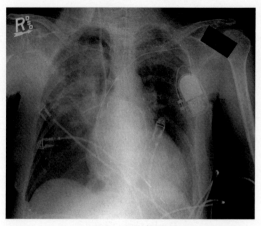

FIG. 3.14. Anteroposterior radiograph of a patient with a pneumothorax in the right apex and a skin fold in the left apex. On the side with the pneumothorax, note the sharp black–white interface medial to the apparent pleural line. In contrast, note that on the side with the skin fold (left side), there is gradual fading from the white pleural line as one moves medially.

not initially detected by the radiologist, and half these patients progressed to tension pneumothorax (49). The most common location for collections of air on the supine film is the anteromedial location because this area is the least dependent pleural recess. The three other locations in which air collects on the supine radiograph are subpulmonically, apicolaterally, and posteromedially. Depending on the size and location of the gas collection, any of the following features can be signs of a pneumothorax in the supine position: an exceptionally deep radiolucent costophrenic sulcus; a lucency over the right or left upper quadrant; or a much sharper than normal appearance of the hemidiaphragm, with or without the presence of a visible visceral pleural line above the diaphragm (1). The interested reader is referred to the review article by Buckner et al. (49) for details concerning the radiologic appearance of air in these locations.

Ultrasound can be used to establish the diagnosis of pneumothorax (18, 50, 51). Normal lung is characterized by having so-called lung sliding and comet tail artifacts on ultrasound. Normally, with real-time sonography, respiratory excursions of the visceral pleura can be discerned from the movement of discrete hypoechoic inhomogeneities within the high-echo band of the pleural reflection (50). This movement has been called pleural sliding or lung sliding (50). In addition, at the boundary between the pleura and the ventilated lung tissue, intensive bandlike reverberation echoes (comet tail artifacts) normally are evoked during breathing movements (51). Lichtenstein et al. (51) performed ultrasound examinations over the anterior chest on 184 hemithoraces including 41 with pneumothorax. They reported that both lung sliding and comet tailar tifacts were absent in all 41 patients with pneumothorax but in only four of the other 142 hemithoraces (3.5%). Ultrasound is particularly useful at diagnosing pneumothorax in the critically ill patient.

Atypical Pneumothorax

As with pleural effusions, the radiologic appearance of a pneumothorax can be atypical. If the parenchyma of the lung is diseased such that the lung does not retain its normal shape, the appearance of the partially collapsed lung is altered. The presence of adhesions between the visceral and the parietal pleura also alters the radiologic appearance of pneumothoraces. Such adhesions are frequently manifested as bandlike structures tethering the partially collapsed lung to the chest wall. Diffuse adhesions between the visceral and the parietal pleura may prevent collapse of an entire lobe (Fig. 3.15).

Clinically and radiologically, it is important to distinguish giant bullae from pneumothoraces because the treatment for the two conditions is different. This differentiation at times is difficult because a large bulla may mimic a large pneumothorax with adhesions. If doubt exists, a CT scan should be obtained because it can unequivocally establish the diagnosis (52).

Tension Pneumothorax

A tension pneumothorax exists when the pressure in the pleural space is positive throughout the respiratory cycle. Because the increased pleural pressure can seriously compromise pulmonary gas exchange and cardiac output (see Chapter 21), it is important to recognize the presence of a tension pneumothorax so treatment

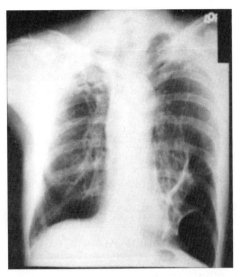

FIG. 3.15. Atypical pneumothorax. Posteroanterior radiograph of a patient with old pulmonary tuberculosis and a secondary spontaneous pneumothorax on the left side. Note that the pleural air is seen only in the lower part of the hemithorax because the visceral and parietal pleura over the upper lung had become fused by the old tuberculosis.

can be undertaken immediately. The radiologic diagnosis of a tension pneumothorax is unreliable from plain radiographic films alone. Although it is frequently stated that enlargement of a hemithorax, flattening of the diaphragm, and contralateral shift of the mediastinum indicate a tension pneumothorax, all three signs occur occasionally with nontension pneumothoraces (1). A definitive diagnosis can be established radiologically only by fluoroscopic examination. With a tension pneumothorax, the increased pleural pressure prevents the shift of the mediastinum toward the involved side on inspiration, as occurs with a nontension pneumothorax, and the movement of the ipsilateral diaphragm is restricted (1). In general, however, it is better to insert a needle into the pleural space to ascertain the presence of a tension pneumothorax than to waste time with radiologic procedures (see Chapter 21) (53).

REFERENCES

1. Fraser RS, Muller NL, Colman N, et al. *Diagnosis of diseases of the chest.* 4th ed. Volume I. Philadelphia: W.B. Saunders, 1999:563–594.

2. Davis S, Gardner F, Qvist G. The shape of a pleural effusion. *Br J Med* 1963;1:436–437.

3. Collins JD, Burwell D, Furmanski S, et al. Minimal detectable pleural effusions. *Radiology* 1972;105: 51–53.

4. Vix VA. Roentgenographic recognition of pleural effusion. *JAMA* 1974;229:695–698.

5. Wang JS, Tseng CH. Changes in pulmonary mechanics and gas exchange after thoracentesis on patients with inversion of a hemidiaphragm secondary to large pleural effusion. *Chest* 1995;107:1610–1614.

6. Mulvey RB. The effect of pleural fluid on the diaphragm. *Radiology*1965;84:1080–1085.

7. Ruskin JA, Gurney JW, Thorsen MK, et al. Detection of pleural effusions on supine chest radiographs. *AJR Am J Roentgenol* 1987;148:681–683.

8. Woodring JH. Recognition of pleural effusion on supine radiographs: How much fluid is required? *AJR Am J Roentgenol* 1984;142:59–64.

9. Emamian SA, Kaasbol MA, Olsen JF, et al. Accuracy of the diagnosis of pleural effusion on supine chest x-ray. *Eur Radiol* 1997;7:57–60.

10. Fleischner FG. Atypical arrangement of free pleural effusion. *Radiol Clin North Am* 1963;1:347–362.

11. Higgins JA, Juergens JL, Bruwer AJ, et al. Loculated interlobar pleural effusion due to congestive heart failure. *Arch Intern Med* 1955;96:180–187.

12. Moskowitz H, Platt RT, Schachar R, et al. Roentgen visualization of minute pleural effusion. *Radiology* 1973; 109:33–35.

13. Kocijancic I, Tercelj M, Vidmar K, et al. The value of inspiratory-expiratory lateral decubitus views in the diagnosis of small pleural effusions. *Clin Radiol* 1999;54:595–597.

14. Moller A. Pleural effusion: use of the semi-supine position for radiograph detection. *Radiology* 1984;150: 245–249.

15. Mathis G. Thoraxsonography–part I: Chest wall and pleura. *Ultrasound Med Biol* 1997;23:1131–1139.

16. McLoud TC, Flower CD. Imaging the pleura: sonography, CT, and MR imaging. *AJR Am J Roentgenol* 1991;156:1145–1153.

17. Yang PC, Luh KT, Chang DB, et al. Value of sonography in determining the nature of pleural effusion: analysis of 320 cases. *AJR Am J Roentgenol* 1992;159:29–33.

18. Wernecke K. Sonographic features of pleural disease. *AJR Am J Roentgenol* 1997;168:1061–1066.

19. Marks WM, Filly RA, Callen PW. Real-time evaluation of pleural lesions: new observations regarding the probability of obtaining free fluid. *Radiology* 1982;142:163–164.

20. Kataoka H, Takada S. The role of thoracic ultrasonography for evaluation of patients with decompensated chronic heart failure. *J Am Coll Cardiol* 2000;35:1638–1646.

21. Wu R-G, Yuan A, Liaw Y-S, et al. Image comparison of real-time gray-scale ultrasound and color Doppler ultrasound for use in diagnosis of minimal pleural effusion. *Am J Respir Crit Care Med* 1994;150:510–514.

22. Ma OJ, Mateer JR, Ogata M, et al. Prospective analysis of a rapid trauma ultrasound examination performed by emergency physicians. *J Trauma*1995;38:879–885.

23. Sisley AC, Rozycki GS, Ballard RB, et al. Rapid detection of traumatic effusion using surgeon-performed ultrasonography. *J Trauma*1998;44:291–296.

24. Lomas DJ, Padley SG, Flower CD. The sonographic appearances of pleural fluid. *Br J Radiol* 1993;66:619–624.

25. Moyers JP, Starnes DL, Bienvenu GL, et al. Thoracentesis performed by radiologist using ultrasound guidance is safe regardless of the amount of fluid withdrawn. *Chest* 1998;114:368S.

26. Henschke CI, Yankelevitz DF, Davis SD. Pleural diseases: multimodality imaging and clinical management. *Curr Prob Diagn Radiol* 1991;20:155–181.

27. Aquino SL, Webb WR, Gushiken BJ. Pleural exudates and transudates: diagnosis with contrast-enhanced CT. *Radiology*1994;192:803–808.

28. Pugatch RD, Spirn PW. Radiology of the pleura. *Clin Chest Med* 1985;6:17–32.

29. Paling MR, Griffin GK. Lower lobe collapse due to pleural effusion: a CT analysis. *J Comput Assist Tomogr* 1985;9:1079–1083.

30. Proto AV, Ball JB Jr. Computed tomography of the major and minor fissures. *AJR Am J Roentgenol* 1983;140:439–448.

31. Gamsu G, Sostman D. Magnetic resonance imaging of the thorax. *Am Rev Respir Dis* 1989;139:254–274.

32. Fisher MR. Magnetic resonance for evaluation of the thorax. *Chest* 1989;95:166–173.

33. Heelan RT, Rusch VW, Begg CB, et al. Staging of malignant pleural mesothelioma: comparison of CT and MR imaging. *AJR Am J Roentgenol* 1999;172:1039–1047.

34. Adams FV, Kolodny E. M-mode ultrasonic localization and identification of fluid-containing pulmonary cysts. *Chest* 1979;75:330–333.

35. Bressler EL, Francis IR, Glazer GM, et al. Bolus contrast medium enhancement for distinguishing pleural from parenchymal lung disease: CT features. *J Comput Assist Tomogr* 1987;11:436–440.

36. Zinn WL, Naidich DP, Whelan CA, et al. Fluid within preexisting pulmonary air-spaces: a potential pitfall in the CT differentiation of pleural from parenchymal disease. *J Comput Assist Tomogr* 1987;11:441–448.

37. Eibenberger KL, Dock WI, Ammann ME, et al. Quantification of pleural effusions: sonography versus radiography. *Radiology* 1994;191:681–684.

38. Blackmore CC, Black WC, Dallas RV, et al. Pleural fluid volume estimation: a chest radiograph prediction rule. *Acad Radiol* 1996;3:103–109.

39. Light RW, Jenkinson SG, Minh V, et al. Observations on pleural pressures as fluid is withdrawn during thoracentesis. *Am Rev Respir Dis* 1980;121:799–804.

40. Maher GG, Berger HW. Massive pleural effusion: malignant and non-malignant causes in 46 patients. *Am Rev Respir Dis* 1972;105:458–460.

41. Liberson M. Diagnostic significance of the mediastinal profile in massive unilateral pleural effusions. *Am Rev Respir Dis* 1963;88:176–180.

42. Yu CJ, Yang PC, Wu HD, et al. Ultrasound study in unilateral hemithorax opacification. Image comparison with computed tomography. *Am Rev Respir Dis* 1993;147:430–434.

43. Renner RR, Markarian B, Pernice NJ, et al. The apical cap. *Radiology* 1974;110:569–573.

44. Hillerdal G. Non-malignant asbestos pleural disease. *Thorax* 1981;36:669–675.

45. Fletcher DE, Edge JR. The early radiological changes in pulmonary and pleural asbestosis. *Clin Radiol* 1970;21:355–365.
46. Katz D, Kreel L. Computed tomography in pulmonary asbestosis. *Clin Radiol* 1979;30:207–213.
47. Carr JJ, Reed JC, Choplin RH, et al. Plain and computed radiography for detecting experimentally induced pneumothorax in cadavers: implications for detection in patients. *Radiology*1992;183:193–199.
48. Glazer HS, Anderson DJ, Wilson BS, et al. Pneumothorax: appearance on lateral chest radiographs. *Radiology*1989;173:707–711.
49. Buckner CB, Harmon BH, Pallin JS. The radiology of abnormal intrathoracic air. *Curr Probl Diagn Radiol*1988;17:37–71.
50. Lichtenstein DA, Menu Y. A bedside ultrasound sign ruling out pneumothorax in the critically ill. Lung sliding. *Chest* 1995;108:1345–1348.
51. Lichtenstein D, Meziere G, Biderman P, et al. The comet-tail artifact: an ultrasound sign ruling out pneumothorax. *Intensive Care Med* 1999;25:383-388.
52. Bourgouin P, Cousineau G, Lemire P, et al. Computed tomography used to exclude pneumothorax in bullous lung disease. *J Can Assoc Radiol* 1985;36:341–342.
53. Light RW. Tension pneumothorax. *Intensive Care Med* 1994;106:1162–1165.

4

Clinical Manifestations and Useful Tests

Normally, the pleural space contains only a few milliliters of pleural fluid. If fluid in the pleural space is detected on a radiologic examination, it is abnormal. Many conditions can be associated with pleural fluid accumulation (see Table 5.1). When pleural fluid is detected, an effort should be made to determine which of the many conditions listed in Table 5.1 is responsible. In this chapter, the clinical manifestations of pleural effusions are first discussed. Then, the various tests used in the differential diagnosis of pleural effusions are reviewed. In Chapter 5, recommendations are given for a systematic approach to the patient with a undiagnosed pleural effusion.

CLINICAL MANIFESTATIONS

The presence of moderate to large amounts of pleural fluid produces symptoms and characteristic changes on physical examination.

Symptoms

The symptoms of a patient with a pleural effusion are mainly dictated by the underlying process causing the effusion. Many patients have no symptoms referable to the effusion. When symptoms are related to the effusion, they arise either from inflammation of the pleura, from compromise of pulmonary mechanics, from interference with gas exchange, or on rare occasions, decreased cardiac output. A pleural effusion associated with pleuritic chest pain indicates inflammation of the pleura, specifically, the parietal pleura as the visceral pleura does not have

pain fibers. Some patients with pleural effusions experience a dull, aching chest pain rather than pleuritic chest pain. This symptom is very suggestive that the patient has pleural malignancy (1). The presence of either pleuritic chest pain or dull, aching chest pain indicates that the parietal pleura is probably involved and that the patient has an exudative pleural effusion.

Ordinarily, the pain associated with pleural disease is well localized and coincides with the affected area of the pleura, because the parietal pleura is innervated mostly by the intercostal nerves. At times, however, pleuritic pain is referred to the abdomen because intercostal nerves are also distributed to the abdomen. A notable exception to the localization of the pain occurs when the central portion of the diaphragmatic pleura is involved. The nerve supply to this portion of the parietal pleura is the phrenic nerve; therefore, inflammation of the central portion of the diaphragm is referred to the tip of the ipsilateral shoulder. Pleuritic pain felt simultaneously in the lower chest and ipsilateral shoulder is pathognomonic of diaphragmatic involvement.

A second symptom of pleural effusion is a dry, nonproductive cough. The mechanism producing the cough is not clear, although it may be related to pleural inflammation. Alternately, lung compression by the fluid may bring opposing bronchial walls into contact, stimulating the cough reflex.

The third symptom of pleural effusion is dyspnea. A pleural effusion acts as a space-occupying process in the thoracic cavity and therefore reduces all subdivisions of lung volumes.

Small-to-moderate-sized pleural effusions displace rather than compress the lung and have little effect on pulmonary function (2). Larger pleural effusions obviously cause a significant reduction in lung volumes, but the improvement in pulmonary function following therapeutic thoracentesis is much less than one would anticipate. We obtained spirometry before and 24 hours after thoracentesis in 26 patients from whom a mean of 1,740 mL pleural fluid was withdrawn (3). In these patients, the mean vital capacity improved 410 ± 390 mL. Patients in this study with higher pleural pressures after the removal of 800 mL pleural fluid and patients with smaller decreases in the pleural pressure after the removal of 800 mL pleural fluid had greater improvements in the forced vital capacity (FVC) after thoracentesis. Associated parenchymal disease probably explains this small increase in pulmonary function following therapeutic thoracentesis. The degree of dyspnea is frequently out of proportion to the size of the pleural effusion. Often, this feature is the result of compromised diaphragmatic function due to the weight of fluid on the diaphragm. At times, the diaphragm becomes inverted and this usually results in disproportionate dyspnea (4). Either pleuritic chest pain, with the resultant splinting, or concomitant parenchymal disease can also be responsible for the disproportionate dyspnea. When the pleural effusion is large, ventricular filling may be impeded leading to a decreased cardiac output and dyspnea (5). Arterial blood gases usually remain at clinically acceptable levels whatever the size of the effusion (6), because of the reflex reduction in perfusion to the lung underlying the effusion.

Physical Examination

When the chest of a patient with or who is suspected of having a pleural effusion is examined, particular attention should be paid to the relative sizes of the hemithoraces and the intercostal spaces. If the pleural pressure is increased on the side of the effusion, that hemithorax will be larger, and the usual concavity of the intercostal spaces will be blunted or even convex. In contrast, if the pleural pressure on the side of the effusion is decreased, as with obstruction of a major bronchus or a trapped lung, the ipsilateral hemithorax will be smaller, and the normal concavity of the intercostal spaces will be exaggerated. In addition, with inspiratory efforts, the intercostal spaces retract. Enlargement of the hemithorax with bulging of the intercostal spaces is an indication for therapeutic thoracentesis to relieve the increased pleural pressure. Signs of decreased pleural pressure are a relative contraindication to therapeutic thoracentesis because the decreased pleural pressure can lead to reexpansion pulmonary edema (7). Of course, in many patients with pleural effusions, the hemithoraces are equal in size, and the intercostal spaces are normal.

Palpation of the chest in patients with pleural effusions is useful in delineating the extent of the effusion. In areas of the chest where pleural fluid separates the lung from the chest wall, tactile fremitus is absent or attenuated because the fluid absorbs the vibrations emanating from the lung. Tactile fremitus is much more reliable than percussion for identifying the upper border of the pleural fluid and the proper place to attempt a thoracentesis. With a thin rim of fluid, the percussion note may still be resonant, but the tactile fremitus is diminished. Palpation may also reveal that the cardiac point of maximum impulse is shifted to one side or the other. With large left pleural effusions, the cardiac point of maximum impulse may not be palpable. In patients with pleural effusions, the position of the trachea should always be ascertained because it indicates the relationship between the pleural pressures in the two hemithoraces.

The percussion note over a pleural effusion is dull or flat. The dullness is maximum at the lung bases where the thickness of the fluid is the greatest. As mentioned earlier, however, the percussion note may not be duller if only a thin rim of fluid is present. Light percussion is better than heavy percussion for identifying small amounts of pleural fluid. If the dullness to percussion shifts as the position of the patient is changed, one can be almost certain that free pleural fluid is present (8).

Auscultation over the pleural fluid characteristically reveals decreased or absent breath sounds.

Near the superior border of the fluid, however, breath sounds may be accentuated and take on a bronchial characteristic. This phenomenon has been attributed to increased conductance of breath sounds through the partially atelectatic lung compressed by the fluid (9). This accentuation of breath sounds does not mean that an associated parenchymal infiltrate is present. Auscultation may also reveal a pleural rub. Pleural rubs are characterized by coarse, creaking, leathery sounds most commonly heard during the latter part of inspiration and the early part of expiration, producing a to-and-fro pattern of sound. Pleural rubs, caused by the rubbing together of the roughened pleural surfaces during respiration, are often associated with local pain on breathing that subsides with breath-holding. Pleural rubs often appear as pleural effusions that diminish in size, either spontaneously or as a result of treatment, because the pleural fluid is no longer present between the roughened pleural surfaces.

It is important to realize that an elevated hemidiaphragm can produce all of the classic physical findings associated with a pleural effusion. Obviously, the chest is not the only structure that should be examined when evaluating a patient with a pleural effusion; clues to the origin of the effusion are often present elsewhere. The effusion is probably due to congestive heart failure if the patient has cardiomegaly, neck vein distension, or peripheral edema. Signs of joint disease or subcutaneous nodules suggest that the pleural effusion is due to rheumatoid disease or lupus erythematosus. An enlarged, nontender nodular liver or the presence of hypertrophic osteoarthropathy suggests metastatic disease, as do breast masses or the absence of a breast. Abdominal tenderness suggests a subdiaphragmatic process, whereas tense ascites suggests cirrhosis and a hepatothorax. Lymphadenopathy suggests lymphoma, metastatic disease, or sarcoidosis.

SEPARATION OF TRANSUDATIVE FROM EXUDATIVE EFFUSIONS

The accumulation of clinically detectable quantities of pleural fluid is distinctly abnormal. A diagnostic thoracentesis (see Chapter 25) should be attempted whenever the thickness of pleural fluid on ultrasound or the decubitus radiograph is greater than 10 mm or whenever loculated pleural fluid is demonstrated with ultrasound unless the patient has typical congestive heart failure. A properly performed diagnostic thoracentesis takes less than 10 minutes and should cause no more morbidity than a venipuncture. The information available from examination of the pleural fluid is invaluable in the management of the patient.

Pleural effusions have classically been divided into transudates and exudates (10). A transudative pleural effusion develops when the systemic factors influencing the formation or absorption of pleural fluid are altered so that pleural fluid accumulates. The pleural fluid is a transudate. The fluid may originate in the lung, the pleura, or the peritoneal cavity (11). The permeability of the capillaries to proteins is normal in the area where the fluid is formed. Examples of conditions producing transudative pleural effusions are left ventricular failure producing increased pulmonary interstitial fluid and a resulting pleural effusion, ascites due to cirrhosis with movement of fluid through the diaphragm, and decreased serum oncotic pressure with hypoproteinemia. In contrast, an exudative pleural effusion develops when the pleural surfaces or the capillaries in the location where the fluid originates are altered such that fluid accumulates. The pleural fluid is an exudate.

The first question to ask in assessing a patient with a pleural effusion is whether that effusion is a transudate or an exudate. If the effusion is a transudate, no further diagnostic pleural procedures are necessary, and therapy is directed to the underlying congestive heart failure, cirrhosis, or nephrosis. Alternately, if the effusion proves to be an exudate, a more extensive diagnostic investigation is indicated to delineate the cause of the effusion.

For many years, a pleural fluid protein level of 3 g per dL was used to separate transudates from exudates, with exudative pleural effusions characterized by a protein level above 3 g per dL (12, 13). Use of this one simple test led to the misclassification of approximately 10% of pleural effusions (12–14). My colleagues and I subsequently demonstrated that with the use of simultaneously obtained serum and pleural fluid protein and lactic acid dehydrogenase (LDH) values, 99% of pleural effusions could be correctly classified as either transudates or exudates (14). Exudative pleural effusions meet at least one of the following criteria, whereas transudative pleural effusions meet none (Light's criteria):

1. Pleural fluid protein divided by serum protein greater than 0.5
2. Pleural fluid LDH divided by serum LDH greater than 0.6
3. Pleural fluid LDH greater than two thirds of the upper limit of normal for the serum LDH

In recent years, other tests have been proposed for the separation of transudates from exudates. The tests that have been proposed to indicate a pleural exudate have included a pleural fluid cholesterol greater than 60 mg per dL (15, 16), a pleural fluid cholesterol greater than 45 mg per dL (17), a gradient of less than 1.2 g per dL for the difference in the pleural fluid and serum albumin level (18), a pleural fluid-to-serum bilirubin ratio above 0.6 (19), and a pleural fluid-to-serum cholinesterase ratio above 0.23 (20).

Two subsequent reports (21, 22) have compared Light's criteria with the other proposed tests and have concluded that Light's criteria best separates exudates and transudates. In the study of Romero et al. (21) of 297 patients including 44 transudates and 253 exudates, Light's criteria were superior to cholesterol in making the distinction. In this study with Light's criteria, 98% of the exudates and 77% of the transudates were correctly classified (21). In a subsequent study of 393 patients including 123 with transudates and 270 with exudates from South Africa (22), Light's criteria were found to be superior to the serum effusion albumin gradient, the effusion cholesterol concentration, and the pleura fluid and serum bilirubin ratio (22). Again in this study, Light's criteria identified 98% of the exudates correctly, but they were less accurate in identifying transudates (22). Two more recent studies have come to similar conclusions (23, 24). It is unlikely that the pleural fluid cholesterol measurement will provide additional information to the ratio of the pleural fluid to the serum protein because the pleural fluid cholesterol level can be accurately predicted from the serum cholesterol and the ratio of the pleural fluid to the serum protein level (25).

In summary, it appears that Light's criteria remain the best biochemical means by which pleural effusions can be classified as transudates or exudates. The primary problem with Light's criteria is that they label some patients with transudative pleural effusions as having exudative pleural effusions. If it is thought that the patient has a transudative pleural effusion clinically but Light's exudative criteria are met, then it is reasonable to measure the serum–pleural fluid albumin gradient. If this gradient is above 1.2 g per dL, then the patient in all probability has a transudative pleural effusion (22). Use of the serum–pleural fluid albumin gradient alone will result in the misclassification of many exudates as transudates (22).

Specific Gravity

The specific gravity of the pleural fluid as measured with a hydrometer was used in the past to separate transudates from exudates (26) because it was a simple and rapid method of estimating the protein content of the fluid. A specific gravity of 1.015 corresponds to a protein content of 3 g per dL, and this value was used to separate transudates from exudates (26). At the present time, refractometers are usually used to estimate the specific gravity of pleural fluid. Unfortunately, the scale on the commercially available refractometers is calibrated for the specific gravity of urine rather than pleural fluid. A reading of 1.020 on the urine specific gravity scale corresponds to a pleural fluid protein level of 3 g per dL. However, there is a scale on the same refractometer for protein levels that is valid for pleural fluid. Because the only reason to measure specific gravity is to estimate the protein level, and because the pleural fluid specific gravity measurement is extraneous and confusing, it should no longer be ordered (27). However, a rapid estimate of the pleural fluid protein content can be obtained at the patient's bedside with the protein scale on the refractometer (27).

Other Characteristics of Transudates

Most transudates are clear, straw colored, nonviscid, and odorless. Approximately 15% have red cell counts above 10,000 per mm^3. Therefore, the discovery of blood-tinged pleural fluid does not mean that the fluid is not a transudate. Because red blood cells contain a large amount of LDH, one might suppose that the LDH level in a blood-tinged or bloody transudative pleural effusion would be so elevated that it would meet the criteria for an exudative pleural effusion. Such does not appear to be the case, however. The LDH isoenzyme present in red blood cells is LDH-1, and in one study of 23 patients with bloody pleural effusions (pleural fluid red cell counts greater than 100,000 per mm^3), the fraction of LDH-1 in the pleural fluid was only slightly increased (28).

The pleural fluid white blood cell count of most transudates is less than 1,000 per mm^3, but about 20% have white blood cell counts that exceed 1,000 per mm^3 (29). Pleural fluid white blood cell counts above 10,000 per mm^3 are rare with transudative pleural effusions. The differential white cell count in transudative pleural effusions may be dominated by polymorphonuclear leukocytes, small lymphocytes, or other mononuclear cells. In a series of 47 transudative effusions, six (13%) had more than 50% polymorphonuclear leukocytes, whereas 16 (34%) had predominantly small lymphocytes, 22 (47%) had predominantly other mononuclear cells, and three (6%) had no one predominant cell type (29). The pleural fluid glucose level is similar to the serum glucose level, but the pleural fluid amylase level is low (30). The pleural fluid pH with transudative pleural effusions is higher than the simultaneously obtained blood pH (31), probably because of active transport of bicarbonate from the blood into the pleural space (32).

GENERAL TESTS FOR DIFFERENTIATING CAUSES OF EXUDATES

Appearance of Fluid

The gross appearance of the pleural fluid frequently yields useful diagnostic information. The color, turbidity, viscosity, and odor should be described. Most transudative and many exudative pleural effusions are clear, straw colored, nonviscid, and odorless. Any deviations should be noted and investigated.

A reddish color indicates that blood is present, and a brownish tinge indicates that the blood has been present for a prolonged period. If the pleural fluid is blood tinged, the pleural fluid red blood cell count is between 5,000 and 10,000 per mm^3. If the pleural fluid appears grossly bloody, a hematocrit should be obtained to determine whether the patient has a hemothorax (see Chapter 22).

Turbid pleural fluid can occur from either increased cellular content or increased lipid content. These two entities can be differentiated if the pleural fluid is centrifuged and the supernatant examined. If turbidity remains after centrifugation, it is in all probability due to increased lipid content, and the fluid should be sent for lipid analysis (see the discussion later in this chapter). Alternately, if the supernatant is clear, the original turbidity was due to increased numbers of cells or other debris. The discovery of pleural fluid that looks like chocolate sauce or anchovy paste is suggestive of amebiasis with a hepatopleural fistula (33). This appearance is due to the presence of a mixture of blood, cytolyzed liver tissue, and small solid particles of liver parenchyma that have resisted dissolution.

A clear or bloody viscous fluid is suggestive of malignant mesothelioma; the high viscosity is secondary to an elevated pleural fluid hyaluronic acid level (34). Of course, the fluid from a pyothorax is also viscid because of the large amounts of cells and debris in the fluid.

The odor of all pleura fluids should be noted. One can immediately establish two diagnoses by smelling the pleural fluid. A feculent odor indicates that the patient has a bacterial infection of his pleural space that is probably anaerobic. If the pleural fluid smells like urine, the patient probably has a urinothorax.

Red Blood Cell Count

Only 5,000 to 10,000 red blood cells per mm^3 need be present to impart a red color to pleural fluid. If a pleural effusion has a total volume of 500 mL and the red blood cell count in the peripheral blood is 5 million per mm^3, a leak of only 1 mL blood into the pleural space will result in a blood-tinged pleural effusion. It is probably for this reason that the presence of blood-tinged or serosanguineous pleural fluid has little diagnostic significance. Over 15% of transudative and over 40% of all types of exudative pleural fluids are blood tinged (29); that is, they have pleural fluid red blood cell counts between 5,000 and 100,000 per mm^3.

Occasionally, pleural fluid obtained by diagnostic thoracentesis appears grossly bloody. In such cases, one can assume that the red blood cell count in the pleural fluid is above 100,000 per mm^3. One should obtain a hematocrit on such pleural fluids to document the amount of blood in the pleural fluid. If the hematocrit of the pleural fluid is greater than 50% of the peripheral hematocrit, a hemothorax is present, and one should consider inserting chest tubes (see Chapter 22). Usually, the hematocrit of bloody pleural fluid is much lower than one would expect from its gross appearance.

The presence of bloody pleural fluid suggests one of three diagnoses, namely, malignant disease, trauma, or pulmonary embolization. In a series of 22 bloody pleural effusions that I observed on medical wards, 12 were due to malignant disease, five to pulmonary embolization, two to trauma, and two to pneumonia, and one was a transudative effusion secondary to cirrhosis (29). The traumatic origin of the pleural effusion may not be obvious, particularly when the patient is on a medical ward. The patient may have broken a rib while coughing or suffered trauma during an episode of inebriation that is not remembered.

At times, it is unclear whether blood in the pleural fluid resulted from or was present before the thoracentesis. If the blood is a result of the thoracentesis, the degree of red discoloration of the fluid should not be uniform throughout the course of aspiration. Examination of the fluid microscopically may also be useful. If the red blood cells were present before the thoracentesis, the macrophages in the pleural fluid usually contain hemoglobin inclusions. If there are no platelets present, the blood is not the result of a traumatic thoracentesis (34). Crenation of the red blood cells in the pleural fluid rarely occurs because the osmotic pressure of the pleural fluid is similar to that of serum.

White Blood Cell Count

Although the white blood cell counts on the pleural fluid have traditionally been performed manually, we have recently shown that the automated counters provide accurate pleural fluid white blood cell counts (35). The pleural fluid for cell counts and differentials should be collected in a test tube with an anticoagulant (35). If the pleural fluid is collected in plastic or glass tubes that are not anticoagulated, the fluid may clot or the cells may clump, providing inaccurate cell counts and differentials (35).

The pleural fluid white blood count is of limited diagnostic use. Most transudates have white cell counts below 1,000 per mm^3, whereas most exudates have white cell counts above 1,000 per mm^3 (14). Pleural fluid white blood cell counts above 10,000 per mm^3 are most commonly seen with parapneumonic effusions, but they are also seen with many other diseases (29), as shown in Table 4.1. I have seen pleural fluid white blood cell counts above 50,000 per mm^3 with both pancreatic disease and pulmonary embolization.

TABLE 4.1. *Etiology of 25 effusions containing more than 10,000 WBC/mm^3*

Diagnosis	Number with >10,000 WBC/mm^3	Total number of effusions	Percentage having >10,000 WBC/mm^3
Parapneumonic effusion	13	26	50
Malignant disease	3	43	7
Pulmonary embolization	3	8	37
Tuberculosis	2	14	14
Pancreatitis	2	5	40
Postmyocardial infarction syndrome	1	3	33
Systemic lupus erythematosus	1	1	100

With grossly purulent pleural fluid, the pleural fluid white blood cell count is frequently much lower than one would anticipate because debris rather than cells accounts for much of the turbidity.

Differential White Cell Count

Examination of a Wright stain of pleural fluid is one of the most informative tests on pleural fluid. Because the pleural fluid white blood cell count is frequently less than 5,000 per mm^3, it is useful to concentrate the cells before staining. This procedure is easily accomplished by centrifuging about 10 mL of fluid and then resuspending the button of cells in about 0.5 mL of supernatant. After thorough mixing, slides are made similarly to those for examining peripheral blood and are stained in the usual way. Occasionally, large amounts of fibrinogen adhere to the cells. In such cases, resuspension in saline solution, followed by centrifugation, is indicated in order to evaluate cellular morphologic features. Automatic cell counters do not provide sufficiently accurate differential cell counts for clinical use (36).

Although most laboratories divide pleural fluid white cells into polymorphonuclear leukocytes and mononuclear cells, I prefer to divide them into four categories: polymorphonuclear leukocytes, lymphocytes, other mononuclear cells and eosinophils, because of the diagnostic significance of small lymphocytes (see "Lymphocytes" later in this chapter). The mononuclear cells include mesothelial cells, macrophages, plasma cells, and malignant cells. Excellent color plates demonstrating the morphologic and staining characteristics of the different cells in pleural effusions are contained in the monograph by Spriggs and Boddington (37).

Neutrophils

Because neutrophils are the cellular component of the acute inflammatory response, they predominate in pleural fluid resulting from acute inflammation such as occurs with pneumonia, pancreatitis, pulmonary embolization, subphrenic abscess, and early tuberculosis. Although over 10% of transudative pleural effusions contain predominantly neutrophils, pleural fluid neutrophilia in transudates has no clinical significance (29). The significance of neutrophils in an exudative pleural effusion is that they indicate acute inflammation of the pleural surface.

Interleukin 8 (IL-8) appears to be one of the primary chemotaxins for neutrophils in the pleural space (38, 39). The number of neutrophils in pleural fluid is correlated with the IL-8 level, and empyemas have the highest levels of IL-8. The addition of IL-8 neutralizing serum decreases the chemotactic activity for neutrophils in empyema fluids (39). The cellular source of IL-8 is unknown (38).

Examination of the pleural fluid neutrophils in patients with parapneumonic effusions is useful in identifying those that are infected. If pleural infection is present, the neutrophils undergo a characteristic degeneration. The nucleus becomes blurred and no longer is stained purple. The cytoplasm shows toxic granulation initially. Subsequently, the neutrophilic granules become indistinct and then are lost. Finally, only a smear cell remains (37).

Eosinophils

Most clinicians believe that significant numbers of eosinophils (>10%) in pleural fluid should be a clue to the origin of the pleural effusion. In most instances, the pleural fluid eosinophilia is due to either air or blood in the pleural space and therefore does not contribute any diagnostic information in these situations. Charcot-Leyden crystals (40), as well as Curschmann's spirals (41), are occasionally found in the pleural fluid of patients with pleural eosinophilia. Their presence appears to have no diagnostic significance.

The factors responsible for pleural fluid eosinophilia have been intensively studied, but there is still no unifying concept and it is likely that multiple factors are involved. In animals, it has been shown that the intrapleural injection of stem cell factor (42), platelet-activating factor (PAF) (43), endotoxin (44, 45), bradykinin (46), and leukotriene B$_4$ (43) all result in pleural fluid eosinophilia. The eosinophil influx is inhibited in some but not all situations by monoclonal antibodies directed against interleukin 5 (IL-5).

In humans, pleural fluid from patients with eosinophilic pleural effusions stimulates bone marrow cells to form colonies of eosinophils (47, 48). In addition, when eosinophils are incubated in the presence of eosinophilic pleural fluid, their survival is prolonged (47). Peripheral blood from patients with eosinophilic pleural effusions does not stimulate the bone marrow to form eosinophil colonies and does not prolong survival of eosinophils. The factor responsible for the increased colony-forming activity and the increased survival appears to be IL-5 (47, 48), although IL-3 and granulocyte or macrophage colony-stimulating factor (GM-CSF) may also play a role (47). In a recent study, we demonstrated that there was a close correlation (r = 0.87) between the levels of IL-5 in the pleural fluid and the numbers of eosinophils in the pleural fluid (49). Both bloody and nonbloody eosinophilic effusions had high levels of IL-5 (49).

The source of the IL-5 appears to be the CD4+ lymphocyte in the pleural fluid (48), but the eosinophils in the pleural fluid may themselves also produce IL-5 (47). The source of the eosinophils in eosinophilic pleural effusions appears to be the bone marrow; no progenitor cells are present in the pleural space. It is not known what stimulates the CD4+ lymphocytes to produce the IL-5. However, it probably results from another cytokine because the intrapleural injection of IL-2 into malignant pleural effusions results in an eosinophilic pleural effusion with a high level of IL-5 (50). There are factors other than IL-5 that recruit eosinophils to the pleural space. Antibodies to IL-5 eliminate the eosinophilic influx to an allergen but not to endotoxin in the mouse (51). However, antibodies to gamma delta lymphocytes eliminate the eosinophilic response to endotoxin (45).

The most common cause of pleural fluid eosinophilia is air in the pleural space. In a series of 127 cases with more than 20% eosinophils in the pleural fluid, 81 (64%) were thought to have pleural fluid eosinophilia secondary to air in the pleural space (37). In a review of 343 pleural effusions with greater than 10% eosinophils, 95 (28%) had air in the pleural space (52). It is likely that the pleural fluid eosinophilia in many other patients

in this series was also due to the introduction of air into the pleural space during a prior thoracentesis. On numerous occasions over the past three decades, I have seen patients who had no pleural fluid eosinophilia at the initial thoracentesis but who had many eosinophils at a subsequent thoracentesis. In each case, a small pneumothorax resulted from the initial thoracentesis. When patients with spontaneous pneumothorax undergo thoracotomy, a reactive eosinophilic pleuritis frequently exists in the resected parietal pleura (53).

The mechanism responsible for the pleural fluid eosinophilia in response to air in the pleural space is unknown but is probably related to IL-5. Smit et al. (54) measured the percentage of eosinophils and the levels of IL-5 in 23 patients with pneumothorax and pleural fluid. They found that IL-5 level and the eosinophil concentration in the pleural fluid were highly correlated (R = 0.84) and that the eosinophil percentage tended to increase with time, with a mean of less than 5% in the first 24 hours, 20% at days 1 to 3, 40% at days 4 to 7, and 50% after day 7 (54). There was no relationship between the PAF level or the monocyte chemotactic protein-1 levels and the eosinophils. In these fluids, IL-8 was not detectable.

The second most common cause of pleural fluid eosinophilia is blood in the pleural space. Following traumatic hemothorax, pleural fluid eosinophils do not usually become numerous until the second week (37). There is frequently an associated peripheral blood eosinophilia that does not disappear until the pleural effusion is completely resolved (55). The pleural effusions associated with pulmonary embolization are frequently bloody and contain numerous eosino-break phils. Bloody pleural fluids due to malignant disease are not usually characterized by eosinophilia (29, 37). In a study conducted by my colleagues and myself of bloody pleural effusions, none of the 11 cases of malignant pleural effusions with pleural fluid red blood cell counts greater than 100,000 per mm^3 had more than 10% eosinophils (29).

If the patient has neither blood nor air in their pleural space, what is the significance of an eosinophilic pleural effusion? Martinez-Garcia et al. (56) retrospectively reviewed 385 consecutive samples of pleural fluid from the initial thoracentesis that were not bloody and found that 45 (12.6%) had more than 10% eosinophils. The leading diagnoses of these patients were parapneumonic effusion (15), malignancy (11), and tuberculosis (7). Rubins and Rubins (57) also reported that malignancy was as common with eosinophilic as with noneosinophilic pleural effusions. It should be noted that these two recent studies differ from older studies that indicated that the presence of pleural fluid eosinophilia made the diagnosis of pleural malignancy or tuberculosis very unlikely (37, 52).

If neither air nor blood is present in the pleural space, several unusual diagnoses should be considered. Pleural eosinophilia is common in patients with asbestos-related pleural effusions. In a review of eosinophilic pleural effusions (52), 15 of 29 (52%) asbestos pleural effusions had more than 10% eosinophils in the pleural fluid. The pleural effusions secondary to drug reactions are frequently eosinophilic. Offending drugs include dantrolene, bromocriptine, and nitrofurantoin (see Chapter 19). Pleural effusions secondary to parasitic diseases such as paragonimiasis (58), hydatid disease (59), amebiasis (37), or ascariasis (37) frequently contain a large percentage of eosinophils. Last, the pleural effusion associated with the Churg-Strauss syndrome is eosinophilic (60).

If none of the foregoing rare diseases is causing the pleural effusion, the following statements are pertinent to patients with eosinophilic pleural effusions. If the patient has pneumonia and pleural effusion, the presence of pleural fluid eosinophilia is a good prognostic sign because such an effusion rarely becomes infected. The origin of approximately 25% of eosinophilic effusions is not established, and these effusions resolve spontaneously. Indeed, no etiology was established for 35% of 343 eosinophilic pleural effusions in the review of Adelman et al. (52). I believe that most of these undiagnosed eosinophilic pleural effusions are due to viral infections or occult pulmonary emboli.

Basophils

Basophilic pleural effusions are distinctly uncommon. I have not seen a pleural effusion that contained more than 2% basophils. A few basophils are usually present in pleural effusions with eosinophils. Basophil counts over 10% are most common with leukemic pleural involvement (37).

Lymphocytes

The discovery that more than 50% of the white blood cells in an exudative pleural effusion are small lymphocytes is important diagnostically because it means that the patient probably has a malignant disease, tuberculous pleuritis, or a pleural effusion after coronary artery bypass graft surgery. In two series (29, 61) studied before the advent of coronary artery bypass graft surgery, 96 of 211 exudative pleural effusions had more than 50% small lymphocytes. Of these 96 effusions, 90 (94%) were due to tuberculosis or malignant disease. When the foregoing series are analyzed, almost all of the effusions secondary to tuberculosis (43 of 46) but only two thirds of the effusions secondary to malignant disease (47 of 70) had predominantly small lymphocytes. In a recent series from our institution (62), 26 patients had chronic pleural effusions postcoronary artery bypass surgery and the mean lymphocyte percentage in these effusions was 61%. Approximately one third of transudative pleural effusions (29) contain predominantly small lymphocytes, and lymphocytosis in these effusions is not an indication for pleural biopsy.

Several papers have assessed the diagnostic utility of separating the pleural lymphocytes into T and B lymphocytes (63–66). In general, this separation has not been useful. With most disease states, the pleural fluid contains a higher percentage of T lymphocytes (70%), a lower percentage of B lymphocytes (10%), and a higher percentage of null cells (20%) than the corresponding peripheral blood (63, 64). The partitioning of lymphocytes may be useful, however, when chronic lymphatic leukemia or lymphoma is suspected. In a report of four such patients, all had more than 80% B lymphocytes in their pleural fluid (65).

The recent development of monoclonal antibodies has permitted a further subdivision of T lymphocytes. In comparison to peripheral blood, in pleural fluid the ratio of the helper and inducer cells (CD4$^+$) to the suppressor and cytotoxic cells (CD8$^+$) is higher regardless of the etiology of the pleural effusion (67–69). Therefore, this subdivision is not useful diagnostically. Natural killer (NK) cells are lymphocytes derived from an unimmunized host that lyse certain tumor cell lines and virus-infected cells. In general, the percentage of T lymphocytes in pleural fluid that are identified as NK cells by either the Leu 7 or Leu 11 monoclonal antibody is much lower than in the peripheral blood whether the patient has tuberculosis or malignancy (69–70). However, there is a discrepancy between the number of NK positive cells and the NK activity of the cells when patients with tuberculosis are compared with patients with malignancy. Although the number of NK cells is comparable in the two populations, there is much more NK activity in the tuberculous pleural effusions (70). The explanation for the functional difference remains unknown.

Mesothelial Cells

Mesothelial cells line the pleural cavities. They frequently become dislodged from the pleural surfaces and are present in the small amount of normal pleural fluid (71). These cells are usually 12 to 30 μm in diameter, but multinucleated forms may have diameters up to 75 μm. Their cytoplasm is light blue (Fig. 4.1A) and often contains a few vacuoles. The nucleus is large (9–22 μ) and stains purplish with a uniform appearance. The nucleus usually contains one to three bright blue nucleoli (37).

Mesothelial cells are significant for two reasons. First, their presence or absence is often useful diagnostically because these cells are uncommon in tuberculous effusions. Spriggs and Boddington (37) analyzed 65 tuberculous effusions and found that only one effusion had more than a single mesothelial cell per 1,000 cells (37). My colleagues and I have confirmed

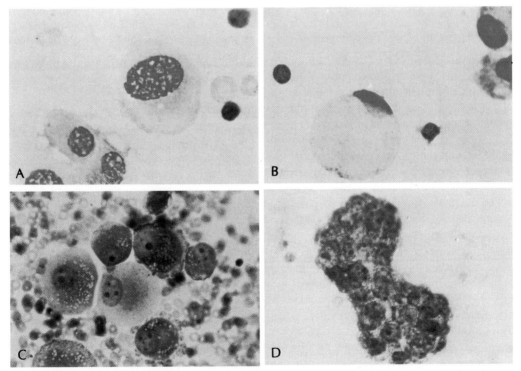

FIG. 4.1. A: Mesothelial cell. Note that the mesothelial cell is large in comparison to the lymphocyte and has light blue cytoplasm and light blue nucleoli of varying shapes and sizes. **B:** Signet ring cell. This macrophage, which has engorged itself with pleural debris, is not a malignant cell. **C:** Malignant cells. Several large cells are similar but vary in size. Note the large, dark nucleoli, which are so different from the nucleoli in the mesothelial cell. **D:** Clump of malignant cells from the pleural fluid of a patient with metastatic adenocarcinoma.

the paucity of mesothelial cells in tuberculous pleural effusions (29), as have Yam (61) and Hurwitz et al. (72). The exception to this observation is the patient with acquired immunodeficiency syndrome (AIDS). Patients with AIDS with a low CD4+ who have tuberculous pleuritis may have numerous mesothelial cells in their pleural fluid (73). The lack of mesothelial cells is not diagnostic of tuberculosis, however. It simply indicates that the pleural surfaces have become extensively involved by the disease process so that the mesothelial cells cannot enter the pleural space. The absence of mesothelial cells is common with complicated parapneumonic effusions and with other conditions in which the pleura becomes coated with fibrin. It is also common with malignant effusions after sclerosing agents have been injected to effect a pleurodesis. Second, mesothelial cells, particularly in their activated form, may be confused with malignant cells. Frequently, an experienced pathologist is required to make the differentiation. Immunohistochemistry is useful in making this distinction (see discussion later in this chapter).

Macrophages

In general, the presence of macrophages in pleural fluid is of limited diagnostic use. By definition, macrophages are cells that store vital dyes. It appears that the origin of the pleural fluid macrophages can be either the circulating monocyte or the mesothelial cell (74). Macrophages vary in diameter from 15 to 50 μm and have irregular nuclei. Their cytoplasm is gray, cloudy, and full of vacuoles. At times, the macrophage may become engorged with debris, taking on the appearance of a "signet-ring" cell, with the nucleus flattened against the side of the cell (Fig. 4.1B). It is important not to confuse these cells with malignant cells. During phagocytosis, macrophages may engulf polymorphonuclear leukocytes or red blood cells. These cells may be evident within the macrophage in various stages of digestion. If red blood cells have been ingested, the iron pigment is retained as dark blue or brown staining material (37). It is important not to confuse macrophages with mesothelial cells because macrophages are sometimes present in tuberculous pleural effusions (37).

Macrophages in the pleural fluid can be definitively identified using the monoclonal antibody CD68 (75). The macrophages in the pleural fluid, in addition to their phagocytic function, also can release interleukin 1 (IL-1) and tumor necrosis factor (TNF) (75). The macrophages in the pleural fluid are also efficient accessory cells for T-cell proliferation (75).

Plasma Cells

The presence of many plasma cells in the pleural fluid suggests multiple myeloma. Smaller numbers of plasma cells are not of any particular diagnostic importance. These cells are of the lymphoid series and produce immunoglobulins. Morphologically, they are larger than small lymphocytes and have an eccentric nucleus and deeply staining basophilic cytoplasm with a clear area at the cell center (Golgi zone) (37). Mature forms have well-defined nuclear chromatin blocks. In a series of 18 effusions with more than 5% plasma cells, four were due to malignant disease, three to tuberculosis, three to congestive heart failure, three to pulmonary embolization, two to pneumonia, one to sepsis, and two were of undetermined origin (37).

Dendritic Cells

Dendritic cells are human leukocyte antigen (HLA) DR–positive accessory cells that play a critical role in the development of cell-mediated immune reactions. Dendritic cells have been identified in the pleural fluid (76). It is unknown whether the dendritic cells in pleural fluid are resident in the pleural space or reach the pleural space from the blood. On light microscopy, dendritic cells from pleural fluid are intermediate in size between lymphocytes and macrophages, do not contain intracytoplasmic inclusions, and have an eccentric nucleus (76).

PROTEIN MEASUREMENTS

The pleural fluid protein levels are generally higher in exudative pleural effusions than in transudative pleural effusions, and this observation serves as a basis for separating transudates from exudates (see the foregoing discussion on this differentiation in this chapter). Pleural fluid

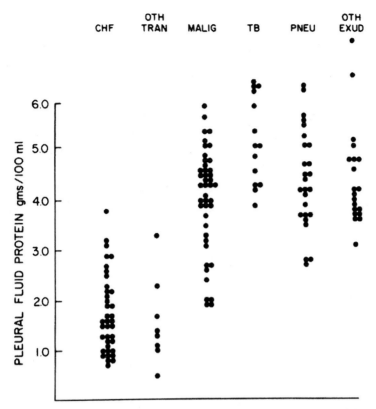

FIG. 4.2. Pleural fluid protein levels in effusion secondary to congestive heart failure (CHF), other transudates (OTH TRAN), malignant disease (MALIG), tuberculosis (TB), pneumonia (PNEU), and other exudates (OTH EXUD). Each point represents one pleural fluid. Note that the distribution of protein levels for all categories of exudative pleural effusions is similar. (From Light RW, MacGregor MI, Luchsinger PC, et al. Pleural effusions: the diagnostic separation of transudates and exudates. *Ann Intern Med* 1972;77:507–513, with permission.)

protein levels are not useful in separating the various types of exudative effusions, however, because the protein level in most exudates is elevated to a comparable degree (Fig. 4.2). At times, a pleural fluid meets the exudative criteria with its LDH, but not with its protein level. Such exudative pleural effusions are almost always parapneumonic effusions or are secondary to malignant pleural disease (14).

Simultaneous electrophoretic studies of serum and pleural fluid demonstrate that the pattern in the pleural fluid is essentially an image of that in the serum, except proportionately more albumin is present in the pleural fluid (77, 78). Along the same lines, the ratio of the pleural fluid to the serum IgG, IgA, and IgM is always below unity and appears to have no diagnostic

value (1, 79). The ratio of the concentration of these proteins is inversely related to their molecular weight (79). The one immunoglobulin measurement that may be diagnostically useful is IgE. Yokogawa et al. (80) measured the pleural fluid and serum IgE levels in five patients with paragonimiasis. In all five patients, the pleural fluid IgE level was above 4,000 IU and exceeded the serum level. A subsequent report, however, measured the pleural fluid and serum IgE levels in seven patients with eosinophilic pleural effusions and seven with noneosinophilic pleural effusions. The pleural fluid levels and the ratio of the pleural fluid and serum IgE concentration were comparable in the two groups, and it was concluded that pleural fluid IgE was the result of passive diffusion from the serum (81). None of the patients in this latter series, however, had paragonimiasis.

GLUCOSE MEASUREMENT

Measurement of the pleural fluid glucose level is useful in the differential diagnosis of exudative pleural effusions because a low pleural fluid glucose level (<60 mg per dL) indicates that the patient probably has one of four disorders, namely, a parapneumonic effusion, malignant disease, rheumatoid disease, or tuberculous pleuritis. Other rare causes of a low glucose pleural effusion include paragonimiasis, hemothorax, Churg-Strauss syndrome, and, occasionally, lupus pleuritis. The pleural fluid glucose level of all transudates and of most exudates parallels that of the serum. In my experience, it is not necessary to obtain pleural fluid glucose levels with the patient fasting or to take the serum glucose level into consideration when evaluating the pleural fluid glucose level.

The pleural fluid glucose level is low in some patients with parapneumonic effusions or empyema (82, 83). The lower the pleural fluid glucose level, the more likely one is dealing with a complicated parapneumonic pleural effusion. If the pleural fluid is thick and purulent, the pleural fluid glucose level is frequently close to zero (82). Even in more serous fluid, the glucose level may be reduced. The presence of a low pleural fluid glucose is a poor prognostic sign in patients with parapneumonic effusion and serves as an indicator that more aggressive therapy such as tube thoracostomy or thoracoscopy with the breakdown of loculations is necessary (84).

Approximately 15% to 25% of patients with malignant pleural effusions have pleural fluid glucose levels below 60 mg per dL (30, 85, 86) and the level may be less than 10 mg per dL. Patients with malignant pleural effusions and a low glucose level have a greater tumor burden in their pleural space than do those with normal pleural fluid glucose levels. In one report of 77 patients with malignant pleural effusion who underwent thoracoscopic examination (86), the extent of the tumor at thoracoscopy was significantly higher in those 16 patients in whom the pleural fluid glucose was less than 60 mg per dL. In addi-

tion, those patients with a low pleural fluid glucose are more likely to have positive pleural fluid cytology and a positive pleural biopsy (87), are less likely to have a good result from chemical pleurodesis (86, 88), and have a shortened life expectancy (88, 89).

The pleural fluid glucose level is also reduced in some patients with tuberculous pleuritis. Indeed, early reports indicated that low pleural fluid glucose levels were seen only with tuberculous pleural effusions (90, 91). Subsequent studies (30, 82, 85, 92), however, revealed that low pleural fluid glucose levels also occurred with malignant and rheumatoid disease and parapneumonic effusion. The distribution of pleural fluid glucose levels for tuberculous and malignant pleural effusions is, in fact, similar (30). The majority of patients with tuberculous pleuritis have a pleural fluid glucose level above 80 mg per dL (30). Accordingly, a low pleural fluid glucose level is compatible with the diagnosis of tuberculous pleuritis, but it is not necessary for the diagnosis.

Pleural effusions due to rheumatoid disease (see Chapter 18) classically have a low pleural fluid glucose level. Carr and Power (92) first reported that rheumatoid pleural effusions had a low pleural fluid glucose level. In a subsequent review of 76 cases of rheumatoid pleural effusions (93), 42% had pleural fluid glucose levels below 10 mg per dL, and 78% had levels below 30 mg per dL. The explanation for the low pleural fluid glucose level in this condition appears to be a selective block to the entry of glucose into the pleural effusion (94). The pleural fluid glucose level in effusions secondary to lupus erythematosus is usually normal. In one report of nine patients, the pleural fluid glucose level exceeded 80 mg per dL in all (95). In a subsequent report (96), the pleural fluid glucose level was below 50 mg per dL in 2 of 14 (14%) of patients with lupus pleuritis.

AMYLASE DETERMINATION

Pleural fluid amylase determinations are useful in the differential diagnosis of exudative pleural effusions because a pleural fluid amylase level above the upper normal limits for serum indicates that the patient has one of three problems:

pancreatic disease, malignant tumor, or esophageal rupture (30). However, it is not cost-effective to obtain an amylase measurement on every undiagnosed pleural fluid; rather, pleural fluid amylase levels should be determined only when esophageal rupture or pancreatic disease is suspected. Approximately 50% of patients with inflammatory pancreatic disease have an accompanying pleural effusion (97). In such patients, the pleural fluid amylase level is usually raised well above the normal upper limits for serum and is also higher than the simultaneously sampled serum (30, 98). On rare occasions, the pleural fluid amylase level is normal at the time of the original thoracentesis, only to become elevated at the time of a subsequent thoracentesis. In some patients with acute pancreatitis with pleural effusion, the chest symptoms of pleuritic chest pain and dyspnea may overshadow the abdominal symptoms. In such instances, an elevated pleural fluid amylase level may be the first hint of a pancreatic problem (30).

Patients with chronic pancreatic disease may also present with a pleural effusion with a high amylase content (99). The effusion results when a sinus tract connects the pancreatic pseudocyst and the pleural space. The patients typically appear chronically ill without abdominal symptoms and look like they have cancer. If a pleural fluid amylase level is not measured, the correct diagnosis may never be established. The key to this diagnosis is a markedly elevated (>1,000 U per L) pleural fluid amylase level (100).

The pleural fluid amylase level is elevated in approximately 10% of malignant pleural effusions (30, 100). The serum amylase level is also elevated in about 50% of patients with malignant pleural effusions and an elevated pleural fluid amylase. The pleural fluid amylase level in malignant pleural effusions is usually only minimally to moderately elevated, in contrast to the marked elevations with pancreatitis or esophageal rupture. The primary site of the tumor in patients with neoplastic pleural effusions and elevated pleural fluid amylase levels is usually not the pancreas (30, 101). Because the amylase in malignant pleural effusions is of the salivary type (102), amylase isoenzyme determinations are useful in distinguishing between malignant

and pancreas-related pleural effusions with high amylase levels.

The pleural fluid amylase level is also elevated with esophageal rupture (30, 103). The origin of the amylase with esophageal rupture has been shown to be the salivary gland rather than the pancreas (104). With the tear in the esophagus, the swallowed saliva with its high amylase content passes into the pleural space. Because the early diagnosis of esophageal perforation is imperative, owing to the high mortality rate without rapid operative intervention, the pleural fluid amylase determination should be performed promptly when this diagnosis is suspected. In animal experiments, the pleural fluid amylase concentration is elevated within 2 hours of esophageal rupture (105).

LACTIC ACID DEHYDROGENASE MEASUREMENT

The pleural fluid LDH level is used to separate transudates from exudates (see discussion earlier in this chapter). Most patients who meet the criteria for exudative pleural effusions with LDH but not with protein levels have either parapneumonic effusions or malignant pleural disease. Although initial reports suggested that the pleural fluid LDH level was increased only in patients with malignant pleural disease (106), subsequent reports demonstrated that the pleural fluid LDH was elevated in most exudative effusions regardless of origin (Fig. 4.3), and therefore, this determination is of no use in the differential diagnosis of exudative pleural effusions (14).

Nevertheless, every time that I perform a thoracentesis, I obtain a pleural fluid LDH level. This is because the level of the pleural fluid LDH is a reliable indicator of the degree of pleural inflammation; the higher the LDH, the more inflamed the pleural surfaces. Serial measurement of the pleural fluid LDH levels are informative when one is dealing with a patient with an undiagnosed pleural effusion. If with repeated thoracenteses the pleural fluid LDH level becomes progressively higher, the degree of inflammation in the pleural space is increasing and one should be aggressive in pursuing a diagnosis. Alternatively, if the pleural fluid LDH level decreases

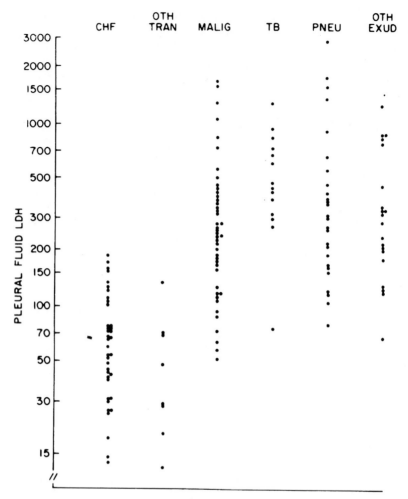

FIG. 4.3. Pleural fluid lactic dehydrogenase (LDH) levels. See the legend of Fig. 4.2 for explanation of abbreviations. Note the similar distributions of the LDH levels for all categories of exudative pleural effusions. (From Light RW, MacGregor MI, Luchsinger PC, et al. Pleural effusions: the diagnostic separation of transudates and exudates. *Ann Intern Med* 1972;77:507–513, with permission.)

with time, the process is resolving and one need not be as aggressive in the approach to the patient.

When bloody pleural fluid is obtained, one might wonder whether the LDH measurement would be useful because red blood cells contain large amounts of LDH. The presence of blood in the pleural fluid, however, usually does not adversely affect the measurement of the LDH. In one study, LDH isoenzyme analysis was performed on 12 pleural fluids that had contained more than 100,000 erythrocytes per mm³. In only one effusion was the LDH-1 percentage-wise

more than 5% above that in the serum, and the total pleural fluid LDH in that effusion was only 107 (28).

Although the total pleural fluid LDH level is not useful in distinguishing among various exudative pleural effusions, one might suppose that LDH isoenzymes would be useful in the differentiation. Three studies have shown that LDH isoenzymes have limited value in the differential diagnosis of exudative pleural effusions (28, 107, 108). All benign effusions with elevated pleural fluid LDH levels and most malignant effusions are characterized by a higher percentage of LDH-4 and LDH-5 in the pleural fluid than in the corresponding serum (28). The increased amounts of LDH-4 and LDH-5 are thought to arise from the inflammatory white blood cells in the pleural effusion (28). Approximately one third of malignant pleural effusions have a different pleural fluid LDH isoenzyme pattern that is characterized by large amounts (>35%) of LDH-2 and less LDH-4 and LDH-5. None of 31 benign exudates in one series had more than 35% LDH-2 (28). No relationship exists between the histologic type of the malignant pleural disease and the pleural fluid LDH-isoenzyme pattern (28). At present, the only situation in which we obtain LDH isoenzyme analysis of pleural fluid is when there is a bloody pleural effusion in a patient who clinically is thought to have a transudative pleural effusion. If the LDH is in the exudative range and the protein is in the transudative range, the demonstration that the majority of the pleural LDH is LDH-1 indicates that the increase in the LDH is due to the blood.

pH AND P_{CO_2} MEASUREMENT

Measurement of the pleural fluid pH and P_{co_2} is useful in the differential diagnosis of exudative pleural effusions. If the pleural fluid pH is less than 7.2, it means that the patient has 1 of 10 conditions: (a) complicated parapneumonic effusion, (b) esophageal rupture, (c) rheumatoid pleuritis, (d) tuberculous pleuritis, (e) malignant pleural disease, (f) hemothorax, (g) systemic acidosis, (h) paragonimiasis, (i) lupus pleuritis, or (j) urinothorax.

The pleural fluid pH is obviously influenced by the arterial pH. With transudative pleural effusions, the pleural fluid pH is usually higher than the simultaneous blood pH (31), presumably because of active transport of bicarbonate from the blood into the pleural space (32). If a low pleural fluid pH is discovered, the arterial pH should be checked to ensure that the patient does not have systemic acidosis. With certain exudative effusions, the pleural fluid pH falls substantially below that of the arterial pH. The explanation for the relative pleural fluid acidosis is as

follows. The relationship between the pleural fluid pH and the blood pH depends on the extent to which the blood and pleural fluid P_{co_2} and bicarbonate are in equilibrium. In conditions associated with pleural fluid acidosis, lactic acid accumulates in the pleural fluid (109, 110), presumably from anaerobic glycolysis in the pleural fluid or tissues. The hydrogen ions associated with the lactic acid combine with bicarbonate to form water and carbon dioxide. Accordingly, the pleural fluid P_{co_2} increases and the pH decreases. Because the addition of 1 mEq of fixed acid to 1 L of pleural fluid results in an increase of 33 mm Hg in the P_{co_2} but in a decrease of only 1 mEq in the bicarbonate concentration (111), pleural fluid acidosis is characterized by a P_{co_2} that is increased proportionately more than the bicarbonate is reduced (31, 109).

The increased pleural fluid P_{co_2} could result from either an increased production of CO_2 or a decreased diffusion of CO_2 from the pleural fluid to blood or a combination of these factors. It is my belief that limited diffusion of CO_2 out of the pleural space is the predominant mechanism. In Fig. 4.4A, it can be seen that changes in the arterial P_{co_2} of a patient with a malignant pleural effusion and mild pleural fluid acidosis were not associated with changes in the pleural fluid P_{co_2}. Similarly, in a second patient, the administration of bicarbonate with an increase in the arterial pH from 7.40 to 7.59 did not change the pleural fluid pH or bicarbonate level (Fig. 4.4B). When pleural fluids are incubated at 37°C *in vitro*, no correlation exists between the rate of acid accumulation *in vitro* and the pleural fluid pH *in vivo* (111, 112), with the possible exception of patients with complicated parapneumonic effusions in whom the rate of acid accumulation is high (112).

The pleural fluid pH is frequently not measured correctly. Chandler et al. (113) surveyed the methods by which pleural fluid pHs were measured at 277 acute care institutions in the southeastern part of the United States in 1998. They reported that the pleural fluid pH was measured with the blood gas machine in only 32% of the institutions, whereas it was measured with dip stick or pH indicator paper in 56% and by a pH

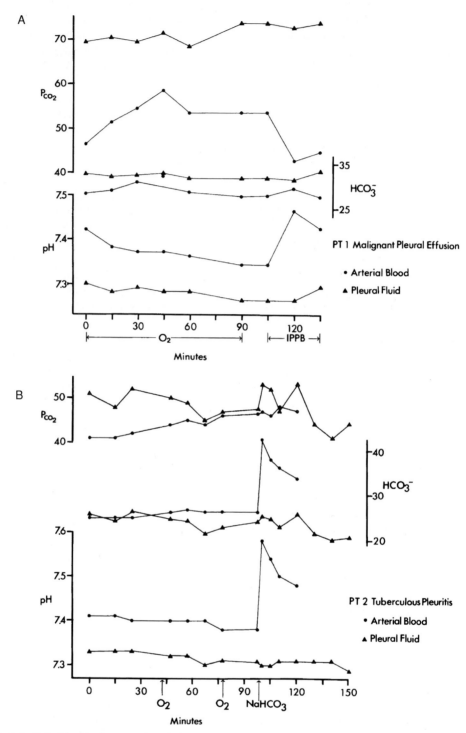

FIG. 4.4. Relationship between pleural fluid and arterial pH, P_{co_2} and HCO_3^-. **A:** Patient with a malignant pleural effusion in whom the administration of supplemental oxygen resulted in an increase in the Pa_{co_2} from 46 to 58. Note that no concomitant change is seen in the pleural fluid P_{co_2}. **B:** Patient with a slightly acidic pleural fluid. The administration of bicarbonate raised the arterial pH from 7.40 to 7.59 but had no influence on the pleural fluid pH.

meter in 12% (113). It has been shown that neither pH indicator strip paper (113–115) nor pH meters (114) are sufficiently accurate for clinical use. The pH meter gives a reading that is approximately 0.20 to 0.30 too high because it measures the pH at room temperature (at which the P_{co_2} is lower) and the sample comes in contact with room air (114). At times, laboratory personnel object to injecting the pleural fluid through blood gas machines for fear of the development of clots. This objection can be overcome if a clot-catching apparatus (Clot Catcher, Bayen Corp., Norwood, MA, USA) is inserted between the syringe and blood gas machine (114).

When the pleural fluid pH is used as a diagnostic test, it must be measured with the same care as arterial pH. The fluid should be collected anaerobically in a heparinized syringe (see Chapter 25). If the fluid is opened to room air, carbon dioxide will leave the fluid and the recorded pH will be falsely high (114). It appears that it is not necessary to put the fluid on ice if the pH is measured within an hour or so (116). Accurate results are also obtained when pleural fluid is transferred from a large syringe to a small heparinized syringe (117). If the effusion is small, injection of the local anesthetic into the pleural fluid may falsely lower the pH (118). If frank pus is obtained at thoracentesis, one should not submit it for pH determination because the thick, purulent fluid may clog the blood gas machine and laboratory personnel may hesitate to analyze subsequent pleural fluids.

In general, pleural fluids with a low pH also have low glucose and high LDH levels (109). If the laboratory reports a low pH with normal glucose and low LDH levels, the pH measurement is probably in error. In like manner, a low glucose level with a normal pH and a low LDH is probably a laboratory error. The only reason to measure the pleural fluid P_{co_2} is to verify the pleural fluid pH because a low pleural fluid pH is almost always associated with a high P_{co_2} (31, 109). The pleural fluid P_{co_2} adds nothing diagnostically.

The pleural fluid pH is most useful in indicating the prognosis of patients with pneumonic effusions (see Chapter 9). If the pleural fluid pH is below 7.0, the patient invariably has a complicated parapneumonic effusion, and attempts should be made to remove all the pleural fluid

with therapeutic thoracentesis or tube thoracostomy (84). If the pleural fluid pH is above 7.2, the prognosis of the patient is excellent and the pleural fluid need not be removed. If the patient has an infection with *Proteus* organisms, the pleural fluid pH may be elevated because these organisms produce ammonia by their urea-splitting ability, which can increase the pH (119). In patients with parapneumonic effusions, the pleural fluid pH may fall before the pleural fluid glucose level becomes depressed (83, 120).

The pleural fluid pH is also decreased with esophageal rupture (103, 121). In fact, Dye and Laforet (121) concluded that a pleural fluid pH of less than 6.0 was highly suggestive of esophageal rupture. These workers attributed the low pleural fluid pH to the reflux of gastric acid through the rent in the esophagus into the pleural space. Subsequent studies in rabbits (122), however, have demonstrated that the pleural fluid pH becomes just as acidic after esophageal rupture if the esophagogastric junction is ligated. It appears that the low pleural fluid pH is due to infection in the pleural space rather than to acid reflux. Over the past few years, we have seen several patients with pleural infection without esophageal rupture in whom the pleural fluid pH was below 6.0. In summary, esophageal rupture is associated with a low pleural fluid pH because of the concomitant pleural infection and not acid reflux. A pleural fluid pH below 6.0 is consistent with but not diagnostic of esophageal rupture.

Patients with pleural effusions secondary to both malignant disease and tuberculosis may have a low pleural fluid pH (31, 109, 123). When my colleagues and I wrote our first paper on pleural fluid pH (31), we concluded that the pleural fluid pH was useful in distinguishing tuberculous from malignant pleural effusions; a pleural fluid pH below 7.3 suggested tuberculosis, whereas a pleural fluid pH above 7.4 suggested malignant disease. Subsequent studies by others (110, 123, 124), however, and my own observations have not supported this conclusion. At present, I consider the pleural fluid pH valueless in distinguishing tuberculous from malignant pleural effusions. The pleural fluid pH does provide information about malignant pleural effusions because patients with a low pleural fluid pH have a shorter life expectancy and are less likely to have a favorable response to pleurodesis (124, 125).

The pleural fluid pH is almost always less than 7.2 with rheumatoid pleural effusions (95). The pleural fluid pH with lupus pleuritis is usually above 7.35 (95), but occasionally, it is less than 7.2 (96). The pleural fluid pH tends to be low with both paragonimiasis (58) and Churg-Strauss syndrome (60), and these are the only two conditions in which a low pleural fluid pH is associated with pleural eosinophilia. Another situation in which the pleural fluid pH may be decreased is with a large hemothorax (31). The metabolism of the many red blood cells in this condition, in conjunction with the atelectatic underlying lung, is the probable explanation for the decreased pH. Finally, the pleural fluid pH may be reduced with urinothorax (126). This is the only situation in which a transudative pleural fluid has a low pH without concomitant systemic acidosis.

TESTS FOR DIAGNOSING PLEURAL MALIGNANCY

Cytologic Examination of Pleural Fluid

Cytologic examination of pleural fluid is one of the most informative laboratory procedures in the diagnosis of pleural effusions because with it a definitive diagnosis can be made in more than 50% of patients with malignant disease involving the pleura. Malignant cells have several characteristics that differentiate them from other cells in the pleural fluid (37). Malignant cells in a given pleural effusion are recognizably similar to each other and are different from any nonmalignant cells in pleural fluid (Fig. 4.1C). Although the overall appearance of the malignant cells is similar, sometimes there is a marked variation in their sizes and shapes; one cell may have many times the diameter of its twin.

Frequently, malignant cells are large. The nuclei of malignant cells may exceed 50 μm diameter, in contrast with mesothelial cell nuclei, which rarely exceed 20 μm in diameter. Small lymphocytes, by comparison, have a diameter of about 10 μm. The nucleoli of malignant cells are often large, exceeding 5 μm in diameter, whereas the nucleoli of nonmalignant

cells in pleural fluid usually do not exceed 3 μm. Malignant cells have a high nucleocytoplasmic ratio. Indeed the nuclear size of the cells in pleural effusions has been used diagnostically. Marchevsky et al. (127) performed a computer-assisted morphometric study of 48 pleural fluids including 20 benign fluids, eight mesotheliomas, and 20 carcinomas. If the mean nuclear diameter exceeded 10.5 μm or the mean nuclear diameter exceeded 9.3 μm and the mean nuclear diameter divided by the cytoplasmic diameter exceeded 0.74, the patient had a malignant pleural effusion. This morphologic analysis was not able to separate carcinomas from mesotheliomas.

There are, however, cytologic characteristics that tend to be different for mesothelioma and adenocarcinomas. Stevens et al. (128) compared the cytologic characteristics of 44 cases of malignant mesothelioma and 46 cases of metastatic adenocarcinomas. They concluded that the following five features separate malignant mesothelioma from adenocarcinoma with better than 95% accuracy. Mesotheliomas tend to have true papillary aggregation, multinucleation with atypia, and cell-to-cell apposition, whereas adenocarcinomas tend to have acinus-like structures and balloon-like vacuolation (128).

Malignant cells sometimes aggregate, and large balls or clumps of cells are characteristic of adenocarcinoma (Fig. 4.1D). Although aggregates of 20 or more benign mesothelial cells occasionally occur, the bizarre, large, vacuolated cells with adenocarcinoma allow for a differentiation between these entities. Small numbers of mitotic figures frequently occur in benign effusions, and, accordingly, the presence of such figures is not indicative of malignant disease. Both malignant cells and macrophages may have vacuolation.

The accuracy of the cytologic diagnosis of malignant pleural effusions has been reported to be anywhere between 40% and 87% (129–131). Several factors influence the percentages in the various reports. First, in many patients with proven malignant disease and pleural effusion, the effusion is not related to malignant involvement of the pleura but rather is secondary to other factors such as congestive heart failure, pulmonary emboli, pneumonia, lymphatic blockade, or hypoproteinemia. In such patients, one cannot expect the pleural fluid cytologic test result to be positive. For example, it is unusual for the results of pleural fluid cytologic tests to be positive in patients with squamous cell carcinoma (29, 37, 132) because the pleural effusions are usually due to bronchial obstruction or lymphatic blockade. Second, the frequency of positive cytologic results depends on the tumor type. For example, with lymphoma, the cytologic examination was positive in 75% of patients with diffuse histiocytic lymphoma but in only 25% of patients with Hodgkin's disease in one series (133). The cytologic test is more frequently positive with adenocarcinomas than with sarcomas (132). Third, the accuracy of the results depends on the way in which the specimens are examined. If both cell blocks and smears are prepared and examined, the percentage of positive diagnoses will be greater than if only one method is used (134). It is recommended that the standard preparation of an effusion should include the preparation of a cell block, and cytospins stained with Diff-Quik and Papanicolaou stains (135). Fourth, the more separate specimens submitted for cytologic examination, the higher the percentage of positive reports (29, 133). In my own experience in patients with proven malignant disease involving the pleural space, the initial pleural fluid cytologic examination is positive in about 60% of patients, and if three separate specimens are submitted, nearly 80% of the patients will have positive results (30). The third specimen frequently contains fresher cells that allow the diagnosis to be made. Fifth, the incidence of positive diagnoses is obviously dependent on the skill of the cytologist. Sixth, the incidence of positive diagnoses is related to the tumor burden in the pleural space. A patient with a large tumor burden is more likely to have a positive pleural fluid cytology than is a patient with a small tumor burden.

In summary, when three separate pleural fluid specimens from a patient with malignant pleural disease are submitted to an experienced cytologist, one should expect a positive diagnosis in about 80% of patients. Because it is important to prevent the pleural fluid specimen from clotting, about 0.5 mL heparin should be added to the syringe during a diagnostic thoracentesis (see Chapter 25). If a larger volume of pleural fluid is obtained during a therapeutic thoracentesis for submission to a cytologist, additional heparin should be added. From the examination of the exfoliated cancer cells, it is usually possible to classify the neoplasm accurately into its histologic type such as adenocarcinoma. Only occasionally is it possible to suggest with confidence the primary site of the neoplasm (132).

Nucleolar Organizer Regions

Nucleolar organizer regions (NOR) are loops of DNA in the nucleus that code for ribosomal RNA and are important in the synthesis of protein (136). These regions are associated with acidic nonhistone proteins that can be visualized by argyrophilic staining (AgNOR). In general malignant cells have more AgNOR staining (136). Although several papers have concluded that AgNOR staining is useful in separating benign and malignant effusions (137–139), there has been no standardization of the technique and there is overlap between benign and malignant cells. Until more research is conducted on AgNOR, it cannot be recommended.

Immunohistochemical Studies

With the development of the necessary technology for monoclonal antibodies (MAb), numerous papers have been published in the past 20 years that have assessed the diagnostic utility of MAb in the diagnosis of pleural malignancy. The basis for this approach is the thought that there are antigens that are unique for benign mesothelial cells, adenocarcinoma cells, and malignant mesothelioma cells. If MAb are developed against these specific antigens, then positive identification of these cells can be made when tissue samples or cytologic preparations are incubated with the antibody and then counterstained with immunoalkaline phosphatase or some similar method.

Several studies have compared the usefulness of the different antibodies in distinguishing the three different cells (140–144). Until the present time, the best markers for adenocarcinoma appear to be carcinoembryonic antigen (CEA), Leu-M1, B72.3, Ber-EP4, and BG-8 (143), whereas the best markers for mesothelioma appear to be calretinin and cytokeratin 5/6. It is important to realize that nonmalignant mesothelial cells will also stain positive for calretinin and cytokeratin 5/6 (145).

When immunohistochemistry is used to differentiate adenocarcinoma from mesothelioma, a panel of monoclonal antibodies should be used. The specific antibodies used depend on the preferences of the local pathologist. If the specimens are sent to a commercial laboratory, the antigens named in the earlier paragraph are recommended. The utility of using such a panel was shown in a study by Brown et al. (142), who evaluated the usefulness of the MAb in a series of 103 adenocarcinomas and 34 mesotheliomas with the CEA, B72.3, and Leu-M1 antibodies. If the specimen were positive for all three, the specificity for adenocarcinoma was 100% and the sensitivity was 70%. If the specimen were positive with two or three of the antibodies, the sensitivity increased to 97%, but there was one false positive. If the specimen were positive with only one of the three antibodies, then two of the patients had adenocarcinoma and two of the patients had mesothelioma. If the specimen were positive for none of the antigens, then the specificity for mesothelioma was 99% and the sensitivity was 91%. However, it must be emphasized that the benign mesothelial cells will also be negative for these antigens.

There are some additional points that need to be made about the immunohistochemical tests. For some of the antibodies, the pattern of the staining is very important. Therefore, it is very important to have an experienced immunohistochemist performing the tests. There are new antibodies being evaluated continuously, and it is hoped that in the near future, antibodies will be developed that are specific for malignant mesothelioma and benign mesothelial cells. Until this time, the immunohistochemical tests are not useful in identifying the origin of the metastatic tumor.

It appears that immunohistochemistry is quite useful in establishing the diagnosis of a lymphomatous pleural effusion. Guzman et al. (146) performed immunocytochemical analysis with the peroxidase-antiperoxidase adhesive slide assay for detection of cell surface antigens using a broad panel of monoclonal antibodies in nine patients with pleural lymphoma.

They were able to recognize clearly six cases of B-cell lymphoma, one case of Hodgkin's disease, and one case of hairy cell leukemia (146).

A role for immunohistochemical tests in establishing the diagnosis of squamous cell carcinoma or small cell carcinoma involving the pleura remains to be demonstrated.

Immunohistochemical tests on cell blocks of pleural fluid or pleural biopsy specimens are available from Impath, Los Angeles, CA, 1-800-447-5816 or www.impath.com at a cost of approximately $75 per antibody.

Electron Microscopic Examination

The diagnosis of mesothelioma and metastatic carcinoma to the pleura is made in most instances by cytology and immunohistochemical assessment, but electron microscopy (EM) still plays a decisive role in some cases with unusual morphology or anomalous histochemical reactions. Accordingly, a portion of the pleural biopsy specimen should be routinely fixed at the time of biopsy for possible subsequent processing for EM (144). Electron microscopy has its greatest utility in differentiating metastatic adenocarcinoma from mesothelioma. The ultrastructural features of mesotheliomas are so characteristic as to be almost diagnostic. These characteristics include the absence of microvillus core rootlets, glycocalyceal bodies, and secretory granules; the presence of intracellular desmosomes, junctional complexes, and intracytoplasmic lumina; and characteristic microvilli. The appearance of the microvilli is the most important diagnostic feature. With adenocarcinoma, they are less abundant and are usually short and stubby, whereas with mesothelioma, they are numerous and are characteristically long and thin (147–148).

Histochemical Studies

Immunohistochemical tests have replaced histochemical tests in distinguishing adenocarcinoma from mesothelioma in many laboratories. However, there are two primary histochemical tests that can be used to differentiate mesotheliomas from adenocarcinomas. The alcian blue stain detects the acid mucins characteristic of mesothelioma (149). In one study, the alcian blue stain was positive in 14 of 29 (47%) mesotheliomas (149), but in none of 44 patients with adenocarcinoma. The periodic acid–Schiff stain after diastase digestion (PAS-D) detects neutral mucins, which are diagnostic of adenocarcinomas. In one study the PAS-D stain was positive in 27 of 44 (61%) patients with adenocarcinoma but in no patients with mesothelioma (149). In summary, if the cells stain positive with PAS-D, the patient in all probability has an adenocarcinoma. If the cells stain positive with alcian blue, the patient in all probability has a mesothelioma. If the cells stain positive with neither, no conclusion can be made.

Tumor Markers in Pleural Fluid

The possibility of establishing the diagnosis of pleural malignancy by demonstrating an elevated level of a tumor marker in the pleural fluid has been the subject of many publications. The tumor markers that have been evaluated have included CEA (150–154), carbohydrate antigens CA 15-3 (150, 154–156), CA 19-9 (150, 154, 157), CA 72-4 (150, 154), cytokeratin 19 fragments (150, 151, 158), sialyl stage-specific antigen (159, 160), neuron-specific enolase (150, 152), and squamous cell carcinoma antigen (150, 152).

In general, I do not recommend that tumor markers be used in the evaluation of patients with undiagnosed pleural effusions. Although an elevated level of any of the tumor markers is very suggestive of malignancy, the specificity is not high enough to establish the diagnosis. Although there is no doubt that the median levels of the different tumor markers are significantly higher in patients with malignancy than in patients with benign pleural effusions, there is always some overlap in the values. If the cutoff level for a tumor marker is set high enough that the level is exceeded by none of the benign effusions, then the test tends to be very insensitive. The same criticism could be made of tests on the pleural fluid for tuberculosis, such as adenosine deaminase or gamma interferon. Nevertheless, I rely

heavily on these tests to establish the diagnosis of tuberculosis. The primary difference in the two situations is that it would be disastrous to wrongly make the diagnosis of malignancy with a tumor marker because the patient is essentially told that he or she has only 90 days to live. If the diagnosis of tuberculosis is wrongly established, the patient is not sentenced to death but rather to taking antituberculous medictions for 6 to 9 months.

In the following section, there are brief discussions of the tumor markers that have been most thoroughly assessed in establishing the diagnosis of pleural effusion.

Carcinoembryonic Antigen

Several articles have concluded that measurement of the CEA levels in pleural fluid is useful in establishing the diagnosis of malignant pleural effusions (161–163). Rittgers et al. (162) reported that 34% of 70 malignant pleural effusions had CEA levels above 12 ng per mL, whereas only 1% of 101 benign effusions had CEA levels this high. Tamura et al. (163) reported that 33 of 66 (50%) patients with a malignant pleural effusion had a pleural fluid CEA level above 10 ng per mL, whereas none of 39 patients with benign disease had pleural fluid CEA levels above this value. Not all the reports have been this positive. Garcia-Pachon et al. (153) measured CEA levels in 273 consecutive patients. They reported that a level of CEA above 10 ng per mL was found in only 43 of 91 (47%) malignant effusions, whereas levels above 10 ng per mL were found in 17 of 182 (9%) nonmalignant effusions including five empyemas, five parapneumonic effusions, and one tuberculous effusion. Some CEA levels in the nonmalignant effusions exceeded 100 ng per mL (153). CEA levels are usually below 10 ng per mL in pleural effusions secondary to lymphomas, sarcomas, and mesotheliomas (150). It appears that a pleural fluid CEA level above 10 ng per mL is suggestive, but not diagnostic, of a malignant pleural effusion. At the present time, routine pleural fluid CEA determinations are not indicated. Cytology, immunohistochemical staining, and pleural biopsy provide a more definite answer.

Carbohydrate Antigens

Three different carbohydrate antigens (CA 15-3, CA 19-9, and CA 72-4) associated with malignancy have been evaluated for their utility is differentiating malignant from benign pleural effusions (150, 154). When the levels of these three antigens are compared in malignant and benign pleural effusions, the overlap between the two groups is substantial (150, 154, 155, 161). If a high enough cutoff level is taken such that only a rare benign effusion is identified, then the tests are not very sensitive. Accordingly, these measurements do not appear to be useful diagnostically.

Sialyl Stage-Specific Antigen

Sialyl stage-specific embryonic antigen-1 is another cancer-associated carbohydrate antigen (159–160). Although cytology-positive pleural fluid from patients with adenocarcinomas have higher mean levels of this cancer-associated antigen than do other pleural fluids (159–160), there is so much overlap that there appears to be no role for the measurement of this antigen in the diagnostic workup of patients with undiagnosed pleural effusions.

Cytokeratin 19 Fragments

Cytokeratin 19 (CYFRA 21-1) is a major component of the cytoskeleton intermediate filaments of simple epithelium cells and is overexpressed in various carcinomas. CYFRA 21-1 is a new tumor marker measuring soluble fragments of cytokeratin. CYFRA 21-1 levels above 100 ng per mL are found in about 60% of patients with carcinoma or mesothelioma (151). CYFRA levels are not elevated in effusions due to lymphomas or sarcomas. However, some patients with benign effusions have pleural fluid CYFRA above 100 ng per mL. In general, there is so much overlap between benign and malignant pleural effusions (158) that the test is not recommended.

Enolase

Enolase is a glycolytic enzyme that is found in extracts of neuroendocrine tumors including small cell lung carcinoma. Pleural effusions due to small cell lung carcinoma tend to have higher levels of enolase than do effusions due to non–small cell lung carcinoma or benign disease (150, 152, 164), but again the overlap is such that the measurement of the enolase levels do not appear to be useful in the differential diagnosis of pleural disease.

Squamous Cell Carcinoma Antigen

Squamous cell carcinoma antigen (SCC) has been used as a serum marker for squamous cell carcinoma. In two studies (150, 152), the pleural fluid levels were low in most patients with malignancy. However, in the study of Miedouge et al. (150), it was positive in 7 of 11 patients (64%) with squamous cell carcinoma. Nevertheless, because SCC is very high in some benign effusions (152), I would not use the pleural fluid SCC to establish the diagnosis of squamous cell carcinoma.

Oncogenes

The development of cancer is a multistep process in which multiple genetic alterations must occur. The transforming genes are collectively called oncogenes. The oncogenes may be related to viruses, environmental carcinogens, or spontaneous mutations. Because the oncogenes are associated with the development of malignancy, one might hypothesize that patients with pleural malignancy would have cells in their pleural fluid containing oncogenes. There have now been several studies testing this hypothesis. Zoppi et al. (165) attempted to detect the p53 protein in 34 embedded blocks of neoplastic fluids and 30 nonneoplastic effusions. They reported that 11 (34%) of the tumor fluids were positive, whereas all the benign fluids were negative (165). Mayall et al. (166) reported similar findings for p53. Tawfik and Coleman (167) reported that benign and malignant effusions did not differ significantly in their expression of the *CMYC* oncogene. Athanassiadou et al. (168) reported that although 21 of 24 malignant effusions (87%) were positive for the *CHARAS* oncogene, the diagnostic usefulness of the test was limited because six of 16 benign effusions (37%) also tested positive.

Hyaluronic Acid

Pleural fluid from patients with mesotheliomas is sometimes abnormally viscid. The increased viscosity in such fluids is due to the presence of increased amounts of hyaluronate, which was previously called hyaluronic acid. Rasmussen and Faber (169) examined the diagnostic usefulness of pleural fluid hyaluronic acid levels in 202 exudates including 19 malignant mesotheliomas. These investigators found that seven of 19 pleural fluids (37%) from patients with malignant mesotheliomas had hyaluronate concentrations above 1 mg per mL, whereas none of the other pleural fluids had hyaluronate levels above 0.8 mg per mL. More recently, Nurminen et al. (170) assayed the levels of hyaluronate in 1,039 pleural effusions including 50 from patients with mesothelioma. They reported that when a cutoff level of 75 mg per mL was used, the assay specificity for malignant mesothelioma was 100% and the sensitivity was 56%. Two more recent papers (171, 172) have reported that the mean levels of hyaluronate are comparable in patients with mesothelioma and metastatic adenocarcinoma. The explanation for the discrepant results appears to be methodologic (173). The measurements of Nurminen were obtained with high-pressure liquid chromatography (HPLC), whereas those of the other two groups were by radioimmunoassay. Unfortunately, the only commercially available measurement in the United States of which I am aware is a radioimmunoassay (Specialty Laboratories, San Diego, CA, USA, and SmithKline Beecham Clinical Laboratories, Philadelphia, PA, USA). Until the results with this assay are verified, it cannot be recommended on a routine basis.

Lectin Binding

Lectins are a class of glycoproteins of nonimmune origin that bind specifically to carbohydrate groups found ubiquitously in various biologic products. Kawai and co-workers (174) investigated lectin binding in 23 pleural mesotheliomas, six effusions with reactive mesothelial cells, and 28 well-differentiated pulmonary adenocarcinomas. In this study, some of the lectins were much more likely to bind to adenocarcino-

mas than to reactive mesothelial cells or mesothelioma cells. These workers could not find significant differences in lectin binding between mesotheliomas and reactive mesothelial cells. Additional research in this area may well demonstrate that studies of lectin binding are useful diagnostically. At the present time, such studies should be considered experimental.

Flow Cytometry

Flow cytometry provides a method for the rapid quantitative measurement of nuclear DNA. It has been proposed as a suitable tool for differentiating between benign and malignant cells because most malignant tumor cells possess an abnormal number of chromosomes (aneuploidy), and consequently an abnormal DNA content (DNA aneuploidy) (175). However, a substantial percentage of metastatic adenocarcinomas and most malignant mesotheliomas are diploid through flow cytometry (136, 176–178). Moreover, a substantial percentage of benign effusions are aneuploid (177). Accordingly, the routine use of flow cytometry to quantitate nuclear DNA levels for the differentiation of benign and malignant effusions cannot be recommended.

Flow cytometry can also be used to identify the surface markers of lymphocytes rapidly and specifically (179) using immunocytometry. Accordingly, the cell lineage (T or B cells) and the clonality of a population of lymphocytes can be determined. These techniques can therefore be used to establish the diagnosis of pleural lymphomas and are recommended in lymphocytic pleural effusions on which the diagnosis of lymphoma is a consideration (179).

Chromosomal Analysis

Abnormalities undoubtedly exist in the chromosome number and structure in some patients with malignant pleural effusions (180, 181). Malignant cells have more chromosomes and marker chromosomes, which are chromosomes with structural abnormalities (translocation, deletion, acentric, dicentric, inversion, isochromosome, or ring) (180). It remains to be demonstrated that there is a place for chromosomal analysis in the routine examination of pleural fluid.

TESTS FOR DIAGNOSING PLEURAL TUBERCULOSIS

Adenosine Deaminase Measurement

Measurement of the adenosine deaminase (ADA) level in pleural fluid is diagnostically useful because ADA levels tend to be higher in tuberculous pleural effusions than in other exudates (161, 182–185). ADA is the enzyme that catalyzes the conversion of adenosine to inosine. In one of the early reports, the ADA levels were evaluated in the pleural fluid of 221 patients. The pleural fluid ADA level exceeded 70 U per L in 33 of 46 (72%) of patients with tuberculous pleuritis. In contrast, none of 173 pleural fluids from patients with other diagnoses had levels this high. Moreover, all 48 pleural fluids from patients with tuberculosis had ADA levels above 45 U per L, whereas only five of the 173 (3%) other pleural fluids had ADA levels above 45 U per L (183). Fontan Bueso et al. (184) reported similar results in a group of 138 pleural effusions including 61 due to tuberculosis and 42 due to malignancy.

Valdés et al. (185) reported their results on 405 pleural fluids including 91 due to tuberculosis, 110 due to malignancy, 58 due to pneumonia, 10 due to empyema, 88 transudates, and 48 miscellaneous. Their results are very similar to those of previous workers with the exception that empyemas also had very high ADA levels (Fig. 4.5). Measurement of the ratio of the pleural fluid to the serum ADA is much less useful diagnostically (185).

From the foregoing three series (183–185), it appears that a pleural fluid ADA level above 70 U per L is highly suggestive of tuberculous pleuritis, whereas a pleural fluid ADA level below 40 U per L virtually rules out this diagnosis. Some caution must be used in relying on ADA levels exclusively to establish the diagnosis of tuberculous pleuritis. The two main diseases that cause an elevated ADA in addition to tuberculosis are rheumatoid pleuritis and empyema (185–186). If the diagnostic criteria for tuberculous pleuritis also includes a pleural fluid lymphocyte-to-neutrophil ratio greater than 0.75, the specificity of the test is increased (187). High pleural fluid ADA levels have also been reported with a very small percent of other neoplasms (188) and with Q fever (189). Patients with lymphocytic pleural effusions after coronary artery bypass graft surgery do not have elevated levels of pleural fluid ADA (190).

Essentially, all the reports from Europe and South Africa have been very positive in finding that the pleural fluid ADA level is useful diagnostically. Interestingly, early reports from Asia were much less positive (161, 163, 191), but more recent reports have shown that the ADA is also very useful diagnostically in Asians (192–194). It is unclear whether the differences in the results are due to ethnic differences or methodologic differences. The distribution of the pleural fluid ADA levels is comparable in human immunodeficiency virus (HIV)–positive and HIV-negative patients with tuberculous pleuritis (192).

Several papers have been written on the diagnostic utility of ADA isoenzymes. ADA has two isoenzymes, ADA1 and ADA2 (194–197). ADA1 is ubiquitous and is produced by lymphocytes, neutrophils, monocytes, and macrophages (195). ADA2 exists only in monocytes and macrophages, and the increase in ADA activity with tuberculous pleuritis is mainly due to ADA2. There is one report in which the use of an ADA1-to-ADA total ratio of less than 0.42 increased the accuracy with which the diagnosis tuberculous pleuritis was established (196). In most cases, ADA isoenzymes are not needed to establish the diagnosis of tuberculosis. However, in certain instances they can be quite useful.

In view of the foregoing information, it is recommended that facilities in which a sizable percentage of the cases of pleural effusions are due to tuberculosis develop the faculty to perform ADA assays on pleural fluid. An ADA level above 70 U per L in a patient who does not have an empyema or rheumatoid arthritis is essentially diagnostic of tuberculous pleuritis. An ADA level above 40 is suggestive of tuberculosis, and the higher the ADA, the more likely the diagnosis of tuberculous pleuritis. In the United States ADA levels can be obtained from Dr. Kent

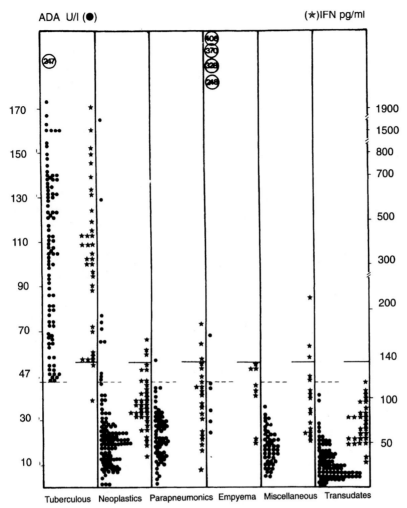

FIG. 4.5. Pleural fluid ADA and interferon-gamma levels in 430 cases. (From Valdés L, San Jose E, Alvarez D, et al. Diagnosis of tuberculous pleurisy using the biologic parameters adenosine deaminase, lysozyme, and interferon gamma. *Chest* 1993;103:458–465, with permission.)

Miller, 55 Circle Creek Way, Armond Beach, Florida 32174, 904-615-0522.

Gamma Interferon

There have been several reports in the past few years that have demonstrated that pleural fluids from patients with tuberculous pleuritis tend to have higher levels of gamma interferon than do other types of exudates (191, 198–200). Pleural fluid gamma interferon levels from the 145 patients reported by Valdés and associates are shown in Fig. 4.5. As can be seen from this figure, 26 of 35 patients (74%) with tuberculous pleurisy had gamma interferon levels above 200 pg per mL, whereas only one effusion out of 110 other effusions that were not empyemas had gamma interferon levels that exceeded this. Villena et al. (200) reported comparable results in 388 pleural fluids including 73 with tuberculous effusions. In this report, a interferon-gamma level of 3.7 U per mL (as measured by radioimmunoassay) had a sensitivity of 0.99 and a specificity of 0.98 (200).

Interferon-gamma is produced by the CD4$^+$ lymphocytes from patients with tuberculous pleuritis (199). The production of interferon-gamma appears to be a useful defense mechanism. Interferon-gamma enhances polymyristate acetate (PMA)–induced hydrogen peroxide production in macrophages, facilitating elimination of intracellular parasites. This lymphokine also inhibits mycobacterial growth in human monocytes (199).

In view of the above-mentioned information, it appears that measurement of the interferon-gamma level is very useful in the diagnosis of tuberculous pleuritis. One must be careful in interpreting the results from a given laboratory, however, since different laboratories report their results in different units. In the United States pleural fluid gamma interferon levels can be obtained from Specialty Laboratories, Santa Monica, CA, 1-800-421-4449. The specimens are assayed only on Mondays and the price is $53.90.

Lysozyme Measurement

The level of lysozyme in the pleural fluid tends to be higher in the pleural fluid from patients with tuberculous pleuritis than in other types of exudates (184, 185, 201, 202). Lysozyme is a bacteriolytic protein with a low molecular weight distributed extensively in organic fluids. In general, the lysozyme levels in tuberculous pleural effusions are greater than those in malignant pleural effusions, but there is so much overlap that the pleural fluid levels themselves are not particularly useful diagnostically. There was one report that suggested that the ratio of the pleural fluid to the serum lysozyme level was useful in separating the two diseases (202). Verea Hernando et al. (202) reported results for 54 patients with tuberculous pleural effusions and 35 patients with malignant pleural effusions. All of the patients with tuberculosis had a ratio above 1.2, whereas only one of the 35 patients (3%) with malignant pleural effusions had ratios above 1.2. A recent study by Valdés et al. (185) did not duplicate these good results; nearly one third of the patients with tuberculous pleuritis had a lysozyme ratio less than 1.1, and many other exudates had ratios that exceeded this value. In this latter ar-

ticle, both the interferon-gamma and the ADA were superior to the lysozyme ratio in differentiating tuberculous from nontuberculous exudates (185). At the present time, the routine measurement of pleural fluid lysozyme to help establish the diagnosis of pleural tuberculosis is not recommended.

Polymerase Chain Reaction

The role of the polymerase chain reaction (PCR) and other nucleic acid amplification–based tests in the diagnosis of tuberculous pleuritis remains to be defined. There are two Food and Drug Administration (FDA)–approved nucleic acid amplification–based tests available for tuberculosis. These tests include a transcription-mediated replication and a hybridization protection assay to detect ribosomal ribonucleic acid (Amplified MTB Direct Test, Gen-Probe, San Diego, CA, USA) and deoxyribonucleic probing of a conserved region of the 16S ribosomal RBNA gene amplified by PCR (Roche Amplicor MTB PCR Test, Roche Molecular Systems, Branchburg, NJ, USA). At present, the FDA limits the use of these tests to acid-fast smear-positive respiratory secretions from previously untreated patients (203). Obviously, most pleural fluids are not acid-fast positive on smear.

Nevertheless, there have been several reports evaluating the utility of PCR for the diagnosis of tuberculous pleuritis. The most positive report was that of Querol et al. (204), who performed PCR on the pleural fluid from 21 patients with pleural tuberculosis and 86 controls. They reported that the sensitivity and specificity of PCR for the diagnosis of tuberculous pleuritis were 81% and 100%, respectively. Comparable results were obtained using pleural fluid ADA with a cutoff level of 45 U per L in which the sensitivity and specificity were 86% and 98%, respectively. Another positive report was presented by Tan et al. (205) who performed PCR on 66 pleural fluid specimens including 16 with tuberculous pleuritis. They reported that PCR was 100% sensitive and 86% specific.

Other investigators have reported poorer results with PCR for the diagnosis of tuberculous pleuritis. Villena et al. (206) reported that the PCR was positive in only 42% of 33 patients with tuberculous pleuritis. Shah et al. (207) reported that the PCR was positive in only 4 of 8 pleural fluids that were culture positive for *Mycoplasma tuberculosis*.

In view of the disparate results in the different studies, the use of the PCR or other nucleic acid amplification–based tests should be considered investigative. Certainly, the expense associated with these tests is much greater than that associated with pleural fluid ADA measurements. In the future, it is likely that these tests will become widely used in the diagnosis of tuberculous pleuritis.

Tuberculous Antigens and Their Antibodies

The possibility of establishing the diagnosis of tuberculous pleuritis by the demonstration of tuberculous antigens or specific antibodies against tuberculous proteins in the pleural fluid has also been investigated. Two reports have evaluated the diagnostic utility of measuring the levels of different tuberculous antigens in the pleural fluid (208–209). Although the mean levels of tuberculous antigens were higher in the pleural fluid of patients with tuberculous pleuritis than in the pleural fluid of other patients, there was so much overlap that the test was of little diagnostic use. In a similar vein, there have been at least six separate reports (210–215) that have indicated that patients with tuberculous pleural effusions tend to have higher levels of specific antituberculous antibodies in their pleural fluid than do patients with other types of exudative effusions. The source of the antibodies, however, is apparently the serum rather than local antibody production in the pleural space (212). Accordingly, it is unlikely that measurement of the antituberculous antibodies in the pleural fluid will add anything diagnostically to measurement of the antituberculous antibodies in the serum (212).

IMMUNOLOGIC STUDIES

Because nearly 5% of patients with rheumatoid arthritis (RA) (216) and 50% of patients with systemic lupus erythematosus (SLE) (217) have pleural effusions sometime during the course of their disease, and because such effusions may be present before the underlying disease is obvious (95, 216), it is important to consider these diagnostic possibilities in patients with exudative pleural effusions of undetermined origin. Numerous papers have assessed the diagnostic utility of various immunologic measurements of the pleural fluid in establishing these diagnoses.

Rheumatoid Factor

Berger and Seckler (218) first reported that rheumatoid factor (RF) was elevated in the pleural fluid of patients with rheumatoid pleuritis. Subsequently, Levine et al. (219) studied pleural fluid RF levels in 65 patients with pleural effusions and found that 41% of patients with bacterial pneumonia and 20% of patients with carcinoma had pleural fluid RF titers equal to or greater than 1:160. In seven of the 65 fluids, the pleural fluid RF titers were greater than the serum titers, but the pleural fluid titer was greater than 1:640 in only one of the patients. These workers concluded that the RF titers in pleural fluid were not useful diagnostically. Halla et al. (95), however, found that the pleural fluid RF was elevated in 11 of 11 seropositive patients with rheumatoid pleural effusions. In each patient, the pleural fluid RF titer was equal to or greater than 1:320 and was equal to or greater than that in the serum. In view of the last-mentioned study, I recommend that RF titers be determined in pleural fluid when the diagnosis of rheumatoid pleuritis is considered. The demonstration of a pleural fluid RF titer equal to or greater than 1:320 and equal to or greater than the serum titer is strong evidence that the patient has a rheumatoid pleural effusion.

Antinuclear Antibodies

In the previous edition of this book, I stated that measurement of the antinuclear antibody (ANA) levels in pleural fluid appeared to be the best test for establishing the diagnosis of lupus pleuritis. Two studies published since the previous edition have cast doubt on this statement. Khare et al. (220) measured pleural fluid ANA levels using the Hep-2 cell line on 82 pleural fluids including eight with systemic lupus erythematosus. Six of the eight patients (75%) with SLE had high (≥1:320) titers of ANA in their pleural fluid with a homogenous staining pattern. In none did the pleural fluid ANA titer differ by more than one dilution from the serum titer. The other two patients with SLE had alternative explanations for their pleural effusions. However, eight of the remaining 74 patients (10.8%) had positive pleural fluid ANA titer ($\geq$1:40) and two had a homogenous pattern. In the patients with SLE, pleural fluid analysis of anti-ssDNA, anti-dsDNA, anti-Sm, anti-SSA, and anti-SSB antibodies reflected the findings in the serum (220). A more recent study evaluated the ANA titers in 126 pleural fluids, again using the HEP-2 cell line as substrate (221). Again all of the pleural fluids from the patients with SLE had a high ANA titer (>1:160), but in this study, the pattern could be either homogenous or speckled (221). Moreover, pleural fluid ANA titers were greater than 1:160 in 13 other patients, 11 of whom had malignant pleural effusions. The pleural fluid and the serum ANA titers were closely correlated in all patients. The explanation for the discrepancy between these two recent studies and two older studies (96, 222) that suggested that the pleural fluid ANA levels were very useful is not known, but it may be related to the cell line used for the assays. Nevertheless, the two more recent studies suggest that measurement of the pleural fluid ANA titer adds essentially nothing to measuring the serum ANA titer in the differential diagnosis of pleural effusions.

Lupus Erythematosus Cells

The demonstration of lupus erythematosus (LE) cells in a pleural effusion was thought to be diagnostic of lupus pleuritis (96). LE cells are formed when polymorphonuclear leukocytes ingest extracellular nuclear material to form a polymorphonuclear leukocyte with a large inclusion of nuclear material. Most pleural effusions secondary to SLE contain LE cells (222). Wang et al. (223) recently reported that LE cells were present in the pleural fluid in eight of 10 patients (80%) with SLE and polyserositis but in none of 112 pleural fluids with other etiologies (223). Noteworthy was the observation that the LE cell test results were identical in the serum and the pleural fluid. This suggests that the diagnosis of SLE can

be established by an LE test on the serum, but an LE test on the pleural fluid adds nothing diagnostically. Moreover, with the development of better immunologic tests for SLE, LE preparations are being performed less and less frequently and laboratories become less proficient in the testing. Testing for LE cells is not recommended unless the laboratory is proficient in this test. It also should be noted that false-positive LE cell results have been reported (224).

Rheumatoid Arthritis Cells

Granular white cells containing cytoplasmic inclusions can be found in the synovial fluid of many patients with RA. These cells are called RA cells only when liberation of RF from the cell can be demonstrated. RA cells have been demonstrated in the pleural fluid of patients with rheumatoid pleuritis (225). Because many pleural fluids contain many white blood cells with cytoplasmic inclusions, because the demonstration of the liberation of RF is time-consuming, and because the diagnosis of rheumatoid pleuritis can usually be established by other means, I do not recommend searching for RA cells in pleural fluid.

Complement Levels

Most patients with pleural effusions secondary to either SLE or RA have reduced pleural fluid complement (Fig. 4.6), whether whole complement (CH50) (226, 227), C3 (95), or C4 (95, 226) is measured. The measurement of pleural fluid complement does not absolutely separate patients with SLE or RA from patients with other exudative pleural effusions, as shown in Fig. 4.6, regardless of whether CH50, C3, or C4 is measured. Nevertheless, a CH50 level below 10 U per mL (226) or a C4 level below 10 times 10^{-5} U per g protein (95) is seen with most patients with either RA or SLE and rarely with other diseases. Because the serum ANA levels and the RF titers appear to be more specific and more sensitive at identifying individuals with pleural effusions due to RA or SLE, it is not recommended that pleural fluid complement levels be obtained routinely.

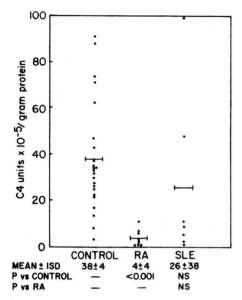

FIG. 4.6. Levels of hemolytic C4 adjusted for total protein in control, rheumatoid arthritis (RA), and systemic lupus erythematosus (SLE) pleural fluids. Note that the pleural fluid from the patients with RA and SLE has lower levels of hemolytic C4. (From Halla JT, Schrohenloher RE, Volanakis JE. Immune complexes and other laboratory features of pleural effusions. *Ann Intern Med* 1980;92:748–752, with permission.)

There have been several recent articles that have evaluated the diagnostic utility of complement activation products in pleural fluid. Two studies have demonstrated that the pleural fluid levels of SC5b-9, which is a product of C3 activation, are elevated in tuberculous pleural fluid as opposed to malignant pleural effusions or transudates (228, 229) and that the SC5b-9 levels are highest in patients with rheumatoid disease (229). However, the overlap between the various groups limits the diagnostic usefulness of this test.

Immune Complexes

Patients with pleural effusions secondary to RA or SLE also have higher pleural fluid levels of immune complexes than patients with effusions due to other causes (95, 230, 231). The differentiation of pleural effusions secondary to SLE and RA from other exudative pleural effusions is less distinct when pleural fluid immune complex levels are used than when pleural fluid complement is used because a substantial percentage of other exudative pleural effusions have elevated pleural fluid immune complex levels (95, 230). The presence of pleural fluid immune complexes also depends on the assay system (95). Patients with SLE have higher levels of immune complexes when the assay is performed with the Clq component of complement or the Raji cell assay than with monoclonal rheumatoid factor. With RA, the level of immune complexes in the pleural fluid is higher than that in the simultaneous serum, whereas in other disease states, the serum level of immune complexes is higher (95). Because measurement of the immune complex level appears to add no information to that obtained from measuring complement levels, it is recommended that pleural fluid immune complex determinations be performed only in research situations.

LIPID STUDIES

Pleural fluid is occasionally milky or opalescent. This opalescence is sometimes mistakenly attributed to myriad white blood cells in the pleural fluid, and the patient is treated for an empyema. This mistake is not made if the supernatant of the centrifuged pleural fluid is examined. In empyema, the supernatant is clear, whereas in a chylous or chyliform effusion, the supernatant remains cloudy or milky. Some pleural fluids with high lipid content also contain numerous red blood cells, and their color is accordingly red or brown. The supernatants of all pleural fluids should be examined for turbidity. Lipid studies of the pleural fluid should be ordered whenever the supernatant is turbid.

The persistent cloudiness of these pleural fluids after centrifugation is due to their high lipid content, which can result from one of three mechanisms. First, the lymphatic duct may be disrupted so that chyle accumulates in the pleural space. The patient is then said to have a chylothorax, and the pleural effusion is called a chylous pleural effusion. Second, large amounts of cholesterol or lecithin-globulin complexes can accumulate for unknown reasons in the pleural fluid. The patient is then said to have a

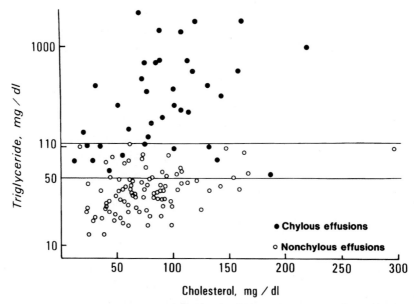

FIG. 4.7. Scattergram of cholesterol and triglyceride values in pleural fluid. Solid dots represent patients whose effusions contained chylomicrons and were considered chylous. Open circles represent patients without chylomicrons whose effusions were considered nonchylous. All patients with triglyceride levels above 110 mg per dL had chylous effusions, whereas no patient with triglyceride levels below 50 mg per dL had a chylous effusion. (From Staats BA, Ellefson RD, Budahn LL, et al. The lipoprotein profile of chylous and nonchylous pleural effusions. *Mayo Clin Proc* 1980;55:700–704, with permission.)

pseudochylothorax and a chyliform pleural effusion. Although some authors have separated pseudochylothoraces into chyliform pleural effusions, characterized by high lecithin-globulin levels, and pseudochylous effusions, characterized by the presence of cholesterol crystals (232, 233), I see no advantage to making this differentiation. Third, if the patient is receiving parenteral nutrition through a central line and the superior vena cava is perforated, the fat emulsion can collect in the pleural space. It is important to distinguish these three entities because the treatment is different for each one.

When milky pleural fluid is discovered, the first question that should be asked is whether the patient is receiving parenteral nutrition through a central line. If the superior vena cava is perforated in such a setting, the intravenous infusion fluid may accumulate rapidly in the pleural space (234). If the patient is receiving a lipid emulsion, the pleural fluid triglyceride level can be very high. However, the pleural fluid glucose

and the potassium levels are usually exceedingly high if the fat emulsion is entering the pleural space (234).

The diagnosis of chylothorax is best made by measuring the triglyceride levels in the pleural fluid. If the pleural fluid triglyceride level exceeds 110 mg per dL, the patient probably has a chylothorax; if the triglyceride level is below 50 mg per dL, the patient does not have a chylothorax (Fig. 4.7). If the triglyceride level is between 50 and 110 mg per dL, the patient may or may not have a chylothorax (235). When the diagnosis is uncertain, lipoprotein analysis of the fluid should be ordered. The demonstration of chylomicrons in the pleural fluid with lipoprotein analysis is diagnostic of chylothorax (235, 236). Most patients with chylothoraces and pleural fluid triglyceride levels below 110 mg per mL are malnourished.

Romero et al. (237) have suggested that the diagnosis of chylothorax should also require a pleural fluid-to-serum cholesterol ratio lower than

1 and a pleural fluid-to-serum triglyceride level less than 1. The first requirement is reasonable because patients with chyliform pleural effusions often have pleural fluid cholesterol levels above 250 mg per dL (238) and this requirement should eliminate them. It should be noted that the clinical picture with chyliform effusion of a long-standing pleural effusion with thickened pleura should be easy to differentiate from that of an acute pleural effusion with normal pleural surfaces seen with chylous effusion. If any doubt exists, lipoprotein analysis of the pleural fluid should be performed. The second criteria proposed by Romero et al. (21) is probably not necessary because in patients without chylothorax, there is no relationship between the serum and the pleural fluid triglyceride level, and the mean pleural fluid triglyceride level is only about 25% of the serum level (25).

Other studies useful for diagnosing turbid pleural fluids are the total lipid content, the cholesterol content, and microscopic examination of the sediment. Most pleural effusions that are cloudy secondary to high lipid levels have a total fat content greater than 400 mg per dL (239). The cholesterol levels in the pleural fluid are elevated in high-lipid pleural effusions due to high numbers of cholesterol crystals or lecithin-globulin complexes (233), but cholesterol levels may also be elevated in chylous pleural effusions (235), as demonstrated in Fig. 4.7. When the turbidity is due to high numbers of cholesterol crystals, examination of the pleural fluid sediment reveals the cholesterol crystals, which are large, rhombic, or polyhedric, as illustrated in Fig. 23.1.

MICROBIOLOGIC STUDIES ON PLEURAL FLUID

Cultures

Pleural fluid from patients with undiagnosed exudative pleural effusions should be cultured for bacteria (both aerobically and anaerobically), mycobacteria, and fungi. For aerobic and anaerobic bacterial cultures, we prefer to inoculate blood culture media right at the bedside because the number of positive cultures will increase with this method (240). For mycobacterial cultures, use of a BACTEC system with bedside inoculation provides higher yields and faster results than do conventional methods. In one study, the median time for the BACTEC cultures to become positive was 18 days (range 3 to 40 days), whereas the median time for conventional cultures was 33.5 days (range 21 to 48 days) (241). If the fluid is not inoculated at the bedside, it should be sent to the laboratory in an anaerobic transport container at room temperature (242). A Gram stain of the fluid should also be obtained. Routine smears for mycobacteria are not indicated because they are almost always negative, unless the patient has a tuberculous empyema or unless the patient is HIV positive.

Culturing pleural fluid from chest tube drainage should be discouraged. Cultures from chest tubes yield inaccurate culture results when compared with direct aspirates (242).

Countercurrent Immunoelectrophoresis

The goal with countercurrent immunoelectrophoresis (CIE) is to identify bacterial antigens in pleural fluid and thus to establish a presumptive bacteriologic diagnosis in patients with parapneumonic pleural effusions. CIE depends on the interaction of an antigen with a negative charge and a specific antibody with a positive charge in an electrical field to form a distinct precipitin line (243, 244). The advantage of CIE over bacterial cultures is that results are available within hours rather than days, so that appropriate antibiotics can be administered sooner. CIE is most useful in the diagnosis of pleural effusions in children, in whom most pleural effusions are due to bacterial infections with *Streptococcus pneumoniae, Staphylococcus aureus,* or *Haemophilus influenza.* These are the three bacteria for which antigens are available to perform CIE studies. In a series of 87 pediatric patients with pleural effusions (243), pleural fluid cultures were positive for one of these three bacteria in 34 patients, and CIE correctly identified the offending organisms in 33 (97%). In about 25% of those patients, the Gram stain of the pleural fluid was negative. In an additional 23 patients, CIE identified antigens in the pleural fluid when the pleural fluid cultures were negative (243).

Another advantage of CIE is that it remains positive for several days after antibiotic therapy is initiated (243, 244). To my knowledge, examination of pleural fluid with CIE has not been performed on a large series of adult patients with pleural effusion. The disadvantage of CIE in the adult patient with a complicated parapneumonic effusion is that many such effusions are due to anaerobic bacteria (83), and antigens for all the anaerobic organisms are not yet available for routine use. Certainly, if CIE is readily available, it should be performed on the pleural fluid from patients with an acute febrile illness and pleural effusion.

Direct Gas-Liquid Chromatography

Most anaerobic bacteria produce volatile fatty acids. Demonstration of such fatty acids by direct gas-liquid chromatography of the pleural fluid has been proposed as a means to establish the diagnosis of anaerobic pleural infections. In one report, pleural fluid from 52 patients, including 14 with anaerobic infections, were analyzed with direct gas-liquid chromatography (245). Multiple volatile fatty acids or succinic acid were present in 13 of the 14 (93%) of the fluids from patients with anaerobic infections. Succinic acid was the major product in 10 patients, and nine of them had infections due to *Bacteroides*. In contrast, pleural fluid from other patients did not contain multiple volatile fatty acids or succinic acid (245). Direct gas-liquid chromatography is a difficult and expensive procedure, however, and it requires specially trained technicians. The resources required for gas-liquid chromatography are probably better spent in upgrading anaerobic culture techniques.

CYTOKINES IN PLEURAL FLUID

Cytokines are soluble peptides secreted by cells that effect the behavior of either the same or other nearby cells through nonenzymatic means. Often they are glycopeptides, and typically they exert their effects at very low concentrations in the picomolar to nanomolar range. Within this broad heading are a number of subclasses, including polypeptide growth factors, interleukins, interferons, and colony-stimulating factors.

In recent years, much research has been devoted toward understanding the role of these peptides. It is not surprising, therefore, that there have been numerous reports assessing the diagnostic utility of the levels of different cytokines in the pleural fluid. In general, with the exception of interferon-gamma, the diagnostic usefulness of cytokine levels in pleural fluid remains to be demonstrated. Nevertheless, I have elected to include a brief discussion of the more commonly studied cytokines because their study has provided clues about the pathogenesis and resolution of pleural injury.

Interleukin-1

IL-1 has an essential role in T-cell activation and is considered a proinflammatory cytokine (246). The highest levels of pleural fluid IL-1 are seen with empyema (247), which is the pleural disease with the most inflammation. Pleural fluid IL-1 and tissue necrosis factor (TNF) are significantly correlated (246). The mean levels of IL-1 are significantly higher in tuberculous than in malignant effusions (246, 248), but there is sufficient overlap that IL-1 levels are not useful diagnostically. The pleural fluid levels of IL-1 are higher than the simultaneous serum levels, suggesting local production (246). Patients with tuberculous pleuritis who develop chronic pleural thickening have significantly higher IL-1 levels than those who do not (246). There is a naturally occurring IL-1 receptor antagonist (IL-1ra). Marie et al. (249) measured the IL-1ra levels in the pleural fluid and serum of 24 patients. They found that the mean plasma level of IL-1ra was significantly higher than the mean pleural fluid level and that patients with infections did not have higher levels than did patients without infections (249).

Interleukin-2

IL-2 plays a crucial role in the mediation of the immune response. It induces and maintains the proliferation of T lymphocytes following mitogen or antigen activation and it also induces production of cytotoxic lymphocytes, NK cells, and lymphokine-activated killer cells. As with IL-1, the pleural fluid levels of IL-2 are higher with tuberculous pleuritis than with malignant pleural effusion, but there is much overlap (248). One of the first events with T-cell activation is the synthesis and surface expression of a receptor of IL-2 (IL-2R), along with the release of a shorter soluble form of IL-2R. The median levels of the soluble IL-2R are higher in tuberculous effusions than in malignant pleural effusions, parapneumonic pleural effusions, and transudative pleural effusions, but again there is substantial overlap (250). The highest pleural fluid IL-2R levels are seen with rheumatoid pleuritis (251). Intrapleural IL-2 has been used to treat malignant pleural effusions because of its ability to induce the production of the various lymphocytes (252). When IL-2 is administered intrapleurally, there are increases in the pleural fluid levels of IL-6, but not of TNF or IL-1 (252).

Interleukin-3

IL-3 induces the proliferation of eosinophils *in vitro* and also prolongs their survival. In patients with eosinophilic pleural effusions, IL-3 appears to help promote the eosinophil proliferation and also prolongs the survival of eosinophils. It appears, however, that IL-3 is less important than IL-5 in promoting these two activities in patients with eosinophilic pleural effusions. Blocking antibodies to IL-5 neutralize more of these activities than do blocking antibodies to IL-3 (47). IL-3 is not detectable by enzyme-linked immunosorbent assay (ELISA) in eosinophilic pleural effusions (48, 49).

Interleukin-4

Human immunity has two major components–cellular and humoral. The T-helper type 1 (Th1) pathway favors cellular immunity, whereas the Th2 pathway favors humoral immunity (253). Early determination toward Th1 and Th2 cells in the immune response is dependent on the balance between interleukin-12 (IL-12), which favors the Th1 response, and IL-4, which favors the Th2 response. In one study of 21 patients with malignant pleural effusions, IL-4 levels in the pleural fluid were below minimal detectable concentrations (253).

Interleukin-5

IL-5 induces the proliferation of eosinophils *in vitro* and prolongs their survival. Pleural fluid IL-5 levels are elevated in patients with posttraumatic eosinophilic pleural effusions (48). The pleural fluid from such individuals acts as a stimulus for eosinophil colony formation, and this stimulatory capability is largely blocked by specific antibodies toward IL-5. In like manner, eosinophilic pleural fluid enhances the survival of eosinophils, and this capability is largely blocked by specific antibodies toward IL-5. We have recently shown in a series of 40 pleural effusions including 30 with more than 10% eosinophils that there was an excellent correlation between the IL-5 levels and the number of eosinophils in the pleural fluid (R = 0.87). Therefore, it appears that IL-5 is one of the primary factors responsible for eosinophilic pleural effusions (47–49).

Interleukin-6

IL-6, also call B-cell stimulatory factor-2 or hepatocyte-stimulating growth factor, is a multifunction cytokine produced by several different cell types such as monocytes, fibroblasts, and endothelial cells (254). IL-6 has a pivotal role in many regulatory functions including maturation of B cells to antibody-producing cells and induction of the synthesis of acute phase proteins. The level of IL-6 in the pleural fluid is significantly correlated with the C-reactive protein level in the serum (255). The levels of IL-6 are much higher in the pleural fluid than they are in the serum (254) and the mean IL-6 levels are much higher in exudates than in transudates (254, 256). Tuberculous effusions contain a significantly higher level of IL-6 than do malignant pleural effusions (256). The pleural fluid from patients with mesothelioma has a significantly higher mean IL-6 level than does the pleural fluid from patients with adenocarcinoma (257). It has been postulated that the thrombocytosis seen in patients with mesothelioma is due to the intrapleural production of large amounts of IL-6 (257). The intrapleural administration of IL-2 results in increased pleural fluid levels of IL-6 (252). One study reported that the levels of soluble IL-6 receptor in pleural fluid were lower than those in the serum and were comparable in different diagnostic categories (255).

Interleukin-8

IL-8 is a powerful neutrophil chemotaxin that contributes to the influx of neutrophils into the pleural space (38, 39, 258). Cultured mesothelial cells produce IL-8 in response to IL-1, TNF-α, or endotoxin (259). Pleural fluid IL-8 levels are most elevated in patients with empyema (38, 39, 259, 260). There are also relatively high levels of IL-8 in the pleural fluid from patients with cancer or tuberculosis, but the levels of IL-8 in the pleural fluid from patients with congestive heart failure are low (261–262). There is a significant correlation between the numbers of neutrophils in empyema fluid and the level of IL-8 in the fluid (38, 39). Neutrophil chemotactic activity is correlated with IL-8 activity, and the majority of the neutrophil chemotactic activity in pleural fluid is neutralized with anti-IL-8 antibodies (38).

IL-8 may also induce lymphocyte chemotaxis into the pleural space (261). Pace et al. (261) demonstrated that in patients with malignant and tuberculous pleural effusions, the lymphocyte count was more closely correlated with the IL-8 level than was the neutrophil count. Moreover, these workers reported that the pleural fluid was chemotactic for lymphocytes and that the chemotactic activity could be eliminated with antibodies to IL-8 (261).

Interleukin-10

IL-10 is the most important antiinflammatory cytokine found within the human immune response (262). An antiinflammatory cytokine by definition is a cytokine that can inhibit the synthesis of IL-1, TNF, or another major proinflammatory cytokine (262). IL-10 is a potent inhibitor of Th1 cytokines, including IL-2 and interferon gamma (262). Chen et al. (253) measured the pleural fluid and serum IL-10 in 21 patients with a malignant pleural effusion. They reported that IL-10 was detectable in 19 of the 21 pleural fluids (90%) and that the levels of IL-10 were higher in the pleural fluid than in the serum (253). They found no correlation with IL-10 levels and lymphocyte subpopulations (253).

Interleukin-12

IL-12 is a recently discovered cytokine with potential for enhancing the cell-mediated immune responses to intracellular pathogens and tumors. Most of the IL-12 biological activity has been described on T and NK cells. IL-12 has an obligatory role for the generation of T-helper type (Th1) cells and for optimal differentiation of cyotoxic T lymphocytes (253). In one study of 21 patients with pleural effusion, IL-12 was below the minimal detectable concentration for all serum and pleural fluid samples (253). It is interesting to note that the intralesional injection of IL-12 into mesotheliomas in the mouse model of mesothelioma leads to tumor regression (263).

Monocyte Chemotactic Peptide

Monocyte chemotactic peptide-1 (MCP-1) is a cytokine that is chemotactic for monocytes. Cultured mesothelial cells in response to IL-1, TNF-α, or endotoxin produce MCP-1 (259). Antony et al. (39) have shown that the pleural fluid levels of MCP-1 are higher in patients with malignant pleural effusions and tuberculous pleural effusions than they are in patients with parapneumonic effusions or congestive heart failure. There is a correlation between the number of monocytes and the pleural fluid MCP-1 levels in patients with malignant pleural effusions. Specific neutralizing antibodies to MCP-1 eliminate approximately 70% of the monocyte chemotactic activity in pleural fluid (39).

Tumor Necrosis Factor-α

TNF-α is a proinflammatory cytokine. In the inflammatory process, TNF-α is one of the first cytokines to appear. Incubation of mesothelial cells in the presence of TNF-α leads to the release of IL-8 and monocyte chemotactic peptide (259). The level of TNF-α in the pleural fluid is a marker of the degree of inflammation. Exudative pleural fluids have higher levels of TNF-α than do transudative pleural effusions (254). The TNF-α levels in the pleural fluid from patients with tuberculosis are significantly greater than in those with pleural malignancy (246, 264). Moreover the TNF-α levels are higher in the pleural fluid than in the serum of the patients with tuberculosis but not those with malignancy (246). In pleural fluid from patients with tuberculosis, the TNF-α levels are significantly correlated with the IL-1 levels (246). The addition of TNF to mesothelial cell cultures results in the mesothelial cells producing plasminogen activator inhibitor type I (PAI-1) and tissue-type plasminogen activator (tPA). Patients with tuberculous pleuritis who go on to develop pleural thickening have higher levels of TNF-α in their pleural fluid than do those who do not develop thickening (246). In rabbits, the administration of polyclonal anti–TNF-α Fab fragments diminishes the pleurodesis induced by talc but not that resulting from doxycycline (265).

Transforming Growth Factor-β

TGF-β is found in inflammatory cells (especially macrophages) and platelets, and is very abundant in the cells of the lung. In mammals, there are three forms of TGF-β; these are TGF-β_1, TGF-β_2, and TGF-β_3 (266). TGF-β is one of the most potent fibrogenic agents ever discovered. Accordingly, TGF-β is an important agent when one considers the response of the pleura to injury. Mesothelial cells express and secrete TGF-β (267). The incubation of human pleural mesothelial cells with TGF-β results in increased levels of plasminogen activator inhibitor 1 (268), which should inhibit the fibrinolytic system.

Both TGF-β_1 and TGF-β_2 are present in pleural fluids from patients (269). The levels of TGF-β_1 and TGF-β_2 both correlate with the pleural fluid LDH level (269). In general, the levels of TGF-β_1 are about 10 times higher that the levels of TGF-β_2 (269). The pleural fluid from patients with mesothelioma tends to have higher levels of TGF-β than does the pleural fluid from patients with metastatic adenocarcinoma (270).

The intrapleural injection of small amounts of TGF-β_2 produces a pleurodesis in both rabbits (271) and sheep (272) that is at least as good as that resulting from tetracycline derivatives or talc. The pleural fluid that results from the intrapleural injection of TGF-β_2 is much less inflammatory than that which results from the intrapleural injection of a tetracycline derivative or talc (271).

Vascular Endothelial Growth Factor

VEGF, also know as vascular permeability factor or vasculotropin, is a multifunctional cytokine that has two primary functions: (a) it increases the permeability of the vasculature, and (b) it is an important angiogenic and lymphogenic factor. In some assays, VEGF is more potent that histamine in increasing vascular permeability (273). The permeability-enhancing capabilities of VEGF are probably most important in regard to pulmonary disease, and it has been hypothesized that VEGF is important in increasing the permeability of the capillaries of the pleura and increasing the rate of pleural fluid formation (274). If this hypothesis proves to be true, pleural effusions in the future may be controlled with inhibitors of VEGF (275).

VEGF receptors are present on mesothelial cells (276). There are detectable levels of VEGF in all pleural effusions (273, 276). The levels of VEGF are higher in exudates than in transudates, but there is significant overlap (273). The levels of VEGF and LDH in the pleural fluid are significantly correlated (273). In patients with malignancy, the pleural fluid VEGF levels are approximately 10 times the serum levels (277).

Platelet-Activating Factor

PAF is a potent lipid mediator that activates platelets, neutrophils, eosinophils, and macrophages, and increases vascular permeability (278). Mesothelial cells synthesize PAF in response to thrombin (278). When PAF in injected intrapleurally, inflammation of the pleura develops associated with neutrophils and eosinophils (278). The relationship between pleural fluid eosinophilia and pleural fluid levels of PAFs is unclear. In one recent report analyzing eosinophilic pleural fluid associated with pneumothorax, there was no correlation between the PAF levels and the numbers of eosinophils (279). However, in a previous report eosinophilic pleural fluids with high levels of eosinophils tended to have high pleural fluid PAF levels (280).

FIBRINOGENESIS AND FIBRINOLYSIS IN THE PLEURAL SPACE

Pleural fibrin deposition is a characteristic of many diseases of the pleura, and fibrin membranes are responsible for the loculations that make the drainage of complicated parapneumonic effusions and empyema difficult. When the pleura is inflamed, the amount of fibrin that is laid down is the result of the balance between fibrinogenesis and fibrinolysis.

Thrombin acts on fibrinogen to produce fibrin. Plasminogen breaks down fibrin and is activated by tPA (268). Human mesothelial cells express tPA but no detectable fibrinolytic activity in a fibrin plate assay. The explanation for the lack of fibrinolytic activity appears to be the production of the plasminogen activator inhibitors (PAI-1). In mesothelial cell cultures, PAI-1 increases in response to both TNF-α and TGF-β (268).

In pleural fluids from humans, patients with tuberculosis have higher levels of PAI-1 than do patients with pleural malignancy, and the levels in the pleural fluid are approximately four times higher than those in the blood (246). In contrast, the pleural fluid levels of tPA are about three times higher in the patients with malignancy than in the patients with tuberculosis (246). This factor possibly explains why there is so much more fibrin deposition in patients with tuberculosis than in patients with pleural malignancy. Patients with pleural TB who develop residual pleural thickening have significantly greater pleural fluid levels of TNF-α and PAI-1 (246).

In certain conditions involving the pleura, for example, parapneumonic effusions, loculations may develop in the pleural space. The loculations are due to fibrin membranes. One might hypothesize that the development of the loculations would depend on the balance between the procoagulant and the fibrinolytic activity in the pleural space. Idell and co-workers (281) measured the procoagulant and fibrinolytic activity in 36 pleural fluids including 21 due to malignancy, three due to empyema, eight due to congestive heart failure, and four due to pneumonia. They found that procoagulant activity was present in some of the exudates, but its presence did not necessarily correlate with loculation and its level did not serve to differentiate the different exudates. The transudates had no active procoagulant. Fibrinolytic activity was absent in all the exudates, whereas five of the eight transudates had fibrinolytic activity (281). In view of the above-mentioned items, measurement of the procoagulant activity in pleural fluids does not appear to be useful either diagnostically or prognostically.

Fibrinogen and Fibrin Degradation Products

The fibrinogen levels in pleural fluid are low in comparison to those in plasma (77, 282). The levels of fibrinogen tend to be low in patients with congestive heart failure and malignancy, and high in patients with tuberculosis and empyema but there is much overlap. The level of d-dimer is comparable in all pleural effusions (282).

MISCELLANEOUS TESTS ON PLEURAL FLUID

Other Proteins

Numerous studies have evaluated the diagnostic usefulness of measuring other proteins in the pleural fluid, including C-reactive protein (283), ferritin (284), mucoproteins (78), fibronectin (285), acid glycosaminoglycans (mucopolysaccharides) (286), beta$_2$-microglobulins (287), and alpha-fetoprotein (287). The pleural fluid levels of these proteins are not useful in the differential diagnosis of exudative pleural effusions.

Other Enzyme Determinations

Many other enzymes, including aldolase (288), glutamic oxaloacetic transaminase, glutamic pyruvic transaminase (288), phosphohexose iso-merase (288), malic dehydrogenase (288), isocitric dehydrogenase (288), glutathione reductase (288), alkaline phosphatase (289), angiotensin-converting enzyme (290), and trans-ketolase, have been measured in the pleural fluid and have been found to give no useful diagnostic information. One report suggested that elevation of the acid phosphatase level in the pleural fluid was diagnostic of metastatic prostatic carcinoma (291), but a second report indicated that approximately 10% of all pleural effusions have acid phosphatase levels above the upper normal limit for serum and higher than in the corresponding serum (292).

REFERENCES

1. Marel M, Stastny B, Melínová L, et al. Diagnosis of pleural effusions–experience with clinical studies 1986–1990. *Chest* 1995;107:1598–1603.
2. Anthonisen NR, Martin RR. Regional lung function in pleural effusion. *Am Rev Respir Dis* 1977;116:201–207.
3. Light RW, Stansbury DW, Brown SE. The relationship between pleural pressures and changes in pulmonary function after therapeutic thoracentesis. *Am Rev Respir Dis* 1986;133:658–661.
4. Wang JS, Tseng CH. Changes in pulmonary mechanics and gas exchange after thoracentesis on patients with inversion of a hemidiaphragm secondary to large pleural effusion. *Chest* 1995;107:1610–1614.
5. Vaska K, Wann LS, Sagar K, et al. Pleural effusion as a cause of right ventricular diastolic collapse. *Circulation* 1992;86:609–617.
6. Brandstetter RD, Cohen RP. Hypoxemia after thoracentesis. A predictable and treatable condition. *JAMA* 1979;242:1060–1061.
7. Pavlin J, Cheney FW Jr. Unilateral pulmonary edema in rabbits after re-expansion of collapsed lung. *J Appl Physiol* 1979;46:31–35.
8. Gilbert VE. Shifting percussion dullness of the chest: a sign of pleural effusion. *South Med J* 1997;90:1255–1256.
9. Bernstein A, White FZ. Unusual physical findings in pleural effusion: intrathoracic manometric studies. *Ann Intern Med* 1952;37:733–738.
10. Paddock FK. The diagnostic significance of serous fluids in disease. *N Engl J Med* 1940;223:1010–1015.
11. Broaddus VC, Light RW. What is the origin of pleural transudates and exudates [Editorial]? *Chest* 1992;102:658.
12. Leuallen EC, Carr DT. Pleural effusion, a statistical study of 436 patients. *N Engl J Med* 1955;252:79–83.
13. Carr DT, Power MH. Clinical value of measurements of concentration of protein in pleural fluid. *N Engl J Med* 1958;259:926–927.
14. Light RW, MacGregor MI, Luchsinger PC, et al. Pleural effusions: the diagnostic separation of transudates and exudates. *Ann Intern Med* 1972;77:507–513.
15. Hamm H, Brohan U, Bohmer R, et al. Cholesterol in pleural effusions: a diagnostic aid. *Chest* 1987;92:296–302.
16. Valdés L, Pose A, Suarez J, et al. Cholesterol: a useful parameter for distinguishing between pleural exudates and transudates. *Chest* 1991;99:1097–1102.
17. Costa M, Quiroga T, Cruz E. Measurement of pleural fluid cholesterol and lactate dehydrogenase. A simple and accurate set of indicators for separating exudates from transudates. *Chest* 1995;108:1260–1263.
18. Roth BJ, O'Meara TF, Cragun WH. The serum-effusion albumin gradient in the evaluation of pleural effusions. *Chest* 1990;98:546–549.
19. Meisel S, Shamiss A, Thaler M, et al. Pleural fluid to serum bilirubin concentration ratio for the separation of transudates from exudates. *Chest* 1990;98:141–144.
20. Garcia-Pachon E, Padilla-Navas I, Sanchez JF, et al. Pleural fluid to serum cholinesterase ratio for the separation of transudates and exudates. *Chest* 1996;110:97–101.
21. Romero S, Candela A, Martin C, et al. Evaluation of different criteria for the separation of pleural transudates from exudates. *Chest* 1993;104:399–404.
22. Burgess LJ, Maritz FJ, Taljaard JJ. Comparative analysis of the biochemical parameters used to distinguish between pleural transudates and exudates. *Chest* 1995;107:1604–1609.
23. Vives M, Porcel JM, De Vera MV, et al. A study of Light's criteria and possible modifications for distinguishing exudative from transudative pleural effusions. *Chest* 1996;109:1503–1507.
24. Gazquez I, Porcel JM, Vives M, et al. Comparative analysis of Light's criteria and other biochemical parameters for distinguishing transudates from exudates. *Respir Med* 1998;92:762–765.
25. Vaz MAC, Teixeira LR, Vargas FS, et al. Relationship between pleural fluid and serum cholesterol levels. *Chest* 2001 (in press).
26. Paddock FK. The relationship between the specific gravity and the protein content in human serous effusions. *Am J Med Sci* 1941;201:569–574.
27. Light RW. Falsely high refractometric readings for the specific gravity of pleural fluid. *Chest* 1979;76:300–301.
28. Light RW, Ball WC. Lactate dehydrogenase isoenzymes in pleural effusions. *Am Rev Respir Dis* 1973;108:660–664.
29. Light RW, Erozan YS, Ball WC. Cells in pleural fluid: their value in differential diagnosis. *Arch Intern Med* 1973;132:854–860.
30. Light RW, Ball WC. Glucose and amylase in pleural effusions. *JAMA* 1973;225:257–260.
31. Light RW, MacGregor MI, Ball WC Jr, et al. Diagnostic significance of pleural fluid pH and P_{co_2}. *Chest* 1973;64:591–596.
32. Rolf LL, Travis DM. Pleural fluid-plasma bicarbonate gradients in oxygen-toxic and normal rats. *Am J Physiol* 1973;224:857–861.
33. Lyche KD, Jensen WA, Kirsch CM, et al. Pleuropulmonary manifestations of hepatic amebiasis. *West J Med* 1990;153:275–278.
34. Judson MA, Lazarchick J, Sahn SA. Pleural fluid platelets: can they help identify traumatic

thoracenteses? *Am J Respir Crit Care* Med 1994;149: A1104.

35. Ayo DS, Lee YC, Conner B, et al. Pleural fluid white blood cell count variation using different sample containers and methods at 4 and 24 hours after collection. *Chest* 1999;116:357S.

36. Conner BD, Ayo DS, Lee YCG, et al. Pleural fluid white blood cell differential variation using different sample containers and methods of analysis. *Am J Respir Dis Crit Care Med* 2000;161:A68.

37. Spriggs AI, Boddington MM. *The cytology of effusions.* 2nd ed. New York: Grune & Stratton, 1968.

38. Broaddus VC, Hebert CA, Vitangcol RV, et al. Interleukin-8 is a major neutrophil chemotactic factor in pleural liquid of patients with empyema. *Am Rev Respir Dis* 1992;146:825–830.

39. Antony VB, Godbey SW, Kunkel SL, et al. Recruitment of inflammatory cells to the pleural space. Chemotactic cytokines, IL-8, and monocyte chemotactic peptide-1 in human pleural fluids. *J Immunol* 1993;151: 7216–7223.

40. Naylor B, Novak PM. Charcot-Leyden crystals in pleural fluids. *Acta Cytol* 1985;29:781–784.

41. Wahl RW. Curschmann's spirals in pleural and peritoneal fluids. Report of 12 cases. *Acta Cytol* 1986;30:147–151.

42. Klein A, Talvani A, Cara DC, et al. Stem cell factor plays a major role in the recruitment of eosinophils in allergic pleurisy in mice via the production of leukotriene B$_4$. *J Immunol* 2000;164:4271–4276.

43. Perez S, Machado J, Cordeiro R, et al. Inhibition by the anti-mitotic drug doxorubicin of platelet-activating-factor-induced late eosinophil accumulation in rats. *Eur J Pharmacol* 1998;356:239–243.

44. Castro-Faria-Neto HC, Penido CM, Larangeira AP, et al. A role for lymphocytes and cytokines on the eosinophil migration induced by LPS. *Mem Inst Oswaldo Cruz* 1997;92(Suppl 2):197–200.

45. Penido C, Castro-Faria-Neto HC, Larangeira AP, et al. The role of gamma-delta T lymphocytes in lipopolysaccharide-induced eosinophil accumulation into the mouse pleural cavity. *J Immunol* 1997;159: 853–860.

46. Pasquale CP, Martins MA, Bozza PT, et al. Bradykinin induces eosinophil accumulation in the rat pleural cavity. *Int Arch Allergy Appl Immunol* 1991;95:244–247.

47. Nakamura Y, Ozaki T, Kamei T, et al. Factors that stimulate the proliferation and survival of eosinophils in eosinophilic pleural effusion: relationship to granulocyte-/macrophage colony-stimulating factor, interleukin-5, and interleukin-3. *Am J Respir Cell Mol Biol* 1993;8:605–611.

48. Schandene L, Namias B, Crusiaux A, et al. IL-5 in post-traumatic eosinophilic pleural effusion. *Clin Exp Immunol* 1993;93:115–119.

49. Mohamed KH, Abdel-Hamid AI, Lee YCG, et al. Pleural fluid levels of IL-5 and eosinophils are closely correlated. *Am J Respir Crit Care Med* 2001 *(in press).*

50. Nakamura Y, Ozaki T, Yanagawa H, et al. Eosinophil colony-stimulating factor induced by administration of interleukine-2 into the pleural cavity of patients with malignant pleurisy. *Am J Respir Cell Mol Biol* 1990;3:291–300.

51. Bozza PT, Castro-Faria-Neto HC, Penido C, et al. IL-5 accounts for the mouse pleural eosinophil accumulation triggered by antigen but not by LPS. *Immunopharmacology* 1994;27:131–136.

52. Adelman M, Albelda SM, Gottlieb J, et al. Diagnostic utility of pleural fluid eosinophilia. *Am J Med* 1984;77:915–920.

53. Askin FB, McCann BG, Kuhn C. Reactive eosinophilic pleuritis. *Arch Pathol Lab Med* 1977;101:187–191.

54. Smit HJ, van den Heuvel MM, Barbierato SB, et al. Analysis of pleural fluid in idiopathic spontaneous pneumothorax; correlation of eosinophil percentage with the duration of air in the pleural space. *Respir Med* 1999;93:262–267.

55. Maltais F, Laberge F, Cormier Y. Blood hypereosinophilia in the course of post-traumatic pleural effusion. *Chest* 1990;98:348–351.

56. Martinez-Garcia MA, Cases-Viedma E, Cordero-Rodriguez PJ, et al. Diagnostic utility of eosinophils in the pleural fluid. *Eur Respir J* 2000;15:166–169.

57. Rubins JB, Rubins HB. Etiology and prognostic significance of eosinophilic pleural effusions. A prospective study. *Chest* 1996;110:1271–1274.

58. Johnson RJ, Johnson JR. Paragonimiasis in Indochinese refugees: roentgenographic findings with clinical correlations. *Am Rev Respir Dis* 1983;128:534–538.

59. Yacoubian HD. Thoracic problems associated with hydatid cyst of the dome of the liver. *Surgery* 1976;79: 544–548.

60. Erzurum SE, Underwood GA, Hamilos DL, et al. Pleural effusion in Churg-Strauss syndrome. *Chest* 1989;95:1357–1359.

61. Yam LT. Diagnostic significance of lymphocytes in pleural effusions. *Ann Intern Med* 1967;66: 972–982.

62. Sadikot RT, Rogers JT, Cheng D-S, et al. Pleural fluid characteristics of patients with symptomatic pleural effusion post coronary artery bypass surgery. *Arch Intern Med* 2000;160:2665–2668.

63. Pettersson T, Klockars MD, Hellstrom P-E, et al. T and B lymphocytes in pleural effusions. *Chest* 1978;73:49–51.

64. Potrykus AM, Steinmann G, Stein E, et al. T- and B-cell responses in patients with malignant pleural effusions. *Br J Cancer* 1981;43:471–477.

65. Domagala W, Emeson EE, Kos LG. T and B lymphocyte enumeration in the diagnosis of lymphocyte-rich pleural fluids. *Acta Cytol* 1981;25:108–110.

66. Moisan T, Chandrasekhar AJ, Robinson J, et al. Distribution of lymphocyte subpopulations in patients with exudative pleural effusions. *Am Rev Respir Dis* 1978;117:507–511.

67. Kockman S, Bernanrd J, Lavaud F, et al. T-lymphocyte subsets in pleural fluids: discrimination according to traditional and monoclonal antibody-defined markers. *Eur J Respir Dis* 1984;65:586–591.

68. Lucivero G, Pierucci G, Bonomo L. Lymphocyte subsets in peripheral blood and pleural fluid. *Eur Respir J* 1988;1:337–340.

69. Guzman J, Bross KJ, Wurtemberger G, et al. Immunocytology in malignant pleural mesothelioma: expression of tumor markers and distribution of lymphocyte subsets. *Chest* 1989;95:590–595.

70. Okubo Y, Nakata M, Kuroiwa Y, et al. NK cells in carcinomatous and tuberculous pleurisy: phenotypic and functional analyses of NK cells in peripheral blood and pleural effusions. *Chest* 1987;92:500–504.

71. Miserocchi G, Agostoni E. Contents of the pleural space. *J Appl Physiol* 1971;30:208–213.
72. Hurwitz S, Leiman G, Shapiro C. Mesothelial cells in pleural fluid: TB or not TB? *S Afr Med J* 1980;57: 937–939.
73. Jones D, Lieb T, Narita M, et al. Mesothelial cells in tuberculous pleural effusions of HIV-infected patients. *Chest* 2000;117:289–291.
74. Antony VB, Sahn SA, Antony AC, et al. Bacillus Calmette-Guérin–stimulated neutrophils release chemotaxins for monocytes in rabbit pleural space in vitro. *J Clin Invest* 1985;76:1514–1521.
75. Gjomarkaj M, Pace E, Melis M, et al. Mononuclear cells in exudative malignant pleural effusions. Characterization of pleural phagocytic cells. *Chest* 1994;106: 1042–1049.
76. Gjomarkaj M, Pace E, Melis M, et al. Dendritic cells with a potent accessory activity are present in human exudative malignant pleural effusions. *Eur Respir J* 1997;10:592–597.
77. Luetscher JA Jr. Electrophoretic analysis of the proteins of plasma and serous effusions. *J Clin Invest* 1941;20:99–106.
78. Zinneman HH, Johnson JJ, Lyon RH. Proteins and mucoproteins in pleural effusions. *Am Rev Tuberc Pulmon Dis* 1957;76:247–255.
79. Telvi L, Jaybert F, Eyquem A, et al. Study of immunoglobulins in pleura and pleural effusions. *Thorax* 1979;34:389–392.
80. Yokogawa M, Kojima S, Araki K, et al. Immunoglobulin E: raised levels in sera and pleural exudates of patients with paragonimiasis. *Am J Trop Med Hyg* 1976:25: 581–586.
81. Nash DR, Wallace RJ Jr. Immunoglobulin E and other immunoglobulins in patients with eosinophilic pleural effusions. *J Lab Clin Med* 1985;106:512–516.
82. Vianna NJ. Nontuberculous bacterial empyema in patients with and without underlying diseases. *JAMA* 1971;215:69–75.
83. Light RW, Girard WM, Jenkinson SG, et al. Parapneumonic effusions. *Am J Med* 1980;69:507–511.
84. Light RW, Rodriguez RM. Management of parapneumonic effusions. *Clin Chest Med* 1998;19:373–382.
85. Berger HW, Maher G. Decreased glucose concentration in malignant pleural effusions. *Am Rev Respir Dis* 1971;103:427–429.
86. Rodriguez-Panadero F, Lopez Mejias J. Low glucose and pH levels in malignant pleural effusions. *Am Rev Respir Dis* 1989;139:663–667.
87. Sahn SA, Good JT Jr. Pleural fluid pH in malignant effusions. *Ann Intern Med* 1988;108:345–349.
88. Sanchez-Armengol A, Rodriguez-Panadero F. Survival and talc pleurodesis in metastatic pleural carcinoma, revisited. Report of 125 cases. *Chest* 1993;104: 1482–1485.
89. Rodriguez-Panadero F, Lopez-Mejias J. Survival time of patients with pleural metastatic carcinoma predicted by glucose and pH studies. *Chest* 1989;95: 320–324.
90. Calnan WL, Winfield BJO, Crowley MF, et al. Diagnostic value of the glucose content of serous pleural effusions. *Br Med J* 1951;1:1239–1240.
91. Barber LM, Mazzadi L, Deakins DO, et al. Glucose level in pleural fluid as a diagnostic aid. *Dis Chest* 1957;31:680–681.
92. Carr DT, Power MH. Pleural fluid glucose with special reference to its concentration in rheumatoid pleurisy with effusion. *Dis Chest* 1960; 37:321–324.
93. Lillington GA, Carr DT, Mayne JG. Rheumatoid pleurisy with effusion. *Arch Intern Med* 1971;128: 764–768.
94. Dodson WH, Hollingsworth JW. Pleural effusion in rheumatoid arthritis. *N Engl J Med* 1966;275: 1337–1342.
95. Halla JT, Schrohenloher RE, Volanakis JE. Immune complexes and other laboratory features of pleural effusions. *Ann Intern Med* 1980;92:748–752.
96. Good JT Jr, King TE, Antony VB, et al. Lupus pleuritis: clinical features and pleural fluid characteristics with special reference to pleural fluid antinuclear antibodies. *Chest* 1983;84:714–718.
97. Lankisch PG, Groge M, Becher R. Pleural effusions: a new negative prognostic parameter for acute pancreatitis. *Am J Gastroenterol* 1994;89:1849–1851.
98. Kaye MD. Pleuropulmonary complications of pancreatitis. *Thorax* 1968;23:297–306.
99. Rockey DC, Cello JP. Pancreaticopleural fistula. Report of 7 cases and review of the literature. *Medicine* 1990;69:332–344.
100. Pottmeyer EW III, Frey CF, Matsuno S. Pancreaticopleural fistulas. *Arch Surg* 1987;122:648–654.
101. Ende N. Studies of amylase activity in pleural effusions and ascites. *Cancer* 1960;13:283–287.
102. Kramer MR, Cepero RJ, Pitchenik AE. High amylase in neoplasm-related pleural effusion. *Ann Intern Med* 1989;110:567–569.
103. Abbott OA, Mansour KA, Logan WC, et al. Atraumatic so-called "spontaneous" rupture of the esophagus. *J Thorac Cardiovasc Surg* 1970;59:67–83.
104. Sherr HP, Light RW, Merson MH, et al. Origin of pleural fluid amylase in esophageal rupture. *Ann Intern Med* 1972;76:985–986.
105. Maulitz RM, Good JT Jr, Kaplan RL, et al. The pleuropulmonary consequences of esophageal rupture: an experimental model. *Am Rev Respir Dis* 1979;120: 363–367.
106. Wroblewski F, Wroblewski R. The clinical significance of lactic dehydrogenase activity of serous effusions. *Ann Intern Med* 1958;48:813–822.
107. Raabo E, Rasmussen KN, Terkildsen TC. A study of the isoenzymes of lactic dehydrogenase in pleural effusions. *Scand J Respir Dis* 1966;47:150– 156.
108. Lossos IS, Intrator O, Berkman N, et al. Lactate dehydrogenase isoenzyme analysis for the diagnosis of pleural effusion in haemato-oncological patients. *Respir Med* 1999;93:338–341.
109. Potts DE, Willcox MA, Good JT Jr, et al. The acidosis of low-glucose pleural effusions. *Am Rev Respir Dis* 1978;117:665–671.
110. Chavalittamrong B, Angsusingha K, Tuchinda M, et al. Diagnostic significance of pH, lactic acid dehydrogenase, lactate and glucose in pleural fluid. *Respiration* 1979;38:112–120.
111. Light RW, Luchsinger P. Metabolic activity of pleural fluid. *J Appl Physiol* 1973;34:97–101.
112. Taryle DA, Good JT Jr, Sahn SA. Acid generation by pleural fluids: possible role in the determination of pleural fluid pH. *J Lab Clin Med* 1979;93: 1041–1046.

113. Chandler TM, McCoskey EH, Byrd RP Jr, et al. Comparison of the use and accuracy of methods for determining pleural fluid pH. *South Med J* 1999;92: 214–217.

114. Cheng DS, Rodriguez RM, Rogers J, et al. Comparison of pleural fluid pH values obtained using blood gas machine, pH meter, and pH indicator strip. *Chest* 1998;114:1368–1372.

115. Lesho EP, Roth BJ. Is pH paper an acceptable, low-cost alternative to the blood gas analyzer for determining pleural fluid pH? *Chest* 1997;112:1291–1292.

116. Sarodia BD, Goldstein LS, Laskowski DM, et al. Does pleural fluid pH change significantly at room temperature during the first hour following thoracentesis? *Chest* 2000;117:1043–1048.

117. Goldstein LS, McCarthy K, Mehta AC, et al. Is direct collection of pleural fluid into a heparinized syringe important for determination of pleural pH? A brief report. *Chest* 1997;112:707–708.

118. Jimenez Castro D, Diaz G, Perez-Rodriguez E, et al. Modification of pleural fluid pH by local anesthesia. *Chest* 1999;116:399–402.

119. Pine JR, Hollman JL. Elevated pleural fluid pH in *Proteus mirabilis* empyema. *Chest* 1983;84:109–111.

120. Potts DE, Levin DC, Sahn SA. Pleural fluid pH in parapneumonic effusions. *Chest* 1976;70:328–331.

121. Dye RA, Laforet EG. Esophageal rupture: diagnosis by pleural fluid pH. *Chest* 1974;66:454–456.

122. Good JT Jr, Taryle DA, Sahn SA. The pathogenesis of the low pleural fluid pH in esophageal rupture. *Am Rev Respir Dis* 1983;127:702–704.

123. Good JT Jr, Taryle DA, Maulitz RM, et al. The diagnostic value of pleural fluid pH. *Chest* 1980;78:55–59.

124. Rodriguez-Panadero F, Lopez-Mejias L. Survival time of patients with pleural metastatic carcinoma predicted by glucose and pH studies. *Chest* 1989;95: 320–324.

125. Sahn SA, Good JT Jr. Pleural fluid pH in malignant effusions. *Ann Intern Med* 1988;108:345–349.

126. Miller KS, Wooten S, Sahn SA. Urinothorax: a cause of low pH transudative pleural effusions. *Am J Med* 1988;85:448–449.

127. Marchevsky AM, Hauptman E, Gil J, et al. Computerized interactive morphometry as an aid in the diagnosis of pleural effusions. *Acta Cytol* 1987;31:131–136.

128. Stevens MW, Leong AS, Fazzalari NL, et al. Cytopathology of malignant mesothelioma: a stepwise logistic regression analysis. *Diagn Cytopathol* 1992; 8:333–342.

129. Jarvi OH, Kunnas RJ, Laitio MT, et al. The accuracy and significance of cytologic cancer diagnosis of pleural effusions. *Acta Cytol* 1972;16:152–157.

130. Grunze H. The comparative diagnostic accuracy, efficiency and specificity of cytologic techniques used in the diagnosis of malignant neoplasm in serous effusions of the pleural and pericardial cavities. *Acta Cytol* 1964;8:150–164.

131. Bueno CE, Clemente G, Castro BC, et al. Cytologic and bacteriologic analysis of fluid and pleural biopsy specimens with Cope's needle. *Arch Intern Med* 1990;150:1190–1194.

132. Naylor B, Schmidt RW. The case for exfoliative cytology of serous effusions. *Lancet* 1964;1:711–712.

133. Melamed MR. The cytological presentation of malignant lymphomas and related diseases in effusions. *Cancer* 1963;16:413–431.

134. Dekker A, Bupp PA. Cytology of serous effusions. An investigation into the usefulness of cell blocks versus smears. *Am J Clin Pathol* 1978;70:855–860.

135. Filie AC, Copel C, Wilder AM, et al. Individual specimen triage of effusion samples: an improvement in the standard of practice, or a waste of resources? *Diagn Cytopathol* 2000;22:7–10.

136. Huang M-S, Tsai M-S, Hwang J-J, et al. Comparison of nucleolar organiser regions and DNA flow cytometry in the evaluation of pleural effusion. *Thorax* 1994;49:1152–1156.

137. Ong KC, Indumathi V, Poh WT, et al. The diagnostic yield of pleural fluid cytology in malignant pleural effusions. *Singapore Med J* 2000;41:19–23.

138. Sujathan K, Kannan S, Pillai KR, et al. Significance of AgNOR count in differentiating malignant cells from reactive mesothelial cells in serous effusions. *Acta Cytol* 1996;40:724–728.

139. Antonangelo L, Saldiva PH, Amaro Junior E, et al. Utility of computerized morphometry combined with AgNOR staining in distinguishing benign from malignant pleural effusions. *Anal Quant Cytol Histol* 1994;16:247–252.

140. Wirth PR, Legier J, Wright GL Jr. Immunohistochemical evaluation of seven monoclonal antibodies for differentiation of pleural mesothelioma from lung adenocarcinoma. *Cancer* 1991;67:655–662.

141. Frisman DM, McCarthy WF, Schleiff P, et al. Immunocytochemistry in the differential diagnosis of effusions: use of logistic regression to select a panel of antibodies to distinguish adenocarcinomas from mesothelial proliferations. *Modern Pathol* 1993;6:179–184.

142. Brown RW, Clark GM, Tandon AK, et al. Multiple-marker immunohistochemical phenotypes distinguishing malignant pleural mesothelioma from pulmonary adenocarcinoma. *Hum Pathol* 1993;24: 347–354.

143. Ordonez NG. The immunohistochemical diagnosis of epithelial mesothelioma. *Hum Pathol* 1999;30:313–323.

144. Corson JM. Pathology of diffuse malignant pleural mesothelioma. *Semin Thorac Cardiovasc Surg* 1997;9:347–355.

145. Barberis MC, Faleri M, Veronese S, et al. Calretinin. A selective marker of normal and neoplastic mesothelial cells in serous effusions. *Acta Cytol* 1997;41:1757–1761.

146. Guzman J, Bross KJ, Costabel U. Malignant lymphoma in pleural effusions: an immunocytochemical cell surface analysis. *Diagn Cytopathol* 1991;7:113–118.

147. Coleman M, Henderson DW, Mukherjee TM. The ultrastructural pathology of malignant pleural mesothelioma. *Pathol Annu* 1989;24:303–353.

148. Jandik WR, Landas SK, Bray CK, et al. Scanning electron microscopic distinction of pleural mesotheliomas from adenocarcinomas. *Modern Pathol* 1993;6:761–764.

149. Warnock ML, Stoloff A, Thor A. Differentiation of adenocarcinoma of the lung from mesothelioma. Periodic acid–Schiff, monoclonal antibodies B72.3, and Leu M1. *Am J Pathol* 1988;133:30–38.

150. Miedouge M, Rouzaud P, Salama G, et al. Evaluation of seven tumour markers in pleural fluid for the diagnosis of malignant effusions. *Br J Cancer* 1999;81: 1059–1065.

151. Salama G, Miedouge M, Rouzaud P, et al. Evaluation

of pleural CYFRA 21-1 and carcinoembryonic antigen in the diagnosis of malignant pleural effusions. *Br J Cancer* 1998;77:472–476.

152. San Jose ME, Alvarez D, Valdés L, et al. Utility of tumour markers in the diagnosis of neoplastic pleural effusion. *Clin Chim Acta* 1997;265:193–205.

153. Garcia-Pachon E, Padilla-Navas I, Dosda D, et al. Elevated level of carcinoembryonic antigen in nonmalignant pleural effusions. *Chest* 1997;111:643–647.

154. Villena V, Lopez-Encuentra A, Echave-Sustaeta J, et al. Diagnostic value of CA 72-4, carcinoembryonic antigen, CA 15-3, and CA 19-9 assay in pleural fluid. *Cancer* 1996;78:736–740.

155. Shimokata K, Totani Y, Nakanishi K, et al. Diagnostic value of cancer antigen 15-3 (CA15-3) detected by monoclonal antibodies (115D8 and DF3) in exudative pleural effusions. *Eur Respir J* 1988;1:341–344.

156. Pinto MM. CA-15.3 assay in effusions: comparison with carcinoembryonic antigen and CA-125 assay and cytologic diagnosis. *Acta Cytol* 1996;40:437–442.

157. Niwa Y, Kishimoto H, Shimokata K. Carcinomatous and tuberculous pleural effusion. Comparison of tumor markers. *Chest* 1985;87:351–355.

158. Lee YC, Knox BS, Garrett JE. Use of cytokeratin fragments 19.1 and 19.21 (Cyfra 21-1) in the differentiation of malignant and benign pleural effusions. *Aust N Z J Med* 1999;29:765–769.

159. Lee YC, Chern JH, Lai SL, et al. Sialyl stage-specific embryonic antigen-1: a useful marker for differentiating the etiology of pleural effusion. *Chest* 1998;114:1542–1545.

160. Ishikawa H, Satoh H, Kamma H, et al. Elevated sialyl Lewis X-i antigen levels in pleural effusions in patients with carcinomatous pleuritis. *Intern Med* 1997;36:685–689.

161. McKenna JM, Chandrasekhar AJ, Henkin RE. Diagnostic value of carcinoembryonic antigen in exudative pleural effusions. *Chest* 1980;78:587–590.

162. Rittgers RA, Loewenstein MS, Feinerman AE, et al. Carcinoembryonic antigen levels in benign and malignant pleural effusions. *Ann Intern Med* 1978;88:631–634.

163. Tamura S, Nishigaki T, Moriwaki Y, et al. Tumor markers in pleural effusion diagnosis. *Cancer* 1988;61:298–302.

164. Shimokata K, Niwa Y, Yamamoto M, et al. Pleural fluid neuron-specific enolase. *Chest* 1989;95:602–603.

165. Zoppi JA, Pellicer EM, Sundblad AS. Diagnostic value of p53 protein in the study of serous effusions. *Acta Cytol* 1995;39:721–724.

166. Mayall F, Heryet A, Manga D, et al. p53 immunostaining is a highly specific and moderately sensitive marker of malignancy in serous fluid cytology. *Cytopathology* 1997;8:9–12.

167. Tawfik MS, Coleman DV. C-myc expression in exfoliated cells in serous effusions. *Cytopathology* 1991;2:83–92.

168. Athanassiadou PP, Veneti SZ, Kyrkou KA, et al. Detection of c-Ha-ras oncogene expression in pleural and peritoneal smear effusions by in situ hybridization. *Cancer Detect Prev* 1993;17:585–590.

169. Rasmussen KN, Faber V. Hyaluronic acid in 247 pleural fluids. *Scand J Respir Dis* 1967;48:366–371.

170. Nurminen M, Dejmek A, Martensson G, et al. Clinical utility of liquid-chromatographic analysis of effusions for hyaluronate content. *Clin Chem* 1994;40:777–780.

171. Hillerdal G, Lindqvist U, Engström-Laurent A. Hyaluronan in pleural effusions and in serum. *Cancer* 1991;67:2410–2414.

172. Pettersson T, Froseth B, Riska H, et al. Concentration of hyaluronic acid in pleural fluid as a diagnostic aid for malignant mesothelioma. *Chest* 1988;94:1037–1039.

173. Martensson G, Thylen A, Lindquist U, et al. The sensitivity of hyaluronan analysis of pleural fluid from patients with malignant mesothelioma and a comparison of different methods. *Cancer* 1994;73:1406–1410.

174. Kawai T, Greenberg SD, Truong LD, et al. Differences in lectin binding of malignant pleural mesothelioma and adenocarcinoma of the lung. *Am J Pathol* 1988;130:401–410.

175. Croonen AM, van der Valk P, Herman CJ, et al. Cytology, immunopathology and flow cytometry in the diagnosis of pleural and peritoneal effusion. *Lab Invest* 1988;58:725–732.

176. Rijken A, Dekker A, Taylor S, et al. Diagnostic value of DNA analysis in effusions by flow cytometry and image analysis. A prospective study on 102 patients as compared with cytologic examination. *Am J Clin Pathol* 1991;95:6–12.

177. Rodriguez de Castro F, Molero T, Acosta O, et al. Value of DNA analysis in addition to cytological testing in the diagnosis of malignant pleural effusions. *Thorax* 1994;49:692–694.

178. Pinto MM. DNA analysis of malignant effusions. Comparison with cytologic diagnosis and carcinoembryonic antigen content. *Anal Quant Cytol Histol* 1992;14:222–226.

179. Moriarty AT, Wiersema L, Snyder W, et al. Immunophenotyping of cytologic specimens by flow cytometry. *Diagn Cytopathol* 1993;9:252–258.

180. Dewald G, Dines DE, Weiland LH, et al. Usefulness of chromosome examination in the diagnosis of malignant pleural effusions. *N Engl J Med* 1976;295:1494–1500.

181. Korsgaard R. Chromosome analysis of malignant human effusions in vivo. *Scand J Respir Dis* 1979; 105(Suppl):1-100.

182. Piras MA, Gakis C, Budroni M, et al. Adenosine deaminase activity in pleural effusions: an aid to differential diagnosis. *Br Med J* 1978;4:1751–1752.

183. Ocana IM, Martinez-Vazquez JM, Seguna RM, et al. Adenosine deaminase in pleural fluids. *Chest* 1983;84:51–53.

184. Fontan Bueso J, Verea H, Perez J, et al. Diagnostic value of simultaneous determination of pleural adenosine deaminase and pleural lysozyme/serum lysozyme ratio in pleural effusion. *Chest* 1988;93:303–307.

185. Valdés L, San Jose E, Alvarez D, et al. Diagnosis of tuberculous pleurisy using the biologic parameters adenosine deaminase, lysozyme, and interferon gamma. *Chest* 1993;103:458–465.

186. Ocana I, Ribera E, Martinez-Vazquez JM, et al. Adenosine deaminase activity in rheumatoid pleural effusion. *Ann Rheum Dis* 1988;47:394–397.

187. Burgess LJ, Maritz FJ, Le Roux I, et al. Combined use of pleural adenosine deaminase with lymphocyte/neutrophil ratio. Increased specificity for the diagnosis of tuberculous pleuritis. *Chest* 1996;109:414–419.

188. Ungerer JP, Grobler SM. Molecular forms of adenosine deaminase in pleural effusions. *Enzyme* 1988;40:7–13.

189. Esteban C, Oribe M, Fernandez A, et al. Increased adenosine deaminase activity in Q fever pneumonia with pleural effusion. *Chest* 1994;105:648.

190. Lee YC, Rogers JT, Rodriguez RM, et al. Adenosine deaminase (ADA) levels in non-tuberculous lymphocytic pleural effusions. *Chest* 2001 *(in press)*.

191. Aoki Y, Katoh O, Nakanishi Y, et al. A comparison study of IFN-gamma, ADA, and CA125 as the diagnostic parameters in tuberculous pleuritis. *Respir Med* 1994;88:139–143.

192. Riantawan P, Chaowalit P, Wongsangiem M, et al. Diagnostic value of pleural fluid adenosine deaminase in tuberculous pleuritis with reference to HIV coinfection and a Bayesian analysis. *Chest* 1999;116:97–103.

193. Teo SK, Chio LF. Adenosine deaminase in pleural fluid—an enzymatic test for tuberculous pleural effusion. *Singapore Med J* 1987;28:220–224.

194. Shibagaki T, Hasegawa Y, Saito H, et al. Adenosine deaminase isozymes in tuberculous pleural effusion. *J Lab Clin Med* 1996;127:348–352.

195. Perez-Rodriguez E, Castro DJ. The use of ADA and ADA isoenzymes in the diagnosis of tuberculous pleuritis. *Curr Opin Pulm Med* 2000;6:259–266.

196. Perez-Rodriguez E, Walton IJ, Hernandez JJ, et al. ADA1/ADAp ratio in pleural tuberculosis: an excellent diagnostic parameter in pleural fluid. *Respir Med* 1999;93:816–821.

197. Valdés L, Alvarez D, San Jose E, et al. Tuberculous pleurisy: a study of 254 patients. *Arch Intern Med* 1998;158:2017–2021.

198. Ribera E, Ocana I, Martinez-Vazquez JM, et al. High level of interferon gamma in tuberculous pleural effusion. *Chest* 1988;93:308–311.

199. Barnes PF, Mistry SD, Cooper CL, et al. Compartmentalization of a CD4 + T lymphocyte subpopulation in tuberculous pleuritis. *J Immunol* 1989;142:1114–1119.

200. Villena V, Lopez-Encuentra A, Echave-Sustaeta J, et al. Interferon-gamma in 388 immunocompromised and immunocompetent patients for diagnosing pleural tuberculosis. *Eur Respir J* 1996;9:2635–2639.

201. Asseo PP, Tracopoulos GD, Kotsovoulou-Fouskak V. Lysozyme (muramidase) in pleural effusions and serum. *Am J Clin Pathol* 1982;78:763–767.

202. Verea Hernando HR, Masa Jimenez JF, Dominguez Juncal L, et al. Meaning and diagnostic value of determining the lysozyme level of pleural fluid. *Chest* 1987;91:342–345.

203. Cockerill FR III, Washington JA II. Microbiologic diagnosis of lower respiratory tract infection. In: Murray JF, Nadel JA, eds. *Textbook of respiratory medicine.* Philadelphia: W.B. Saunders, 2000:607–631.

204. Querol JM, Minguez J, Garcia-Sanchez E, et al. Rapid diagnosis of pleural tuberculosis by polymerase chain reaction. *Am J Respir Crit Care Med* 1995;152;1977–1981.

205. Tan MF, Ng WC, Chan SH, et al. Comparative usefulness of PCR in the detection of *Mycobacterium* tuberculosis in different clinical specimens. *J Med Microbiol* 1997;46:164–169.

206. Villena V, Rebollo MJ, Aguado JM, et al. Polymerase chain reaction for the diagnosis of pleural tuberculosis in immunocompromised and immunocompetent patients. *Clin Infect Dis* 1998;26:212–214.

207. Shah S, Miller A, Mastellone A, et al. Rapid diagnosis of tuberculosis in various biopsy and body fluid specimens by the AMPLICOR *Mycobacterium* tuberculosis polymerase chain reaction test. *Chest* 1998;113:1190–1194.

208. Baig MME, Pettengell KE, Simgee AE, et al. Diagnosis of tuberculosis by detection of mycobacterial antigens in pleural effusions and ascites. *S Afr Med J* 1986;69:101–102.

209. Yew WW, Chan CY, Kwan SY, et al. Diagnosis of tuberculous pleural effusion by the detection of tuberculostearic acid in pleural aspirates. *Chest* 1991;100:1261–1263.

210. Banchuin N, Pumprueg U, Pimolpan V, et al. Anti-PPD IgG responses in tuberculous pleurisy. *J Med Assoc Thai* 1987;70:321–325.

211. Dhand R, Gangul NK, Vaishnavi C, et al. False-positive reactions with enzyme-linked immunosorbent assay of *Mycobacterium* tuberculosis antigens in pleural fluid. *J Med Microbiol* 1988;26:241–243.

212. Levy H, Wayne LG, Anderson BE, et al. Antimycobacterial antibody levels in pleural fluid reflect passive diffusion from serum. *Chest* 1990;97:1144–1147.

213. Caminero JA, Rodriguez de Castro F, Carrillo T, et al. Diagnosis of pleural tuberculosis by detection of specific IgG anti-antigen 60 in serum and pleural fluid. *Respiration* 1993;60:58–62.

214. Van Vooren JP, Farber CM, De Bruyn J, et al. Antimycobacterial antibodies in pleural effusions. *Chest* 1990;97:88–90.

215. Murate T, Mizoguchi K, Amano H, et al. Antipurified-protein–derivative antibody in tuberculous pleural effusions. *Chest* 1990;97:670–673.

216. Walker WC, Wright V. Rheumatoid pleuritis. *Ann Rheum Dis* 1967;26:467–474.

217. Winslow WA, Ploss LN, Loitman B. Pleuritis in systemic lupus erythematosus: its importance as an early manifestation in diagnosis. *Ann Intern Med* 1958;49:70–88.

218. Berger HW, Seckler SG. Pleural and pericardial effusions in rheumatoid disease. *Ann Intern Med* 1966;64:1291–1297.

219. Levine H, Szanto M, Brieble HG, et al. Rheumatoid factor in non-rheumatoid pleural effusions. *Ann Intern Med* 1968;69:487–492.

220. Khare V, Baethge B, Lang S, et al. Antinuclear antibodies in pleural fluid. *Chest* 1994;106:866–871.

221. Wang DY, Yang PC, Yu WL, et al. Serial antinuclear antibodies titre in pleural and pericardial fluid. *Eur Respir J* 2000;15:1106–1110.

222. Leechawengwong M, Berger HW, Sukumaran M. Diagnostic significance of antinuclear antibodies in pleural effusion. *Mt Sinai J Med* 1979;46:137–139.

223. Wang DY, Yang PC, Yu WL, et al. Comparison of different diagnostic methods for lupus pleuritis and pericarditis: a prospective three-year study. *J Formos Med Assoc* 2000;99:375–380.

224. Chao TY, Huang SH, Chu CC. Lupus erythematosus cells in pleural effusions: diagnostic of systemic lupus erythematosus? *Acta Cytol* 1997;41:1231–1233.

225. Carmichael DS, Golding DN. Rheumatoid pleural effusion with "RA cells" in the pleural fluid. *Br Med J* 1967;1:814.

226. Hunder GG, McDuffie FC, Hepper NGG. Pleural fluid complement in systemic lupus erythematosus and rheumatoid arthritis. *Ann Intern Med* 1972;76:357–362.

227. Glovsky MM, Louie JS, Pitts WH Jr, et al. Reduction of pleural fluid complement activity in patients with systemic lupus erythematosus and rheumatoid arthritis. *Clin Immunol Immunopathol* 1976;6:31–41.

228. Porcel JM, Vives M, Gazquez I, et al. Usefulness of pleural complement activation products in differentiating tuberculosis and malignant effusions. *Int J Tuberc Lung Dis* 2000;4:76–82.

229. Salomaa ER, Viander M, Saaresranta T, et al. Complement components and their activation products in pleural fluid. *Chest* 1998;114:723–730.

230. Andrews BS, Arora NS, Shadforth MF, et al. The role of immune complexes in the pathogenesis of pleural effusions. *Am Rev Respir Dis* 1981;124:115–120.

231. Hunder GG, McDuffie FC, Huston KA, et al. Pleural fluid complement, complement conversion, and immune complexes in immunologic and nonimmunologic diseases. *J Lab Clin Med* 1977;90:971–980.

232. Bruneau R, Rubin P. The management of pleural effusions and chylothorax in lymphoma. *Radiology* 1965;85:1085–1092.

233. Hughes RL, Mintzer RA, Hidvegi DF, et al. The management of chylothorax. *Chest* 1979;76:212–218.

234. Wolthuis A, Landewe RB, Theunissen PH, et al. Chylothorax or leakage of total parenteral nutrition? *Eur Respir J* 1998;12:1233–1235.

235. Staats BA, Ellefson RD, Budahn LL, et al. The lipoprotein profile of chylous and nonchylous pleural effusions. *Mayo Clin Proc* 1980;55:700–704.

236. Seriff NS, Cohen ML, Samuel P, et al. Chylothorax: diagnosis by lipoprotein electrophoresis of serum and pleural fluid. *Thorax* 1977;32:98–100.

237. Romero S, Martin C, Hernandez L, et al. Chylothorax in cirrhosis of the liver: analysis of its frequency and clinical characteristics. *Chest* 1998;114:154–159.

238. Coe JE, Aikawa JK. Cholesterol pleural effusion. *Arch Intern Med* 1961;108:763–774.

239. Roy PH, Carr DT, Payne WS. The problem of chylothorax. *Mayo Clin Proc* 1967;42:457–467.

240. Xiol X, Castellvi JM, Guardiola J, et al. Spontaneous bacterial empyema in cirrhotic patients: a prospective study. *Hepatology* 1996;23:719–723.

241. Maartens G, Bateman ED. Tuberculous pleural effusions: increased culture yield with bedside inoculation of pleural fluid and poor diagnostic value of adenosine deaminase. *Thorax* 1991;46:96–99.

242. Everts RJ, Reller LB. Pleural space infections: microbiology and antimicrobial therapy. *Semin Respir Infect* 1999;14:18–30.

243. Lampe RM, Chottipitayasunondh T, Sunakorn P. Detection of bacterial antigen in pleural fluid by counterimmunoelectrophoresis. *J Pediatr* 1976;88:557–560.

244. Coonrod JD, Wilson HD. Etiologic diagnosis of intrapleural empyema by counterimmunoelectrophoresis. *Am Rev Respir Dis* 1976;113:637–641.

245. Thadephalli H, Gangopadhyay PK. Rapid diagnosis of anaerobic empyema by direct gas-liquid chromatography of pleural fluid. *Chest* 1980;77:507–513.

246. Hua CC, Chang LC, Chen YC, et al. Proinflammatory cytokines and fibrinolytic enzymes in tuberculous and malignant pleural effusions. *Chest* 1999;116:1292–1296.

247. Silva-Mejias C, Gamboa-Antinolo F, Lopez-Cortes LF, et al. Interleukin-1 beta in pleural fluids of different etiologies. Its role as inflammatory mediator in empyema. *Chest* 1995;108:942–945.

248. Shimokata K, Saka H, Murate T, et al. Cytokine content in pleural effusion. *Chest* 1991;99:1103–1107.

249. Marie C, Losser MR, Fitting C, et al. Cytokines and soluble cytokine receptors in pleural effusions from septic and nonseptic patients. *Am J Respir Crit Care Med* 1997;156:1515–1522.

250. Chang SC, Hsu YT, Chen YC, et al. Usefulness of soluble interleukin 2 receptor in differentiating tuberculous and carcinomatous pleural effusions. *Arch Intern Med* 1994;154:1097–1101.

251. Pettersson T, Soderblom T, Nyberg P, et al. Pleural fluid soluble interleukin 2 receptor in rheumatoid arthritis and systemic lupus erythematosus. *J Rheumatol* 1994;21:1820–1824.

252. Yanagawa H, Sone S, Munekata M, et al. IL-6 in malignant pleural effusions and its augmentation by intrapleural instillation of IL-2. *Clin Exp Immunol* 1992;88:207–212.

253. Chen YM, Yang WK, Whang-Peng J, et al. Elevation of interleukin-10 levels in malignant pleural effusion. *Chest* 1996;110:433–436.

254. Alexandrakis MG, Coulocheri SA, Bouros D, et al. Evaluation of ferritin, interleukin-6, interleukin-8 and tumor necrosis factor alpha in the differentiation of exudates and transudates in pleural effusions. *Anticancer Res* 1999;19:3607–3612.

255. Yokoyama A, Kohno N, Fujino S, et al. Soluble interleukin-6 receptor levels in pleural effusions. *Respir Med* 1996;90:329–332.

256. Yokoyama A, Maruyama M, Ito M, et al. Interleukin 6 activity in pleural effusion. *Chest* 1992;102:1055–1059.

257. Nakano T, Chahinian AP, Shinjo M, et al. Interleukin 6 and its relationship to clinical parameters in patients with malignant pleural mesothelioma. *Br J Cancer* 1998;77:907–912.

258. Miller EJ, Idell S. Interleukin-8: an important neutrophil chemotaxin in some cases of exudative pleural effusions. *Exp Lung Res* 1993;19:589–601.

259. Antony VB, Hott JW, Kunkel SL, et al. Pleural mesothelial cell expression of C-C (monocyte chemotactic peptide) and C-X-C (interleukin 8) chemokines. *Am J Respir Cell Mole Biol* 1995;12:581–588.

260. Segura RM, Alegre J, Varela E, et al. Interleukin-8 and markers of neutrophil degranulation in pleural effusions. *Am J Respir Cell Mol Biol* 1997;157:1565–1572.

261. Pace E, Gjomarkaj M, Melis M, et al. Interleukin-8 induces lymphocyte chemotaxis into the pleural space. Role of pleural macrophages. *Am J Respir Crit Care Med* 1999;159:1592–1599.

262. Opal SM, DePalo VA. Anti-inflammatory cytokines. *Chest* 2000;117:1162–1172.

263. Caminschi I, Venetsanakos E, Leong CC, et al. Interleukin-12 induces an effective antitumor response in malignant mesothelioma. *Am J Respir Cell Mol Biol* 1998;19:738–746.

264. Gursel G, Gokcora N, Elbeg S, et al. Tumor necrosis factor-alpha (TNF-alpha) in pleural fluids. *Tubercle Lung Dis* 1995;76:370–371.

265. Cheng D-S, Rogers J, Wheeler A, et al. The effects of intrapleural polyclonal anti-tumor necrosis factor alpha (TNF) Fab fragments on pleurodesis in rabbits. *Lung* 2000;178:19–30.

266. Perkett EA. Role of growth factors in lung repair and diseases. *Curr Opin Pediatr* 1995;7:242–249.
267. Gerwin BI, Lechner JF, Reddel RR, et al. Comparison of production of transforming growth factor-beta and platelet-derived growth factor by normal human mesothelial cells and mesothelioma cell lines. *Cancer Res* 1987;47:6180–6184.
268. Idell S, Zwieb C, Kumar A, et al. Pathways of fibrin turnover of human pleural mesothelial cells in vitro. *Am J Respir Cell Mol Biol* 1992;7:414–426.
269. Cheng D-S, Lee YC, Rogers JT, et al. Vascular endothelial growth factor level correlates with transforming growth factor-β isoform levels in pleural effusions. *Chest* 2000;118:1747–1753.
270. Maeda J, Ueki N, Ohkawa T, et al. Transforming growth factor-beta 1 (TGF-beta 1)–and beta 2–like activities in malignant pleural effusions caused by malignant mesothelioma or primary lung cancer. *Clin Exp Immunol* 1994;98:319–322.
271. Light RW, Cheng DOS, Lee YC, et al. A single intrapleural injection of transforming growth factor-2 produces excellent pleurodesis in rabbits. *Am J Respir Crit Care Med* 2000;162:98–104.
272. Lee YC, Lane KB, Parker RE, et al. Transforming growth factor beta-2 (TGF2) produces effective pleurodesis in sheep with no systemic complications. *Thorax* 2000;55:1058–1062.
273. Cheng C-S, Rodriguez RM, Perkett EA, et al. Vascular endothelial growth factor in pleural fluid. *Chest* 1999;115:760–765.
274. Light RW, Hamm H. Malignant pleural effusion: would the real cause please stand up? *Eur Respir J* 1997;10:1701–1702.
275. Zebrowski BK, Yano S, Liu W, et al. Vascular endothelial growth factor levels and induction of permeability in malignant pleural effusions. *Clin Cancer Res* 1999;5:3364-3368.
276. Thickett DR, Armstrong L, Millar AB. Vascular endothelial growth factor (VEGF) in inflammatory and malignant pleural effusions. Thorax 1999;54:707–710.
277. Kraft A, Weindel K, Ochs A, et al. Vascular endothelial growth factor in the sera and effusions of patients with malignant and nonmalignant disease. *Cancer* 1999;85:178–187.
278. Kimura I, Sakamoto Y, Shibasaki M, et al. Release of endothelins and platelet-activating factor by a rat pleural mesothelial cell line. *Eur Respir J* 2000;15:170–176.
279. Smit HJ, van den Heuvel MM, Barbierato SB, et al. Analysis of pleural fluid in idiopathic spontaneous pneumothorax; correlation of eosinophil percentage with the duration of air in the pleural space. *Respir Med* 1999;93:262–267.
280. Oda M, Satouchi K, Ikeda I, et al. The presence of platelet-activating factor associated with eosinophil and/or neutrophil accumulations in the pleural fluids. *Am Rev Respir Dis* 1990;141:1469–1473.
281. Idell S, Girard W, Koenig KB, et al. Abnormalities of pathways of fibrin turnover in the human pleural space. *Am Rev Respir Dis* 1991;144:187–194.
282. Philip-Joet F, Alessi MC, Philip-Joet C, et al. Fibrinolytic and inflammatory processes in pleural effusions. *Eur Respir J* 1995;8:1352–1356.
283. Yilmaz Turay U, Yildirim Z, Turkoz Y, et al. Use of pleural fluid C-reactive protein in diagnosis of pleural effusions. *Respir Med* 2000;94:432–435.
284. Demirkazik A, Dincol D, Hasturk S, et al. Diagnostic value of ferritin in the differential diagnosis of malignant effusions. *Cancer Biochem Biophys* 1998;16:243–251.
285. Delpuech P, Desch G, Fructus F. Fibronectin is unsuitable as a tumor marker in pleural effusions. *Clin Chem* 1989;35:166–168.
286. Arai H, Endo M, Yokosawa A, et al. On acid glycosaminoglycans (mucopolysaccharides) in pleural effusion. *Am Rev Respir Dis* 1975;111:37–42.
287. Vladutiu AO, Brason FW, Adler RH. Differential diagnosis of pleural effusions: clinical usefulness of cell marker quantitation. *Chest* 1981;79:297–301.
288. Brauer MJ, West M, Zimmerman HJ. Comparison of glycolytic and oxidative enzyme and transaminase values in benign and malignant effusions with those in serums. *Cancer* 1963;16:533–541.
289. Feldstein AM, Samachson J, Spencer H. Levels of calcium, phosphorus, alkaline phosphatase and protein in effusion fluid and serum in man. *Am J Med* 1963;35:530–535.
290. Bedrossian CWM, Stein DA, Miller WC, et al. Levels of angiotensin-converting enzyme in pleural effusion. *Arch Pathol Lab Med* 1981;105:345–346.
291. Veran P, Moigneteau C, Lasausse G, et al. Les phosphatases desépanchements pleuraux de diverses natures. Leur intérêt dans le cancer de la prostate. *J Fr Med Chir Thorac* 1965;19:621–643.
292. Migueres J, Jovger A, About P. Valuer theorique et pratique de certains dosages enzymatiques au cours des épanchements pleuraux (amylase, phosphatases, lacticodeshydrogenase). A propos de 129 observations. *J Fr Med Chir Thorac* 1969;23:443–458.

5

Approach to the Patient

Whenever a patient with an abnormal chest radiograph is evaluated, the possibility of a pleural effusion should be considered. Increased densities on the chest radiograph are frequently attributed to parenchymal infiltrates when they actually represent pleural fluid. Most patients with pleural effusions have blunting of the posterior costophrenic sulcus on the lateral chest radiograph. If this angle is blunted, bilateral decubitus chest radiographs should be obtained to ascertain whether free pleural fluid is present (see Chapter 3). Alternatively, the fluid can be demonstrated by ultrasound or chest computed tomography (CT) scan. This chapter provides a guide to the approach to a patient with an undiagnosed pleural effusion. The management of patients with pleural effusions due to specific diseases is discussed in the chapters dealing with those diseases.

FREQUENCIES OF VARIOUS DIAGNOSES

Pleural effusions can occur as complications of many different diseases (Table 5.1). The vigor with which various diagnoses are pursued depends on the likelihood that the individual has that particular disease. Table 5.2 shows the approximate annual incidence for the most common causes of pleural effusions. These data are rough estimates of the incidence of the various types of pleural effusions. An epidemiologic study from the Czech Republic found that the four leading causes of pleural effusions in order of incidence were congestive heart failure, malignancy, pneumonia, and pulmonary embolism (1). Congestive heart failure and cirrhosis cause almost all transudative pleural effusions, whereas malignant disease, pneumonia, and pulmonary embolization are the three main causes of exudative pleural effusions. Two other frequent causes of exudative pleural effusions are viral infections and the effusion that occurs after coronary artery bypass graft surgery.

SEPARATION OF EXUDATES FROM TRANSUDATES

If free pleural fluid is demonstrated on the decubitus film, with ultrasound or with a CT scan, one should consider performing a diagnostic thoracentesis (Fig. 5.1). It has been my experience that diagnostic thoracentesis is difficult if the thickness of the fluid on the decubitus radiograph or the CT scan is less than 10 mm. If the thickness of the fluid is greater than 10 mm, however, consideration should be given to performing a diagnostic thoracentesis (see Chapter 25). If the patient has obvious congestive heart failure, I perform a diagnostic thoracentesis if any of the following three conditions are met: (a) the effusions are not bilateral and comparably sized, (b) the patient has pleuritic chest pain, or (c) the patient is febrile. Otherwise, treatment of the congestive heart failure is initiated. If the pleural effusions do not rapidly disappear, I then perform a diagnostic thoracentesis several days later. It must be remembered, however, that the characteristics of the pleural fluid may occasionally change from those of a transudate to those of an exudate with diuresis. Chakko et al. (2) treated nine patients with congestive heart failure for a mean of 6 days and found that in three of the nine patients, a pleural fluid that was a transudate initially developed

TABLE 5.1. *Differential diagnosis of pleural effusion*

I. Transudative pleural effusions
  A. Congestive heart failure
  B. Cirrhosis
  C. Nephrotic syndrome
  D. Superior vena caval obstruction
  E. Fontan procedure
  F. Urinothorax
  G. Peritoneal dialysis
  H. Glomerulonephritis
  I. Myxedema
  J. Cerebrospinal fluid leaks to pleura
  K. Hypoalbuminemia
  L. Pulmonary emboli
  M. Sarcoidosis
II. Exudative Pleural Effusions
  A. Neoplastic diseases
    1. Metastatic disease
    2. Mesothelioma
    3. Body cavity lymphoma
    4. Pyothorax associated lymphoma
  B. Infectious diseases
    1. Bacterial infections
    2. Tuberculosis
    3. Fungal infections
    4. Parasitic infections
    5. Viral infections
  C. Pulmonary embolization
  D. Gastrointestinal disease
    1. Pancreatic disease
    2. Subphrenic abscess
    3. Intrahepatic abscess
    4. Intrasplenic abscess
    5. Esophageal perforation
    6. Postabdominal surgery
    7. Diaphragmatic hemia
    8. Endoscopic variceal sclerosis
    9. Postliver transplant
  E. Heart diseases
    1. Postcoronary artery bypass graft surgery
    2. Postcardiac injury (Dressler's) syndrome
    3. Pericardial disease
  F. Obstetric and gynecological disease
    1. Ovarian hyperstimulation syndrome
    2. Fetal pleural effusion
    3. Postpartum pleural effusion
    4. Megis' syndrome
    5. Endometriosis
  G. Collagen vascular diseases
    1. Rheumatoid pleuritis
    2. Systemic lupus erythematosus
    3. Drug-induced lupus
    4. Immunoblastic lymphadenopathy
    5. Sjögren's syndrome
    6. Familial Mediterranean fever
    7. Churg-Strauss syndrome
    8. Wegener's granulomatosis
  H. Drug-induced pleural disease
    1. Nitrofurantoin
    2. Dantrolene
    3. Methysergide
    4. Ergot alkaloids
    5. Amiodarone
    6. Interleukin-2
    7. Procarbazine
    8. Methotrexate
    9. Clozapine
  I. Miscellaneous diseases and conditions
    1. Asbestos exposure
    2. Postlung transplant
    3. Postbone marrow transplant
    4. Yellow nail syndrome
    5. Sarcoidosis
    6. Uremia
    7. Trapped lung
    8. Therapeutic radiation exposure
    9. Drowning
    10. Amyloidosis
    11. Milk of calcium pleural effusion
    12. Electrical burns
    13. Extramedullary hematopoiesis
    14. Rupture of mediastinal cyst
    15. Acute respiratory distress syndrome
    16. Whipple's disease
    17. Iatrogenic pleural effusions
  J. Hemothorax
  K. Chylothorax

the characteristics of an exudate with diuresis. We performed a similar study (3) on 12 patients in whom the repeat thoracentesis was performed 12 to 48 hours after diuresis was initiated. In this later study, the characteristics of the pleural fluid in only one patient changed from transudative to exudative.

One of the main purposes of the diagnostic thoracentesis is to determine whether the patient has a transudative or an exudative pleural effusion. This distinction is made by analysis of the levels of protein and lactate dehydrogenase (LDH) in the pleural fluid and in the serum (4). If none of the criteria in Fig. 5.1 are met, the patient has a transudative pleural effusion. Therefore, the pleural surfaces can be ignored while the congestive heart failure, cirrhosis, or nephrosis, for example, is treated. Alternately, if any of the three criteria in Fig. 5.1 are met, the patient probably has an exudative pleural fluid. The exudative nature indicates that the pleural effusion resulted from local disease where the fluid originated, and further investigation should be directed toward the genesis of the local disease

TABLE 5.2. *Approximate annual incidence of various types of pleural effusions in the United States*

Type	Incidence (number of persons)
Congestive heart failure	500,000
Parapneumonic effusion	300,000
Malignant pleural effusion	200,000
Lung	60,000
Breast	50,000
Lymphoma	40,000
Other	60,000
Pulmonary embolization	150,000
Viral disease	100,000
Cirrhosis with ascites	50,000
Postcoronary artery bypass graft surgery	50,000
Gastrointestinal disease	25,000
Tuberculosis	2,500
Mesothelioma	2,300
Asbestos exposure	2,000

(5). It should be remembered, however, that 15% to 20% of patients with congestive heart failure or cirrhosis will meet these exudative criteria. If a patient has congestive heart failure or cirrhosis but the pleural fluid meets exudative criteria, the difference between the serum albumin and pleural fluid albumin (the pleural fluid albumin gradient) should be measured. If this difference exceeds 1.2 g per dL, the patient should be classified as having a transudative pleural effusion and no further diagnostic tests are indicated (6).

If there is a significant likelihood that the patient has a transudative pleural effusion, the most cost-effective utilization of the laboratory is to only obtain the protein and LDH levels of the pleural fluid at the initial diagnostic thoracentesis. Pleural fluid can be set aside for other tests if the fluid proves to be an exudate. Peterman and Speicher (7) reviewed the charts of 83 patients whose pleural fluid was a transudate by protein and LDH levels during a 1-year period. They found that 725 additional studies were performed on these 83 pleural fluids. Only nine of the 725 studies yielded a positive result, and the positive result was eventually proven to be false in seven of the nine patients. If no tests other than the protein and LDH had been obtained in these 83 patients, there would have been a mean cost savings of $185 per patient.

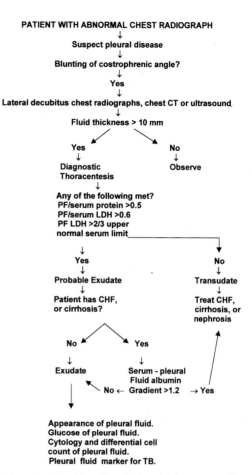

FIG. 5.1. Algorithm for distinguishing transudative from exudative pleural effusions.

DIFFERENTIATING AMONG VARIOUS EXUDATIVE PLEURAL EFFUSIONS

In order to differentiate among the various causes of exudative pleural effusions, one should initially examine the gross appearance of the fluid, obtain a pleural fluid differential cell count and cytologic examination, measure the levels of glucose and LDH in the pleural fluid, and obtain a test for a pleural fluid marker for tuberculosis. Other tests can then be ordered on an individual basis.

Appearance of Pleural Fluid

The gross appearance of the pleural fluid should always be noted and evaluated as outlined in

Fig. 5.2. If the pleural fluid appears bloody, a hematocrit should be obtained on the fluid. The hematocrit is frequently much lower than one would expect from the appearance of the pleural fluid. The blood in the pleural fluid is not significant if the pleural fluid hematocrit is less than 1% (8). If the pleural fluid hematocrit is greater than 1%, the patient most likely has malignant pleural disease, a pulmonary embolus, or a traumatically induced pleural effusion (8). If the hematocrit is greater than 50% of that of the peripheral blood, the patient has a hemothorax, and one should consider performing a tube thoracostomy (see Chapter 22).

If the pleural fluid is turbid or milky or if it is bloody, the supernatant of the pleural fluid should be examined to see whether it is cloudy. If the pleural fluid was turbid when originally withdrawn, but the turbidity clears with centrifugation, the turbidity was due to cells or debris in the pleural fluid. Most patients who have very turbid pleural fluid that clears with centrifugation have a pleural infection. If the turbidity persists after centrifugation, the patient probably has a chylothorax or a pseudochylothorax (see Chapter 23). These two entities can be differentiated by the patient's history, examination of the sediment for cholesterol crystals, and lipid analysis of the supernatant (Fig. 5.2). Pseudochyloraces usually occur when the pleural effusion has been present for many years. Cholesterol crystals may be found in the sediment, and high levels of triglycerides are not usually present in the pleural fluid. In contrast, chylothoraces are more acute, do not contain cholesterol crystals, and are characterized by high levels of triglycerides. The management of a patient with a chylothorax or a pseudochylothorax is discussed in Chapter 23.

Routine Measurements on Exudative Pleural Fluids

When a patient has an undiagnosed exudative effusion, there are several tests that should be routinely obtained, namely, a pleural fluid cell count and differential, a pleural fluid glucose and LDH level, cytologic examination of the pleural fluid, and a pleural fluid marker for tuberculosis. In previous editions of this book, I recommended that a pleural fluid amylase also be obtained, However, the pleural fluid amylase only occasionally helps in making a diagnosis and, therefore, it should not be obtained on a routine basis (9). It should be obtained if acute pancreatitis, esophageal

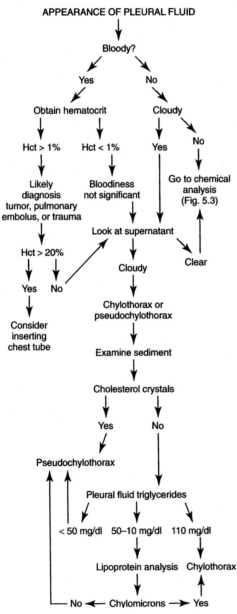

FIG. 5.2. Algorithm for evaluating the appearance of pleural fluid.

rupture, or chronic pancreatic pleural effusion is suspected (9).

Pleural Fluid Differential Cell Count

In patients with exudative pleural effusions, the cell count and the differential provide clues about the etiology of the pleural effusion. When neutrophils predominate in the pleural fluid, an acute process is affecting the pleural surfaces, and the chest radiograph should be evaluated for parenchymal infiltrates. The presence of an infiltrate indicates that the patient probably has a parapneumonic effusion although pulmonary embolus and bronchogenic carcinoma should also be considered. The diagnosis of a parapneumonic effusion is likely if purulent sputum is present. When purulent sputum or peripheral leukocytosis is not seen, the patient should have a spiral CT scan to rule out pulmonary embolus. In the event of a negative scan, a bronchoscopy with transbronchial biopsy should be performed to determine the cause of the parenchymal infiltrate. If after all these studies the diagnosis is still not clear, video-assisted thoracoscopy (see Chapter 27) should be performed if the infiltrate is worsening or the effusion is increasing in size.

The patient with an exudative pleural effusion with predominantly polymorphonuclear leukocytes and without parenchymal infiltrates most likely has pulmonary embolus, viral infection, gastrointestinal disease, asbestos pleural effusion, malignant pleural disease, or acute tuberculous pleuritis. Accordingly, the patient should undergo a spiral CT scan or a lung scan for evaluation of pulmonary embolus. A gastrointestinal etiology of the pleural effusion can be evaluated with an abdominal CT scan or ultrasound. A careful history should be taken for asbestos exposure. The marker for tuberculosis (adenosine deaminase [ADA] or interferon-gamma) will indicate whether the patient has tuberculosis, and the cytology will provide the first evaluation for pleural malignancy.

The patient with an exudative pleural effusion with predominantly mononuclear cells in the pleural fluid has a chronic process involving the pleural space. Malignant disease, pulmonary embolization, pleural effusions following CABG, and tuberculosis are the four most common causes of this picture. Again, the cytology on the pleural fluid is the first step in evaluating the possibility of malignancy. The history will demonstrate a CABG within the previous months or years. An elevated level of ADA interferon-gamma in the pleural fluid essentially establishes the diagnosis of tuberculous pleuritis (see Chapter 10). If none of the above tests are positive, the possibility of pulmonary embolus should be assessed with a spiral CT scan or a lung scan.

Pleural Fluid Glucose

The routine measurement of the pleural fluid glucose level is recommended because the presence of a reduced (<60 mg per dL) pleural fluid glucose dramatically reduces the spectrum of diagnostic possibilities. Most patients with a reduced pleural fluid glucose level (<60 mg per dL) have one of four conditions: parapneumonic effusion, malignant pleural effusion, tuberculous pleuritis, or rheumatoid pleural effusion (10). Other rare causes of a low glucose pleural effusion include paragonimiasis, hemothorax, Churg-Strauss syndrome, urinothorax, and occasionally lupus pleuritis. Most patients with a reduced pleural fluid glucose level also have a reduced pleural fluid pH and an increased pleural fluid LDH level. Laboratory errors in the performance of one of these three tests should be suspected when these relationships are not maintained.

Patients with either parapneumonic effusions or tuberculous pleuritis may have an acute illness characterized by fever, cough, and pleuritic chest pain and a low pleural fluid glucose level. Patients with parapneumonic effusions usually have radiologically evident parenchymal infiltrates, whereas most of those with tuberculous pleuritis have no infiltrates. The differential cell count on the pleural fluid is also useful in making the differentiation because most patients with parapneumonic effusions have predominantly neutrophils in their pleural fluid, whereas most patients with tuberculous pleuritis have predominantly lymphocytes.

Patients with subacute or chronic symptoms and a low pleural fluid glucose level may have malignant pleural disease, rheumatoid disease, tuberculosis, or even a chronic bacterial infection. The diagnosis of rheumatoid pleuritis (see Chapter 19) is usually easy. The differentiation among tuberculosis, malignant disease, and chronic bacterial infection may be more difficult. The pleural fluid cytology is usually positive for malignant cells in patients with a malignant pleural effusion and a low pleural fluid glucose. The pleural fluid marker for tuberculosis should be positive with tuberculous pleuritis, and neutrophils should predominate in the pleural fluid if a chronic bacterial infection is present.

Pleural Fluid Lactate Dehydrogenase

Although the level of LDH in the pleural fluid is not particularly useful in the differentiation of the various exudative pleural effusions, a pleural fluid LDH should be obtained every time that a thoracentesis is performed on a patient with an undiagnosed pleural effusion. The pleural fluid LDH is a reliable indicator of the degree of pleural inflammation. If, with repeated thoracenteses, the pleural fluid LDH level increases, the degree of inflammation in the pleural space is becoming progressively worse and one should be aggressive in pursuing a diagnosis. Alternatively, if the pleural fluid LDH level decreases with repeated thoracentesis, the degree of inflammation in the pleural space is becoming progressively less and one need not be as aggressive in the approach to the patient (11).

Pleural Fluid Cytology

If a patient has malignancy, cytologic examination of the pleural fluid is a fast, efficient, and minimally invasive means by which to establish the diagnosis. The percentage of malignant pleural effusions that are diagnosed with cytology has been reported to be anywhere between 40% and 87%. There are several factors that influence the diagnostic yield with cytology. Almost all adenocarcinomas are diagnosed with cytology, but the yield is less with squamous cell carcinoma,

Hodgkin's disease, and sarcomas. Obviously, the yield will also depend on the skill of the cytologist. The yield also depends on the extent of the tumor—the greater the tumor burden in the pleural space, the more likely the cytology is to be positive.

Pleural Fluid Markers for Tuberculosis

Over the past 40 years, the diagnosis of tuberculous pleuritis has usually been established with needle biopsy of the pleura. However, it is now possible to make the diagnosis of pleural tuberculosis by measuring the level of ADA or the level of interferon-gamma in the pleural fluid.

Pleural Fluid ADA Level

The diagnosis of tuberculosis is virtually established if the pleural fluid ADA level is above 50 U per L and the patient has predominantly lymphocytes in the pleural fluid. The higher the pleural fluid ADA level, the more likely the patient is to have tuberculous pleuritis. In one recent study, the ADA was above 47 U per L in 253 of 254 patients with tuberculous pleuritis (12). In a second report, only five of 173 patients (3%) with pleural effusions due to other etiologies, including 46 with malignancy and 30 with pneumonia, had ADA levels that exceeded 45 U per mL (13). The two other disease entities that tend to have a high pleural fluid ADA level are empyema and rheumatoid pleuritis (13), and both of these conditions are easily distinguished from pleural tuberculosis by the clinical picture.

Pleural Fluid Interferon-Gamma Levels

Pleural fluid interferon-gamma levels are also elevated with tuberculous pleuritis. Pleural fluid interferon-gamma levels are very efficient at differentiating tuberculous from nontuberculous pleural effusion. Using a cutoff level of 3.7 U per mL, Villena et al. (14) demonstrated that this test resulted in a sensitivity of 0.99 and a specificity of 0.98 in a series of 388 pleural effusions including 73 tuberculous effusions. These results were better than the same group reported with ADA (11).

OPTIONS WHEN NO DIAGNOSIS OBTAINED AFTER INITIAL THORACENTESIS

When no diagnosis has been obtained after an initial thoracentesis that includes a pleural fluid marker for tuberculosis and cytology, what are the options? The first thing that we recommend is a spiral CT scan. With the spiral CT scan, the possibility of pulmonary embolus can be evaluated and the presence of pulmonary infiltrates or mediastinal lymphadenopathy can be evaluated as well (15). If the spiral CT scan does not demonstrate a pulmonary embolus, then there are five options available to the physician, namely, observation, needle biopsy of the pleura, bronchoscopy, thoracoscopy, or thoracotomy with open biopsy.

Observation

This is probably the best option if the patient is improving and there are no parenchymal infiltrates. Remember that no diagnosis is ever established in approximately 15% of patients with exudative pleural effusion. If the patient has malignancy, spontaneous improvement probably will not occur. If the patient has pulmonary embolism, the diagnosis should have been made by spiral CT scan, whereas if the patient has tuberculous pleuritis, one of the pleural fluid markers for tuberculosis should have been positive.

Bronchoscopy

Bronchoscopy is useful in the diagnosis of pleural effusion only if one or more of the following four conditions are present (16). (a) A pulmonary infiltrate is present on the chest radiograph or the chest CT scan. In this situation, particular attention should be paid to the area that contains the infiltrate. (b) Hemoptysis is present–hemoptysis in the presence of a pleural effusion is very suggestive of an endobronchial lesion. (c) The pleural effusion is massive, that is, it occupies more than three fourths of the hemithorax. (d) The mediastinum is shifted toward the side of the effusion–an endobronchial lesion is probable. In patients with pleural effusions with positive

cytology but no hemoptysis or no parenchymal infiltrates, bronchoscopy will not identify the primary tumor (17).

Thoracoscopy

In the diagnosis of pleural disease, thoracoscopic procedures should be used only when the less invasive diagnostic methods such as thoracentesis with cytology and markers for tuberculosis have not yielded a diagnosis. In one series of 620 patients with pleural effusions, only 48 (8%) remained without a diagnosis after less invasive procedures and were subjected to thoracoscopy (18). If the patient has malignancy, thoracoscopy will establish the diagnosis more than 90% of the time and the diagnosis of mesothelioma is probably best made with thoracoscopy. Thoracoscopy can also establish the diagnosis of tuberculosis (19, 20). An advantage to thoracoscopy in the diagnosis of pleural disease is that pleurodesis can also be performed at the time of the procedure. It should be emphasized, however, that thoracoscopy rarely establishes the diagnosis of benign disease (21). Thoracoscopy is indicated in the patient with an undiagnosed pleural effusion who is not improving spontaneously and in whom there is a significant likelihood that malignancy or tuberculosis is present.

Needle Biopsy of the Pleura

The primary use of needle biopsy of the pleura over the past 40 years has been to diagnose tuberculous pleuritis. However, as outlined earlier, markers for tuberculosis obtained from the pleural fluid are very efficient at establishing this diagnosis. In recent years, with the emergence of multidrug-resistant tuberculosis, cultures for *Mycoplasma tuberculosis* have become important in guiding the therapy of tuberculosis. Some have advocated performing a needle biopsy of the pleura so that a specimen of the pleura could be cultured. However, only about 33% of patients with tuberculous pleuritis have a positive pleural biopsy culture and a negative pleural fluid culture (22). In addition, to my knowledge, no patient has developed disseminated multidrug-resistant tuberculosis after presenting with a pleural effusion without parenchymal infiltrates and receiving a standard course of antituberculous drugs. In view of the above-mentioned factors, pleural biopsy is usually not indicated for the diagnosis of tuberculous pleuritis.

Pleural biopsy can also establish the diagnosis of malignant pleural disease. However, in most series, cytology of the pleural fluid is much more sensitive in establishing the diagnosis. If the cytology of the fluid is negative, the pleural biopsy is usually nondiagnostic. In one series, the pleural biopsy was positive in only 20 of 118 (17%) of patients with pleural malignancy and negative cytology (23). Because thoracoscopy is diagnostic in more than 90% of patients with pleural malignancy and negative cytology, it is the preferred diagnostic procedure in the patient with a cytology-negative pleural effusion who is suspected of having malignancy. Needle biopsy of the pleura is indicated if the patient has an undiagnosed pleural effusion that is not improving and thoracoscopy is not available. Needle biopsy of the pleural is also indicated if pleural tuberculosis is suspected and a pleural fluid marked for tuberculosis is unavailable or equivocal.

Open Pleural Biopsy

Open thoracotomy with direct biopsy of the pleura has been supplanted by video-assisted thoracoscopy in many institutions. The main indication for open pleural biopsy (or for thoracoscopy) is progressive undiagnosed pleural disease. If both procedures are available, thoracoscopy is usually preferred because it is associated with less morbidity.

It should be emphasized that open pleural biopsy does not always provide a diagnosis in a patient with an undiagnosed pleural effusion. Douglass et al. (24) reported that thoracotomy failed to provide a specific diagnosis for seven of 21 patients with pleural effusion. The group at the Mayo Clinic reviewed their experience with open pleural biopsy for undiagnosed pleural effusion between 1962 and 1972 and reported that during this time period no diagnosis was established in 51 such patients (25). In 31 of the patients (61%), there was no recurrence of the pleural effusion,

and no cause ever became apparent. However, 13 of the patients were eventually proven to have malignant disease (six patients with lymphoma, four patients with mesothelioma, and three with other malignancy).

REFERENCES

1. Marel M, Arustova M, Stasny B, et al. Incidence of pleural effusion in a well-defined region: epidemiologic study in central Bohemia. *Chest* 1993;104:1486–1489.
2. Chakko SC, Caldwell SH, Sforza PP. Treatment of congestive heart failure: its effect on pleural fluid chemistry. *Chest* 1989;95:978–982.
3. Shinto RA, Light RW. The effects of diuresis upon the characteristics of pleural fluid in patients with congestive heart failure. *Am J Med* 1990;88:230–233.
4. Light RW, MacGregor MI, Luchsinger PC, et al. Pleural effusions: the diagnostic separation of transudates and exudates. *Ann Intern Med* 1972;77:507–513.
5. Broaddus VC, Light RW. What is the origin of pleural transudates and exudates [Editorial]? *Chest* 1992;102:658.
6. Burgess LJ, Maritz FJ, Taljaard JJ. Comparative analysis of the biochemical parameters used to distinguish between pleural transudates and exudates. *Chest* 1995;107:1604–1609.
7. Peterman TA, Speicher CE. Evaluating pleural effusion: a two-stage laboratory approach. *JAMA* 1984;252:1051–1053.
8. Light RW, Erozan YS, Ball WC. Cells in pleural fluid: their value in differential diagnosis. *Arch Intern Med* 1973;132:854–860.
9. Branca P, Rodriguez RM, Rogers JT, et al. Routine measurement of pleural fluid amylase is not indicated. *Arch Intern Med* 2001;161:228–232.
10. Light RW, Ball WC. Glucose and amylase in pleural effusions. *JAMA* 1973;225:257–260.
11. Villena V, Navarro-Gonzalvez JA, Garcia-Benayas C, et al. Rapid automated determination of adenosine deaminase and lysozyme for differentiating tuberculous and nontuberculous pleural effusions. *Clin Chem* 1996;42:218–221.
12. Valdes L, Alvarez D, San Jose E, et al. Tuberculous pleurisy: a study of 254 patients. *Arch Intern Med* 1998;158:2017–2021.
13. Ocana IM, Martinez-Vazquez JM, Seguna RM, et al. Adenosine deaminase in pleural fluids. *Chest* 1983;84:51–53.
14. Villena V, Lopez-Encuentra A, Echave-Sustaeta J, et al. Interferon-gamma in 388 immunocompromised and immunocompetent patients for diagnosing pleural tuberculosis. *Eur Respir J* 1996;9:2635–2639.
15. Johnson PT, Wechsler RJ, Salazar AM, et al. Spiral CT of acute pulmonary thromboembolism: evaluation of pleuroparenchymal abnormalities. *J Comput Assist Tomogr* 1999;23:369–373.
16. Chang S-C, Perng RP. The role of fiberoptic bronchoscopy in evaluating the causes of pleural effusions. *Arch Intern Med* 1989;149:855–857.
17. Feinsilver SH, Barrows AA, Braman SS. Fiberoptic

bronchoscopy and pleural effusion of unknown origin. *Chest* 1986;90:514–515.

18. Kendall SW, Bryan AJ, Large SR, et al. Pleural effusions: is thoracoscopy a reliable investigation? A retrospective review. *Respir Med* 1992;86:437–440.

19. de Groot M, Walther G. Thoracoscopy in undiagnosed pleural effusions. *S Afr Med J* 1998;88:706–711.

20. Emad A, Rezaian GR. Diagnostic value of closed percutaneous pleural biopsy vs pleuroscopy in suspected malignant pleural effusion or tuberculous pleurisy in a region with a high incidence of tuberculosis: a comparative, age-dependent study. *Respir Med* 1998;92:488–492.

21. Daniel TM. Diagnostic thoracoscopy for pleural disease. *Ann Thorac Surg* 1993;56:639–640.

22. Light RW. Closed needle biopsy of the pleura is a valuable diagnostic procedure. Con closed needle biopsy. *J Bronchol* 1999;5:332–336.

23. Prakash URS, Reiman HM. Comparison of needle biopsy with cytologic analysis for the evaluation of pleural effusion: analysis of 414 cases. *Mayo Clin Proc* 1985;60:158–164.

24. Douglass BE, Carr DT, Bernatz PE. Diagnostic thoracotomy in the study of "idiopathic" pleural effusion. *Am Rev Tuberc* 1956;74:954–957.

25. Ryan CJ, Rodgers RF, Unni KK, et al. The outcome of patients with pleural effusion of indeterminate cause at thoracotomy. *Mayo Clin Proc* 1981;56:145–149.

6

Transudative Pleural Effusions

Transudative pleural effusions occur when the systemic factors influencing the formation and absorption of pleural fluids are altered so that pleural fluid accumulates. In this chapter, the various causes of transudative pleural effusions are discussed.

CONGESTIVE HEART FAILURE

Congestive heart failure is probably the most common cause of pleural effusion. The reason for the low incidence of pleural effusions secondary to heart failure in most studies is that researchers interested in pleural effusions usually do not see most patients with pleural effusions of this origin. In an epidemiologic study from the Czech Republic, congestive heart failure was the most common cause of pleural effusion (1). The incidence of pleural effusions in patients with congestive heart failure is high. In a recent study from Japan, Kataoka et al. (2) studied 60 patients admitted to a Japanese hospital for an exacerbation of stable congestive heart failure with computed tomography (CT) scan, ultrasound, and chest radiograph. They reported that by CT scan, 50 patients (83%) had a right-sided pleural effusion, whereas 46 patients (77%) had a left-sided pleural effusion. Approximately one third of the effusions had a volume that exceeded 700 mL (2).

Race et al. (3) reviewed the autopsies at the Mayo Clinic between 1948 and 1953 of 402 patients who had congestive heart failure during life. The researchers found that 290 of the patients (72%) had pleural effusions with volumes greater than 250 mL. Of the patients with pleural effusions, 88% had bilateral pleural effusions, whereas 8% and 4% had unilateral right-sided and left-sided effusions, respectively (3).

Pathophysiology

In recent years, concepts of pleural fluid formation and reabsorption in patients with heart failure have undergone significant modifications. In the past, it was believed that the pleural fluid that accumulated in patients with congestive heart failure was due to increased pressure in the capillaries in the visceral or the parietal pleura. These increased pressures were thought to result in an increased entry of fluid into the pleural space from the parietal pleura and a decreased removal of fluid through the visceral pleura, according to Starling's equation.

The current theories on pleural fluid formation and reabsorption give us a different entry pathway and a different exit pathway for pleural fluid in patients with congestive heart failure. It appears that the majority of the fluid that enters the pleural space in patients with congestive heart failure comes from the alveolar capillaries rather than the pleural capillaries (4). When the pressure in the pulmonary capillaries is elevated, increased amounts of fluid enter the interstitial spaces of the lung. The increased fluid in the interstitial spaces results in an increased interstitial pressure in the subpleural interstitial spaces (5). The fluid then moves from the pulmonary interstitial spaces across the visceral pleura into the pleural space. There appears to be relatively little resistance to fluid movement from the pulmonary interstitial spaces across the visceral pleura (4). When pulmonary edema is produced in sheep with volume overloading, approximately 25% of the pulmonary edema fluid exits the lung through the visceral pleura (6).

At present, it is believed that almost all fluid exits the pleural space through the lymphatics in the parietal pleura rather than by passively diffusing across the visceral pleura (see Chapter 2). Pleural fluid accumulates in patients with congestive heart failure when the rate of entry of fluid into the pleural space exceeds the capability of the lymphatics in the parietal pleura to remove the fluid. In normal sheep, the capacity of the lymphatics to remove fluid is approximately 0.28 mL per kg per hour (7). If there is elevated pressure in the systemic veins, the lymphatic clearance is decreased (8).

In the clinical situation, it appears that the accumulation of pleural fluid in patients with congestive heart failure is related more to left ventricular failure than to right ventricular failure. Wiener-Kronish et al. (9) prospectively evaluated 37 patients with congestive heart failure secondary to ischemic heart disease or to cardiomyopathy who were admitted to a coronary care unit. Nineteen patients had a pleural effusion. The mean wedge pressure in the patients with an effusion (24.1 ± 1.3 mm Hg) was significantly higher than in those without an effusion (17.2 ± 1.5 mm Hg). There also was a greater likelihood of finding pleural effusions if severe rather than mild pulmonary edema was found roentgenographically. In a subsequent study (10), these same researchers were unable to demonstrate any pleural effusions in 27 patients with chronic pulmonary hypertension or chronically elevated right atrial pressures.

In summary, it appears that pleural fluid accumulates in patients with congestive heart failure when they have left ventricular failure. The high pressures in the pulmonary capillaries lead to increased amounts of fluid in the interstitial spaces. The fluid in the interstitial spaces enters the pleural space through the highly permeable visceral pleura. Fluid accumulates when the entry of fluid into the pleural space overwhelms the capacity of the lymphatics in the parietal pleura to remove the fluid. Small amounts of fluid may enter the pleural space from the capillaries in either pleural surface. Elevation of the systemic venous pressure may decrease the lymphatic clearance from the pleural space.

Clinical Manifestations

Pleural effusions due to congestive heart failure are usually associated with other manifestations of that disease. The patient often has a history of increasing dyspnea on exertion, increasing peripheral edema, and orthopnea or paroxysmal nocturnal dyspnea. The dyspnea is frequently out of proportion to the size of the effusion. Physical examination usually reveals signs of both right-sided heart failure with distended neck veins and peripheral edema and left-sided heart failure with rales and an S3 ventricular gallop as well as signs of the pleural effusions.

The chest radiograph almost always reveals cardiomegaly and usually bilateral pleural effusions. Congestive heart failure is by far the most common cause of bilateral pleural effusions, but if cardiomegaly is not present, an alternate explanation should be sought. In one series of 78 patients with bilateral pleural effusions but a normal-sized heart, only three (4%) were due to congestive heart failure (11). Although in the past it was thought that pleural effusions due to congestive heart failure were commonly unilateral on the right or at least were much larger on the right side, such does not appear to be the case. In the autopsy series of Race et al. (3), 88% of the patients studied had bilateral pleural effusions. Moreover, the mean volume of pleural fluid in the right pleural space (1,084 mL) was only slightly greater than the mean volume of pleural fluid in the left pleural space (913 mL). In this series, 35 patients had unilateral pleural effusions, and of these 35 patients, 16 (46%) had either pulmonary embolism or pneumonia (3). When two series (12, 13) comprising 124 patients are combined, 100 patients (81%) had bilateral pleural effusions, 15 (12%) had unilateral right-sided effusions, and nine (7%) had unilateral left-sided effusions. Therefore, the presence of a unilateral pleural effusion or bilateral pleural effusions of disparate size is an indication to search for other causes of the effusion.

Diagnosis

The diagnosis of pleural effusions secondary to congestive heart failure comes readily to mind every time a patient is seen with congestive heart failure. One must be careful to avoid the trap of ascribing the pleural effusion to congestive heart failure when it has another cause. In the series of Race et al. (3), over 25% of the patients with congestive heart failure and pleural effusions had either pulmonary emboli or pneumonia at autopsy. Certainly, if the patient is febrile, has pleural effusions that are greatly disparate in size, has a unilateral pleural effusion, has pleuritic chest pain, or does not have cardiomegaly, a diagnostic thoracentesis should be performed.

If the patient has cardiomegaly and bilateral pleural effusions, is afebrile, and does not have pleuritic chest pain, we initiate treatment of the congestive heart failure and observe the patient to determine whether the pleural fluid is reabsorbed. If the effusions do not disappear within a few days, we then perform a diagnostic thoracentesis. One problem with this approach is that with diuresis, the characteristics of the pleural fluid may change from those of a transudate to those of an exudate. Chakko and co-workers (14) treated nine patients with congestive heart failure for a mean of 6 days and found that in three of the nine patients, a pleural fluid that was a transudate initially, developed the characteristics of an exudate. We performed a similar study (15) on 12 patients in whom the repeat thoracentesis was performed 12 to 48 hours after diuresis was initiated and found that in only one patient had the characteristics of the pleural fluid become exudative. In those patients whose pleural fluid developed exudative characteristics the protein ratio was 0.62 or less, the lactate dehydrogenase (LDH) ratio was less then 1.0, and the LDH level was less than 85% the upper normal limit for serum.

The pleural fluid from a patient with congestive heart failure is typically a transudate with a ratio of pleural fluid to serum protein below 0.5, a ratio of pleural fluid to serum LDH under 0.6, and an absolute pleural fluid LDH level below two thirds of the upper limit of normal for serum (Light's criteria) (16). If the foregoing criteria are satisfied in a patient with congestive heart failure, the patient has a transudative pleural effusion that can be ascribed to the congestive heart failure, and no further diagnostic studies are indicated. Such transudative pleural effusions may be blood tinged, and the pleural fluid differential cell count may reveal predominantly polymorphonuclear leukocytes, small lymphocytes, or other mononuclear cells (17).

The pleural fluid from approximately 15% to 20% of patients with congestive heart failure will be classified as exudates by Light's criteria (18). Most of the patients who are misclassified are receiving diuretics (18). If the pleural fluid meets exudative criteria but the effusion is thought to be due to congestive heart failure, the pleural fluid to serum albumin gradient should be examined. If this gradient is greater than 1.2 g per dL, the pleural effusion in all probability is due to the congestive heart failure and additional diagnostic studies are not indicated (18). If the protein and LDH criteria are not met and the albumin gradient is less than 1.2 g per dL, the pleural effusion is not due to the heart failure. Rather, the patient has an exudative pleural effusion, and further diagnostic tests such as pleural fluid cytologic study and spiral CT scan of the chest should be obtained.

Treatment

The preferred treatment of pleural effusion secondary to heart failure is with digitalis, diuretics, and afterload reduction. When the heart failure is successfully managed, the pleural effusion disappears. Occasionally, large pleural effusions cause patients to be very dyspneic. The removal of 500 to 1,000 mL of pleural fluid from such persons may rapidly relieve the dyspnea.

Patients with large pleural effusions and refractory heart failure sometimes receive symptomatic relief from therapeutic thoracentesis. In such patients, pleurodesis with a sclerosing agent may be considered (19). At the present time, we recommend 500 mg of doxycycline as the sclerosing agent in this situation. Bleomycin is not recommended in this situation because it is not an effective agent in the rabbit model with normal pleura (20).

An alternative approach is to use a pleuroperitoneal shunt. The shunt consists of two catheters connected with a valved pump chamber. The two one-way valves in the pump chamber are positioned such that fluid can only flow from the pleural space to the peritoneal cavity through the pump chamber. Because the pleural pressure is almost always more negative than the peritoneal pressure, the pumping chamber must be used to move fluid from the pleural cavity to the peritoneal cavity. Little et al. (21) reported that two patients with refractory pleural effusions secondary to congestive heart failure were managed successfully with the pleuroperitoneal shunt.

HEPATIC HYDROTHORAX

Pleural effusions occur occasionally as a complication of hepatic cirrhosis. Pleural effusions usually occur only when ascitic fluid is present. Lieberman et al. (22) reviewed 330 patients with cirrhosis and ascites, and found that 18 (5.5%) had pleural effusions; Johnston and Loo (23) found that 6.0% of 200 patients with cirrhosis had pleural effusions. In the second series, none of the 54 patients with cirrhosis without ascites had a pleural effusion (23). In some patients, the ascites is not clinically evident, but it can almost always be demonstrated with ultrasonography (24). The pleural effusion in patients with cirrhosis and ascites is usually right sided (67%), but occasionally it is left sided (16%) or bilateral (16%) (22, 23).

Pathophysiology

Patients with cirrhosis frequently have decreased plasma oncotic pressure (23), and from Fig. 2.1, one might hypothesize that the pleural effusions arise because of it. Indeed, in the experimental animal, the induction of decreased plasma oncotic pressure leads to the accumulation of pleural fluid (25). This mechanism does not appear to be the predominant cause of pleural effusions in patients with cirrhosis and ascites, however. Rather, the pleural effusions appear to be produced by movement of the ascitic fluid from the peritoneal cavity into the pleural cavity.

Johnston and Loo (23) demonstrated that after the intraperitoneal injection of India ink, cells in the pleural fluid contained many carbon particles, whereas cells in the peripheral blood contained none. In addition, after the intravenous injection of radiolabeled albumin, the albumin first appeared in the peritoneal fluid and then in the pleural fluid. Following the intraperitoneal injection of radiolabeled albumin, the concentration of the labeled protein was greater in the pleural fluid than in the plasma; after intrapleural injection, the labeled protein appeared in the plasma before it appeared in the peritoneal fluid (23). Because no air entered the pleural space following the intraperitoneal injection of carbon dioxide in one patient, these researchers concluded that the pleural effusion arose from the transfer of ascitic fluid from the peritoneal to the pleural space by the lymphatic vessels. This conclusion appears to have been incorrect. Datta and colleagues (26) injected radiolabeled human serum albumin into the peritoneal cavity of a patient with ascites and a large pleural effusion. They were able to demonstrate that when the labeled protein was picked up by the lymphatic system in the diaphragm, it flowed into normal mediastinal lymphatic channels and from them into the subclavian vein. It did not enter the pleural space.

Studies by Lieberman et al. (22) suggest that fluid passes directly from the peritoneal to the pleural cavity through pores in the diaphragm. These researchers introduced 500 to 1,000 mL of air into the peritoneal cavity of five patients with cirrhosis, ascites, and pleural effusions. In all five patients, a pneumothorax developed 1 to 48 hours after the induction of the pneumoperitoneum. Thoracoscopic examination was performed in three other patients after the induction of the pneumoperitoneum, and in one of these patients, air bubbles were seen coming through an otherwise undetectable diaphragmatic defect (22). At postmortem examination, diaphragmatic defects were demonstrated in two of the patients (22). More recently, Mouroux et al. (27) were able to visualize the defects in four patients during thoracoscopy.

From the foregoing studies, it is evident that the pleural fluid in these patients originates from the ascitic fluid. It is probable that the fluid passes directly into the pleural space through defects in the diaphragm. In the patient with tense ascites and increased intraabdominal pressure, the diaphragm may be stretched, causing microscopic defects. The increased hydrostatic pressure in the ascitic fluid results in a one-way transfer of fluid from the peritoneal to the pleural cavity. In some patients, transfer of ascitic fluid across the diaphragm by the lymphatic vessels may be important in the production of the pleural effusion. My experience with the placement of chest tubes in such patients leads me to believe that the direct movement of fluid is the dominant mechanism. In order to control the symptoms from large hydrothoraces in several patients with cirrhosis and ascites, I have performed tube thoracostomy, followed by the injection of a sclerosing agent. In each instance, the placement of the chest tube was followed by rapid (within minutes) diminution in the amount of ascites.

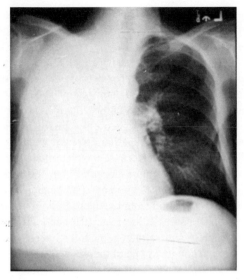

FIG. 6.1. Posteroanterior chest radiograph demonstrating a large right pleural effusion. This patient with massive ascites suddenly developed shortness of breath. A previous chest radiograph (see Fig. 3.4) had suggested a subpulmonic pleural effusion.

Clinical Manifestations

Patients with pleural effusions from cirrhosis and ascites have clinical pictures dominated by the cirrhosis and ascites. At times, these patients develop acute dyspnea in association with large pleural effusions. Although the pleural effusions may be small to moderate in size, frequently they are large and occupy the entire hemithorax (Fig. 6.1). The large effusions probably occur because the diaphragmatic defect permits fluid to flow from the peritoneal into the pleural cavity until the pleural pressure approaches the peritoneal pressure. Indeed, the pleural pressures in patients with pleural effusions secondary to ascites are higher than in patients with other transudative pleural effusions (28).

Hepatic hydrothorax is much more common on the right side than on the left side (29). On rare occasions, hepatic hydrothorax may be bilateral. It is thought that hepatic hydrothorax is more common on the right side because the right hemidiaphragm is more likely to have embryologic developmental defects (29).

Diagnosis

The diagnosis of pleural effusion secondary to cirrhosis and ascites is usually easy. Both a paracentesis and a thoracentesis should be performed to ascertain that the ascites and pleural fluid are compatible with the diagnosis and do not have high polymorphonuclear cell counts. The pleural fluid protein level is usually higher than the ascitic fluid protein level (22), but is still below 3.0 g per dL, and the pleural fluid LDH is low. The pleural fluid is occasionally blood tinged or is frankly bloody, but such findings have no significance and are probably due to the patient's poor coagulation status. The differential cell count may reveal predominantly polymorphonuclear leukocytes, small lymphocytes, or other mononuclear cells. Amylase levels should be determined and cytologic examination should be performed on both fluid specimens to rule out pancreatic ascites or malignant disease.

An occasional patient with cirrhosis will develop a hepatic hydrothorax and not have clinically evident ascites. Kakizaki et al. (30)

reviewed the literature on this subject and were able to find 28 cases. Twenty-seven cases were on the right side and only one case was on the left side, and this occurred in a patient who had a tear in the left diaphragm as a result of a splenectomy (30). The diagnosis can be established with the intraperitoneal injection of technetium 99m (^{99m}Tc)–sulfur colloid and the subsequent demonstration of radioactivity in the thorax (31).

In patients with cirrhosis, ascites, and pleural effusion, it is important to be aware of the possibility of spontaneous pleural infection, which is somewhat analogous to the spontaneous bacterial peritonitis that occurs in these patients (32). Xiol et al. (32) originally reported on 11 episodes of spontaneous pleural infection in eight patients. They used the term spontaneous bacterial empyema (32). Because the fluid does not look like pus, I prefer to use the term spontaneous bacterial pleuritis (34) to emphasize its similarity with spontaneous bacterial peritonitis. In a subsequent study, Xiol et al. (33) prospectively studied 24 episodes of spontaneous bacterial pleuritis in 16 of 120 patients (13%) admitted with a diagnosis of hepatic hydrothorax. Patients were said to have spontaneous bacterial pleuritis if they had cirrhosis along with a positive bacterial culture of the pleural fluid and a neutrophil count greater than 250 cells per mm^3 or negative culture and a neutrophil count greater than 500 cells per mm^3. Patients with pneumonia were excluded. In 14 of the 24 episodes, there was concomitant spontaneous bacterial peritonitis (33). The pleural-fluid cultures were positive in 18 patients and included eight patients with *Escherichia coli*, four patients with streptococcus species, three patients with enterococcus species, and two patients with *Streptococcus pneumoniae*. The treatment of choice is an antibiotic to which the cultured bacteria are susceptible. Tube thoracostomy is not indicated (33).

Treatment

The management of pleural effusions associated with cirrhosis and ascites should be directed toward treatment of the ascites because the hydrothorax is an extension of the peritoneal fluid. The patient should be put on a low-salt diet, and diuretics should be administered. The best diuretic therapy appears to be the combination of furosemide and spironolactone. The initial starting dose is 40 mg of furosemide and 100 mg of spironolactone. This combination appears to have the optimal ratio for the two diuretics. The doses can be increased up to 160 mg of furosemide and 400 mg of spironolactone daily (35). Serial therapeutic thoracenteses are not indicated because the pleural fluid rapidly reaccumulates.

Certain patients are refractory to salt restriction and diuretics and remain symptomatic from the presence of the large pleural effusion. In such patients, the treatment of choice is liver transplantation. The next best treatment is to implant a transjugular intrahepatic portal systemic shunt (TIPS). A recent randomized controlled study demonstrated that TIPS was a superior treatment to serial thoracentesis in patients with refractory ascites (36). In this study, 60 patients were randomly assigned to TIPS or serial thoracentesis and there was a significant survival advantage with the TIPS procedure (36). The largest series on the use of TIPS with hepatic hydrothorax was reported by Gordon and colleagues (37). In this series, 24 patients were treated and 14 of the patients had complete relief of symptoms after shunt placement and did not require further thoracentesis (37). Five additional patients required fewer thoracenteses, but the remaining five patients developed worsening liver function and died within 45 days (37).

If neither TIPS nor liver transplantation is feasible, the best alternative treatment is probably video-thoracoscopy with closure of the diaphragmatic defects and pleurodesis. In a recent report, 18 patients were subjected to 21 thoracoscopies with talc insufflation (three patients were subjected to a second procedure after the first failed) (38). Diaphragmatic defects were detected and closed in five of the 18 patients (28%). The procedure was effective in 10 of 21 patients (48%). The median hospital stay was 15 days. The precarious medical condition of patients with hepatothorax is reflected in the 30% mortality in the 3 months following the surgery (38).

Mouroux et al. (39) performed this procedure in eight patients using talc insufflation. Diaphragmatic defects were found and closed in six of the patients, and none had a recurrent pleural effusion. No defects were found in the remaining two patients, but after talc insufflation, the effusions occupied only the lower one third of the hemithorax. I do not recommend talc insufflation for the reasons discussed in Chapter 7 but would recommend pleural abrasion instead.

Although implantation of a peritoneojugular shunt might at first glance appear to be a good alternative in the management of hepatic hydrothorax, shunts frequently do not control the pleural effusion. The explanation for the ineffectiveness of the shunt is related to the pressure differences between the peritoneal cavity, the pleural space, and the systemic veins. Because the pleural pressure is less than the central venous pressure, fluid will preferentially move to the pleural space rather than to the central veins (40).

PLEURAL EFFUSION AS A COMPLICATION OF PERCUTANEOUS TRANSHEPATIC CORONARY VEIN OCCLUSION

Patients with bleeding esophageal varices are sometimes managed by injecting Gelfoam or other materials transhepatically into the coronary vein, in the hope that the injected material will lodge in the esophageal veins and will stop the bleeding. To perform this procedure, the liver is entered through the diaphragm (41). In a least one patient, a large pleural effusion requiring tube thoracostomy developed following this procedure (41). On several occasions I have observed that pleural fluid rapidly accumulates after this procedure in patients who had ascites before the procedure. I hypothesize that the pleural effusion arose because the iatrogenic diaphragmatic defect allowed the ascitic fluid to flow into the pleural space. Pleural effusions may also appear by the same mechanism after percutaneous transhepatic cholangiography.

PERITONEAL DIALYSIS

During the past 20 years, there has been an increasing use of continuous ambulatory peritoneal dialysis (CAPD) in the treatment of chronic renal failure. Pleural effusions can result from CAPD owing to the movement of the dialysate from the peritoneal cavity into the pleural cavity through a mechanism similar to that with cirrhosis and ascites. Nomoto et al. (42) reviewed 3,195 patients from 161 medical centers in Japan on CAPD. They reported that 1.6% developed this complication secondary to movement of the dialysate from the peritoneal cavity through the diaphragm into the pleural space (42). The effusion developed within 30 days of initiating the dialysis in 50% of the patients, but 18% had been on dialysis for more than a year before the effusion developed (42). The pleural effusion occurs on the right side about 90% of the time, but it can be bilateral or left sided (42). Pleural effusions can also develop as a complication of acute peritoneal dialysis (43).

The diagnosis of a pleural effusion secondary to peritoneal dialysis is usually very easy. The pleural fluid in these patients is characterized by a glucose level intermediate between that of the dialysate and the serum, a protein level below 1 g per dL, and a low LDH.

When a patient on peritoneal dialysis develops a pleural effusion, the dialysis usually must be stopped. If further peritoneal dialysis is deemed appropriate, there are two approaches. First, a tube thoracostomy can be performed with instillation of a sclerosing agent such as doxycycline (44). If this approach is taken, small-volume peritoneal dialysis can be performed for 10 to 14 days during which the pleurodesis is done (44). The second approach is to attempt to close the pleuroperitoneal communication surgically. The communications have been closed successfully using both a thoracotomy (45) and video-assisted thoracoscopy (46).

OTHER CAUSES OF TRANSUDATIVE PLEURAL EFFUSIONS

Nephrotic Syndrome

Pleural effusion is common in patients with the nephrotic syndrome. In a study of 52 patients (47), 21% had pleural effusions. With the nephrotic syndrome, the pleural effusions are usually bilateral and are frequently infrapulmonary in location (47). The mechanism responsible for the transudative pleural effusion associated with the nephrotic syndrome is probably the combination of decreased plasma oncotic pressure and increased hydrostatic pressure. The increased hydrostatic pressure is due to salt retention producing hypervolemia (48).

The diagnosis of pleural effusion secondary to the nephrotic syndrome is not difficult in the typical clinical situation. A diagnostic thoracentesis should be performed to ascertain that the pleural fluid is indeed a transudate. One should always consider the possibility of pulmonary emboli in patients with the nephrotic syndrome and pleural effusion. In one series of 36 patients with the nephrotic syndrome, 22% had pulmonary emboli (49). In addition, the nephrotic syndrome may be due to or complicated by renal vein thrombosis, and in such instances, the incidence of pulmonary emboli is high (49). A lung scan or a spiral CT scan should be obtained in all patients with the nephrotic syndrome and pleural effusion. If the lung scan or spiral CT scan is equivocal, evidence for deep venous thrombosis should be sought with venograms, impedance plethysmograms, or a pulmonary arteriogram.

The treatment of the pleural effusion associated with the nephrotic syndrome should be aimed at decreasing the protein loss in the urine to increase the plasma protein. This is best accomplished by administering angiotensin-converting enzyme inhibitors, lowering the protein content of the diet, and using nonsteroidal antiinflammatory agents cautiously (50). Serial therapeutic thoracenteses should not be performed because they only further deplete the protein stores. In selected individuals who are symptomatic from the pleural effusion, one should consider a pleurodesis with a sclerosing agent.

Superior Vena Caval Obstruction

In sheep, elevation of the pressure in the superior vena cava leads to the accumulation of pleural fluid. Allen et al. (8) demonstrated that once the pressure in the superior vena cava was elevated above 15 mm Hg, pleural fluid accumulated. The higher the pressure in the superior vena cava, the greater the fluid accumulation. The fluid was transudative in that the ratio of the pleural fluid

to serum protein was less than 0.5. These workers attributed the pleural fluid formation to either lymph leakage out of the lymphatics that pass through the chest or obstruction of lung or chest lymphatics with subsequent leakage of interstitial fluid into the pleural space.

In the clinical situation, most patients that have superior vena caval obstruction do not have a pleural effusion. If such a patient has a pleural effusion, one should try to exclude other causes such as malignant disease involving the pleura. In neonates, however, superior vena caval thrombosis is associated with the development of bilateral pleural effusions. Dhande et al. (51) reported a series of five babies who developed superior vena caval obstruction as a complication of the use of central venous catheters. The effusions occurred 7 to 19 days after the initial placement or change of a central venous catheter. All required repeated thoracenteses to remove pleural fluid that accumulated at a rate of approximately 200 mL per kg per day. The fluid was a clear transudate (protein level 1.2 to 2.2 g per dL) but became chylous when feedings were given. These workers attributed the pleural fluid accumulation to obstruction of thoracic lymph flow into the venous system. The incidence of superior vena cava thrombosis in infants who receive central venous catheters for total parenteral nutrition is about 10% (52). The infusion of urokinase is usually ineffective in treating these individuals (52).

Fontan Procedure

With the Fontan procedure, the right ventricle is bypassed by an anastomosis between the superior vena cava, the right atrium, or the inferior vena cava and the pulmonary artery (53). The procedure is typically performed for tricuspid atresia or univentricular heart. Pleural effusion is a significant problem after the Fontan procedure. Persistent pleural drainage is the primary cause of prolonged postoperative hospital stay in patients who have had a Fontan procedure (54). Zellers et al. (55) analyzed pleural fluid formation after this procedure on 46 patients. They reported that median amount of pleural drainage was 3,220 mL, with a range of 155 to 31,000 mL. Most of the patients had pleural drainage from both sides. The mean duration of the pleural fluid drainage was 14 days (54, 55).

The pathogenesis of the formation of the large amounts of pleural fluid postoperatively in these patients is not definitely known. It is probably related to the increased systemic venous pressure. It is unclear, however, whether increased pleural fluid transudation from the parietal pleura, lymphatic leakage into the pleural space (56), or hormonal changes are responsible for the large accumulations of pleural fluid. Spicer et al. (57) analyzed the factors that were related to the development of pleural effusions after the Fontan procedure in 71 patients. They found that patients with significant aortopulmonary collateral vessels evidenced by angiographic opacification of the pulmonary arteries or veins had more prolonged pleural drainage. They believed that the aortopulmonary collateral vessels contributed to volume loading of the systemic ventricle and to elevation of the pulmonary artery, and right atrial and caval pressures, all of which increase the rate of formation of the pleural fluid. When 13 patients were subjected to preoperative embolization of these vessels, the median duration of the effusion postoperatively was only 6.5 days (57).

It has been hypothesized that alterations in the hormones that regulate fluid and electrolyte homeostasis may also play a role (58). Indeed in one study, patients who developed effusions following surgery had an elevated serum renin and angiotensin compared with those who did not (58). However, the administration of captopril had no effect on pleural fluid formation in a subsequent study (54).

The optimal treatment for the patient who has prolonged pleural drainage after a Fontan procedure remains to be determined. The intrapleural administration of tetracycline at the end of the surgical procedure had no effect on the amount or the duration of the fluid drainage (55). In patients who have markedly prolonged pleural fluid drainage, consideration should be given to the implantation of a pleuroperitoneal shunt (59). Some patients have been managed successfully with medium-chain triglycerides or with pleurectomy and ligation of the thoracic duct (56).

Urinothorax

Pleural effusion can develop when there is retroperitoneal urinary leakage secondary to urinary obstruction, trauma, retroperitoneal inflammatory or malignant processes, failed nephrostomy, or kidney biopsy (60, 61). Such a pleural fluid accumulation is called a urinothorax. This is a rare cause of pleural effusions; only 21 cases had been reported by 1986 (61). The pleural effusion tends to develop within hours after the precipitating event and dissipates rapidly once the obstruction is relieved. It is believed that the urine moves retroperitoneally into the pleural space.

The diagnosis is usually easy if it is considered. The pleural fluid looks and smells like urine, and has the biochemical characteristics of a transudate. Confirmation of the diagnosis can be obtained with simultaneous measurements of the pleural fluid and creatinine levels. Only with urinothorax is the pleural fluid creatinine greater than the serum creatinine (62). The pleural fluid with a urinothorax at times has a low pH (63) or a low glucose level (62), both uncommon features with a transudative pleural effusion.

Glomerulonephritis

Patients with acute glomerulonephritis frequently have pleural effusions. In a series of 76 children, 42 (55%) had pleural effusions (64). The pleural effusions are transudative and are probably due to increased intravascular pressures because most patients have cardiomegaly or peripheral edema in addition to the pleural effusions.

Myxedema

Pleural effusions occasionally occur as a complication of myxedema. In one review of 128 patients with hypothyroidism from the Massachusetts General Hospital and the Medical University of South Carolina, pleural effusion occurred in 28 patients, but the pleural effusion was believed to be due to the hypothyroidism in only six patients (65). In one of these six patients the pleural effusion was believed to be secondary to a myxedematous pericardial effusion, whereas in the other five patients, there was no evidence of pericardial disease. When the pleural effusion occurs simultaneously with a pericardial effusion, the pleural fluid is usually a transudate (66). The isolated pleural effusion secondary to hypothyroidism can be either an exudate or a transudate (65). The diagnosis is one of exclusion in a patient with hypothyroidism. The obvious treatment for pleural effusions associated with myxedema is thyroid replacement.

Cerebrospinal Fluid Leaks to the Pleura

On rare occasions cerebrospinal fluid (CSF) can collect in the pleural space and produce a pleural effusion. This most commonly occurs following ventriculopleural shunting (67), but it can also occur when a ventriculoperitoneal shunt migrates to the pleural cavity. Traumatic subarachnoid pleural fistulas can occur with penetrating injuries and fractures of the thoracic spine. Subarachnoid pleural fistulae can also occur following thoracic spinal surgery (68, 69). The diagnosis is suggested by the characteristics of the pleural fluid, which appears to be CSF. The fluid is clear and colorless, and the protein level is very low (68, 69). At times, the diagnosis can be made by radionuclide cisternography (69).

Hypoalbuminemia

From Starling's equation (Equation 2.1), hypoalbuminemia would decrease the oncotic pressure of the blood and would increase the rate of pleural fluid formation. It is unclear how frequently hypoalbuminemia causes a pleural effusion. In patients with cirrhosis and hypoalbuminemia, the pleural effusions are related to the transdiaphragmatic transfer of ascitic fluid rather than hypoproteinemia. Eid et al. (70) reviewed the prevalence of pleural effusions in patients with serum protein levels above 3.5 g per dL, between 2.1 and 3.5 g per dL, 1.0 and 2.0 g per dL, or lower. They found that the incidence of pleural effusions was comparable in each group. In the group with serum albumin levels less than 2.0 g per dL, three of 21 had a pleural effusion and there were alternative explanations for the pleural effusions in each of these three cases. These researchers concluded that hypoalbuminemia per se is an uncommon

cause of pleural effusion. In contrast, Mattison et al. (71) attributed 8% of 62 effusions occurring in patients in a medical intensive care unit to hypoalbuminemia. However, most of these patients had other possible explanations for their pleural effusion (71).

Meigs' Syndrome

Although the pleural fluid associated with Meigs' syndrome (benign ovarian tumors with ascites and pleural effusion) is often considered a transudate (72), the pleural fluid protein levels are usually above 3.5 g per dL, (73, 74) and therefore the effusions are exudates. Accordingly, this syndrome is further discussed in Chapter 17.

Pulmonary Embolus

About 20% of the pleural effusions that occur with pulmonary embolization are transudates. This condition is discussed in detail in Chapter 14.

Sarcoidosis

This condition is occasionally accompanied by a transudative rather than an exudative pleural effusion (see Chapter 20).

REFERENCES

1. Marel M, Stastny B, Light RW. Incidence of pleural effusion in the central Bohemia region. *Chest* 1993;104:1486–1489.
2. Kataoka H, Takada S. The role of thoracic ultrasonography for evaluation of patients with decompensated chronic heart failure. *J Am Coll Cardiol* 2000;35:1638–1646.
3. Race GA, Scheifley CH, Edwards JE. Hydrothorax in congestive heart failure. *Am J Med* 1957;22:83–89.
4. Wiener-Kronish JP, Broaddus VC. Interrelationship of pleural and pulmonary interstitial liquid. *Annu Rev Physiol* 1993;55:209–226.
5. Bhattacharya J, Gropper MA, Staub NC. Interstitial fluid pressure gradient measured by micropuncture in excised dog lung. *J Appl Physiol* 1984;56:271–277.
6. Broaddus VC, Wiener-Kronish JP, Staub NC. Clearance of lung edema into the pleural space of volume-loaded anesthetized sheep. *J Appl Physiol* 1990;68;2623–2630.
7. Broaddus VC, Wiener-Kronish JP, Berthiaume Y, et al. Removal of pleural liquid and protein by lymphatics in awake sheep. *J Appl Physiol* 1988;64:384–390.

8. Allen SJ, Laine GA, Drake RE, et al. Superior vena caval pressure elevation causes pleural effusion formation in sheep. *Am J Physiol* 1988;255:H492-H495.

9. Wiener-Kronish JP, Matthay MA, Callen PW, et al. Relationship of pleural effusions of pulmonary hemodynamics in patients with congestive heart failure. *Am Rev Respir Dis* 1985;132:1253–1256.

10. Wiener-Kronish JP, Goldstein R, Matthay RA, et al. Lack of association of pleural effusion with chronic pulmonary arterial and right atrial hypertension. *Chest* 1987;92:967–970.

11. Rabin CB, Blackman NS. Bilateral pleural effusion: its significance in association with a heart of normal size. *J Mt Sinai Hosp* 1957;24:45–63.

12. Peterman TA, Brothers SK. Pleural effusions in congestive heart failure and in pericardial disease. *N Engl J Med* 1983;309:313.

13. Weiss JM, Spodick DH. Laterality of pleural effusions in chronic congestive heart failure. *Am J Cardiol* 1984;53:951.

14. Chakko SC, Caldwell SH, Sforza PP. Treatment of congestive heart failure: its effect on pleural fluid chemistry. *Chest* 1989;95:978–982.

15. Shinto RA, Light RW. The effects of diuresis upon the characteristics of pleural fluid in patients with congestive heart failure. *Am J Med* 1990;88:230–233.

16. Light RW, MacGregor MI, Luchsinger PC, et al. Pleural effusions: the diagnostic separation of transudates and exudates. *Ann Intern Med* 1972;77:507–513.

17. Light RW, Erozan YS, Ball WC. Cells in pleural fluid: their value in differential diagnosis. *Arch Intern Med* 1973;132:854–860.

18. Burgess LJ, Maritz FJ, Taljaard JJ. Comparative analysis of the biochemical parameters used to distinguish between pleural transudates and exudates. *Chest* 1995;107:1604–1609.

19. Glazer M, Berkman N, Lafair JS, et al. Successful talc slurry pleurodesis in patients with nonmalignant pleural effusion. *Chest* 2000;117:1404–1409.

20. Vargas FS, Wang N-S, Lee HM, et al. Effectiveness of bleomycin in comparison to tetracycline as pleural sclerosing agent in rabbits. *Chest* 1993;104:1582–1584.

21. Little AG, Kodowaki MH, Ferguson MK, et al. Pleuroperitoneal shunting. Alternative therapy for pleural effusions. *Ann Surg* 1988;208:443–450.

22. Lieberman FL, Hidemura R, Peters RL, et al. Pathogenesis and treatment of hydrothorax complicating cirrhosis with ascites. *Ann Intern Med* 1966;64:341–351.

23. Johnston RF, Loo RV. Hepatic hydrothorax: studies to determine the source of the fluid and report of thirteen cases. *Ann Intern Med* 1964;61:385–401.

24. Rubinstein D, McInnes IE, Dudley FJ. Hepatic hydrothorax in the absence of clinical ascites: diagnosis and management. *Gastroenterology* 1985;88:188–191.

25. Mellins RB, Levine OR, Fishman AP. Effect of systemic and pulmonary venous hypertension on pleural and pericardial fluid accumulation. *J Appl Physiol* 1970;29:564–569.

26. Datta N, Mishkin FS, Vasinrapee P, et al. Radionuclide demonstration of peritoneal-pleural communication as a cause for pleural fluid. *JAMA* 1984;252:210.

27. Mouroux J, Hebuterne X, Perrin C, et al. Treatment of pleural effusion of cirrhotic origin by videothoracoscopy. *Br J Surg* 1994;81:546–547.

28. Light RW, Jenkinson SG, Minh V, et al. Observations on pleural pressures as fluid is withdrawn during thoracentesis. *Am Rev Respir Dis* 1980;121:799–804.

29. Lazaridis KN, Frank JW, Krowka MJ, et al. Hepatic hydrothorax: pathogenesis, diagnosis, and management. *Am J Med* 1999;107:262-267.

30. Kakizaki S, Katakai K, Yoshinaga T, et al. Hepatic hydrothorax in the absence of ascites. *Liver* 1998;18:216–220.

31. Daly JJ, Potts JM, Gordon L, et al. Scintigraphic diagnosis of peritoneo-pleural communication in the absence of ascites. *Clin Nucl Med* 1994;19:892–894.

32. Xiol X, Castellote J, Baliellas C, et al. Spontaneous bacterial empyema in cirrhotic patients: analysis of eleven cases. *Hepatology* 1990;11:365–370.

33. Xiol X, Castellvi JM, Guardiola J, et al. Spontaneous bacterial empyema in cirrhotic patients: a prospective study. *Hepatology* 1996;23:719–723.

34. Light RW, Broaddus VC. Pleural effusion. In: Murray JF, Nadel JA, eds. *Textbook of respiratory medicine.* Philadelphia: W.B. Saunders, 2000:2013–2042.

35. Runyon BA. Care of patients with ascites. *N Engl J Med* 1994;330:337–342.

36. Rossle M, Ochs A, Gulberg V, et al. A comparison of paracentesis and transjugular intrahepatic portosystemic shunting in patients with ascites. *N Engl J Med* 2000;342:1701–1707.

37. Gordon FD, Anastopoulos HT, Crenshaw W, et al. The successful treatment of symptomatic, refractory hepatic hydrothorax with transjugular intrahepatic portosystemic shunt. *Hepatology* 1997;25:1366–1369.

38. Milanez de Campos JR, Filho LOA, Werebe EC, et al. Thoracoscopy and talc poudrage in the management of hepatic hydrothorax. *Chest* 2000;118:13–17.

39. Mouroux J, Perrin C, Venissac N, et al. Management of pleural effusion of cirrhotic origin. *Chest* 1996;109:1093–1096.

40. Ikard RW, Sawyers JL. Persistent hepatic hydrothorax after peritoneojugular shunt. *Arch Surg* 1980;115:1125–1127.

41. Widrich WC, Johnson WC, Robbins AH, et al. Esophagogastric variceal hemorrhage: its treatment by percutaneous transhepatic coronary vein occlusion. *Arch Surg* 1978;113:1331–1338.

42. Nomoto Y, Suga T, Nakajima K, et al. Acute hydrothorax in continuous ambulatory peritoneal dialysis—a collaborative study of 161 centers. *Am J Nephrol* 1989;9:363–367.

43. Rudnick MR, Coyle JF, Beck LH, et al. Acute massive hydrothorax complicating peritoneal dialysis, report of 2 cases and a review of the literature. *Clin Nephrol* 1979;12:38–44.

44. Chow CC, Sung JY, Cheung CK, et al. Massive hydrothorax in continuous ambulatory peritoneal dialysis: diagnosis, management and review of the literature. *N Z Med J* 1988;27:475–477.

45. Allen SM, Matthews HR. Surgical treatment of massive hydrothorax complicating continuous ambulatory peritoneal dialysis. *Clin Nephrol* 1991;36:299–301.

46. Di Bisceglie M, Paladini P, Voltolini L, et al. Videothoracoscopic obliteration of pleuroperitoneal fistula in continuous peritoneal dialysis. *Ann Thorac Surg* 1996;62:1509–1510.

47. Cavina C, Vichi G. Radiological aspects of pleural effusions in medical nephropathy in children. *Ann Radiol Diagn* 1958;31:163–202.

48. Kinasewitz GT. Transudative effusions. *Eur Respir J* 1997;10:714–718.
49. Llach F, Arieff AI, Massry SG. Renal vein thrombosis and nephrotic syndrome: a prospective study of 36 adult patients. *Ann Intern Med* 1975;83:8–14.
50. Palmer BF. Southwestern internal medicine conference: nephrotic edema—pathogenesis and treatment. *Am J Med Sci* 1993;306:53–67.
51. Dhande V, Kattwinkel J, Alford B. Recurrent bilateral pleural effusions secondary to superior vena cava obstruction as a complication of central venous catheterization. *Pediatrics* 1983;72:109–113.
52. Swaniker F, Fonkalsrud EW. Superior and inferior vena caval occlusion in infants receiving total parenteral nutrition. *Am Surg* 1995;61:877–881.
53. Laks H, Milliken JC, Perloff JK, et al. Experience with the Fontan procedure. *J Thorac Cardiovasc Surg* 1984;88:939–951.
54. Heragu N, Mahony L. Is captopril useful in decreasing pleural drainage in children after modified Fontan operation? *Am J Cardiol* 1999;84:1109–1112.
55. Zellers TM, Driscoll DJ, Humes RA, et al. Glenn shunt: effect on pleural drainage after modified Fontan operation. *J Thorac Cardiovasc Surg* 1989;98:725–729.
56. van de Wal HJ, Tanke RF, Roef MJ. The modified Senning operation for cavopulmonary connection with autologous tissue. *J Thorac Cardiovasc Surg* 1994;108:377–380.
57. Spicer RL, Uzark KC, Moore JW, et al. Aortopulmonary collateral vessels and prolonged pleural effusions after modified Fontan procedures. *Am Heart J* 1996;131:1164–1168.
58. Mainwaring RD, Lamberti JJ, Carter TL Jr, et al. Renin, angiotensin II, and the development of effusions following bidirectional Glenn and Fontan procedures. *J Card Surg* 1995;10:111–118.
59. Sade RM, Wiles HB. Pleuroperitoneal shunt for persistent pleural drainage after Fontan procedure. *J Thorac Cardiovasc Surg* 1990;100:621–623.
60. Belie JA, Milan D. Pleural effusion secondary to ureteral obstruction. *Urology* 1979;14:27–29.
61. Sulcate JR. Urinothorax: report of 4 cases and review of the literature. *J Urol* 1986;135:805–808.
62. Stark D, Shades J, Baron RL, et al. Biochemical features of urinothorax. *Arch Intern Med* 1982;142:1509–1511.
63. Miller KS, Wooden S, Sahn SA. Urinothorax: a cause of low pH transudative pleural effusions. *Am J Med* 1988;85:448–449.
64. Kirkpatrick JA Jr, Fleisher DS. The roentgen appearance of the chest in acute glomerulonephritis in children. *J Pediatr* 1964;64:492–498.
65. Gottehrer A, Roa J, Stanford GG, et al. Hypothyroidism and pleural effusions. *Chest* 1990;98:1130–1132.
66. Smolar EN, Rubin JE, Avramides A, et al. Cardiac tamponade in primary myxedema and review of the literature. *Am J Med Sci* 1976;272:345–352.
67. Beach C, Manthey DE. Tension hydrothorax due to ventriculopleural shunting. *J Emerg Med* 1998;16:33–36.
68. Monla-Hassan J, Eichenhorn M, Spickler E, et al. Duropleural fistula manifested as a large pleural transudate: an unusual complication of transthoracic diskectomy. *Chest* 1998;114:1786–1789.
69. Gupta SM, Frias J, Garg A, et al. Aberrant cerebrospinal fluid pathway. Detection by scintigraphy. *Clin Nucl Med* 1986;11:593–594.
70. Eid AA, Keddissi JI, Kinasewitz GT. Hypoalbuminemia as a cause of pleural effusions. *Chest* 1999;115:1066–1069.
71. Mattison LE, Coppage L, Alderman DF, et al. Pleural effusion in the medical ICU. Prevalence, causes and clinical implications. *Chest* 1997;111:1018–1023.
72. Lowell JR. *Pleural effusions. A comprehensive review.* Baltimore: University Park Press, 1977.
73. Neustadt JE, Levy RC. Hemorrhagic pleural effusion in Meigs' syndrome. *JAMA* 1968;204:179–180.
74. Solomon S, Farber SJ, Caruso LJ. Fibromyomata of the uterus with hemothorax. Meigs' syndrome? *Arch Intern Med* 1971;127:307–309.

7

Pleural Effusions Related to Metastatic Malignancies

INCIDENCE

Malignant disease involving the pleura is the second leading cause of exudative pleural effusions after parapneumonic effusions. Because many parapneumonic effusions are small and are not subjected to thoracentesis, malignancy is probably the leading cause of exudative effusions subjected to thoracentesis. In our series from Baltimore, 42% of 102 exudative pleural effusions were due to malignant disease (1). In an epidemiologic study from the Czech Republic, malignancy accounted for 24% of all the pleural effusions (2).

Carcinomas of the lung and breast and lymphomas account for approximately 75% of malignant pleural effusions (Table 7.1). Metastatic ovarian carcinoma is the fourth leading cause of malignant pleural effusions, whereas sarcomas, particularly melanoma, account for a small percentage of malignant pleural effusions. No other single tumor accounts for more than 1% of malignant pleural effusions. In about 6% of patients with malignant pleural effusions, the primary tumor is not identified (3, 4).

Lung Cancer

In most series, lung cancer is the leading cause of malignant pleural effusion (5). When patients with lung cancer are first evaluated, about 15% have a pleural effusion (6). During the course of this disease, however, at least 50% of patients with disseminated lung cancer develop a pleural effusion. Pleural effusions occur with all the cell types of lung carcinoma but appear to be most frequent with adenocarcinoma (5, 7). The incidence of pleural effusions in patients with small cell lung carcinoma is about 10% (8). Patients with lung cancer who have anti-p53 antibodies are more likely to have pleural effusions. In one series, nine of 10 patients (90%) with this antibody had pleural effusions, whereas 42 of 115 patients (36%) without the antibody had a pleural effusion (9).

At times, pleural effusions develop in patients who have undergone resection for adenocarcinoma. The incidence of pleural effusion is higher if there is either lymph node or pleural involvement by tumor at the time of surgery (10). In one series 18 of 19 patients who developed a cytology positive pleural effusion after resection had either lymph node metastases, pleural involvement, or both (10). The median time from resection to diagnosis of malignant pleural effusion was 8 months. Most effusions that develop more than 24 months after surgery are due to another primary (10).

It is important to emphasize that the presence of a pleural effusion in a patient with lung cancer almost always indicates that the patient is not curable with surgery whether or not the cytology is positive. Sugiura and associates (11) reviewed 197 patients with stage IIIB or IV non–small cell lung cancer. They reported that the survival for stage IIIB without effusion, stage IIIB with effusion and stage IV were 15.3, 7.5, and 5.5 months, respectively (11). The survival was similar whether the pleural fluid cytology was positive or negative (11). It has been suggested that patients with lung cancer and pleural

TABLE 7.1. *Causes of malignant pleural effusions in two different series*

Tumor	Spriggs and Boddington[a]		Anderson et al.[b]	
	n	%	*n*	%
Lung carcinoma	275	43	32	24
Breast carcinoma	157	25	35	26
Lymphoma and leukemia	52	8	34	26
Ovarian carcinoma	27	4	9	7
Sarcoma (including melanoma)	13	2	5	4
Uterine and cervical carcinoma	6	1	3	2
Stomach carcinoma	18	3	1	1
Colon carcinoma	9	1	0	0
Pancreatic carcinoma	7	1	0	0
Bladder carcinoma	7	1	0	0
Other carcinoma	23	4	6	4
Primary unknown	40	6	8	6
Total	634		133	

[a]From Spriggs AI, Boddington MM. *The cytology of effusions,* 2nd ed. New York: Grune & Stratton, 1968, with permission.
[b]From Anderson CB, Philpott GW, Ferguson TB. The treatment of malignant pleural effusions. *Cancer* 1974;33:916–922, with permission.

effusion be classified as stage IV (12). Another study also demonstrated that with multivariate analysis, the presence of a pleural effusion at the time of diagnosis adversely affected prognosis (6).

How should the patient with bronchogenic carcinoma and an ipsilateral cytology-negative pleural effusion be evaluated? Rodriguez-Panadero (13) performed thoracoscopy on 21 patients with lung cancer and an ipsilateral cytology-negative pleural effusion. At thoracoscopy, only five patients were believed to be potentially resectable, but when these five were subjected to thoracotomy, their tumors were found to be unresectable due to mediastinal invasion (13). In another older study from the Mayo Clinic, five of 73 patients with bronchogenic carcinoma and ipsilateral cytology-negative pleural effusions had long-term survival after the lung cancer was resected (14). In view of the above-mentioned two studies, it is recommended that patients with bronchogenic carcinoma and an ipsilateral cytology-negative pleural effusion undergo thoracoscopy. If the thoracoscopy is negative, a computed tomography (CT) scan of the chest should be obtained to evaluate the mediastinal lymph nodes. If the CT scan demonstrates lymph node enlargement, a mediastinoscopy should be performed. If the CT scan demonstrates no lymph node enlargement and the thoracoscopy is negative, consideration should be given to an exploratory thoracotomy if the patient has no other contraindication to curative resection.

Breast Carcinoma

The second leading cause of malignant pleural effusion is metastatic breast carcinoma. Fracchia et al. (15) reviewed 601 patients with disseminated breast carcinoma and found that 48% had pleural effusions. The effusions were large enough to warrant therapeutic intervention in 48% of the patients. Goldsmith et al. (16) reviewed the autopsies of 365 patients who had died of disseminated breast carcinoma and reported that 46% had pleural effusions. Pleural effusions were more common with lymphangitic spread (63%) than without lymphangitic spread (41%) (16). In this series, the pleural effusions were on the same side as the primary breast carcinoma in 58% of these patients, on the opposite side in 26%, and on both sides in 16% (16). In a second series, the effusion was ipsilateral in 70%, contralateral in 20%, and bilateral in 10% (17). Ipsilateral effusions are less common if radiotherapy was part of the initial treatment (18). With breast carcinoma, the mean interval between the development of the primary tumor and the appearance of the pleural effusion is about 2 years (18), but this interval can be as long as 20 years (19). In patients with pleural effusions secondary to breast carcinoma, determination of the steroid receptors in the effusion does not appear to be useful in planning therapy (20).

Lymphomas

Lymphomas, including Hodgkin's disease, are the third leading cause of malignant pleural effusions. The incidence of pleural effusion with Hodgkin's disease at presentation is about 7% (21). During the course of the disease the incidence of pleural effusion is about 16% (22). Patients with Hodgkin's disease who have pleural effusions almost invariably have intrathoracic lymph node involvement, frequently without microscopic pleural involvement (23). Most patients with Hodgkin's disease and pleural effusion have the nodular sclerosis type (24). Only about 3% of the effusions present with Hodgkin's disease are chylothoraces.

The incidence of pleural effusion at presentation in non-Hodgkin's lymphoma is 6% to 13% (21, 25). With this neoplasm, 20% to 70% have evidence of mediastinal disease and 90% have evidence of disease elsewhere. For non-Hodgkin's lymphoma, large cell lymphomas more frequently have associated pleural disease than do small cell lymphomas (24). The presence of a pleural effusion at the time of presentation does not adversely affect complete remission or survival rates with non-Hodgkin's lymphoma (26). The cytology on the pleural fluid is positive in almost all cases (25, 26). Approximately 20% of the effusions present with non-Hodgkin's lymphomas are chylothoraces (25).

Vieta and Craver (22) also reported that 12% of 158 patients with lymphatic leukemia and 4% of 52 patients with myelogenous leukemia had pleural effusions. Parietal pleural involvement was uncommon at autopsy with leukemia, however.

PATHOPHYSIOLOGIC FEATURES

A malignant tumor can directly or indirectly lead to a pleural effusion in several different ways (Table 7.2). Although it is frequently written that

TABLE 7.2. *Mechanisms by which malignant disease leads to pleural effusions*

Direct result
  Pleural metastases with increased permeability
  Pleural metastases with obstruction of pleural lymphatic vessels
  Mediastinal lymph node involvement with decreased pleural lymphatic drainage
  Thoracic duct interruption (chylothorax)
  Bronchial obstruction (decreased pleural pressures)
  Pericardial involvement

Indirect result
  Hypoproteinemia
  Postobstructive pneumonitis
  Pulmonary embolism
  Postradiation therapy

lymphatic obstruction is the primary pathophysiologic abnormality responsible for the pleural effusion with malignancy, this appears to not be true (27). The basis for the contention that lymphatic obstruction is responsible is the observation that at postmortem studies, the presence of pleural effusions is correlated with metastases to the lymph nodes (28). However, the normal rate of pleural fluid formation is thought to be only 15 mL per day. Therefore, if there were complete blockage of the lymphatics, the rate of pleural fluid accumulation should only be 15 mL per day. Certainly, the rate of pleural fluid accumulation with pleural malignancy frequently exceeds this (29). Moreover, if the fluid accumulation was solely due to lymphatic obstruction, one would expect the fluid to be a transudate rather than an exudate, which it almost always is.

We believe that the most common explanation for the pleural effusion with metastatic disease to the pleura is increased permeability of the pleura (27). Indeed, in the series of Leckie and Tothill (30), a patient with bronchogenic carcinoma had the second highest amount of protein entering the pleural space of the 40 patients studied. The mechanism by which pleural metastases increase the permeability of the pleura is not definitely known. However, we postulate that it is due to the production of vascular endothelial growth factor (VEGF) by the tumor (27). Indeed, the median level of VEGF in pleural effusions secondary to malignancy is much higher than that in patients with effusions secondary to congestive heart failure (31). VEGF is one of the most potent agents known for increasing vascular permeability (32). Yano et al. have developed an animal model of a malignant pleural effusion by injecting human adenocarcinoma cells into the pleural space of nude mice (33). The formation of pleural fluid in this model is markedly reduced if the animals are given an inhibitor of the VEGF receptor (33).

It is likely that lymphatic blockade and the resulting decreased clearance of fluid from the pleural space contributes to the accumulation of pleural fluid, although for the reasons outlined earlier, this is not the predominant mechanism in most cases. Leckie and Tothill (30) reported that the mean amount of protein leaving the pleural space in patients with malignant pleural effusions was less than that leaving the pleural space in patients with tuberculosis, pulmonary embolism, or congestive heart failure. This decreased lymphatic drainage can occur through two separate mechanisms. First, because the fluid leaves the pleural space through stomas in the lymphatic vessels in the parietal pleura (34), metastases to the parietal pleura that obstruct these stomas can decrease fluid clearance. Second, the lymphatic vessels of the parietal pleura drain mainly through the mediastinal lymph nodes. Therefore, neoplastic involvement of the mediastinal lymph nodes can decrease the lymphatic clearance of the pleural space.

Malignant tumors can also produce pleural effusions by obstructing the thoracic duct, in which case the resulting pleural effusion is a chylothorax. In fact, most chylothoraces that are not traumatic in origin are secondary to neoplastic involvement of the thoracic duct. Lymphomas are responsible for 75% of chylothoraces secondary to malignant disease (see Chapter 23).

Another mechanism by which malignant tumors produce pleural effusion is through bronchial obstruction. When a neoplasm obstructs the mainstem bronchus or a lobar bronchus, the lung distal to the obstruction becomes atelectatic. Therefore, the remaining lung must overexpand or the ipsilateral hemithorax must contract to compensate for the loss of volume of the atelectatic lung. These events result in a more negative pleural pressure, and it is easy to see from Fig. 2.1 that such a negative pleural pressure causes pleural fluid to accumulate. My associates and I studied a patient with obstruction of the bronchus intermedius in whom the pleural pressure dropped from -12 to -48 cm H_2O as 200 mL pleural fluid was removed (35).

Pericardial involvement is frequent with metastatic malignant diseases. When a pericardial effusion is caused by such involvement and hydrostatic pressures become elevated in the systemic and pulmonary circulation, transudative pleural effusions may result.

Not all pleural effusions in patients with malignant disease are related to intrathoracic involvement by the neoplasm. Pulmonary infection distal to a partially or totally occluded bronchus may produce a parapneumonic effusion (see Chapter 9). The incidence of pulmonary embolization is higher in patients with malignant disease, and emboli can cause pleural effusions (see Chapter 14). Patients with intrathoracic neoplasms frequently receive radiotherapy for their tumors, and this treatment can also result in pleural effusions (see Chapter 20), as can some types of chemotherapy (see Chapter 19). Many patients with malignant disease are malnourished and have hypoproteinemia, and this disorder can lead on rare occasions to the formation of transudative pleural effusions (see Chapter 6).

AUTOPSY STUDIES

The most detailed autopsy series on pleural involvement in malignant disease are those of Meyer (28) and Rodriguez-Panadero et al. (36). It appears that pleural metastases with bronchogenic carcinoma are usually due to pulmonary arterial emboli to the ipsilateral pleura. Virtually all patients with metastatic pleural involvement from lung carcinoma have involvement of the visceral pleura (28, 36). In the series of Rodriguez-Panadero and associates, pulmonary vascular invasion by the tumor was found in 19 of the 24 cases (36). Parietal pleural metastases result from direct extension from the visceral pleura (28, 36).

In patients with nonbronchogenic carcinoma, the visceral pleural is almost always involved also. Involvement of the parietal pleura again appears to result from direct extension from the visceral pleura (28, 36). The origin of these metastases is controversial. Meyer attributed them to tertiary spread from secondary hepatic tumors (28). In his series of 23 patients with pleural metastases, 19 (83%) had hepatic metastases. In the series by Rodriguez-Panadero et al., however, hepatic metastases could be demonstrated only in 71% of the patients and they attributed the visceral pleural metastases to blood-borne metastases from the primary (36). The latter explanation appears more plausible to me. The presence of pleural metastases does indicate systemic dissemination of the disease and renders the patient incurable with surgery alone.

Not all patients with pleural metastases have pleural effusions. In Meyer's series, only 60% of patients with pleural metastases had pleural effusion (28). In Rodriguez-Panadero's study only 30 of 55 patients (55%) with metastatic disease to the pleura had pleural effusion (36). Meyer found that the presence of a pleural effusion was more closely related to neoplastic invasion of the mediastinal lymph nodes than to the extent of pleural involvement by nodular metastases (28).

CLINICAL MANIFESTATIONS

The most common symptom reported by patients with malignant pleural effusions is dyspnea, which occurs in more than 50% (7). Symptoms attributable to the tumor itself are also frequent. In one series, weight loss occurred in 32%, malaise in 21%, and anorexia in 14% of patients (7). When patients with malignant pleural effusions are compared with those with benign pleural effusions, patients with malignant pleural effusions are more likely to have dull chest pain (34% versus 11%), whereas patients with benign disease are more likely to have pleuritic chest pain (51% versus 24%) (37). Temperature elevations are significantly more common in patients with benign disease (73%) than in patients with malignant disease (37%) (37).

Chest Radiographs

The size of a malignant pleural effusion varies from a few milliliters to several liters, with the fluid occupying the entire hemithorax and shifting the mediastinum to the contralateral side.

Malignant disease is the most common cause of a massive pleural effusion and accounted for 31 of 46 (67%) of effusions occupying an entire hemithorax in one series (38).

Almost all patients with pleural effusions secondary to bronchogenic carcinoma have radiographically demonstrable pulmonary abnormalities besides the effusion. At times, a therapeutic thoracentesis must be performed before the pulmonary abnormality is evident. Although almost all patients with pleural effusions secondary to lymphoma have mediastinal lymph node involvement at autopsy, this involvement is not always evident in chest radiographs (22). In a series of 22 patients with chylothorax due to lymphoma, only five patients (23%) had hilar or mediastinal adenopathy demonstrable on routine chest radiographs (39). In another series, however, 71% of 21 patients with pleural effusions secondary to lymphoma had visible mediastinal lymph node involvement on chest radiographs (40). In a third series of 19 patients with non-Hodgkin's lymphoma, only four patients had mediastinal lymphadenopathy (41). The chest radiographs of patients with pleural effusions due to malignant tumors other than lung carcinoma or lymphoma often reveal only a pleural effusion. In a series of 105 patients with pleural effusion due to breast carcinoma (19), only 9% had radiographically evident pulmonary metastases.

In certain instances, the chest CT scan is useful in patients with malignant pleural effusion. O'Donovan and Eng (42) reviewed the CT findings in 86 patients with documented malignant effusions. They reported the following incidences of concurrent abnormalities: pericardial effusion, 3%; pericardial thickening, 14%; mediastinal adenopathy, 43%; chest wall involvement, 12%; lymphangitic carcinoma, 7%; and suspicious lung masses, nodules, or infiltrates, 53%.

Pleural Fluid

The pleural fluid from a malignant pleural effusion is almost always an exudate (43, 44). Ashchi et al. (45) reviewed the medical records of 171 patients with malignant pleural effusion and found that in eight of the cases, the fluid was transudative. There were alternative explanations for the transudative effusions in seven of the eight cases (45). In another study, 97 of 98 patients with malignant pleural effusions had exudates (44). The ratio of the pleural fluid to the serum protein level is less than 0.5 in about 20% of malignant pleural effusions (7, 43), but the lactic dehydrogenase (LDH) ratio exceeds 0.6 or the absolute pleural fluid LDH meets exudative criteria in this 20% (43). Most pleural effusions that meet exudative criteria by the LDH level but not by the protein level are malignant pleural effusions (43).

The presence of grossly bloody pleural fluid (red blood cell count greater than 100,000 per mm^3) suggests malignant pleural disease. In our series of 22 such effusions, 12 (55%) of the bloody pleural effusions were due to malignant disease (1). Nearly 50% of malignant pleural effusions, however, have red blood cell counts under 10,000 per mm^3 and do not appear bloody (1). The pleural fluid white blood cell count with malignant pleural effusion is variable, with the usual count between 1,000 and 10,000 per mm^3 (1). The predominant cells in the pleural fluid differential white cell count of these effusions are lymphocytes in about 45%, other mononuclear cells in about 40%, and polymorphonuclear leukocytes in about 15% (1). Although in the past it was stated that pleural fluid eosinophilia (>10%) made pleural malignancy unlikely, two recent studies suggest that the presence of pleural fluid eosinophilia does not decrease the likelihood that the patient has malignancy (46, 47).

The pleural fluid glucose level is reduced to below 60 mg per dL in approximately 15% to 20% of malignant pleural effusions (48–50). A low pleural fluid glucose in association with a malignant pleural effusion indicates that the patient has a high tumor burden in the pleural space. Rodriguez-Panadero and Lopez-Mejias (50) performed thoracoscopy on 77 patients with a malignant pleural effusion and found that the extent of the tumor was significantly greater in those with a low pleural fluid glucose. Cytology and pleural biopsy are more likely to be positive in patients with low-glucose pleural effusions (50). Because of the large tumor burden, patients with a low pleural fluid glucose level have a poorer prognosis (51). It appears that the low glucose

levels with malignant pleural effusion are due to impaired glucose transfer from blood to pleural fluid (52). Increased glucose utilization by the pleural tumor probably also plays a role in producing the low pleural fluid glucose.

Approximately one third of patients with malignant pleural effusions have a pleural fluid pH below 7.3 (50, 53, 54). Patients with a low pleural fluid pH also tend to have a low pleural glucose (50, 54). As one might anticipate, they have a greater tumor burden, are more likely to have positive pleural fluid cytology and pleural biopsy, and have a shorter survival than individuals with malignant pleural effusions and a pH level above 7.3 (50, 54). The pathogenesis of the low pH with malignant pleural effusions appears to be due to the combination of acid production by the pleural fluid or the pleura and a block to the movement of carbon dioxide out of the pleural space (52).

Approximately 10% of patients with malignant pleural effusions have an elevated pleural fluid amylase level (49). Usually, the primary tumor is not in the pancreas in these patients (49, 55). Analysis of the amylase isoenzymes has demonstrated that the amylase in malignant effusions is the salivary isoenzyme rather than the pancreatic isoenzyme (56), and therefore amylase isoenzyme analysis can be used to differentiate pancreatic effusions from malignant effusions.

DIAGNOSIS

The diagnosis of a malignant pleural effusion is established by demonstrating malignant cells in the pleural fluid or in the pleura itself. In most cases, this is done by cytologic examination of the pleural fluid or biopsy of the pleura.

Cytologic Examination

The characteristics of malignant cells in pleural fluid are described in Chapter 4. The percentage of cases in which cytologic study of the pleural fluid establishes the diagnosis of a malignant pleural effusion ranges from 40% to 87% (57–61). The reasons for this variability in the diagnostic yield with cytologic study are discussed in Chapter 4. When three separate pleural fluid specimens from a patient with malignant pleural disease are submitted to an experienced cytologist, one should expect a positive diagnosis in about 80% of patients. The incidence of positive results depends on the primary tumor. Most cases of metastatic adenocarcinoma can be diagnosed by pleural fluid cytology. Positive results are uncommon with squamous cell carcinoma because the pleural effusions are usually due to bronchial obstruction or lymphatic blockade (1, 3, 62). With lymphoma, the cytologic test is positive in about 25% of patients with Hodgkin's disease and in 50% to 60% of patients with non-Hodgkin's lymphoma. By cytologic examination, the neoplasm can usually be classified into a histologic type such as adenocarcinoma, but the primary site of the tumor cannot usually be identified (62).

Immunohistochemical Tests

The use of monoclonal antibodies directed against various antigens is useful in distinguishing malignant from benign pleural effusions (63). Metastatic adenocarcinomas tend to stain positive with carcinoembryonic antigen (CEA), MOC-3,1, B72.3, and BG-8 (63), whereas reactive mesothelial cells or malignant mesothelial cells do not stain positive with any of these monoclonal antibodies (see Chapter 4). Over 95% of adenocarcinomas will stain positive for at least two of the above-mentioned four antigens, whereas almost no mesotheliomas stain positive for more than one (64). The technology with these monoclonal antibodies is likely to improve, and it is recommended that all laboratories that deal with significant numbers of pleural fluids develop the capability to perform these immunohistochemical tests.

Tumor Markers in Pleural Fluid

In the past decade, there have been many articles purporting to show the usefulness of tumor markers in establishing the diagnosis of malignant pleural effusions. Tumor markers evaluated have included CEA; carbohydrate antigens 15-3, 19-9, and 72-4 (65); neuron-specific enolase (65); squamous cell carcinoma (SCC) antigen; cytokeratin 19 fragments (CYFRA21-1) (65, 66); and sialyl state-specific mouse embryonic antigen (SSEA-1) (67). Although the levels of tumor markers in the pleural fluid are significantly higher in malignant effusions than in benign effusions, there is almost always some overlap (65). In order for tumor markers to be useful in the diagnosis of malignant effusions, they have to be 100% specific. One does not want to misdiagnose a benign pleural effusion as a malignant effusion and inform the patient that they only have several months to live. In view of the above-mentioned reasons, the use of tumor markers for the diagnosis of pleural malignancy is not recommended.

Pleural Biopsy

Needle biopsy of the pleura can establish the diagnosis of a malignant pleural effusion. The percentage of positive pleural biopsies in patients with malignant pleural disease ranges from 39% to 75% (60, 68, 69). In general, pleural fluid cytology is superior to pleural biopsy in establishing the diagnosis of pleural malignancy. Pleural biopsy has a lower diagnostic yield than pleural fluid cytologic examination because, in about 50% of patients with malignant pleural disease, the costal parietal pleura is not involved (70). In one large series of 281 patients with malignant pleural disease, the cytology was positive for malignant cells in 162 patients (58%), whereas the pleural biopsy was positive in 123 (44%) (60). The diagnosis of malignancy was established by pleural biopsy alone in only 20 of the 281 patients (7.1%) (60). Another way to look at this series is to consider the 118 patients with malignancy but negative cytology. Pleural biopsy established the diagnosis of malignancy in only 20 of these 118 patients (17%).

What is the role of needle biopsy of the pleura in establishing the diagnosis of malignant pleural effusion in the twenty-first century? Because thoracoscopy is very effective at establishing this diagnosis and because the needle biopsy is diagnostic in less than 20% of patients with malignancy and negative cytology, I rarely perform needle biopsy of the pleura. Certainly, if the cytology is negative and thoracoscopy is unavailable or an outpatient procedure is desired, consideration can be given to performing needle biopsy of the pleura.

Observation Thoracoscopy or Open Thoracotomy?

In many patients with exudative pleural effusions, no diagnosis is apparent after the initial diagnostic thoracentesis including pleural fluid cytology and a marker in the pleural fluid for tuberculosis. In such instances, a spiral CT scan of the chest is recommended. If pulmonary emboli are demonstrated with the CT scan, the etiology of the effusion is established. If parenchymal abnormalities are present, a bronchoscopy should be performed. If the CT scan suggests mesothelioma, then thoracoscopy should be performed to establish this diagnosis.

If the CT scan shows nothing other than the pleural effusion, the approach to the patient should be governed by the clinical picture. If there is nothing in the patient's history to suggest carcinoma and if the patient's symptoms are improving, then it is probably best to observe the patient for several weeks because only a small percentage of these patients have malignant pleural disease (71). Alternatively, if the symptoms of the patient are worsening or if there is something in the clinical picture that suggests malignancy, the patient should undergo thoracoscopy. Thoracoscopy will establish the diagnosis of malignancy in about 90% of patients with malignancy (72, 73). If facilities for thoracoscopy are not available, an alternative approach is to peform a thoracotomy with open biopsy of the pleura or to perform a needle biopsy of the pleura. If thoracoscopy or thoracotomy is performed, a procedure such as a pleural abrasion should be performed to prevent recurrence of the pleural effusion.

Mesothelioma?

The possibility of a malignant mesothelioma (see Chapter 8) should be considered whenever a patient's pleural fluid cytologic study or pleural biopsy suggests metastatic adenocarcinoma, because the epithelial form of malignant mesothelioma is frequently misinterpreted as adenocarcinoma on cytologic examination or pleural biopsy (74). If no primary tumor is evident, a CT scan of the thorax should be obtained. If the CT scan suggests mesothelioma, one should consider thoracoscopy or exploratory thoracotomy for staging and possible radical pleuropneumonectomy (see Chapter 8).

As discussed early in this chapter and in Chapter 8, electron microscopy and immunohistochemical tests are useful in making this differentiation. In addition, histochemical tests using periodic acid–Schiff stain (PAS) or alcian blue and electron microscopy are very useful in differentiating metastatic adenocarcinoma from mesothelioma (see Chapter 8).

Lipid Analysis

The possibility of a chylothorax should be considered in every patient with malignant disease and a pleural effusion. If a chylothorax is present, the mediastinal lymph nodes are probably involved, and the treatment of choice is radiation to the mediastinum or chemotherapy. The supernatant of the pleural fluid from patients with malignant pleural effusions should be examined. If the supernatant is turbid, a chylothorax should be suspected, and the triglyceride level in the pleural fluid should be determined. If the pleural fluid triglyceride level exceeds 110 mg per dL, the patient probably has a chylothorax; if the level is below 50 mg per dL, the patient does not have a chylothorax (75). If the level is between 50 and 110 mg per dL, lipoprotein electrophoresis should be performed (75) (see Chapter 23).

Other Diagnostic Tests

Numerous articles have recommended various diagnostic tests such as flow cytometry, chromosomal analysis of pleural fluid cells, or LDH isoenzymes in the diagnosis of malignant pleural effusions. These various tests are discussed in Chapter 4. In general, they are not recommended. Flow cytometry with immunophenotyping is useful in making the diagnosis of lymphoma (41).

Unknown Primary

Most patients who are diagnosed with a malignant pleural effusion already are known to have a malignancy. However, if the patient presents with a malignant pleural effusion, where is its likely origin? A recent article reviewed 42 consecutive patients referred to the Royal Marsden Hospital with a malignant pleural effusion and no known primary. The patients included 27 men and 15 women. Despite CT scans of chest and abdomen and mammography and pelvic ultrasound in 10 patients, a primary was determined in only 15 (10 men and five women), and the primary was in the lung in all cases (76). The median survival in this group was 12 months from diagnosis (76).

In view of the above-mentioned findings, it is recommended that patients with a malignant pleural effusion and an unknown primary tumor have a CT of the chest, abdomen, and pelvis. If pulmonary parenchymal abnormalities are discovered, then a bronchoscopy is indicated with special attention to the area of abnormality. If there are no parenchymal abnormalities, then bronchoscopy will probably be nondiagnostic (76). Masses in the abdomen should be evaluated. If the patient has symptoms referable to a specific organ, that organ should be evaluated. If the patient is a woman, mammography and a careful pelvic examination should be performed. If the foregoing sequence of tests does not identify the site of the primary tumor, it is recommended that further tests not be undertaken (76).

PROGNOSIS

The prognosis of patients with malignant pleural effusions is not good. In a recent report, the median survival of 417 patients with malignant pleural effusions was only 4.0 months (51). This 4.0-month median survival is on the optimistic side because all 417 patients were judged to be fit enough to undergo pleurodesis (51). The most important factor influencing the life expectancy in patients with malignant pleural effusion is the source of the tumor. In the aforementioned study, the median survivals were 3.0 months for 146 patients with lung cancer, 2.3 months for 18 patients with gastrointestinal primaries, 5.0 months for 60 patients with breast carcinoma and 51 patients with unknown primary, and 6.0 months for 29 patients with mesothelioma (51). A second factor that is very important in determining the prognosis of patients is their Karnofsky Performance Scale (KPS) score. Burrows and

associates reported that the median survival of patients with a KPS less than 30 was 34 days, whereas the median survival of patients with a KPS score greater than 70 was 395 days (77).

Other factors associated with a poor prognosis are a pleural fluid pH below 7.28, a pleural fluid glucose level below 60 mg per dL, or a pleural fluid LDH more than twice the upper limit of normal for serum. All of the above-mentioned poor prognostic factors probably reflect a greater tumor burden in the pleural space. None of the above-mentioned factors are really accurate at predicting survival (51, 77).

TREATMENT

A simplified algorithm for the management of patients with malignant pleural effusion is given in Fig. 7.1. The initial step is to identify the location of the primary lesion. Frequently, the location of the primary is already known when the pleural effusion is first identified. If the primary is unknown, then the procedures outlined in the previous paragraph should be followed.

Systemic Chemotherapy

The main reason to identify the primary tumor is to decide whether systemic chemotherapy is indicated. The presence of a malignant pleural effusion usually indicates disseminated tumor, at least for nonbronchogenic carcinoma (28). Therefore, the only hope for cure or prolonged palliation is with systemic chemotherapy. Fentiman and co-workers (19) reported that pleural effusions were controlled in seven of 22 patients (32%) with metastatic breast carcinoma who were given systemic chemotherapy, whereas Jones et al. (78) reported positive responses in six of eight patients (75%) given systemic chemotherapy. Livingston et al. (79) reported that 36% of 53 patients with small cell lung carcinoma had complete disappearance of their pleural effusions with chemotherapy. The median survival of patients with small cell lung carcinoma with limited disease and a pleural effusion is 13.9 months, compared with a median survival of 18.3 months if no pleural effusion is present (80). In addition,

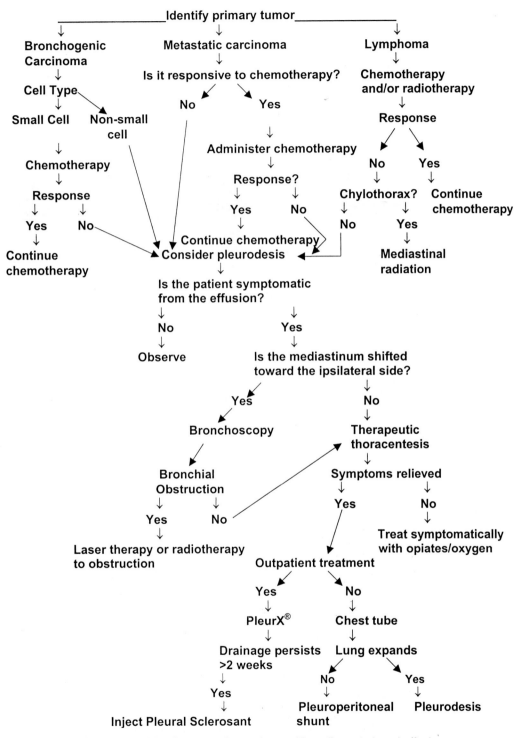

FIG. 7.1. Algorithm for managing patients with malignant pleural effusions.

pleural effusions in lymphomas frequently respond to chemotherapy (26).

In patients undergoing systemic chemotherapy, pleural effusions should be aspirated before chemotherapy is given because the antineoplastic drugs may accumulate in the pleural space and lead to increased systemic toxicity (8).

Mediastinal Radiation

When a patient with a malignant pleural effusion has a chylothorax, the thoracic duct is usually involved by the neoplastic process. Therefore, it is logical to administer radiotherapy to the mediastinum in such patients who have tumor types against which primary chemotherapy is not effective. In one series, mediastinal radiation resulted in adequate control of the chylothorax for the remainder of the patient's life in 68% of those with lymphomas and in 50% of those with metastatic carcinoma (81).

Chemical Pleurodesis

Chemical pleurodesis should be considered in patients with malignant pleural effusions who are not candidates for systemic chemotherapy and who do not have a chylothorax. This procedure should also be considered in those for whom systemic chemotherapy or mediastinal radiotherapy has failed. When managing such a patient, the first question to answer is whether the patient is symptomatic from the effusion. The only symptom likely to be relieved with pleurodesis is dyspnea. If the patient does not have symptoms attributable to the pleural effusion, it does not make sense to insert a chest tube and to attempt a pleurodesis just to make the chest radiograph look better. In a similar vein, if the patient is moribund from disseminated tumor, he or she should not be tortured for the last few days of his or her life with chest tubes. If a patient's quality of life is diminished by dyspnea and he or she has a life expectancy of more than a few weeks, however, one should consider pleurodesis. This local therapy probably does not improve the duration of the patient's life, but it can improve the quality of life.

Before a pleurodesis is attempted, the position of the mediastinum on the chest radiograph

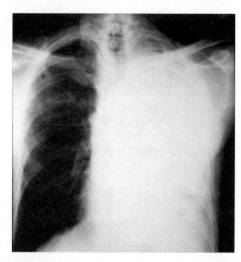

FIG. 7.2. Posteroanterior chest radiograph from a patient with a malignant pleural effusion. Note that the mediastinum is shifted toward the side of the effusion.

should be evaluated, because its position tells much about the pleural pressure on the side of the effusion. If the mediastinum is shifted toward the side of the effusion (Fig. 7.2), the pleural pressure is more negative on the side of the effusion. Pleurodesis is then unlikely to be successful because the ipsilateral lung is unable to expand. In such patients, a bronchoscopic examination should be performed to assess the patency of the major bronchi. If neoplastic obstruction of the bronchi is discovered, radiotherapy, laser therapy, or an endobronchial stent should be considered for relief of the bronchial obstruction. If no obstructing lesion is found, the lung is probably encased by the tumor, and a pleurectomy (discussed later in this chapter) should be considered.

If the mediastinum is in midline position or has shifted to the contralateral side (Fig. 7.3), then a therapeutic thoracentesis should be performed. The purpose of this procedure is to determine whether it relieves the dyspnea of the patient. Only those patients who experience significant symptomatic improvement from this thoracentesis should be considered to be candidates for chemical pleurodesis. The exercise tolerance does not increase in a substantial fraction of patients with a malignant pleural effusion after

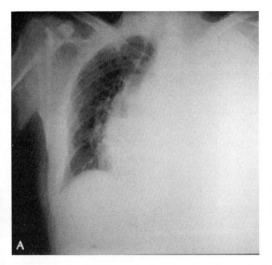 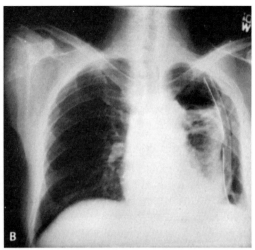

FIG. 7.3. A: Posteroanterior chest radiograph from a patient with a malignant pleural effusion. Note that the mediastinum is shifted away from the side with the pleural effusion. **B:** Posteroanterior chest radiograph from same patient after insertion of a chest tube into the left pleural space. Note that the left lung is not well expanded. Accordingly, a sclerosing agent should not be injected into the pleural space.

a therapeutic thoracentesis (82, 83). In like manner, there is no decrease in the level of dyspnea at a given workload in many patients (82, 83). If over 1,000 mL of pleural fluid are removed during this procedure, pleural pressures should be monitored (35).

Prognostic Factors for Successful Chemical Pleurodesis

In the past, it has been shown that if the pleural fluid pH or glucose levels are reduced, pleurodesis is less likely to be successful (54, 84). In one large series in which pleurodesis was attempted with talc insufflation during thoracoscopy, pleurodesis failed in six of 14 patients (43%) if the pH was below 7.2 but only in eight of 92 patients (9%) if the pleural fluid pH was above 7.2 (84). Comparable findings have been reported when the pleurodesis was attempted with intrapleural tetracycline (54). Similar results are reported when a glucose measurement of less than 60 mg per dL was used as a predictor of pleurodesis failure. A recent review of 433 patients undergoing pleurodesis found that the pleural fluid pH was the only independent predictor of pleurodesis failure (51). Interestingly, the receiver operator curves (ROC) for the pleural fluid pH, pleural fluid glucose, and pleural fluid LDH level were virtually superimposable (51). Nevertheless, a low pleural fluid pH should not be taken as an absolute contraindication to chemical pleurodesis because 40% of patients with a pleural fluid pH below 7.00 will still have a successful pleurodesis and 68% of the patients with pleural fluid pH below 7.3 will have a successful pleurodesis. Interestingly, in this large series, there was no association between pleurodesis success and the pleurodesis technique (thoracoscopy versus tube thoracostomy), pleurodesis agent (talc, bleomycin, or tetracycline derivative), or tumor type (51).

It appears that the pleurodesis is related to the changes in pleural pressure during thoracentesis. Lan et al. (85) measured the change in pleural pressure after 500 mL of pleural fluid had been withdrawn in 65 patients with a malignant pleural effusion. Then they inserted a chest tube and continued to drain the lung until (a) the drainage was less than 150 mL per day, (b) the drainage was less than 250 mL per day for 4 consecutive days, or (c) the drainage had continued for 10 days. At this time, they attempted pleurodesis if the lung had expanded. They found that

14 patients had a pleural elastance greater than 19 cm H_2O, that is, the pleural pressure decreased by more than 9.5 cm H_2O when the 500 mL of pleural fluid was withdrawn. They found that 11 of the 14 patients had a lung that had not expanded. Pleurodesis was attempted in the remaining three patients with bleomycin and failed in all. In contrast, only three of the 51 patients with pleural elastance less than 19 cm H_2O had a trapped lung and bleomycin pleurodesis was successful at 1 month in 42 of 43 (98%) of the patients who returned for reevaluation.

The results of the above-mentioned study could have been anticipated because pleurodesis will fail if the two pleural surfaces cannot be brought into approximation. The rapid fall in the pleural pressure is an indication that the underlying lung is unlikely to expand with the removal of the pleural fluid.

Mechanisms for Pleurodesis

Originally, antineoplastic agents such as nitrogen mustard (86) or radioisotopes (87) were injected into the pleural space in the hope that these agents would kill the tumor cells and control the pleural effusion. It was subsequently shown that the injection of these agents often controlled the pleural effusion when tumor cells persisted and that the effectiveness of intrapleural therapy was related more to the creation of a pleurodesis that prevented the accumulation of the pleural fluid than to any antineoplastic effect of the agent administered (88, 89). The effectiveness of intracavitary nitrogen mustard is much greater when the instillation of this agent is combined with tube thoracostomy (4), because the apposition of the two pleural surfaces allows the fibrotic process to obliterate the pleural space.

Subsequent to the demonstration of the importance of the chemical pleuritis in controlling pleural effusions, nonspecific irritants such as talc (90), tetracycline derivatives (91), silver nitrate, and quinacrine (92) were combined with tube thoracostomy in an attempt to control malignant effusions. The initial event in the production of a pleurodesis by these agents without question is an injury to the pleura. An acute exudative pleural effusion develops within 12 hours of the instillation of essentially all of the agents that are currently used for pleurodesis including talc (93), tetracycline derivatives (94), quinacrine (95), mitoxantrone (96), and bleomycin (95). The pleural fluid that accumulates after the intrapleural injection of these agents is initially characterized by relatively high protein, LDH, and neutrophil counts (97). However, injury to the pleura, as evidenced by the production of an acute exudative pleural effusion, is not sufficient to induce a pleurodesis because many agents, when injected intrapleurally, produce an acute exudative effusion but do not produce a pleurodesis (95).

The response of the pleura to an injury is a complex and poorly understood multifactorial process that can result in the development of fibrosis with the obliteration of the pleural space, or it can result in restoration of the pleura to its normal state. The mechanisms of pleurodesis seem to differ from agent to agent. The histologic appearance is much different with mitoxantrone (96) than it is with talc (93) or tetracycline derivatives (94). The pleurodesis that follows talc, but not tetracycline, can be blocked if corticosteroids are given systemically (98) or if tumor necrosis factor alpha–blocking antibodies (99) are given intrapleurally immediately after talc is administered.

The balance between the procoagulant system and the fibrinolytic system may also be important in determining whether a pleurodesis will result after the intrapleural injection of a substance. If the procoagulant system dominates, then pleurodesis will result, whereas if the fibrinolytic system dominates, no pleurodesis will result. When rabbits are given tetracycline intrapleurally, the number of pleural adhesions that occur is reduced if the rabbits are given either heparin or urokinase intrapleurally (100). In humans, pleurodesis occurs after talc insufflation only if the intrapleural fibrinolytic activity decreases (101).

Cytokines and Pleurodesis (The Future?)

Without a doubt, cytokines are involved in the production of a pleurodesis, but the importance of various cytokines in inducing either fibrosis or repair remains to be determined. In the future, it is likely that pleurodesis will be produced by the intrapleural injection of cytokines. One cytokine that is an excellent candidate as an effective pleurodesis-producing agent is transforming growth factor β (TGF-β). TGF-β has several characteristics that would be important for a pleurodesis agent. (a) TGF-β is a potent fibrogenic cytokine that regulates extracellular matrix production. In situations in which there is too much TGF-β, fibrosis results (102). The transient overexpression of TGF-β in the rat lung leads to marked pleural and interstitial fibrosis (103). (b) Once present, TGF-β can induce its own transcription (104), which suggests that a single injection may be sufficient. (c) Mesothelial cells express and secrete TGF-β; therefore, one intrapleural injection of TGF-β might result in prolonged secretion of TGF-β, which could result in pleurodesis. (d) The incubation of human pleural mesothelial cells with TGF-β results in secretion of increased levels of plasminogen activator inhibitor 1 (PAI-1) (105). This could facilitate pleurodesis because inhibition of the fibrinolytic system is thought to be necessary for the production of a pleurodesis (101).

Our preliminary studies in both rabbits (97) and sheep (106) demonstrate that the intrapleural injection of small amounts of TGF-β results in a better pleurodesis than does the intrapleural injection of either doxycycline or talc slurry. Moreover, the pleural fluid that results from the intrapleural injection of TGF-β is characterized by a much lower white blood cell count and LDH level than is the fluid that results from the intrapleural injection of doxycycline or talc slurry (97). We believe that TGF-β produces a fibrotic reaction in the pleural space without the necessity for a pleural injury. If indeed this is the situation, TGF-β will be an ideal agent for pleurodesis. However, the effectiveness and safety of TGF-β as an agent for pleurodesis in humans has yet to be evaluated.

Choice of Sclerosing Agent

At the present time, the agents that are most commonly recommended are the tetracycline derivatives (minocycline or doxycycline), talc (either insufflated or as a slurry), the antineoplastic agents bleomycin or mitoxantrone, and silver

nitrate. A brief discussion of these four categories of agents follows.

Tetracycline Derivatives

During the 1980s, tetracycline was probably the agent most commonly used for creating a pleurodesis. Tetracycline, 35 mg per kg, is effective in creating a pleurodesis in rabbits (95). Tetracycline is also effective in treating malignant pleural effusions. Sherman et al. (107) reported that tetracycline, 1,500 mg, effectively controlled 94.4% of 108 malignant pleural effusions. In a review of 11 reports involving 359 patients, the success rate with tetracycline was 67% (108).

Parenteral tetracycline is no longer available in the United States, although it remains available in some countries such as Germany (109). Accordingly, the tetracycline derivatives minocycline and doxycycline have been evaluated. In the rabbit, minocycline, 7 mg per kg (110), or doxycycline, 10 mg per kg, (94) produces a pleurodesis that is comparable to that produced by tetracycline, 35 mg per kg. One disturbing aspect of the intrapleural administration of tetracycline derivatives in animals is that it is associated with a high incidence of hemothorax, which is frequently fatal (110). The hemothoraces and the mortality, however, are prevented if chest tubes are inserted into the animals (94).

Doxycycline and minocycline are effective at producing pleurodesis in patients with malignant pleural effusion. When five reports (111–115) with a total of 110 patients are combined, there was control of the effusion at 30 days in 91 of the patients (83%). The usual dose of doxycycline is 500 mg. There has also been one report in which the administration of minocycline, 300 to 500 mg, produced a complete response at 30 days in 62.5% of patients and a partial response (no need for further thoracentesis) in an additional 25% (116). The primary side effect when pleurodesis is performed with a tetracycline derivative is severe chest pain (117). Although the chest pain tends to be worse in patients who receive the tetracycline derivative for a pneumothorax, at times, it is still very severe in patients with malignant pleural effusions. It is recommended that patients who receive a tetracycline derivative for pleurodesis be given lorazepam or midazolam in addition to systemic pain medications before the injection.

Talc

Talc can be instilled into the pleural space either as an aerosol (insufflation) or suspended in saline (slurry). The disadvantage of the insufflation methods is that it must be done in conjunction with either thoracoscopy or thoracotomy, whereas the talc slurry can be administered through chest tubes. Insufflated talc was first used in 1935 by Bethune (118) to produce a pleurodesis. Subsequent studies have shown that insufflated talc is very effective for creating a pleurodesis.

Animal studies have demonstrated that either insufflated talc or talc slurry can produce a pleurodesis if the pleura is normal. However, there is no convincing evidence that talc is superior to other agents. In our rabbit model, talc slurry at a dose of 400 mg per kg produces a pleurodesis (119), but doxycycline, 10 mg per kg, is at least as effective (97). Moreover, it should be noted that the dose of talc slurry necessary to produce a pleurodesis in rabbits (400 mg per kg) is much higher than that typically used in patients (~100 mg per kg) (119). Bresticker et al. (120) reported that talc insufflation (1 g) and mechanical abrasion were essentially equivalent in producing pleurodesis, whereas Jerram et al. (121) reported that mechanical abrasion was superior to talc slurry in producing a pleurodesis.

Insufflated talc is very effective at creating a pleurodesis in patients with malignant pleural effusion. Ribas-Milanez de Campos et al. (122) treated 383 patients with malignant pleural effusions with 2 g of insufflated talc and reported a success rate of 93.4%. Hartman et al. (123) reported that the intrapleural insufflation of 3 to 6 g of aerosolized talc controlled malignant pleural effusions in 37 of 39 (95%) patients for 90 days.

It appears that talc in a slurry is also very effective in producing a pleurodesis (90, 124–126). Adler and Sayek (90) treated 44 hemithoraces with malignant pleural effusion with 10 g of talc in 250 mL of saline and reported control of the effusion in 41 (93%). Webb et al. (125) reported a 100% success rate in 28 patients with malig-

nant effusions who were given 5 g talc and 3 g of thymol iodine in 50 mL of saline. Kennedy et al. (126) reported that 10 g of talc mixed in 150 to 250 mL of normal saline solution effectively controlled 38 of 47 (81%) malignant pleural effusions.

Since the last edition of this book in which I stated that talc was the agent of choice for pleurodesis, there have been increasing concerns about its safety. In the literature, there are at least 32 reported cases of the acute respiratory distress syndrome (ARDS) occurring after talc is administered either as a slurry (126–129) or insufflated (130–134). In some cases, the patients presented with respiratory failure and required mechanical ventilation. In eight instances (127, 129–131, 133), the patients died. The extent of the problem is illustrated by my experience at the 1999 annual meeting of the American College of Chest Physicians. At that meeting, I cochaired a symposium with Dr. John Heffner and we polled the audience concerning their experience with talc. The majority of the approximately 50 physicians, who were present and had experience with talc, had seen patients with ARDS following the intrapleural administration of talc. When the same question was presented concerning ARDS after either tetracycline derivatives or bleomycin, none of the audience had seen such cases.

The incidence of ARDS following intrapleural talc has varied markedly from series to series, and most of the reported cases have been from the United States. The highest incidence was that reported by Rehse and associates (131), who retrospectively reviewed their experience of 89 talc pleurodesis procedures in 78 patients after one patient developed fulminant pneumonia after receiving talc. They reported that 9% of their patients developed ARDS requiring mechanical ventilation, and one of their patients died (131). All of their patients received 5 g of talc, and three patients had received insufflated talc, while four received talc slurry. In contrast Weissberg and Ben-Zeev (135) observed no cases of ARDS in 360 cases who received 2 g talc intrapleurally and concluded that the ARDS was dose related. This does not appear to be the case, however, because of the four fatal cases reported by Campos et al. (130) all had received 2 g of insufflated talc.

The mechanism responsible for the ARDS after intrapleural talc is not definitely known. The acute lung injury could be due either to talc itself or its contaminants such as bacteria, fungi, endotoxin, dolomite, quartz, kaolinite, calcite, or chlorite. One hypothesis is that the acute pneumonitis is related to the systemic absorption of talc with the subsequent elaboration of inflammatory mediators. This hypothesis is supported by the observations in the case reported by Rinaldo et al. (127) in which there were large quantities of talc in the bronchoalveolar fluid of their patient. Talc particles were also found in the bronchoalveolar lavage in all four of the patients reported by Ribas-Milanez de Campos et al. In addition, one of the patients reported by Ribas-Milanez de Campos et al. died, and this patient had talc crystals present in almost every organ at autopsy, including the ipsilateral and contralateral lung, brain, liver, kidney, heart, and skeletal muscle. Animal studies have also demonstrated the extrapleural dissemination of talc administered intrapleurally (136, 137). A possible explanation for the different incidences is that the median size of the talc particles vary markedly from one preparation to another (138).

Antineoplastics Including Bleomycin, Nitrogen Mustard, and Mitoxantrone

Bleomycin is another agent that has become popular recently as a sclerosing agent for malignant pleural effusions. The popularity of bleomycin is due in part to a controlled study by Ruckdeschel et al. comparing the results with 60 units of bleomycin and 1,000 mg tetracycline (139) in 44 patients. The rate of success with bleomycin at 30 days (64%) was significantly better than that with tetracycline (33%). It should be noted that less than an optimal dose of tetracycline was used in this study, and the rate of success with tetracycline was much less than that generally reported.

Overall, it appears that bleomycin is less effective than talc or the tetracycline derivatives in producing a pleurodesis. In a review of eight reports with a total of 199 patients using bleomycin to treat malignant pleural effusions, the overall success rate was only 54% (108). In a recent randomized controlled study, bleomycin failed in 41% of patients at 30 days, 59% at 90 days, and 65% at 180 days (140). In the rabbit model, bleomycin is ineffective in producing a pleurodesis (141). Last, bleomycin is much more expensive ($1,000) than the tetracycline derivatives or talc. Therefore, it cannot be recommended.

Nitrogen mustard was one of the first antineoplastic agents to be used intrapleurally to treat malignant pleural effusions. Interestingly, the results with nitrogen mustard on the average are better than those with bleomycin. For example, Leininger et al. (142) administered 10 mg of nitrogen mustard through the chest tube to 18 patients and reported that the treatment was effective in 17 (94%). Kinsey et al. (143) administered 30 mg of nitrogen mustard through a tube thoracostomy in 62 patients and reported that the effusion was completely controlled in 57 (87%). Interestingly, nitrogen mustard is the only antineoplastic agent other than mitoxantrone that is effective in producing pleurodesis in animals (144). Because nitrogen mustard is at least as effective as bleomycin and costs less than $100, it is the agent of choice if an antineoplastic agent is going to be used.

Another antineoplastic agent that has shown some promise as a pleural sclerosant is mitoxantrone. In one report, the intrapleural administration of 40 mg mitoxantrone to 21 patients with malignant pleural effusions resulted in complete control of the effusions in all cases at 60 days (145). Another article found that mitoxantrone was comparable to bleomycin in controlling malignant pleural effusions (146). One advantage of mitoxantrone over bleomycin is that mitoxantrone binds to cell membranes and therefore is likely to remain in the pleural space longer (147). Interestingly, the intrapleural injection of mitoxantrone leads to proportionately more inflammation than does the intrapleural injection of tetracycline derivatives or talc (96). In the animal model, the intrapleural administration of high doses of mitoxantrone produces a pleurodesis, but there is a significant amount of cardiotoxicity (96). Cardiotoxicity has also been reported in patients who have received mitoxantrone intrapleurally. At the present time, mitoxantrone is not recommended as a sclerosing agent because it is no more effective than talc or the tetracycline derivatives, is associated with more toxicity (96), and is very expensive ($4,000).

Other antineoplastic agents such as cisplatin, doxorubicin, etoposide, fluorouracil, and mitomycin-C have been evaluated for the treatment of pleural effusions, and the response rates have been less than 50% for almost all (108). Therefore, their use cannot be recommended.

Silver Nitrate

Silver nitrate was probably the first agent used to produce a pleurodesis and is very effective (147). In the 1980s, silver nitrate was replaced by tetracycline probably because of severe side effects seen after the intrapleural injection of high concentrations of this agent. Subsequent studies in rabbits demonstrated that a lower concentration of silver nitrate (0.5%) was as effective as tetracycline, 35 mg per kg, in producing a pleurodesis (148). Moreover, this dose of silver nitrate is superior to talc, 400 mg per kg, in producing pleurodesis in rabbits (149). Although there are only limited studies in humans, one recent study demonstrated that the intrapleural injection of 20 mL of 0.5% silver nitrate produced control of the pleural effusion in 22 of 23 patients (95.6%) (147).

Other Agents

Over the years, there have been many other articles evaluating the capability of various other agents to produce a pleurodesis. Several agents that presumably work by being immune modulators have been evaluated. Dried killed *Corynebacterium parvum,* an anaerobic gram-positive bacterium, has been evaluated in nine reports involving a total of 169 patients and has an overall success rate of 76% (108). The availability of *C. parvum* worldwide is very limited and is becoming more limited. OK-432 is obtained from the SU strain of *Streptococcus pyogenes* and has properties similar to *C. parvum* in that it is both immunostimulating and cytotoxic. In Japan, it is considered by some to be the sclerosing agent of choice (150). Response rates as high as 75% have been obtained. To my knowledge, OK-432 is

available only in Asia. Interferon-gamma (151), tumor necrosis factor, (152) and interleukin-2 (152) have all been tried in small numbers of patients with results that are not particularly impressive.

Agent of Choice

The following recommendations for the selection of an agent for pleurodesis in patients with malignant pleural effusions are made based on the above-mentioned information. If a patient has a malignant pleural effusion and is being treated with tube thoracostomy, the agent of choice at the present time is doxycycline, 500 mg. Alternative tetracycline derivatives are tetracycline, 1,500 mg, or minocycline, 300 mg. If a tetracycline derivative is unavailable, 20 mL of 0.5% silver nitrate or 40 mg of nitrogen mustard are reasonable alternatives. If a patient has a malignant pleural effusion diagnosed during thoracoscopy or at thoracotomy, the patient should be subjected to pleural abrasion or parietal pleurectomy. Talc would be recommended if it were not associated with the development of the acute respiratory distress syndrome.

Intrapleural Injection of Sclerosing Agent

Once a patient has been selected to undergo pleurodesis, a decision must be made as to whether the procedure should be performed on an inpatient or an outpatient basis. Pleurodesis accomplished on an outpatient basis has two advantages: First, it allows the patient to remain at home. Because the mean hospitalization time of patients treated in hospital is about 6.5 days (153) and the patient has a life expectancy of only about 90 days, this hospitalization represents 5% and probably the best days of the patient's remaining life. Second, it decreases the cost of the treatment because there are no hospitalization costs. In one study, the costs associated with the outpatient management of malignant pleural effusions were $2,000, whereas the costs associated with inpatient management were $7,000 (154).

Since the last edition of this book, there have been several articles on the treatment of malignant pleural effusions on an outpatient basis (153–155). The method that uses the PleurX catheter is discussed in detail in the section on alternative therapies for pleural sclerosis. The alternative system is that developed by Patz (155). With this system, a small-bore (10.3 F) all-purpose drainage catheter is placed with imaging guidance. Then up to 1,000 mL of pleural fluid is drained and then the catheter is connected to a 600-mL bag (Tru-Close; UreSil Lp; Skokie, IL, USA) for gravity drainage. After a baseline chest radiograph is obtained, the patient is sent home and asked to return if he or she experiences increasing pain, shortness of breath, or fever. When the drainage is less than 100 mL per day, the patient returns for outpatient sclerotherapy. The following day, the patient returns for tube removal. Patz (155) treated 19 patients with 60 units of bleomycin. At 30 days, 79% of the patients had either a total (53%) or partial (26%) pleurodesis response.

When the PleurX catheter is compared with the gravity drainage system of Patz, the PleurX appears to have several advantages. It appears to be safer. If the gravity system of the Patz system becomes disconnected, there is a greater likelihood of pneumothorax or pleural infection. The gravity system is less acceptable to the patient because they are saddled with the drainage bag. The primary disadvantage of the PleurX catheter is that it is more expensive.

For the reasons mentioned earlier, pleural sclerosis should be performed on an outpatient basis whenever feasible. When pleural sclerosis is performed on an outpatient basis, there is no hurry to perform the injection because there are no daily hospital costs. Therefore, the pleural effusion is drained for 7 to 10 days and then a radiograph is obtained to confirm that there is not a significant amount of fluid in the pleural space. If successful reexpansion of the lung cannot be accomplished with pleural drainage, as shown in Fig. 7.3B, sclerosing agents should not be injected into the pleural space. Their injection can only thicken the visceral pleura and allow even less lung expansion. If the lung does not expand with tube thoracostomy, the pleural fluid can be drained on a chronic basis with the PleurX catheter or a pleuroperi-toneal shunt can be placed (discussed later in this chapter). One of these options should definitely be performed if the mediastinum is shifted away from the side of the effusion (Fig. 7.3A). If the patient is in excellent condition, pleurectomy can be considered (discussed later in this chapter).

Because the injection of any of the tetracycline derivatives produces an intense pleuritis that can be very painful, some authors (156) have suggested that the patient should be given local anesthesia such as lidocaine hydrochloride intrapleurally. There are no controlled studies evaluating the efficacy of intrapleural lidocaine, and at the present time, no intrapleural anesthetic is recommended. However, patients should be given systemic medication to control the pain. We currently use lorazepam or midazolam to produce conscious sedation.

After the sclerosant is injected, the catheter is flushed with an additional 50 to 100 mL of saline solution and then no drainage is performed for a couple of hours. Although in the past it has been recommended that the patient be moved into different positions so that the sclerosant contacts all the pleural surfaces, this does not appear to be necessary. In animals, the dispersal of radioisotopes injected intrapleurally is similar whether the animals are rotated or not (157). In humans the dispersal of the injected radioisotopes is similar whether or not the patients are rotated (158). Rotation did not have a statistically significant effect on the results of pleurodesis in one randomized study with tetracycline derivatives (159). The rate of success with rotation was 73.7% while the rate of success with no rotation was 61.9% (159). However, because rotating the patient certainly does not decrease the likelihood of pleurodesis and because the patient has much less pain with rotation if the small catheters are used, it is recommended that all patients be rotated unless it is particularly uncomfortable for the patient.

After a couple of hours, the patient is sent home with instructions to drain the pleural space daily with the PleurX catheter, and continuously with the gravity system. The patient records the drainage on a daily basis. When the total drainage over a 3-day period is less than 50 mL, the patient is instructed to return to the clinic. A chest radiograph is obtained, and the catheter is removed if there is no pleural effusion. If there was no drainage and there is a significant amount of pleural fluid, then either the pleural fluid is loculated or the catheter is obstructed. The intrapleural administration of 150,000 U of streptokinase is often effective treatment for both of these conditions.

Inpatient pleural sclerosis is very similar to outpatient pleural sclerosis. One option available if the pleural sclerosis is performed as an inpatient is thoracoscopy. The results with thoracoscopy overall are probably better than the results with tube thoracostomy because patients with trapped lungs can be identified (and therefore do not receive a pleural sclerosant), and loculated pleural effusions can be completely drained. Indeed, if thoracoscopy is performed and no pleural sclerosis is attempted, 62% of the patients have no recurrence of their pleural effusion for the remainder of their life (160, 161). Nevertheless, thoracoscopy is not recommended if a diagnosis is already established. In an analysis performed by Heffner et al. (51), the results with thoracoscopy were not significantly better than those with tube thoracostomy. Yim et al. (162) randomized 28 patients to pleurodesis through thoracoscopy and talc insufflation, and 27 patients to pleurodesis with tube thoracostomy and talc slurry. They found that there was no significant differences in the results with the two different methods (162). Moreover, thoracoscopy adds significantly to the expense of the procedure. Of course, if thoracoscopy is performed for diagnosis and a pleural malignancy is found, a procedure such as a pleural abrasion should be performed to create a pleurodesis.

If the pleurodesis is performed on an inpatient basis, one has the option of using larger tubes. There is no evidence that the use of a large tube provides better results than does the use of a small tube. Clementsen et al. (163) randomized 18 patients to either a no. 10 F or a no. 24 F catheter and reported that there was no difference in the response rates. Patients accepted the small catheter more readily (163). Marom et al. (164) treated 32 patients using a 14-F self-retaining vanSonneberg catheter, which was inserted with the Seldinger technique. They reported that 23 of 32 (72%) patients had a complete response, four (12%) had a partial response, and pleurodesis failed in five (16%).

The chest tube is connected to a water-sealed drainage system, and the effusion is allowed to drain (142). Negative pressure should not be applied to the chest tube in this situation because the combination of a chronic pleural effusion and the application of negative pleural pressure can cause reexpansion pulmonary edema (see Chapter 21). If the lung has not expanded within 24 hours, then negative pressure should be applied to the chest tube.

Once the chest tube has been inserted, how long should one wait before injecting the sclerosing agent? It is important to make certain that the underlying lung has fully expanded before the injection is made. If the underlying lung has not expanded, then the injection of a sclerosing agent will lead to only additional thickening of the visceral pleura, which will further compromise the function of the underlying lung. Some authors have advocated that the sclerosing agent not be injected until the drainage from the chest tube is less than 150 mL (139). However, there is no supporting data for this practice. Villanueva et al. (165) randomly assigned patients to a group in which tetracycline was not instilled until the drainage was less than 150 mL per day and a group in which tetracycline was instilled as soon as the lung had reexpanded. The rate of success was the same in each group (80%), but the duration of the chest tubes was much less in the latter group (2 days) than in the former group (7 days). In view of this study, it is recommended that the sclerosant be injected as soon as the lung has reexpanded.

After the sclerosant is injected, the chest tube is clamped for 2 hours. Then the chest tube is unclamped and negative pressure (-15 to -20 cm H_2O) is applied to the chest tube. Suction is maintained for at least 24 hours and until the pleural drainage is less than 150 mL per day. The keys to the success of this procedure are the pleuritis produced by the sclerosant and the approximation of the visceral and the parietal pleura by the chest tubes so that a pleural symphysis can occur. There appears to be no advantage if the sclerosant is injected twice. In one study (166), 25 patients received one injection of tetracycline, 20 mg per kg, and 25 patients received instillations of tetracycline, 20 mg per kg, on 2 consecutive days. Effusions recurred in four patients in each group (166).

Alternatives to Pleurodesis

If the patient is not a good candidate for chemical pleurodesis, there are several options available that include implantation of a PleurX catheter, symptomatic treatment, the implantation of a pleuroperitoneal shunt, serial thoracentesis, pleurectomy, and pleural radiotherapy.

Indwelling (PleurX) Catheter

The PleurX catheter was developed as a means by which patients with malignant pleural effusions could have their pleural fluid drained repeatedly without having to return to the hospital. The PleurX catheter is a 15.5 F silicone rubber catheter, 66 cm in length, with fenestrations along the proximal 24 cm (PleurX, Denver Biomaterials, Golden, CO, USA, 800-824-8454). It is inserted into the pleural space using the Seldinger technique under local anesthesia by pulmonologists, interventional radiologists, or surgeons. The catheter is maintained in place with a chest wall tunnel 5 to 8 cm in length (153, 154). This particular catheter has a special valve on its distal end that is designed to enhance the safety of the product. The valve prevents fluid or air from passing in either direction through the catheter unless the catheter is accessed with the matched drainage line. The pleural fluid is drained on a daily basis by inserting the access tip of the drainage line into the valve of the catheter and then draining the fluid via an external tube into vacuum bottles.

In the initial multicenter study using this catheter to treat malignant pleural effusions, the efficacy and safety of the catheter were compared with those of doxycycline pleurodesis through tube thoracostomy. All patients were initially hospitalized. The median hospitalization for the 94 patients who received the PleurX catheter was 1 day, whereas the median hospitalization for the 41 patients who had doxycycline pleurodesis was 6.5 days. Of the 94 patients who received the PleurX catheter, the effusion was initially controlled by the catheter in 91 (97%). The presence of the catheter leads to a spontaneous pleurodesis in about 50% of patients with a median time to pleurodesis of 28 days (167). Patients who experienced a pleurodesis tended to have a gradual decrease in the amount of pleural fluid formed daily (29). Several of the patients had the catheter in place for more than 1 year.

The morbidity from the catheter is relatively low (153). Early (in-hospital) morbidity occurred in 10 of 96 patients with the indwelling catheter, and it included fever (three patients), pneumothorax (three patients), misplacement of the catheter (two patients), reexpansion pulmonary edema (one patient), and hypercapnic respiratory failure secondary to oversedation (one patient). In the 90-day follow-up period, three patients developed tumor seeding of the catheter tract that did not require therapy. Six patients developed local cellulitis around the catheter tract that responded to oral antibiotic treatment, and seven patients reported pain during fluid drainage.

Putnam et al. (154) subsequently compared their experience with the indwelling pleural catheter and pleurodesis with doxycycline or talc at M.D. Anderson Hospital. In this study 60/100 patients who were treated with the indwelling catheter were treated as outpatients (154). This study documented that the total cost was much less when patients could be treated as an outpatient.

The PleurX catheter is an advance in the management of patients with malignant pleural effusions because it allows patients to be treated easily as outpatients and obviates the necessity for return visits for a repeat thoracentesis. However, it should be noted that about 50% of the patients never experience a spontaneous pleurodesis and therefore are burdened with the catheter the remainder of their lives. Because there are complications associated with prolonged use of the catheter (e.g., empyema, tumor seeding of catheter tract, loculation of the effusion), it is recommended that patients who have weekly pleural fluid production of more than 1,000 mL fluid after the catheter has been in place for 7 to 14 days have an attempt at chemical pleurodesis through the PleurX catheter.

Symptomatic Treatment

The two primary symptoms associated with a malignant pleural effusion are chest pain and shortness of breath. If the patient has chest pain, sufficient analgesics should be given to control the pain. There is no reason to worry about narcotic addiction because the life expectancy of the patient is so short.

If the primary symptom is dyspnea, the patient should be given opiates or oxygen, or both. Both opiates and oxygen relieve the dyspnea. The disadvantage of opiates is that their administration can be associated with an increase in the Pa_{CO_2}, which, in turn, will lead to a decrease in the Pa_{O_2}. The disadvantage of oxygen is that it is very expensive and is not very portable. Opiates are probably underused in the treatment of dyspnea associated with pleural effusions.

Pleuroperitoneal Shunt

An alternative approach to the management of patients with malignant pleural effusions is the placement of a pleuroperitoneal shunt (167–170), which is marketed commercially by Denver Biomaterials (Golden, CO, USA, [800] 824-8454). This device consists of two catheters connected with a valved pump chamber (Fig. 7.4). The two

one-way valves in the pump chamber are positioned such that fluid can only flow from the pleural space to the pump chamber to the peritoneal cavity. These valves open at a positive pressure of about 1 cm H_2O. Because the pleural pressure is almost always more negative than the peritoneal pressure, the pumping chamber must be used to move fluid from the pleural cavity to the peritoneal cavity. The capacity of the pump chamber is approximately 1.5 mL. When the pump chamber is compressed, fluid is forced from the chamber into the peritoneal cavity. Then when the pump chamber is released, negative pressure created in the pump chamber draws fluid from the pleural cavity to the pump chamber.

Little et al. (168) reported their experience with the insertion of these shunts into 29 patients, 22 of whom had malignant pleural disease. Eight of the patients had previously had chest tube placement with attempted sclerosis with tetracycline. In most instances, shunt implantation was performed in the operating room using general anesthesia, but in four patients, local anesthesia was used. When the pleuroperitoneal shunt was first released, the pump chamber was always placed in a subcutaneous pocket caudal to a skin incision in the lateral part of the inframammary crease and fixed to the tissues with sutures through the sewing holes in the base of the pump chamber. Subsequently, a modification of the shunt has been developed in which the pumping chamber is placed exteriorly

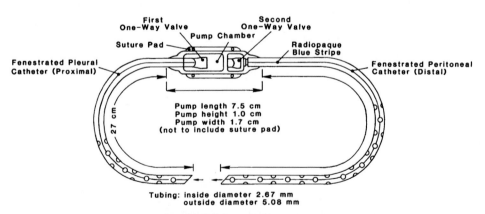

FIG. 7.4. Diagram of the Denver Pleuro-Peritoneal Shunt, which consists of a fenestrated pleural catheter, a flexible pump chamber containing two one-way valves, and a fenestrated peritoneal catheter. The one-way valves open at a positive pressure of about 1 cm H_2O.

and the volume of the chamber is 2.5 mL rather than 1.5 mL. Therefore, less pumping is required. The pleural catheter is inserted at the lateral and superior aspect of the incision with a Seldinger-type introducer kit. The abdominal catheter is tunneled subcutaneously across the costal margin and inserted, through a 3-cm skin incision, into the peritoneal cavity through a small incision in the peritoneum. Pump compression by physicians and nurses is initiated in the recovery room and is then started by the patient or the patient's family on the first postoperative day. Within 3 days of shunt placement, pump compression usually causes no discomfort. Most patients are ready for discharge from the hospital within 48 hours of the operation. Selected patients can have the procedure performed on an outpatient basis.

The first sizable series of patients receiving the pleuroperitoneal shunt was reported by Little et al. (168) in 1988. They inserted shunts into 29 patients with excellent results overall. Three patients never pumped on their shunts, one obese patient was unable to localize the pump chamber, a 90-year-old man suffering from senility was simply unable to comply, and one patient developed a cancer phobia and refused to touch her shunt. Two patients died shortly after implantation from disseminated malignant disease. Excellent results were obtained in 20 of the remaining 24 patients. The 14 patients with malignant effusions had a median survival of 4 months, and there were no instances of peritoneal tumor seeding. In five patients, the shunts became occluded by fibrinous debris between 3 weeks and 2 months after the operation. Replacement was uneventful in all five instances.

Since this original report (168), there have been several additional reports (169–172). In these latter four studies, a total of 84 patients with malignancy were treated and 76 had either failed pleurodesis or had a trapped lung. Alleviation of dyspnea and control of the effusion was obtained in more than 90% of the patients. These results are particularly impressive when one realizes that previous treatment failed in more than 90% of the patients in these four series. The primary complication with the pleuroperitoneal shunt is that in about 15% of patients, the shunt becomes occluded. In such a situation, it should be replaced (173).

What should be the place of the pleuroperitoneal shunt in the management of patients with malignant pleural effusions? The shunt should certainly be used in the patient in whom the lung does not expand after tube thoracostomy. Petrou and associates inserted pleuroperitoneal shunts into 63 patients who had a trapped lung at thoracoscopy and reported effective palliation in more than 95% (174). The pleuroperitoneal shunt should also be considered in patients in whom pleurodesis has failed.

There are no studies comparing the efficacy of the shunt and chemical pleurodesis. The advantages of the shunt include the following: (a) the total hospitalization time is less than with chemical pleurodesis, (b) the amount of pain is probably less than with pleurodesis, (c) the procedure can be performed on an outpatient basis, and (d) the patient may benefit psychologically from using the pump when he or she is dyspneic. The disadvantages of the shunt include the following: (a) The shunt becomes obstructed in some patients, (b) insertion frequently requires general anesthesia, and (c) the patient must use the pump daily.

At the present time, when outpatient therapy of malignant pleural effusions is undertaken, the PleurX catheter is recommended because it is easier to insert. However, if a chylothorax is present, the recommended therapeutic method is the pleuroperitoneal shunt because the nutritional status of the patient is preserved with this method. The pleuroperitoneal shunt is also preferred in patients in whom the underlying lung is trapped because in this instance, the patient will require some type of pleural drainage for the rest of his or her life.

Pleurectomy

In carefully selected individuals, pleurectomy can be of use in controlling malignant pleural effusions. Pleurectomy may be attempted in two different situations (175). The first is in the patient who undergoes a diagnostic thoracotomy for an undiagnosed pleural effusion. If malignant disease is found, an immediate parietal pleurectomy is useful to prevent recurrence of the effusion (175). Parietal pleurectomy consists of stripping all of the parietal pleura from the rib cage and the mediastinum. The second situation is in the symptomatic patient with a persistent pleural effusion and trapping of the ipsilateral lung so that the injection of sclerosing agents is contraindicated. The surgical procedure involves decortication of the trapped lung in conjunction with parietal pleurectomy. Pleurectomy controls the pleural effusion in more than 90% of cases (175). It is a substantial operation with a mortality rate of about 10%, however (175). A pleurectomy combined with decortication is recommended only in a patient who is symptomatic from the pleural effusion, who is in good overall condition, and whose primary tumor either is under control or is progressing slowly. I have yet to see such a patient, but an occasional patient with breast carcinoma meets these criteria.

Thoracentesis

In the past, many patients with malignant pleural effusion were managed with repeated therapeutic thoracenteses for symptomatic relief. This regimen has several drawbacks. After therapeutic thoracentesis, malignant pleural effusions reaccumulate rapidly, usually within 1 to 3 days (4). Repeated thoracenteses lead to protein depletion; the removal of 2,000 mL pleural fluid containing 4 g per dL protein deprives the patient of 80g protein. The patient must visit the physician frequently for the procedure. In addition, repeated thoracenteses often lead to loculation of the pleural fluid, which makes subsequent pleurodesis difficult (4). In view of these disadvantages, serial therapeutic thoracentesis should be performed only in moribund patients in whom the procedure offers symptomatic relief.

REFERENCES

1. Light RW, Erozan YS, Ball WC. Cells in pleural fluid: their value in differential diagnosis. *Arch Intern Med* 1973;132:854–860.
2. Marel M, Arustova M, Stasny B, et al. Incidence of pleural effusion in a well-defined region: epidemiologic study in central Bohemia. *Chest* 1993;104:1486–1489.
3. Spriggs AI, Boddington MM. *The cytology of effusions,* 2nd ed. New York: Grune & Stratton, 1968.
4. Anderson CB, Philpott GW, Ferguson TB. The treatment of malignant pleural effusions. *Cancer* 1974; 33:916–922.
5. Johnston WW. The malignant pleural effusion: a review of cytopathologic diagnoses of 584 specimens from 472 consecutive patients. *Cancer* 1985;56:905–909.
6. Naito T, Satoh H, Ishikawa H, et al. Pleural effusion as a significant prognostic factor in non-small cell lung cancer. *Anticancer Res* 1997;17:4743–4746.
7. Chernow B, Sahn SA. Carcinomatous involvement of the pleura. *Am J Med* 1977;63:695–702.
8. Herrstedt J, Clementsen P, Hansen OP. Increased myelosuppression during cytostatic treatment and pleural effusion in patients with small cell lung cancer. *Eur J Cancer* 1992;28A:1070–1073.
9. Lai CL, Tsai CM, Tsai TT, et al. Presence of serum anti-p53 antibodies is associated with pleural effusion and poor prognosis in lung cancer patients. *Clin Cancer Res* 1998;4:3025–3030.
10. Renshaw AA, Madge R, Sugarbaker DJ, et al. Malignant pleural effusions after resection of pulmonary adenocarcinoma. *Acta Cytol* 1998;42:1111–1115.
11. Sugiura S, Ando Y, Minami H, et al. Prognostic value of pleural effusion in patients with non-small cell lung cancer. *Clin Cancer Res* 1997;3:47–50.
12. Leong SS, Lima CM, Sherman CA, et al. The 1997 International Staging System for non-small cell lung cancer: have all the issues been addressed? *Chest* 1999;115:242–248.
13. Rodriguez-Panadero F. Lung cancer and ipsilateral pleural effusion. *Ann Oncol* 1995;6[Suppl 3]:S25–S27.
14. Decker DA, Dines DE, Payne WS, et al. The significance of a cytologically negative pleural effusion in bronchogenic carcinoma. *Chest* 1978;74:640–642.
15. Fracchia AA, Knapper WH, Carey JT, et al. Intrapleural chemotherapy for effusion from metastatic breast carcinoma. *Cancer* 1970;26:626–629.
16. Goldsmith HS, Bailey HD, Callahan EL, et al. Pulmonary lymphangitic metastases from breast carcinoma. *Arch Surg* 1967;94:483–488.
17. Banerjee AK, Willetts I, Robertson JF, et al. Pleural effusion in breast cancer: a review of the Nottingham experience. *Eur J Surg Oncol* 1994;20:33–36.
18. Apffelstaedt JP, Van Zyl JA, Muller AG. Breast cancer complicated by pleural effusion: patient characteristics and results of surgical management. *J Surg Oncol* 1995;58:173–175.
19. Fentiman IS, Millis R, Sexton S, et al. Pleural effusion in breast cancer: a review of 105 cases. *Cancer* 1981;47:2087–2092.
20. Brankovic-Magic M, Neskovic-Konstantinovic Z, Nikolic-Vukosavljevic D, et al. Steroid receptors in pleural effusions of advanced breast cancer patients. *Intern J Biol Markers* 1995;10:143–148.
21. Romano M, Libshitz HI. Hodgkin disease and non-Hodgkin lymphoma: plain chest radiographs and chest computed tomography of thoracic involvement in previously untreated patients. *Radiol Med (Torino)* 1998;95:49–53.
22. Vieta JO, Craver LF. Intrathoracic manifestations of the lymphomatoid diseases. *Radiology* 1941;37: 138–158.
23. Stolberg HO, Patt NL, MacEwen KF, et al. Hodgkin's disease of the lung: roentgenologic-pathologic correlation. *AJR Am J Roentgenol* 1964;92:96–115.

24. Berkman N, Breuer R, Kramer MR, et al. Pulmonary involvement in lymphoma. *Leuk Lymphoma* 1996;20:229–237.

25. Xaubet A, Diumenjo MC, Marin A, et al. Characteristics and prognostic value of pleural effusions in non-Hodgkin's lymphomas. *Eur J Respir Dis* 1985;66: 135–140.

26. Elis A, Blickstein D, Mulchanov I, et al. Pleural effusion in patients with non-Hodgkin's lymphoma: a case-controlled study. *Cancer* 1998;83:1607–1611.

27. Light RW, Hamm H. Malignant pleural effusion: would the real cause please stand up? *Eur Respir J* 1997;10:1701–1702.

28. Meyer PC. Metastatic carcinoma of the pleura. *Thorax* 1966;21:437–443.

29. Light RW, Rodriguez RM. Factors predicting spontaneous pleurodesis in patients with indwelling pleural catheters. *Chest* 2001 (*in press*).

30. Leckie WJH, Tothill P. Albumin turnover in pleural effusions. *Clin Sci* 1965;29:339–352.

31. Cheng C-S, Rodriguez RM, Perkett EA, et al. Vascular endothelial growth factor in pleural fluid. *Chest* 1999;115:760–765.

32. Collins PO, Connolly DT, Williams TJ. Characterization of increase in vascular permeability induced by vascular permeability factor in vivo. *Br J Pharmacol* 1993;109:195–199.

33. Yano S, Herbst RS, Shinohara H, et al. Treatment for malignant pleural effusion of human lung adenocarcinoma by inhibition of vascular endothelial growth factor receptor tyrosine kinase phosphorylation. *Clin Cancer Res* 2000;6:957–965.

34. Wang NS. The preformed stomas connecting the pleural cavity and the lymphatics in the parietal pleura. *Am Rev Respir Dis* 1975;111:12–20.

35. Light RW, Jenkinson SG, Minh V, et al. Observations on pleural pressures as fluid is withdrawn during thoracentesis. *Am Rev Respir Dis* 1980;121:799–804.

36. Rodriguez-Panadero F, Borderas Naranjo F, Lopez Mejias J. Pleural metastatic tumours and effusions. Frequency and pathogenic mechanisms in a post-mortem series. *Eur Respir J* 1989;2:366–369.

37. Marel M, Stastny B, Melínová L, et al. Diagnosis of pleural effusions: experience with clinical studies, 1986–1990. *Chest* 1995;107:1598–1603.

38. Maher GG, Berger HW. Massive pleural effusion: malignant and nonmalignant causes in 46 patients. *Am Rev Respir Dis* 1972;105:458–460.

39. Weick JK, Kiely JM, Harrison EG Jr, et al. Pleural effusion in lymphoma. *Cancer* 1973;31:848–853.

40. Bruneau R, Rubin P. The management of pleural effusions and chylothorax in lymphoma. *Radiology* 1965;85:1085–1092.

41. Celikoglu F, Teirstein AS, Krellenstein DJ, et al. Pleural effusion in non-Hodgkin's lymphoma. *Chest* 1992;101:1357–1360.

42. O'Donovan PB, Eng P. Pleural changes in malignant pleural effusions: appearance on computed tomography. *Cleve Clin J Med* 1994;61:127–131.

43. Light RW, MacGregor MI, Luchsinger PC, et al. Pleural effusions: the diagnostic separation of transudates and exudates. *Ann Intern Med* 1972;77:507–513.

44. Assi Z, Caruso JL, Herndon J, et al. Cytologically proved malignant pleural effusions: distribution of transudates and exudates. *Chest* 1998;113:1302–1304.

45. Ashchi M, Golish J, Eng P, et al. Transudative malignant pleural effusions: prevalence and mechanisms. *South Med J* 1998;91:23–26.

46. Martinez-Garcia MA, Cases-Viedma E, Cordero-Rodriguez PJ, et al. Diagnostic utility of eosinophils in the pleural fluid. *Eur Respir J* 2000;15:166–169.

47. Rubins JB, Rubins HB. Etiology and prognostic significance of eosinophilic pleural effusions. A prospective study. *Chest* 1996;110:1271–1274.

48. Martinez-Moragon E, Aparicio J, Sanchis J, et al. Malignant pleural effusion: prognostic factors for survival and response to chemical pleurodesis in a series of 120 cases. *Respiration* 1998;65:108–113.

49. Light RW, Ball WC. Glucose and amylase in pleural effusions. *JAMA* 1973;225:257–260.

50. Rodriguez-Panadero F, Lopez-Mejias J. Low glucose and pH levels in malignant pleural effusions. *Am Rev Respir Dis* 1989;139:663–667.

51. Heffner JE, Nietert PJ, Barbieri C. Pleural fluid pH as a predictor of survival for patients with malignant pleural effusions. *Chest* 2000;117:79–86.

52. Good JT Jr, Taryle DA, Sahn SA. The pathogenesis of low glucose, low pH malignant effusions. *Am Rev Respir Dis* 1985;131:737–741.

53. Light RW, MacGregor MI, Ball WC Jr, et al. Diagnostic significance of pleural fluid pH and P_{co_2}. *Chest* 1973;64:591–596.

54. Sahn SA, Good JT Jr. Pleural fluid pH in malignant effusions. *Ann Intern Med* 1988;108:345–349.

55. Ende N. Studies of amylase activity in pleural effusions and ascites. *Cancer* 1960;13:283–287.

56. Kramer MR, Saidana MJ, Cepero RJ, et al. High amylase levels in neoplasm-related pleural effusion. *Ann Intern Med* 1989;110:567–569.

57. Jarvi OH, Kunnas RJ, Laitio MT, et al. The accuracy and significance of cytologic cancer diagnosis of pleural effusions. *Acta Cytol* 1972;16:152–157.

58. Grunze H. The comparative diagnostic accuracy, efficiency and specificity of cytologic techniques used in the diagnosis of malignant neoplasm in serous effusions of the pleural and pericardial cavities. *Acta Cytol* 1964;8:150–164.

59. Dekker A, Bupp PA. Cytology of serous effusions. An investigation into the usefulness of cell blocks versus smears. *Am J Clin Pathol* 1978;70:855–860.

60. Prakash URS, Reiman HM. Comparison of needle biopsy with cytologic analysis for the evaluation of pleural effusion: analysis of 414 cases. *Mayo Clin Proc* 1985;60:158–164.

61. Bueno CE, Clemente G, Castro BC, et al. Cytologic and bacteriologic analysis of fluid and pleural biopsy specimens with Cope's needle. *Arch Intern Med* 1990;150:1190–1194.

62. Naylor B, Schmidt RW. The case for exfoliative cytology of serous effusions. *Lancet* 1964;1:711–712.

63. Ordonez NG. Role of immunohistochemistry in differentiating epithelial mesothelioma from adenocarcinoma. Review and update. *Am J Clin Pathol* 1999; 112:75–89.

64. Brown RW, Clark GM, Tandon AK, et al. Multiple-marker immunohistochemical phenotypes distinguishing malignant pleural mesothelioma from pulmonary adenocarcinoma. *Hum Pathol* 1993;24:347–354.

65. Miedouge M, Rouzaud P, Salama G, et al. Evaluation of seven tumour markers in pleural fluid for the

diagnosis of malignant effusions. *Br J Cancer* 1999;81: 1059–1065.

66. Lee YC, Knox BS, Garrett JE. Use of cytokeratin fragments 19.1 and 19.21 (Cyfra 21-1) in the differentiation of malignant and benign pleural effusions. *Aust N Z J Med* 1999;29:765–769.

67. Lee YC, Chern JH, Lai SL, et al. Sialyl stage-specific embryonic antigen-1: a useful marker for differentiating the etiology of pleural effusion. *Chest* 1998;114:1542–1545.

68. Salyer WR, Eggleston JC, Erozan YS. Efficacy of pleural needle biopsy and pleural fluid cytopathology in the diagnosis of malignant neoplasm involving the pleura. *Chest* 1975;67:536–539.

69. Frist B, Kahan AV, Koss LG. Comparisons of the diagnostic values of biopsies of the pleura and cytologic evaluation of pleural fluids. *Am J Clin Pathol* 1979;72:48–51.

70. Canto A, Rivas J, Saumench J, et al. Points to consider when choosing a biopsy method in cases of pleurisy of unknown origin. *Chest* 1983;84:176–179.

71. Poe RH, Ortiz C, Israel RH, et al. Sensitivity, specificity, and predictive values of closed pleural biopsy. *Arch Intern Med* 1984;144:325–328.

72. Hucker J, Bhatnagar NK, al-Jilaihawi AN, et al. Thoracoscopy in the diagnosis and management of recurrent pleural effusions. *Ann Thorac Surg* 1991;52:1145–1147.

73. Menzies R, Charbonneau M. Thoracoscopy for the diagnosis of pleural disease. *Ann Intern Med* 1991;114:271–276.

74. Antman KH. Clinical presentation and natural history of benign and malignant mesothelioma. *Semin Oncol* 1981;8:313–320.

75. Staats BA, Ellefson RD, Budahn LL, et al. The lipoprotein profile of chylous and nonchylous pleural effusions. *Mayo Clin Proc* 1980;55:700–704.

76. Bonnefoi H, Smith IE. How should cancer presenting as a malignant pleural effusion be managed? *Br J Cancer* 1996;74:832–835.

77. Burrows CM, Mathews WC, Colt HG. Predicting survival in patients with recurrent symptomatic malignant pleural effusions: an assessment of the prognostic values of physiologic, morphologic, and quality of life measures of extent of disease. *Chest* 2000;117:73–78.

78. Jones SE, Durie BGM, Salmon SE. Combination chemotherapy with adriamycin and cyclophosphamide for advanced breast cancer. *Cancer* 1975;36:90–97.

79. Livingston RB, McCracken JD, Trauth CJ, et al. Isolated pleural effusion in small cell lung carcinoma: favorable prognosis. *Chest* 1982;81:208–211.

80. Albain KS, Crowley JJ, LeBlanc M, et al. Determinants of improved outcome in small-cell lung cancer: an analysis of the 2,580-patient Southwest Oncology Group data base. *J Clin Oncol* 1990;8:1563–1574.

81. Roy PH, Carr DT, Payne WS. The problem of chylothorax. *Mayo Clin Proc* 1967;42:457–467.

82. Shinto RA, Stansbury DW, Brown SE, et al. Does therapeutic thoracentesis improve the exercise capacity of patients with pleural effusion? *Am Rev Respir Dis* 1987;135:A244.

83. Shinto RA, Stansbury DW, Fischer CE, et al. The effect of thoracentesis on central respiratory drive in patients with large pleural effusions. *Am Rev Respir Dis* 1988;137:A112.

84. Sanchez-Armengol A, Rodriguez-Panadero F. Survival and talc pleurodesis in metastatic pleural carcinoma, revisited. Report of 125 cases. *Chest* 1993;104:1482–1485.

85. Lan RS, Lo SK, Chuang ML, et al. Elastance of the pleural space: a predictor for the outcome of pleurodesis in patients with malignant pleural effusion. *Ann Intern Med* 1997;126:768–774.

86. Weisberger AS, Levine B, Storaasli JP. Use of nitrogen mustard in treatment of serous effusions of neoplastic origin. *JAMA* 1955;159:1704–1706.

87. Ariel IM, Oropeza R, Pack GT. Intracavitary administration of radioactive isotopes in the control of effusions due to cancer. *Cancer* 1966;19:1096–1101.

88. Austin EH, Flye MW. The treatment of recurrent malignant pleural effusion. *Ann Thorac Surg* 1979;28:190–203.

89. Izbicki R, Weyhing BT, Baker L, et al. Pleural effusion in cancer patients: a prospective randomized study of pleural drainage with the addition of radio-active phosphorous to the pleural space vs. pleural drainage alone. *Cancer* 1975;36:1511–1518.

90. Adler RH, Sayek I. Treatment of malignant pleural effusion: a method using tube thoracostomy and talc. *Ann Thorac Surg* 1976;22:8–15.

91. Rubinson RM, Bolooki H. Intrapleural tetracycline for control of malignant pleural effusion: a preliminary report. *South Med J* 1972;65:847–849.

92. Dollinger MR, Krakoff IH, Karnofsky DA. Quinacrine (Atabrine) in the treatment of neoplastic effusions. *Ann Intern Med* 1967;66:249–257.

93. Xie C, Teixeira LR, Wang N-S, et al. Serial observations after high dose talc slurry in the rabbit model for pleurodesis. *Lung* 1998;176:299–307.

94. Wu W, Teixeira LR, Light RW. Doxycycline pleurodesis in rabbits. Comparison of results with and without chest tube. *Chest* 1998;114:563–568.

95. Sahn SA, Good JT. The effect of common sclerosing agents on the rabbit pleural space. *Am Rev Respir Dis* 1981;124:65–67.

96. Vargas FS, Teixeira LR, Antonangelo L, et al. Acute and chronic pleural changes after the intrapleural instillation of mitoxantrone in rabbits. *Lung* 1998;176:227–236.

97. Light RW, Cheng D-S, Lee YC, et al. A single intrapleural injection of transforming growth factor-2 produces excellent pleurodesis in rabbits. *Am J Respir Crit Care Med* 2000;162:98–104.

98. Xie C, Teixeira LR, McGovern JP, et al. Systemic corticosteroids decrease the effectiveness of talc pleurodesis. *Am J Respir Crit Care Med* 1998;157:1441–1444.

99. Cheng D-S, Rogers J, Wheeler A, et al. The effects of intrapleural polyclonal anti-tumor necrosis factor alpha (TNF) Fab fragments on pleurodesis in rabbits. *Lung* 2000;178:19–30.

100. Strange C, Baumann MH, Sahn SA, et al. Effects of intrapleural heparin or urokinase on the extent of tetracycline-induced pleural disease. *Am J Respir Crit Care Med* 1995;151:508–515.

101. Rodriguez-Panadero F, Segado A, Martin Juan J, et al. Failure of talc pleurodesis is associated with increased pleural fibrinolysis. *Am J Respir Crit Care Med* 1995;151:785–790.

102. Grande, JP. Role of transforming growth factor-β in tissue injury and repair. *P.S.E.B.M.* 1997;214:27–40.

103. Sime PJ, Xing Z, Graham FL, et al. Adenovector-mediated gene transfer of active transforming growth factor-beta₁ induces prolonged severe fibrosis in rat lung. *J Clin Invest* 1997;100;768–776.

104. Perkett EA. Role of growth factors in lung repair and diseases. *Curr Opin Pediatr* 1995:7:242–249.

105. Idell S, Zwieb C, Kumar A, et al. Pathways of fibrin turnover of human pleural mesothelial cells in vitro. *Am J Respir Cell Mol Biol* 1992;7:414–426.

106. Lee YCG, Lane KB, Parker RE, et al. Transforming growth factor (TGF)-β_2 produces effective pleurodesis in sheep with no systemic complications. *Thorax* 2000;55:1058–1062.

107. Sherman S, Grady KJ, Seidmen JC. Clinical experience with tetracycline pleurodesis of malignant pleural effusions. *South Med J* 1987;80:716–719.

108. Walker-Renard PB, Vaughan LM, Sahn SA. Chemical pleurodesis for malignant pleural effusions. *Ann Intern Med* 1994;120:56–64.

109. Costabel U. Adieu, tetracycline pleurodesis; (but not in Germany). *Chest* 1993;103:984.

110. Light RW, Wang NS, Sassoon CS, et al. Comparison of the effectiveness of tetracycline and minocycline as pleural sclerosing agents in rabbits. *Chest* 1994;106:577–582.

111. Robinson LA, Fleming WH, Galbraith TA. Intrapleural doxycycline control of malignant pleural effusions. *Ann Thorac Surg* 1993;55:1115–1121.

112. Heffner JE, Standerfer RJ, Torstveit J, et al. Clinical efficacy of doxycycline for pleurodesis. *Chest* 1994;105:1743–1747.

113. Mansson T. Treatment of malignant pleural effusion with doxycycline. *Scand J Infect Dis* 1988;53 [Suppl]:29–34.

114. Seaton KG, Patz EF Jr, Goodman PC. Palliative treatment of malignant pleural effusions: value of small-bore catheter thoracostomy and doxycycline sclerotherapy. *AJR Am J Roentgenol* 1995;164:589–591.

115. Pulsiripunya C, Youngchaiyud P, Pushpakom R, et al. The efficacy of doxycycline as a pleural sclerosing agent in malignant pleural effusion: a prospective study. *Respirology* 1996;1:69–72.

116. Peng M-J, Kuo H-T, Chen P-J, et al. Minocycline pleurodesis for malignant pleural effusions. *Thorac Med* 1995;10:243–248.

117. Light RW, O'Hara VS, Moritz TE, et al. Intrapleural tetracycline for the prevention of recurrent spontaneous pneumothorax. *JAMA* 1990;264:2224–2230.

118. Bethune N. Pleural poudrage: new technique for deliberate production of pleural adhesions as preliminary to lobectomy. *J Thorac Cardiovasc Surg* 1935;4: 251–261.

119. Light RW, Wang N-S, Sassoon CSH, et al. Talc slurry is an effective pleural sclerosant in rabbits. *Chest* 1995;107:1702–1706.

120. Bresticker MA, Oba J, LoCicero J III, et al. Optimal pleurodesis: a comparison study. *Ann Thorac Surg* 1993;55:364–366.

121. Jerram RM, Fossum TW, Berridge BR, et al. The efficacy of mechanical abrasion and talc slurry as methods of pleurodesis in normal dogs. *Vet Surg* 1999;28: 322–332.

122. Ribas-Milanez de Campos J, Vargas FS, de Campos Werebe E, et al. Thoracoscopic talc poudrage: 15 years experience. *Chest* 2001 (*in press*).

123. Hartman DL, Gaither JM, Kesler KA, et al. Comparison of insufflated talc under thoracoscopic guidance with standard tetracycline and bleomycin pleurodesis for control of malignant pleural effusions. *Cardiovasc Surg* 1993;105:743–748.

124. Noppen M, Degreve J, Mignolet M, et al. A prospective, randomized study comparing the efficacy of talc slurry and bleomycin in the treatment of malignant pleural effusions. *Acta Clin Belg* 1997;52:258–262.

125. Webb WR, Ozmen V, Moulder PV, et al. Iodized talc pleurodesis for the treatment of pleural effusions. *J Thorac Cardiovasc Surg* 1992;103:881–886.

126. Kennedy L, Rusch VW, Strange C, et al. Pleurodesis using talc slurry. *Chest* 1994;106:342–346.

127. Rinaldo JE, Owens GR, Rogers RM. Adult respiratory distress syndrome following intrapleural instillation of talc. *J Thorac Cardiovasc Surg* 1983;85:523–526.

128. Bouchama A, Chastre J, Gaudichet A, et al. Acute pneumonitis with bilateral effusion after talc pleurodesis. *Chest* 1984;86:795–797.

129. Marel M, Skácel Z, Bednár M, et al. *Corynebacterium parvum,* bleomycin and talc in the treatment of malignant pleural effusions. *J Buon* 1998;1:165–170.

130. Campos JR, Werebe EC, Vargas FS, et al. Respiratory failure due to insufflated talc. *Lancet* 1997;349: 251–252.

131. Rehse DH, Aye RW, Florence MG. Respiratory failure following talc pleurodesis. *Am J Surg* 1999;177: 437–440.

132. Todd TR, Delarue NC, Ilves R, et al. Talc poudrage for malignant pleural effusion. *Chest* 1980;78:542–543.

133. Nandi P. Recurrent spontaneus pneumothorax; an effective method of talc poudrage. *Chest* 1980;77:493–495.

134. Migueres J, Jover A. Indications du talcage de plévresous pleursocopie au cours des pleurésies malignes récidivantes. A propos de 26 observations. *Poumon-Coeur* 1981;37:295–297.

135. Weissberg D, Ben-Zeev I. Talc pleurodesis. Experience with 360 patients. *J Thorac Cardiovasc Surgery* 1993;106:689–695.

136. Werebe EC, Pazetti R, De Campos JRM, et al. Systemic distribution of talc after intrapleural administration in rats. *Chest* 1999;115:190–193.

137. Kennedy L, Harley RA, Sahn SA, et al. Talc slurry pleurodesis. Pleural fluid and histologic analysis. *Chest* 1995;107:1707–1712.

138. Ferrer J, Villarino MA, Tura JM, et al. Comparison of size and composition of nine different talcs. Its relevance for pleurodesis. *Am J Respir Crit Care Med* 1998;57:A66.

139. Ruckdeschel JC, Moores D, Lee JY, et al. Intrapleural therapy for malignant pleural effusions. A randomized comparison of bleomycin and tetracycline. *Chest* 1991;100:1528–1535.

140. Diacon AH, Wyser C, Bollinger CT, et al. Prospective randomized comparison of thoracoscopic talc poudrage under local anaestheia vs. bleomycin instillation for pleurodesis in malignant pleural effusions. *Am J Resp Dis Crit Care Med* 2000;162:1445–1449.

141. Vargas FS, Wang NS, Despars JA, et al. Effectiveness of bleomycin in comparison to tetracycline as pleural sclerosing agent in rabbits. *Chest* 1993;104:1582–1584.

142. Leininger BJ, Barker Wl, Lanstron HT. A simplified method for management of malignant pleural effusion. *J Thoracic Cardiovasc Surg* 1969;58:758–763.

143. Kinsey DL, Carter D, Klassen KP. Simplified management of malignant pleural effusion. *Arch Surg* 1964;89:389–391.

144. Marchi E, Vargas FS, Teixeira LR, et al. Comparison of nitrogen mustard, cytarabine and dacarbazine as pleural sclerosing agents in rabbits. *Eur Respir J* 1997;10:598–602.

145. Morales M, Exposito MC. Intrapleural mitoxantrone for the palliative treatment of malignant pleural effusions. *Support Care Cancer* 1995;3:147–149.

146. Maiche AG, Virkkunen P, Kontkanen T, et al. Bleomycin and mitoxantrone in the treatment of malignant pleural effusions. *Am J Clin Oncol* 1993;16:50–53.

147. Vargas FS, Carmo AO, Teixeira LR. A new look at old agents for pleurodesis. Nitrogen mustard, sodium hydroxide and silver nitrate. *Curr Opin Pulm Med* 2000;6:281–286.

148. Vargas FS, Teixeira LR, Silva LMMF, et al. Comparison of silver nitrate and tetracycline as pleural sclerosing agents in rabbits. *Chest* 1995;108:1080–1083.

149. Vargas FS, Teixeira LR, Vaz MAC, et al. Silver nitrate is superior to talc slurry in producing pleurodesis in rabbits. *Chest* 2000;118:808–813.

150. Kataoka M, Morishita R, Hiramatsu J, et al. OK-432 induces production of neutrophil chemotactic factors in malignant pleural effusion. *Intern Med* 1995;34:352–356.

151. Sartori S, Trevisani L, Nielsen I, et al. Intracavitary bleomycin vs interferon in the management of malignant pleural effusions. *Chest* 1998;113:1145–1146.

152. Lissoni P, Barni S, Tancini G, et al. Intracavitary therapy of neoplastic effusions with cytokines: comparison among interferon alpha, beta and interleukin-2. *Support Care Cancer* 1995;3:78–80.

153. Putnam JB Jr, Light RW, Rodriguez RM, et al. A randomized comparison of indwelling pleural catheter and doxycycline pleurodesis in the management of malignant pleural effusions. *Cancer* 1999;86:1992–1999.

154. Putnam JB Jr, Walsh GL, Swisher SG, et al. Outpatient management of malignant pleural effusion by a chronic indwelling pleural catheter. *Ann Thorac Surg* 2000;69:369–375.

155. Patz EF Jr. Malignant pleural effusions: recent advances and ambulatory sclerotherapy. *Chest* 1998;113[Suppl 1]:74S–77S.

156. Sherman S, Ravikrishnan KP, Patel AS, et al. Optimum anesthesia with intrapleural lidocaine during chemical pleurodesis with tetracycline. *Chest* 1988;93:533–536.

157. Vargas FS, Teixeira LR, Coelho IJC, et al. Distribution of pleural injectate: effect of volume of injectate and animal rotation. *Chest* 1994;106:1246–1249.

158. Lorch DG, Gordon L, Wooten S, et al. Effect of patient positioning on distribution of tetracycline in the pleural space during pleurodesis. *Chest* 1988;93:527–529.

159. Dryzer SR, Allen ML, Strange C, et al. A comparison of rotation and nonrotation in tetracycline pleurodesis. *Chest* 1993;104:1763–1766.

160. Groth G, Gatzemeier U, Haubingen K, et al. Intrapleural palliative treatment of MPEs with mitoxantrone versus placebo (pleural tube alone). *Ann Oncol* 1991;2:213–215.

161. Sorensen PG, Svendsen TL, Enk B. Treatment of MPE with drainage, with and without instillation of talc. *Eur J Respir Dis* 1984;65:131–135.

162. Yim AP, Chan AT, Lee TW, et al. Thoracoscopic talc insufflation versus talc slurry for symptomatic malignant pleural effusion. *Ann Thorac Surg* 1996;62:1655–1658.

163. Clementsen P, Evald T, Grode G, et al. Treatment of malignant pleural effusion: pleurodesis using a small percutaneous catheter. A prospective randomized study. *Respir Med* 1998;92:593–596.

164. Marom EM, Patz EF Jr, Erasmus JJ, et al. Malignant pleural effusions: treatment with small-bore catheter thoracostomy and talc pleurodesis. *Radiology* 1999;210:277–281.

165. Villanueva AG, Gray AW Jr, Shahian DM, et al. Efficacy of short term versus long term tube thoracostomy drainage before tetracycline pleurodesis in the treatment of malignant effusions. *Thorax* 1994;49:23–25.

166. Landvater L, Hix WR, Mills M, et al. Malignant pleural effusion treated by tetracycline sclerotherapy: a comparison of single vs repeated instillation. *Chest* 1988;93:1196–1198.

167. Cimochowski GE, Joyner LR, Fardin R, et al. Pleuroperitoneal shunting for recalcitrant pleural effusion. *J Thorac Cardiovasc Surg* 1986;92:866–870.

168. Little AG, Kadowaki MH, Ferguson MK, et al. Pleuroperitoneal shunting: alternative therapy for pleural effusions. *Ann Surg* 1988;208:443–450.

169. Tzeng E, Ferguson MK. Predicting failure following shunting of pleural effusions. *Chest* 1990;98:890–893.

170. Lee KA, Harvey JC, Reich H, et al. Management of malignant pleural effusions with pleuroperitoneal shunting. *J Am College Surg* 1994;178:586–588.

171. Tsang V, Fernando HC, Goldstraw P. Pleuroperitoneal shunt for recurrent malignant pleural effusion. *Thorax* 1990;45:369–372.

172. Ponn RB, Blancaflor J, D'Agostino RS, et al. Pleuroperitoneal shunting for intractable pleural effusions. *Ann Thorac Surg* 1991;51:605–609.

173. al-Kattan KM, Kaplan DK, Goldstraw P. The non-functioning pleuro-peritoneal shunt: revise or replace? *Thorac Cardiovasc Surg* 1994;42:310–312.

174. Petrou M, Kaplan D, Goldstraw P. Management of recurrent malignant pleural effusions. The complementary role talc pleurodesis and pleuroperitoneal shunting. *Cancer* 1995;75:801–805.

175. Martini N, Bains MS, Beattie EJ Jr. Indications for pleurectomy in malignant effusion. *Cancer* 1975;35:734–738.

Primary Tumors of the Pleura

Malignant Mesotheliomas, Solitary Fibrous Tumors, Body Cavity Lymphoma, and Pyothorax-Associated Lymphoma

MALIGNANT MESOTHELIOMAS

Malignant mesotheliomas are thought to arise from the mesothelial cells that line the pleural cavities. Individuals with a history of exposure to asbestos have a much greater risk of developing these neoplasms. Malignant mesothelioma with its dismal prognosis should be differentiated from the solitary fibrous tumor of the pleura with its excellent prognosis, which is discussed later in this chapter. A small percentage of mesotheliomas (less than 10%) arise in the peritoneal cavity (1), but only pleural mesotheliomas are discussed in this chapter.

Etiologic Factors

The occurrence of mesothelioma in many persons is related to previous exposure to asbestos. Asbestos is a fibrous silicate of various chemical types. The main types of asbestos are chrysotile and the amphiboles, which include crocidolite, amosite, tremolite, actinolite, and anthophyllite. The different types of asbestos vary in their ability to induce mesothelioma (2). Fibers with the greatest length-to-diameter ratio are the most carcinogenic (2). At the present time, chrysotile constitutes 99% of current global asbestos production, and can be related to the development of mesothelioma only when the level of exposure is high (1). One of the possible reasons for the lower risk of malignancy from chrysotile exposure is due to the fact that it is cleared from the lungs in a matter of weeks, whereas the amphiboles are cleared only in a matter of decades (3). Crocidolite and amosite are the most carcinogenic amphiboles. Tremolite is a potent inducer of mesothelioma when the fibers have a high length-to-diameter ratio such as occurs in some areas of Greece (4), but the tremolite that contaminates chrysotile ore has a short length and appears to be a low-grade mesothelial carcinogen (4). No case of mesothelioma has been reported to date among Finnish miners exposed to anthophyllite asbestos, although there is a high incidence of pleural calcification as a result of this exposure.

Epidemiologic studies have implicated asbestos in the pathogenesis of malignant mesothelioma (5). In a recent study from Australia, nine of 247 patients with the highest estimated cumulative exposure to asbestos had mesothelioma. The percentage of patients with mesothelioma who have a history of occupational exposure to asbestos ranges from 10% in a series from the Mayo Clinic (6) to 70% in New England, England, and South Africa (7), where shipyards or asbestos mines are located. The risk of developing mesothelioma from asbestos exposure appears to be higher in manufacturing industries than in mining and milling. Because asbestos is found in a variety of industrial products, including insulation, roofing and ceiling tiles, brake linings, and numerous small appliances, many individuals are unaware of their exposure to this substance.

Further evidence implicating asbestos as an etiologic agent in mesotheliomas comes from animal studies. The intrapleural injection of any of the different types of asbestos (including chrysotile) results in the production of mesotheliomas in 8% to 66% of animals, depending upon the dose. Mesotheliomas can also be induced after the inhalation of various types of asbestos (8). These mesotheliomas are histologically identical to the human tumor (9, 10).

The incidence of mesotheliomas following asbestos exposure increases linearly with intensity of exposure but exponentially (to the 3rd or 4th power) with time from first asbestos exposure. The risk of malignant mesothelioma can be estimated from the following mathematical equation:

$$R = K \times F \times T^p$$

where R is the risk of mesothelioma, K is a coefficient dependent on the fiber size and type (highest for crocidolite and lowest for chrysotile), F is the number of fibers per milliliter, T is the time after the first exposure, and p is the exponent that is thought to be between 3 and 4 (1).

At times, the asbestos exposure may not be obvious. In one report (11), five cases of mesothelioma developed in a Native American pueblo of approximately 2,000 persons. Epidemiologic investigation revealed that asbestos mats were used to insulate worktables against the intense heat of brazing torches and molten metal in the preparation of silver jewelry. In addition, the villagers scrubbed leather with cakes of asbestos to make their leggings and moccasins a brilliant white.

The mechanism by which asbestos fibers induce malignant changes is not known. The asbestos fiber appears to have two major sources of genotoxicity: generation of reactive oxygen species and mechanical effects such as interference with mitotic spindle formation and the segregation of chromosomes (12). Exposure to asbestos can also damage the cellular DNA and if the cells with the damaged DNA either do not undergo apoptosis or undergo cell cycle arrest, a malignant transformation may occur. It should be noted, however, that so far no consistent abnormalities in oncogenes or suppressor genes have been found in human mesothelioma (1).

Mineral fibers other than asbestos can induce mesotheliomas. In one area of Turkey, about 1% of the population dies each year of malignant mesothelioma (13). Villagers are usually aged 40 to 60 years when the mesotheliomas develop. Asbestos does not occur in the local soil or rocks, nor is it handled in the village. The atmosphere in the area does contain increased amounts of erionite, a mineral of the zeolite family. This mineral is a major contributor to the clouds in the area. This report suggests that the inhalation of airborne respirable fibers other than asbestos can be associated with the subsequent development of pleural mesotheliomas (13). Indeed when erionite fibers are administered intrapleurally to rats, they are two orders of magnitude more carcinogenic than crocidolite (14).

There are probably other factors related to the development of pleural mesothelioma. Antman et al. (15) reported that mesothelioma developed in proximity to a field of therapeutic radiation administered 10 to 31 years previously in four patients. Roviaro et al. (16) reviewed 35 cases of pleural mesothelioma and found that three of the patients had calcified posttuberculous fibrothorax. There is no clear evidence of a familial tendency to develop mesothelioma (17), and there is no definite evidence that smoking increases the risk of mesothelioma (1).

One factor that has received much attention in the past decade as a possible etiologic factor in the development of malignant mesothelioma is the simian virus 40 (SV40). The impetus for these investigations was the observation that the intrapleural injection of SV40 would induce mesotheliomas in hamsters (18). Early poliomyelitis vaccines contaminated with SV40 were a potential source for the SV40 DNA in humans (1). Subsequent studies demonstrated that there were SV40 DNA large T antigen sequences in pleural malignant mesotheliomas (19). For example, in one recent study, specific SV40 sequences were present in 57% of epithelial invasive malignant mesotheliomas but not in sarcomatous or mixed malignant mesotheliomas (19).

Lung cancers lacked SV40 sequences, as did nonmalignant tissues adjacent to malignant mesotheliomas (19). The accumulated evidence only points to SV40 as a possible cofactor in the pathogenesis of malignant mesothelioma. In humans, the SV40 may represent a bystander or passenger, or the tumor tissue may represent a favorable milieu for the replication of preexisting latent SV40 (1). It is interesting that SV40 virus was not present in any of 29 mesotheliomas in Turkey, a country where SV40-contaminated vaccines were not administered (20).

Incidence

The annual incidence of malignant mesotheliomas in the United States has been increasing over the past few decades and is expected to peak in approximately the year 2000, with an annual incidence of 2,300 (21). In comparison, the annual incidence of mesothelioma in Western Europe in the year 2000 is 5,000 and is expected to peak around the year 2018 with an annual incidence of 9,000 (22). The difference in the incidence in the two locations is due to the fact that the maximal exposure to asbestos in Europe occurred in approximately 1970, whereas the maximum exposure in the United States occurred from the 1930s to the 1960s (21). The incidence of mesothelioma in men is approximately eight times that in women (21). The higher incidence in men is due for the most part to higher occupational exposure to asbestos. The seriousness of the problem with mesothelioma attributed to asbestos exposure is emphasized by the observation that, in Sweden, there are more deaths annually from mesothelioma due to asbestos exposure than to all fatal occupational accidents (23).

Pathologic Features

Malignant mesotheliomas in the earliest stages appear grossly as multiple white or gray granules, nodules, or flakes on normal or opaque parietal pleura (24). As the tumor progresses, the pleural surface becomes progressively thicker and nodular in appearance. The growing tumor extends in all directions to form a continuous layer encasing the lung and leading to contraction of the involved hemithorax. In advanced cases, the diaphragm, liver, pericardium, heart, contralateral pleura, and other mediastinal structures may be involved. At autopsy, hematogenously disseminated metastases are present in one third to one half of patients. In contrast to other sarcomas, however, the hematogenous metastases are usually clinically silent, and death generally results from complications arising from the primary lesion (7).

Microscopically, malignant mesotheliomas are characterized by marked structural variation within a single tumor or among different tumors with a similar gross appearance (25). Histologically, malignant mesotheliomas are classified as epithelial, fibrous, or biphasic, as recommended by the World Health Organization (26). Other classifications with more subtypes have also been developed (26). In a compilation of 819 cases from the literature, 50% were epithelial, 34% were biphasic, and 16% were fibrous (27). The neoplastic cells of the epithelial form may show various epithelial arrangements such as papillary, tubular, tubulopapillary, cordlike, and sheetlike patterns. The epithelial cells may take various shapes but most commonly are cuboidal and uniform in size with vesicular nuclei. The fibrous (sarcomatous) form resembles a spindle cell sarcoma in that the cells are spindle shaped with a parallel arrangement and have ovoid or elongated nuclei with well-developed nucleoli (28). The biphasic type has features of both the epithelial and fibrous forms.

Clinical Manifestations

Two thirds of patients with malignant mesothelioma are between the ages of 40 and 70 years (7, 29), and many have a history of exposure to asbestos 20 or more years in the past. Most patients initially experience the insidious onset of chest pain or shortness of breath (2). Patients usually have had symptoms for several months before they see a physician (2). The chest pain is usually nonpleuritic and is frequently referred to the upper abdomen or shoulder because of diaphragmatic involvement. As the disease progresses, the patients lose weight and develop a dry, hacking cough and progressive dyspnea. Some patients have irregular episodes of low-grade fever (29). Physical examination may reveal clubbing. Examination of the chest reveals that the involved hemithorax is sometimes reduced in size, and, at times, there is retraction of the intercostal spaces. In addition, there are the physical signs of a pleural effusion.

Radiographic Manifestations

The chest radiograph (Fig. 8.1) reveals a pleural effusion in about 75% to 90% of patients (30, 31). This effusion is frequently large, occupying 50% or more of the hemithorax and obscuring the pleural tumor. In about one third of patients, pleural plaques are evident in the opposite hemithorax (32). With progression of the disease, the tumor encases the ipsilateral lung and thereby produces a mediastinal shift to the side of the effusion and results in a loculated pleural effusion. In the late stages of the disease, the chest radiograph may show mediastinal widening, enlargement of the cardiac shadow due to infiltration of the pericardium, and destruction of the ribs or soft tissue masses (33). At times, rounded atelectasis is present (see Chapter 24).

Because routine chest radiographs often underestimate the extent of the disease, chest computed tomography (CT) scans are invaluable in delineating the extent of the disease (30–33). Chest CT scans should be obtained for all patients in whom a malignant mesothelioma is considered (Fig. 8.1C). With mesothelioma, the disease is unilateral in almost all cases (31). On CT scan, the pleura is thickened, with an irregular, often

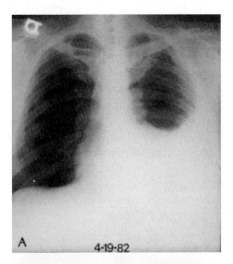

4-19-82

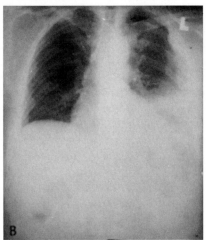

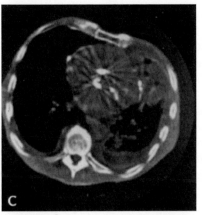

FIG. 8.1 Malignant mesothelioma. **A:** Posteroanterior chest radiograph demonstrating left pleural effusion and thickening of the pleura over the upper left lung. **B:** Posteroanterior chest radiograph from the same patient after therapeutic thoracentesis revealing a small left lung and marked pleural thickening. **C:** CT scan of the chest demonstrating shrunken left hemithorax and shift of the mediastinum toward the left. Pericardial calcifications due to previous asbestos exposure are also present.

nodular internal margin that serves to distinguish this tumor from other types of pleural thickening. These changes are most pronounced at the base of the lung. The CT scan usually reveals marked thickening of the major fissure due to a combination of fibrosis, tumor, and associated fluid. The fissure may also appear nodular because of tumor infiltration (32). At times, pleural thickening is seen predominantly along the mediastinum. In such cases, the pulmonary margin is irregular, and separate nodules representing either metastases or lymph node infiltration may be seen in the juxtamediastinal tissue.

The volume of the hemithorax with malignant mesothelioma is quite varied. If the patient has a pleural effusion with pleural thickening and decreased volume of the ipsilateral hemithorax, it is very suggestive of mesothelioma. In one series, the volume of the hemithorax was reduced in 42% of 50 cases of mesothelioma (30), whereas in another case, the volume of the hemithorax was reduced in 30% of 50 cases (31). It should be emphasized, however, that contralateral mediastinal shift is seen in about 15% to 25% of cases, and this is usually due to a large effusion (30, 31).

The CT scan is also useful in demonstrating disease beyond the pleura and thereby is quite useful in staging the disease. It often reveals intrapulmonary nodules that are not apparent on the standard chest radiograph (32). The CT scan may reveal chest wall invasion, diaphragmatic invasion, or extension of the tumor to the liver or retroperitoneal space. CT scans are not without their problems with mesothelioma; CT fails to identify chest wall and mediastinal invasion in some patients who undergo surgical resections (34). In addition, it is often very difficult to distinguish pleural disease alone from associated pericardial disease, and extensive pleural disease often envelops and obscures the nodal anatomy in the hilar and middle mediastinal nodal groups (30).

Another imaging modality that may prove useful in the diagnosis of malignant mesothelioma is fluorodeoxyglucose (FDG) positron emission tomography (PET) (35). In one series, 28 patients with pleural thickening, including 24 with malignant and four with benign disease, were subjected to FDG-PET scanning. The uptake of FDG was significantly higher in the malignant lesions than in the benign lesions. In addition, the FDG-PET images provided excellent delineation of the extent of the disease (35). However, it does not appear that metastatic adenocarcinoma can be differentiated from malignant mesothelioma with this imaging technique.

Pleural Fluid

The pleural fluid with mesotheliomas is yellow in about 50% of patients and serosanguineous in the remainder. This fluid is exudative. In approximately one third of patients, the pleural fluid glucose is below 50 mg per dL and the pleural fluid pH is below 7.20 (36). Patients with a low pleural fluid pH or low pleural fluid glucose level tend to have a poorer prognosis (36). The pleural fluid generally is cellular and contains a mixture of normal mesothelial cells, differentiated and undifferentiated malignant mesothelial cells, and varying numbers of lymphocytes and polymorphonuclear leukocytes (37).

At times, the pleural fluid of patients with malignant mesothelioma is viscid, owing to the presence of large amounts of hyaluronate, which was previously called hyaluronic acid. Nurminen et al. (38) assessed the diagnostic utility of hyaluronate levels by assaying the levels in 1,039 pleural fluids including 50 from mesothelioma. They found that with a cutoff of 75 mg per L for hyaluronate, the assay specificity for malignant mesothelioma was 100% and the sensitivity was 56% (38). It should be noted that another study (39) demonstrated that the hyaluronate measurements were much less useful. It appears that the poor results in the latter study are probably attributable to procedural mistakes (40). The results by Nurminen (38) were obtained by high-pressure liquid chromatography (HPLC), and this assay is not generally available in the United States.

Diagnosis

The diagnosis of malignant mesothelioma should be considered in all patients with exudative pleural effusions. The suspicion of mesothelioma should be higher in middle-aged or older patients with persistent chest pain or shortness of breath, particularly if there is a history of asbestos exposure. The chest CT scan is frequently suggestive of the diagnosis. Although a diagnosis of malignancy can be established by cytologic smears or needle biopsies of the pleura, these procedures usually cannot distinguish between a metastatic adenocarcinoma and a mesothelioma. In one series (41), 80 patients with mesothelioma had pleural fluid cytology. In 20 patients (25%), cytologic examination of the pleural fluid established that the patient had malignant disease, but in none could the diagnosis of mesothelioma be established definitely with only cytology.

There are, however, certain cytologic features that assist in making this differentiation. One report (42) compared the cytologic features of 44 cases of malignant mesothelioma and 46 cases of metastatic adenocarcinomas, and the authors concluded that the following five features separate malignant mesothelioma from adenocarcinoma with better than 95.4% accuracy. Mesotheliomas tend to have true papillary aggregation, multinucleation with atypia, and cell-to-cell apposition, whereas adenocarcinomas tend to have acinus-like structures and balloon-like vacuolation (42). In addition, immunohistochemical studies on cell blocks from pleural fluid are useful in distinguishing mesothelioma from adenocarcinoma (43–45) (see Chapter 4).

Needle biopsy of the pleura is usually not diagnostic of mesothelioma. In one report (41), the needle biopsy was diagnostic of mesothelioma in only 18 of 84 cases (21%). Also, there is poor concordance among different pathologists when the diagnosis of mesothelioma is based on specimens from needle biopsy (46).

Accordingly, more invasive procedures are necessary to provide a larger tissue sample so that a definitive diagnosis can be made. If the patient has skin deposits, these should be biopsied. However, usually the diagnosis must be made with thoracoscopy or open biopsy. Thoracoscopy establishes the diagnosis of mesothelioma more than 90% of the time. When two recent series (47, 48) are combined, the diagnosis was established in 51 of the 56 (90%) patients. These results are similar to those with thoracotomy and open biopsy (29). Thoracoscopy is therefore the procedure of choice because its diagnostic yield is similar to that of open thoracotomy, but the procedure is less invasive (49).

Malignant mesothelioma often infiltrates needle tracts, thoracotomy scars, and chest tube drainage sites after diagnostic or therapeutic procedures. These tumor deposits can be quite bothersome to the patient (50). It appears that such seeding can be prevented with small amounts of irradiation after the procedure. Boutin et al. (50) randomized 40 consecutive patients to receive three treatments of 7 Gy each 10 to 15 days after thoracoscopy when the wounds had healed. They reported that the incidence of entry tract metastases was 40% in the control group but zero in the treatment group. In view of this, consideration should be given to postprocedure radiation in patients with malignant mesothelioma.

Histologic examination of hematoxylin and eosin (H&E)–stained tissue section remains the primary method by which the diagnosis of malignant mesothelioma is established. However, it is frequently difficult to distinguish malignant mesothelioma from metastatic adenocarcinomas on the H&E-stained slides (24, 51). At present, immunohistochemical procedures have gained widespread acceptance as valuable adjuncts in establishing the diagnosis of malignant mesothelioma (24, 51). Some of the immunohistochemical markers are positive with adenocarcinomas, whereas others are positive with malignant mesotheliomas. When one wishes to differentiate metastatic adenocarcinoma from malignant mesothelioma, the tissue sections should be stained with a panel of immunohistochemical markers (see Chapter 4). At the present time, the best markers for mesothelioma appear to be calretinin and cytokeratin 5/6, whereas the best markers for adenocarcinoma appeared to be carcinoembryonic antigen (CEA), MOC-31, and BG-8 (51). However, it is important to realize that nonmalignant mesothelial cells also stain positive for calretinin and cytokeratin 5/6 (52). It is anticipated that over the next decade, markers that are more sensitive and more specific will be developed.

The diagnosis of malignant mesotheliomas is usually established by the combination of the histology and the immunohistochemical stains. However, when doubt exists, two tests that have been used for decades can at times still be useful. The periodic acid–Schiff stain can still be used to distinguish mesotheliomas from adenocarcinomas. The presence of strongly positive vacuoles after diastase digestion effectively establishes the diagnosis of adenocarcinoma, although not all adenocarcinomas have this staining characteristic. In addition, most mesotheliomas contain large amounts of hyaluronate that stain positively with colloidal iron or alcian blue stains. To be unequivocally positive, absence or attenuation of blue staining after pretreatment of a serial section with bovine testicular hyaluronidase overnight is required (53).

The diagnosis of pleural mesothelioma is made accurately in most cases without resorting to electron microscopic (EM) examination (24). However, because EM still plays a decisive role in some cases with unusual morphology or anomalous histochemical or immunohistochemical reactions, a portion of the pleural specimen should be routinely fixed at the time of pleural biopsy for possible subsequent processing for EM (24). Epithelial mesotheliomas are characterized by the presence of tonofilaments, desmosomes, and microvilli. The appearance of the microvilli is important in distinguishing mesotheliomas from adenocarcinomas. With mesothelioma, the microvilli are numerous and are characteristically long and thin, whereas in adenocarcinoma they are typically much less frequent and are usually short and stubby (24, 54). In one study (54), the mean length-to-diameter ratio of the microvilli of mesotheliomas with scanning electron micro-scopy was 19.7:1 (range 13.7 to 23.5:1), whereas that for adenocarcinomas was 2.5:1 (range 1.3 to 4:1). Scanning electron microscopy can be used when glutaraldehyde-fixed, plastic-embedded tissue is not available for transmission electron microscopy (54). A number of subcellular structures, such as mucin granules, myclino-somes, microvilli coated by a filamentous glycocalyx, and microvillous rootlets, may be observed in some adenocarcinomas. The presence of any of these features excludes mesothelioma (25).

Flow cytometry does not appear to be particularly useful in establishing the diagnosis of malignant mesothelioma. Burmer et al. (55) performed flow cytometry on 46 cases of malignant pleural mesothelioma and 31 nonmesothelioma malignancies of the pleural space. They reported that 65% of the mesotheliomas were diploid in DNA content, with intermediate to low proliferative rates. In contrast, 85% of the nonmesothelial malignant neoplasms were aneuploid.

Management and Prognosis

The prognosis of patients with pleural mesothelioma is more dependent on so-called pretreatment factors than on the effect of therapeutic intervention. In general, the prognosis of patients with malignant mesothelioma is not good, with median survival time overall of about 8 to 12 months after diagnosis (56, 57). It should be noted, however, that the life expectancy is higher in patients with mesothelioma than in patients with metastatic malignancy, in which case, the median survival is about 3 months after diagnosis. The prognosis is better with the epithelial type as compared with the fibrous type mesothelioma (56–58). Patients with the tubulopapillary type of epithelial mesothelioma have the best prognosis, with a median survival of more than 2 years after symptoms begin (58). Patients with larger tumor volumes and more advanced stages of the disease also have shorter survival times (59). Survival time varies inversely with age, with the longest survival time occurring in the youngest age group (56, 60). Survival is also better in women and in patients with a better performance status. Survival time is also poorer in patients with regional lymph node involvement.

Staging

When a patient is suspected of having a mesothelioma, the extent of the disease should be staged because the stage of the disease dictates the therapeutic approach. There have been several different staging systems proposed. The staging scheme recommended by the Cancer Committee of the College of American Pathologists is

TABLE 8.1. *TNM and stage grouping for mesothelioma*

Primary Tumor (T)
T0   No evidence of primary tumor
T1   Tumor limited to ipsilateral parietal or visceral pleura
T2   Tumor invades any of the following: ipsilateral lung, endothoracic fascia, diaphragm, or pericardium
T3   Tumor invades any of the following: ipsilateral chest wall muscle, ribs, or mediastinal organs or tissues
T4   Tumor directly extends to any of the following: contralateral pleural, contralateral lung, peritoneum, intraabdominal organs, or cervical tissue

Regional Lymph Nodes (N)
N0   No regional lymph node metastasis
N1   Metastasis in ipsilateral peribronchial or ipsilateral hilar lymph nodes, including intrapulmonary nodes involved by direct extension of the primary tumor
N2   Metastasis in ipsilateral mediastinal or subcarinal lymph nodes
N3   Metastasis in contralateral mediastinal, contralateral hilar, ipsilateral or contralateral scalene, or supraclavicular lymph nodes.

Distant Metastasis (M)
M0   No evidence of distant metastasis
M1   Distant metastasis

AJCC/UICC TNM Stage Groupings

Stage I	T1	N0	M0
	T2	N0	M0
Stage II	T1	N1	M0
	T2	N1	M0
Stage III	T1	N2	M0
	T2	N2	M0
	T3	N0,1,2	M0
Stage IV	Any T	N3	M0
	T4	Any N	M0
	Any T	Any N	M1

TNM, primary tumor, regional lymph nodes, and distant metastasis.

TABLE 8.2. *Pathologic staging of diffuse malignant mesothelioma of the pleura*

Stage	Manifestation
I	Tumor confined within the capsule of the parietal pleura, i.e., involving only the ipsilateral pleura, lung, pericardium, and diaphragm
II	Tumor involving chest wall or mediastinal structures; possible lymph node involvement inside the chest
III	Tumor penetrating diaphragm to involve the peritoneum; contralateral pleural involvement; lymph node involvement outside the chest
IV	Distant bloodborne metastases

Modified from Butchart EG, Ashcroft T, Barnsley WC, et al. The role of surgery in diffuse malignant mesothelioma of the pleura. *Semin Oncol* 1981;8:321–328, with permission from Grune & Stratton.

that developed by the American Joint Committee on Cancer (AJCC) and the International Union Against Cancer (UICC) tumor, nodes, and metastases (TNM) staging system as shown in Table 8.1. To stage the disease, the following studies are required: a barium swallow to assess esophageal involvement; a bronchoscopic examination to assess involvement of the tracheobronchial tree; a chest CT scan to assess mediastinal or chest wall involvement; brain, liver, and bone scans to look for distant metastases; and possibly, a pneumoperitoneogram to look for di-

aphragmatic penetration (61). Rusch and Venkatraman investigated prognostic factors in 231 patients who underwent thoracotomy between 1983 and 1998. They found that the median survival time for stage I tumors was 29.9 months; for stage II, 19 months; for stage III, 10.4 months; and for stage IV, 8 months (62). A recent study demonstrated that magnetic resonance imaging (MRI) did not add significantly to CT in staging mesothelioma (63). A simpler staging system devised by Butchart is shown in Table 8.2.

Palliative Therapy

No satisfactory treatment exists for malignant mesothelioma. The beneficial effects of treatment of malignant mesothelioma are moot (64). There are no controlled studies that demonstrate that any treatment is effective in prolonging survival. It is unclear whether any of the available treatments prolong life. Law et al. (65) compared the survival rates in 64 untreated patients and 52 treated patients seen at the Brompton and the Royal Marsden Hospitals between 1971 and 1980. The two groups of patients had comparable clinical conditions at the time of presentation. Whether or not the patient received treatment depended on the attending physician; some treated all patients, whereas others managed all patients symptomatically. The survival curves for the 64 untreated patients and the 12 patients who received radiotherapy, the 28 patients who received decortication, and the 12 patients who received chemotherapy were virtually identical. The median survival time was about 18 months; 10% of patients survived more than 4 years, including seven of the 64 (11%) untreated patients (65). These results indicate that controlled cooperative studies are needed to assess the effectiveness of the various treatment modalities proposed for malignant mesothelioma.

Shortness of breath and chest pain are the two most troublesome symptoms in patients with malignant mesothelioma. The shortness of breath can be due either to the presence of a large pleural effusion or to invasion of the lung or mediastinum by the tumor. If the patient is breathless and has a pleural effusion, a therapeutic thoracentesis should be performed. If the shortness of breath is relieved by the thoracentesis, a pleurodesis should be attempted (41) or a pleuroperitoneal shunt inserted. Details concerning both these procedures are delineated in Chapter 7. If the shortness of breath is not relieved by the thoracentesis, then oxygen or opiates should be prescribed.

The other main symptom in patients with malignant mesothelioma is chest pain, frequently caused by tumor invasion of the chest wall. In such persons, local palliative radiotherapy may relieve the symptoms (33), but frequently, the response is minimal or nonexistent (31, 66). More often, strong analgesics must be administered to control the pain. If the pain is severe, consideration should be given to performing a percutaneous cervical cordotomy. In one recent series, this procedure was performed on 52 patients with intractable chest pain who were taking a median of 100 mg morphine per day (67). After the procedure, 38% of the patients were able to stop taking morphine and another 37% were able to reduce their morphine by more than 50%. Two patients experienced troublesome dysesthesia following the procedure, and four had persistent motor weakness. No patient became hemiplegic or was unable to walk.

Another troublesome symptom in approximately one third of patients is intermittent fever and sweating (41). Law et al. (41) reported that the administration of prednisolone was of some benefit in alleviating the fever and sweating, and usually improved the appetite and the well-being of the patient.

Surgical Treatment

Surgical management appears to be the only form of therapy that offers the patient any hope for cure. Butchart et al. (61) operated on 29 patients with malignant mesothelioma between 1959 and 1972 and reported that two patients (7%) were alive, without evidence of recurrence, 3.5 and 6 years after operation. The surgical resections performed by this group were extensive, with removal of the pleura, lung, lymph nodes, ipsilateral pericardium, and diaphragm. The in-hospital postoperative mortality rate was 31%. These workers concluded that radical pleuropneumonectomy was only indicated for patients younger than the age of 60 who are fit and who have stage I tumors of the epithelial type.

In recent years, Sugarbaker et al. (68) have reported good results in a series of 183 patients who underwent extrapleural pneumonectomy, followed by chemotherapy and radiotherapy. Patients were operated on only if they had a Karnofsky performance status greater than 70%, a creatinine level and liver function tests within normal limits, and a tumor that was judged to be completely resectable on the basis of CT and MRI scan. The extrapleural pneumonectomy entailed resection of the pleura, lung, diaphragm, and pericardium en bloc (68).

In this series, there were seven (3.8%) perioperative deaths and the median postoperative length of stay was 9 days. Overall, the median survival for these patients was 19 months and the 2- and 5-year survival rates were 38% and 15%, respectively. The subset of 31 patients with epithelial cell type, negative resection margins, and negative extrapleural nodal status had a median survival of 51 months, a 2-year survival rate of 68%, and a 5-year survival rate of 46% (68).

It should be emphasized that the series reported by Sugarbaker represents a very select group of patients and the median survival overall of 19 months was disappointing. Less than 15% of patients with malignant mesothelioma are candidates for extrapleural pneumonectomy. There is no evidence that patients with fibrous mesotheliomas are benefited. Based on the above-mentioned series, it is recommended that patients in relatively good health who have stage I disease of the epithelial type be considered for this radical surgery. There is no definite proof, however, that their life expectancies will be extended by the procedure, and the combination of surgery, radiotherapy, and chemotherapy is expensive, time-consuming, and usually requires that the patients be away from home for considerable periods of time.

Other researchers have recommended that only pleurectomies be performed (29, 69). Wanebo et al. (69) performed pleurectomies on 33 patients with malignant mesothelioma, of whom 17 had the epithelial variant and 16 the mesenchymal variant. Four of the 17 patients with the epithelial variant (23%) and three of the 16 patients with the mesenchymal type (19%) were disease-free at 17 to 69 months postoperatively. These authors followed their surgical procedures with high-dose radiotherapy or systemic chemotherapy because tumor was left behind when pneumonectomies were not performed. The regimens of chemotherapy and radiotherapy were not consistent, and, therefore, their roles in combination with resection remain to be defined. The large advantage that this surgery has over the extrapleural pneumonectomy is that it has a much lower rate of associated morbidity and mortality (29). However, it appears less likely to cure the patient because tumor is left behind.

Rusch and Venkatraman (62) compared the survival rate in 115 patients who had extrapleural pneumonectomy and 59 patients with pleurectomy and decortication who had participated in various trials. They could find no difference in the survival rates with the two surgical methods (62). It should be noted that in most series, surgery is combined with another therapeutic modality. Controlled studies are needed to compare the extrapleural pneumonectomy with the pleurectomy with no surgery.

Chemotherapy

The role of chemotherapy in the treatment of malignant mesothelioma remains to be defined. No chemotherapy trials have stratified patients according to histologic form or stage of the disease. Moreover, until recently, most patients with mesothelioma did not have objective parameters to follow, in that the extent of the disease could not be gauged accurately from the chest radiographs. The availability of CT scan of the chest has partially corrected this deficiency. However, it is difficult to separate fluid and inflammatory reactions from tumor and the CT scan is also subject to intercut variations.

No single drug has consistently induced a response rate greater than 20% (70). Agents that produce response rates in 10% to 20% of patients include doxorubicin, epirubicin, mitomycin, cyclophosphamide, ifosfamide, cisplatin, and carboplatin (70). In general, combination chemotherapy trials do not demonstrate a consistently greater response rate than single-agent trials. Because no study has demonstrated a survival benefit with chemotherapy compared with palliative therapy, chemotherapy is not currently recommended for malignant mesothelioma unless the patient is in a controlled clinical trial.

Intrapleural chemotherapy probably has more promise than systemic chemotherapy. It has been shown that when drugs are administered intrapleurally, there is a threefold to fivefold advantage on a logarithmic scale for pleural versus plasma area under the concentration–time curves for cisplatin and mitomycin (70). However, the results of clinical studies have been disappointing (71).

Radiotherapy

The results with radiotherapy in the treatment of malignant mesothelioma have been disappointing (72). External radiotherapy does not control mesotheliomas locally and is associated with severe toxicity in the underlying lung (73). It is not recommended at the present time (72). There may be a place for internal radiation therapy in the management of malignant mesothelioma (74). In one report from the Memorial Sloan-Kettering Cancer Center, 33 patients were treated with the implantation of permanent radioactive iodine-125 sources in residual tumor. This report concluded that local radiotherapy improved the length of survival (74).

Novel Therapies for Malignant Mesothelioma

Because the current therapies for mesothelioma are so ineffective, the search for newer therapies continues. Although none of the following therapies has been proven to be effective, significant advances in the therapy for mesothelioma may arise from one or more of these therapies. Astoul et al. (75) administered interleukin 2 (IL-2) to 22 patients with malignant mesothelioma and reported 11 partial responses and one complete response. However, the median survival time of these patients was only 18 months. Marzo et al. demonstrated that antisense oligonucleotides specific for transforming growth factor-2 inhibited the growth of malignant mesothelioma both in vitro and in vivo (76). Several phase I studies using gene therapy have been reported (77, 78). Rubins et al. have shown that lovastatin induces apoptosis in malignant mesothelioma cells and suggest that its effectiveness should be assessed in clinical trials (79).

SOLITARY FIBROUS TUMORS OF THE PLEURA

In the literature, there is a great diversity in the nomenclature of benign fibrous tumors of the pleura; these tumors have also been called localized mesothelioma, benign fibrous mesothelioma, benign localized fibroma, and submesothelial fibroma (80). The term solitary fibrous tumor is preferred for several reasons: (a) although the neoplasm is usually histologically and biologically benign, malignant forms clearly exist, and, in some cases, the histologic distinction between the two is difficult, if not impossible; (b) the neoplasm often shows evidence of fibroblastic differentiation; and (c) the results

of ultrastructural, immunohistochemical, and experimental studies suggest that the tumor originates in the submesothelium itself (81). In contrast to malignant mesothelioma, the prognosis with benign fibrous tumors of the pleural is excellent (80). These tumors are uncommon; over a 25-year period, 52 cases were seen at the Mayo Clinic (82). Most patients with benign fibrous tumors of the pleura have no history of asbestos exposure (80, 81).

Pathologic Features

Grossly benign fibrous tumors appear as firm, encapsulated yellow tumors, which may be vascular with prominent veins over their external surfaces (83). About two thirds of these fibrous tumors arise from the visceral pleura, whereas one third arise from the parietal pleura. At times, these tumors invade the lung and chest wall locally (84). Solitary fibrous tumors are characterized histologically by uniform, elongated spindle cells and varied amounts of collagen and reticulum fibers in bundles of many sizes (82). The cell of origin of this tumor is not yet known; most believe that the tumor arises from the multipotential subpleural fibroblasts (81, 84, 85), but some believe that the tumor arises from the mesothelial cell (86). An absolute distinction between a localized benign fibrous tumor and a localized malignant mesothelioma is not always possible (86).

Clinical Manifestations

This tumor is evenly distributed between the sexes, and the median age of presentation is 57 years (84). Approximately 50% of patients with benign fibrous tumors are asymptomatic, and the tumor is detected on routine chest radiographs (82, 85). In the remaining patients, cough, chest pain, and dyspnea are the most frequent symptoms, each occurring in about 40% of symptomatic patients. About 25% of symptomatic patients are febrile without any evidence of infection (85). The incidence of hypertrophic pulmonary osteoarthropathy in patients with benign fibrous tumors is high. Approximately 20%

of patients with this tumor have hypertrophic pulmonary osteoarthropathy, and the incidence is much higher with larger tumors. In one series, 10 of 11 patients (91%) with lesions larger than 7 cm in diameter had hypertrophic pulmonary osteoarthropathy, whereas none of 41 patients with smaller lesions had the syndrome (82). When the tumors are surgically removed, the symptoms of hypertrophic pulmonary osteoarthropathy are relieved immediately in almost all patients (82).

Another paraneoplastic syndrome that sometimes accompanies solitary fibrous tumors of the pleura is hypoglycemia (Doege-Potter syndrome). Of the approximately 150 extrapancreatic tumors causing hypoglycemia reported by 1975, 10 were benign fibrous tumors of the pleura. In a review of 360 cases of solitary fibrous tumors of the pleura, symptomatic hypoglycemia was reported in 4% (85). The mechanism responsible

for the hypoglycemia appears to be the production of high levels of insulin-like growth factor II (IGF-II) by the tumor (87). The increased production of this insulin-like substance leads to an increased use of glucose by peripheral tissues and decreased production of glucose by the liver. Tumors that are associated with hypoglycemia tend to be large. The hypoglycemia is relieved with surgical removal of the tumor.

Radiologically, these tumors are manifested as solitary, sharply defined, discrete masses located at the periphery of the lung or related to a fissure (7, 83). At times, the mass may become very large, occupying most of the hemithorax (Fig. 8.2). The mass is frequently lobulated (7). The mass has an associated pleural effusion about 10% of the time (82, 88), but the presence or absence of an effusion apparently has no effect on the patient's prognosis (7). In one case, more than

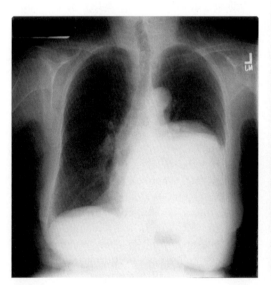
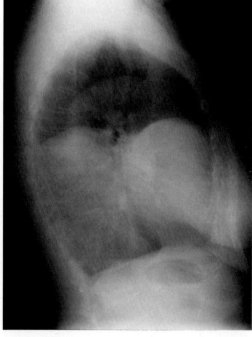

FIG. 8.2. Solitary fibrous tumor of the pleura. **A:** Posteroanterior chest radiograph demonstrating a large mass in the left hemithorax. **B:** Lateral radiograph demonstrating a large lobulated mass. These radiographs were from a 90-year-old lady who presented with severe hypoglycemia. At thoracotomy, the mass was found to be a solitary fibrous tumor of the pleura and it was completely removed. The patient became asymptomatic postoperatively with resolution of the hypoglycemia.

170 L of transudative pleural fluid was produced by a solitary fibrous tumor (88). Calcifications are occasionally evident within the mass (83).

The appearance of the solitary fibrous tumors on CT scan is characteristic (81, 89). The tumors are large, noninvasive and tend to enhance with intravenous contrast material, but the enhancement is frequently nonhomogeneous. The intense enhancement of these tumors appears to be due to their high vascularity, while areas of low attenuation are due to foci of myxoid or cystic degeneration and hemorrhage in the lesion (89). There is no associated mediastinal lymphadenopathy.

Diagnosis

A thoracotomy is usually necessary for diagnosis, although the diagnosis has been established by transthoracic cutting needle biopsy in some patients (90). However, because the appropriate treatment for the solitary fibrous tumor is surgical removal, most patients should be subjected to thoracotomy for diagnosis and excision. The existence of benign tumors, such as solitary fibrous tumors of the pleura, that can produce systemic symptoms underscores the importance of obtaining histologic proof of malignant disease in patients suspected of having malignant tumors before instituting radiotherapy or chemotherapy. Obviously, bronchoscopic and sputum cytologic tests are negative with solitary fibrous tumors.

Treatment and Prognosis

The treatment of choice for solitary fibrous tumors is surgical removal. If the tumor originates in the visceral pleura, substantial amounts of lung parenchyma may also have to be removed (82). Surgical resection cures about 90% of these patients (82, 85), but recurrent disease occurs in the remaining 10%. The recurrences may occur more than 10 years after the initial resection. It is recommended that annual chest radiographs be obtained postoperatively in patients with solitary fibrous tumors to detect recurrences early so that they can be surgically removed.

PRIMARY EFFUSION LYMPHOMA

Primary effusion lymphoma is an uncommon non-Hodgkin's lymphoma that grows in the liquid phase in the serous body cavities in the absence of solid tumors (91, 92). Primary effusion lymphoma is also known as body cavity lymphoma and is associated with human herpes virus 8 (HHV-8) or Kaposi's sarcoma–associated herpes virus (KSHV) (93). HHV-8 is a gamma herpes virus with sequence homology to the Epstein-Barr virus (94). The presence of the HHV-8 virus appears to be specific for primary effusion lymphoma. Uphoff et al. (94) searched for the presence of HHV-8 sequences by polymerase chain reaction using a panel of 133 human cell lines from a variety of solid tumors, 114 hematopoietic cell lines including 50 B-cell leukemia-lymphoma-derived cell lines, and seven cell lines established from patients with primary effusion lymphoma. All of the cell lines from the patients with primary effusion lymphoma were strongly positive for HHV-8, whereas none of the other cell lines were positive for HHV-8. This observation suggests an etiologic role for HHV-8 in primary effusion lymphoma. Many of these tumors are also characterized by the presence of the Epstein-Barr virus (92).

Primary effusion lymphoma usually occurs in homosexual patients with acquired immunodeficiency syndrome (AIDS) (91). These tumors occasionally occur in patients who are not infected with the human immunodeficiency virus (HIV), particularly in elderly men (93). The tumors have a large cell morphology, and their immunophenotype is null. Nevertheless, they do have a B-cell genotype (93). It has been shown that the normal counterpart of the primary effusion lymphoma tumor cells is the mature B-cell or preplasma cell.

The chest radiographs and CT scans show thickening of the parietal pleura and a pericardial thickening in many patients. Many patients also have pericardial effusions, and some patients also have ascites (93). The pleural fluid is a lymphocytic exudate characterized by a very high lactate dehydrogenase level. The diagnosis can usually be established with pleural fluid cytology. The primary effusion lymphoma has a distinctive morphology bridging large cell immunoblastic lymphoma and anaplastic large cell lymphoma. The optimal treatment for these lymphomas remains to be established (95), but the median survival is only 4 to 6 months.

PYOTHORAX-ASSOCIATED
LYMPHOMA

Pyothorax-associated lymphoma is a new entity, and only about 60 cases have been reported, mostly in Japan (96). Pyothorax-associated lymphoma occurs almost exclusively in patients who, several decades earlier, received artificial pneumothorax for the treatment of long-standing pleural tuberculosis. Therefore, the name should probably be pneumothorax-associated lymphoma rather than pyothorax-associated lymphoma. However, there have been cases that developed after empyema (97). Most of these lymphomas are of B-cell lineage. The Epstein-Barr virus genome has been detected in all of the tumors tested (98).

Patients with pyothorax-associated lymphoma commonly present with chest pain, productive cough, fever, or dyspnea. Some patients present with a tumor of the chest wall. The male-to-female ratio of patients with this disease is 5.2:1. The CT scan reveals pleural masses without effusions in the majority of patients (99). The treatment of choice appears to be aggressive wide-field radiation therapy of 50 Gy (99). If the patient can tolerate surgery, pleuropneumonectomy may be curative (99). Results with chemotherapy have been disappointing (99).

REFERENCES

1. Lee YC, de Klerk NH, Henderson DW, et al. Malignant mesothelioma. In: Hendrick D, Burge S, Beckett B, Churg A, eds. *Occupational disorders of the lung.* Philadelphia: WB Saunders, 2001.
2. Pisani RJ, Colby TV, Williams DE. Malignant mesothelioma of the pleura. *Mayo Clin Proc* 1988;63:1234–1244.
3. Churg A. Asbestos-related disease in the workplace and the environment: controversial issues. *Monogr Pathol* 1993;36:52–77.
4. Churg A. Chrysotile, tremolite, and malignant mesothelioma in man. *Chest* 1988;93:621–628.
5. Hansen J, de Klerk NH, Musk AW, et al. Environmental exposure to crocidolite and mesothelioma: exposure-response relationships. *Am J Respir Crit Care Med* 1998;157:69–75.
6. Oels HC, Harrison EG Jr, Carr DT, et al. Diffuse malignant mesothelioma of the pleura: a review of 37 cases. *Chest* 1971;60:564–570.
7. Antman KH. Clinical presentation and natural history of benign and malignant mesothelioma. *Semin Oncol* 1981;8:313–320.
8. Berman DW, Crump KS, Chatfield EJ, et al. The sizes, shapes, and mineralogy of asbestos structures that induce lung tumors or mesothelioma in AF/HAN rats following inhalation. *Risk Anal* 1995;15:181–195.
9. Wagner JC, Berry G, Timbrell V. Mesothelioma in rats after inoculation with asbestos and other materials. *Br J Cancer* 1973;28:173–185.
10. Shabad LM, Pylev LN, Krivosheeva LV, et al. Experimental studies on asbestos carcinogenicity. *J Nat Cancer Inst* 1974;52:1175–1187.
11. Driscoll RJ, Mulligan WJ, Schultz D, et al. Malignant mesothelioma: a cluster in a Native American pueblo. *N Engl J Med* 1988;318:1437–1438.
12. Broaddus VC. Asbestos, the mesothelial cell and malignancy: a matter of life or death. *Am J Respir Cell Mol Biol* 1997;17:657–659.
13. Baris YI, Saracci R, Simonato L, et al. Malignant mesothelioma and radiological chest abnormalities in two villages in central Turkey. An epidemiological and environmental investigation. *Lancet* 1981;1:984–987.
14. Carthew P, Hill RJ, Edwards RE, et al. Intrapleural administration of fibers induces mesothelioma in rats in the same relative order of hazard as occurs in man after exposure. *Hum Exp Toxicol* 1992;11:530–534.
15. Antman KH, Corson JM, Li FP, et al. Malignant mesothelioma following radiation exposure. *J Clin Oncol* 1983;1:695–700.
16. Roviaro GC, Sartori F, Calabro F, et al. The association of pleural mesothelioma and tuberculosis. *Am Rev Respir Dis* 1982;126:569–571.
17. Huncharek M. Genetic factors in the aetiology of malignant mesothelioma. *Eur J Cancer* 1995;31A:1741–1747.
18. Cicala C, Pompetti F, Carbone M. SV40 induces mesotheliomas in hamsters. *Am J Pathol* 1993;142:1524–1533.
19. Shivapurkar N, Wiethege T, Wistuba II, et al. Presence of simian virus 40 sequences in malignant mesotheliomas and mesothelial cell proliferations. *J Cell Biochem* 2000;76:181–188.
20. Emri S, Kocagoz T, Olut A, et al. Simian virus 40 is not a cofactor in the pathogenesis of environmentally induced malignant pleural mesothelioma in Turkey. *Anticancer Res* 2000;20:891–894.
21. Price B. Analysis of current trends in United States mesothelioma incidence. *Am J Epidemiol* 1997;145:211–218.
22. Peto J, Decarli A, La Vecchia C, et al. The European mesothelioma epidemic. *Br J Cancer* 1999;79:666–672.
23. Jarvholm B, Englund A, Albin M. Pleural mesothelioma in Sweden: an analysis of the incidence according to the use of asbestos. *Occup Environ Med* 1999;56:110–113.
24. Branscheid D, Krysa S, Bauer E, et al. Diagnostic and therapeutic strategy in malignant pleural mesothelioma. *Br J Cardiothorac Surg* 1991;5:466–472.
25. Corson JM. Pathology of diffuse malignant pleural mesothelioma. *Semin Thorac Cardiovasc Surg* 1997;9:347–355.

26. Corson JM. Pathology of malignant mesothelioma. In: Antman K, Aisner J, eds: *Asbestos-related malignancy.* Orlando, FL: Grune & Stratton, 1987:179–199.
27. Nash G, Otis CN. Protocol for the examination of specimens from patients with malignant pleural mesothelioma: a basis for checklists. Cancer Committee, College of American Pathologists. *Arch Pathol Lab Med* 1999;123:39–44.
28. Hillerdal G. Malignant mesothelioma 1982: review of 4710 published cases. *Br J Dis Chest* 1983;77:321–343.
29. Suzuki Y: Pathology of human malignant mesothelioma. *Semin Oncol* 1981;8:268–282.
30. Kawashima A, Libshitz HI. Malignant pleural mesothelioma: CT manifestations in 50 cases. *Am J Roentgenol* 1990;155:965–969.
31. Yilmaz UM, Utkaner G, Yalniz E, et al. Computed tomographic findings of environmental asbestos-related malignant pleural mesothelioma. *Respirology* 1998;3:33–38.
32. Kreel L. Computed tomography in mesothelioma. *Semin Oncol* 1981;8:302–312.
33. Aisner J, Wiernik PH. Malignant mesothelioma: current status and future prospects. *Chest* 1978;74:438–444.
34. Ng CS, Munden RF, Libshitz HI. Malignant pleural mesothelioma: the spectrum of manifestations on CT in 70 cases. *Clin Radiol* 1999;54:15–21.
35. Benard F, Sterman D, Smith RJ, et al. Metabolic imaging of malignant pleural mesothelioma with fluorodeoxyglucose positron emission tomography. *Chest* 1998;114:713–722.
36. Gottehrer A, Taryle DA, Reed CE, et al. Pleural fluid analysis in malignant mesothelioma. *Chest* 1991;100:1003–1006.
37. Klempman S. The exfoliative cytology of diffuse pleural mesothelioma. *Cancer* 1962;15:691–704.
38. Nurminen M, Dejmek A, Martensson G, et al. Clinical utility of liquid-chromatographic analysis of effusions for hyaluronate content. *Clin Chem* 1994;40:777–780.
39. Hillerdal G, Lindquist U, Engstrôm-Laurent A. Hyaluronan in pleural effusions and in serum. *Cancer* 1991;67:2410–2414.
40. Martensson G, Thylen A, Lindquist U, et al. The sensitivity of hyaluronan analysis of pleural fluid from patients with malignant mesothelioma and a comparison of different methods. *Cancer* 1994;73:1406–1410.
41. Law MR, Hodson ME, Turner-Warwick M. Malignant mesothelioma of the pleura: clinical aspects and symptomatic treatment. *Eur J Respir Dis* 1984;65:162–168.
42. Stevens MW, Leong AS, Fazzalari NL, et al. Cytopathology of malignant mesothelioma: a stepwise logistic regression analysis. *Diagn Cytopathol* 1992;8:333–342.
43. Wirth PR, Legier J, Wright GL Jr. Immunohistochemical evaluation of seven monoclonal antibodies for differentiation of pleural mesothelioma from lung adenocarcinoma. *Cancer* 1991;67:655–662.
44. Frisman DM, McCarthy WF, Schleiff P, et al. Immunocytochemistry in the differential diagnosis of effusions: use of logistic regression to select a panel of antibodies to distinguish adenocarcinomas from mesothelial proliferations. *Mod Pathol* 1993;6:179–184.
45. Brown RW, Clark GM, Tandon AK, et al. Multiple-marker immunohistochemical phenotypes distinguishing malignant pleural mesothelioma from pulmonary adenocarcinoma. *Hum Pathol* 1993;24:347–354.
46. Andrion A, Magnani C, Betta PG, et al. Malignant mesothelioma of the pleura: interobserver variability. *J Clin Pathol* 1995;48:856–860.
47. Menzies R, Charbonneau M. Thoracoscopy for the diagnosis of pleural disease. *Ann Intern Med* 1991;114:271–276.
48. Hucker J, Bhatnagar NK, Al-Jilaihawi AN, et al. Thoracoscopy in the diagnosis and management of recurrent pleural effusions. *Ann Thorac Surg* 1991;114:271–276.
49. Boutin C, Rey F. Thoracoscopy in pleural malignant mesothelioma: a prospective study of 188 consecutive patients. Part 1: diagnosis. *Cancer* 1993;72:389–393.
50. Boutin C, Rancoise R, Viallat J-R. Prevention of malignant seeding after invasive diagnostic procedures in patients with pleural mesothelioma. *Chest* 1995;108:754–758.
51. Ordonez NG. The immunohistochemical diagnosis of epithelial mesothelioma. *Hum Pathol* 1999;30:313–323.
52. Barberis MC, Faleri M, Veronese S, et al. Calretinin. A selective marker of normal and neoplastic mesothelial cells in serous effusions. *Acta Cytol* 1997;41:1757–1761.
53. Warnock ML, Stoloff A, Thor A. Differentiation of adenocarcinoma of the lung from mesothelioma: periodic acid–Schiff, monoclonal antibodies B72.3, and Leu M1. *Am J Pathol* 1988;133:30–38.
54. Jandik WR, Landas SK, Bray CK, et al. Scanning electron microscopic distinction of pleural mesotheliomas from adenocarcinomas. *Mod Pathol* 1993;6:761–764.
55. Burmer GC, Rabinovitch PS, Kulander BG, et al. Flow cytometric analysis of malignant pleural mesotheliomas. *Hum Pathol* 1989;20:777–783.
56. Van Gelder T, Damhuis RA, Hoogsteden HC. Prognostic factors and survival in malignant pleural mesothelioma. *Eur Respir J* 1994;7:1035–1038.
57. Curran D, Sahmoud T, Therasse P, et al. Prognostic factors in patients with pleural mesothelioma: the European Organization for Research and Treatment of Cancer experience. *J Clin Oncol* 1998;16:145–152.
58. Johansson L, Linden CJ. Aspects of histopathologic subtype as a prognostic factor in 85 pleural mesotheliomas. *Chest* 1996;109:109–114.
59. Pass HI, Temeck BK, Kranda K, et al. Preoperative tumor volume is associated with outcome in malignant pleural mesothelioma. *J Thorac Cardiovasc Surg* 1998;115:310–317.
60. Edwards JC, Abrams KR, Leverment JN, et al. Prognostic factors for malignant mesothelioma in 142 patients: validation of CALGB and EORTC prognostic scoring systems. *Thorax* 2000;55:731–735.
61. Butchart EG, Ashcroft T, Barnsley WC, et al. The role of surgery in diffuse malignant mesothelioma of the pleura. *Semin Oncol* 1981;8:321–328.
62. Rusch VW, Venkatraman ES. Important prognostic factors in patients with malignant pleural mesothelioma, managed surgically. *Ann Thorac Surg* 1999;68:1799–1804.
63. Heelan RT, Rusch VW, Begg CB, et al. Staging of malignant pleural mesothelioma: comparison of CT and MR imaging. *AJR Am J Roentgenol* 1999;172:1039–1047.
64. Jett JR. Malignant pleural mesothelioma. A proposed new staging system *Chest* 1995;108:895–897.
65. Law MR, Gregor A, Hodson ME, et al. Malignant mesothelioma of the pleura: a study of 52 treated and 64 untreated patients. *Thorax* 1984;39:255–259.
66. Elmes PC, Simpson MJC. The clinical aspects of mesothelioma. *Q J Med* 1976;179:427–449.

67. Jackson MB, Pounder D, Price C, et al. Percutaneous cervical cordotomy for the control of pain in patients with pleural mesothelioma. *Thorax* 1999;54:238–241.
68. Sugarbaker DJ, Flores RM, Jaklitsch MT, et al. Resection margins, extrapleural nodal status, and cell type determine postoperative long-term survival in trimodality therapy of malignant pleural mesothelioma: results in 183 patients. *J Thorac Cardiovasc Surg* 1999;117:54–65.
69. Wanebo HJ, Martini N, Melamed MR, et al. Pleural mesothelioma. *Cancer* 1976;38:2481–2488.
70. Ong ST, Vogelzang NJ. Chemotherapy in malignant pleural mesothelioma. A review. *J Clin Oncol* 1996;14:1007–1017.
71. Lee JD, Perez S, Wang HJ, et al. Intrapleural chemotherapy for patients with incompletely resected malignant mesothelioma: the UCLA experience. *J Surg Oncol* 1995;60:262–267.
72. de Perrot M, Kurt AM, Robert JH, et al. Clinical behavior of solitary fibrous tumors of the pleura. *Ann Thorac Surg* 1999;67:1456–1459.
73. Mattson K, Holsti LR, Tammilehto L, et al. Multimodality treatment programs for malignant pleural mesothelioma using high-dose hemithorax irradiation. *Int J Radiat Oncol Biol Phys* 1992;24:643–650.
74. McCormack PM, Nagasaki F, Hilaris BS, et al. Surgical treatment of pleural mesothelioma. *J Thorac Cardiovasc Surg* 1982;84:834–842.
75. Astoul P, Picat-Joossen D, Viallat JR, et al. Intrapleural administration of interleukin-2 for the treatment of patients with malignant pleural mesothelioma: a Phase II study. *Cancer* 1998;83:2099–2104.
76. Marzo AL, Fitzpatrick DR, Robinson BW, et al. Antisense oligonucleotides specific for transforming growth factor beta 2 inhibit the growth of malignant mesothelioma both in vitro and in vivo. *Cancer Res* 1997;57:3200–3207.
77. Sterman DH, Kaiser LR, Albelda SM. Gene therapy for malignant pleural mesothelioma. *Hematol Oncol Clin North Am* 1998;12:553–568.
78. Caminschi I, Venetsanakos E, Leong CC, et al. Cytokine gene therapy of mesothelioma. Immune and antitumor effects of transfected interleukin-12. *Am J Respir Cell Mol Biol* 1999;21:347–356.
79. Rubins JB, Greatens T, Kratzke RA, et al. Lovastatin induces apoptosis in malignant mesothelioma cells. *Am J Respir Crit Care Med* 1998;157:1616–1622.
80. Sandvliet RH, Heysteeg M, Paul MA. A large thoracic mass in a 57-year-old patient. *Chest* 2000;117:897–900.
81. Pleural neoplasms. In: Fraser RS, Muller NL, Colman N, et al., eds. *Diagnosis of diseases of the chest,* 4th ed. Philadelphia: WB Saunders, 1999:2807–2847.
82. Okike N, Bernatz PE, Woolner LB. Localized mesothelioma of the pleura: benign and malignant variants. *J Thorac Cardiovasc Surg* 1978;75:363–372.
83. Hutchinson WB, Friedenberg MJ. Intrathoracic mesothelioma. *Radiology* 1963;80:937–945.
84. England DM, Hochholzer L, McCarthy MJ. Localized benign and malignant fibrous tumors of the pleura. A clinicopathologic review of 223 cases. *Am J Surg Pathol* 1989;13:640–658.
85. Briselli M, Mark EJ, Dickerson GR. Solitary fibrous tumors of the pleura: eight new cases and review of 360 cases in the literature. *Cancer* 1981;47:2678–2689.
86. Ellis K, Wolff M. Mesotheliomas and secondary tumors of the pleura. *Semin Roentgenol* 1977;12:303–311.
87. Le Roith D. Tumor induced hypoglycemia. *N Engl J Med* 1999;341:757–758.
88. Ulrik CS, Viskum K. Fibrous pleural tumour producing 171 litres of transudate. *Eur Respir J* 1998;12:1230–1232.
89. Lee KD, Im JG, Choe KO, et al. CT findings in benign fibrous mesothelioma of the pleura: pathologic correlation in nine patients. *AJR Am J Roentgenol* 1992;158:983–986.
90. Weynand B, Noel H, Goncette L, et al. Solitary fibrous tumor of the pleura: a report of five cases diagnosed by transthoracic cutting needle biopsy. *Chest* 1997;112:1424–1428.
91. Ibrahimbacha A, Farah M, Saluja J. An HIV-infected patient with pleural effusion. *Chest* 1999;116:1113–1115.
92. Nador RG, Cesarman E, Chadburn A, et al. Primary effusion lymphoma: a distinct clinicopathologic entity associated with the Kaposi's sarcoma–associated herpes virus. *Blood* 1996;88:645–656.
93. Ascoli V, Scalzo CC, Danese C, et al. Human herpes virus-8 associated primary effusion lymphoma of the pleural cavity in HIV-negative elderly men. *Eur Respir J* 1999;14:1231–1234.
94. Uphoff CC, Carbone A, Gaidano G, et al. HHV-8 infection is specific for cell lines derived from primary effusion (body cavity–based) lymphomas. *Leukemia* 1998;12:1806–1809.
95. Light RW, Hamm H. Pleural disease and the acquired immune deficiency syndrome. *Eur Respir J* 1997;10:2638–2643.
96. Taniere P, Manai A, Charpentier R, et al. Pyothorax-associated lymphoma: relationship with Epstein-Barr virus, human herpes virus-8 and body cavity-based high grade lymphomas. *Eur Respir J* 1998;11:779–783.
97. Cheung C, Schonell M, Manoharan A: A variant of pyothorax-associated lymphoma. *Postgrad Med J* 1999;75:613–614.
98. Kanno H, Ohsawak M, Iuchi K, et al. Appearance of a different clone of Epstein-Barr virus genome in recurrent tumor of pyothorax-associated lymphoma (PAL) and a mini-review of PAL. *Leukemia* 1998;12:1288–1294.
99. Aruga T, Itami J, Nakajima K, et al. Treatment for pyothorax-associated lymphoma. *Radiother Oncol* 2000;56:59–63.

9

Parapneumonic Effusions and Empyema

Despite the advent of potent antibiotics, bacterial pneumonia still results in significant morbidity and mortality in the American population. The annual incidence of bacterial pneumonia is estimated to be 4 million, with approximately 20% of patients requiring hospitalization (1). Because as many as 40% of hospitalized patients with bacterial pneumonia have an accompanying pleural effusion (2), effusions associated with pneumonia account for a large percentage of pleural effusions. The morbidity and mortality rates in patients with pneumonia and pleural effusions are higher than in patients with pneumonia alone. In one study, the relative risk of mortality in patients with community-acquired pneumonia was 7.0 times higher for patients with bilateral pleural effusions and 3.4 times higher for patients with unilateral pleural effusion of moderate or greater size compared with other patients with community-acquired pneumonia alone (3). In assessing risks of patients with community-acquired pneumonia, the presence of a pleural effusion is given the same weight as a Po_2 less than 60 mm Hg (4).

Most pleural effusions associated with pneumonia resolve without any specific therapy directed toward the pleural fluid (2), but about 10% of patients require operative intervention for their resolution. Delay in instituting proper therapy for these effusions is responsible for much of the morbidity. In one series of 39 patients from San Francisco General Hospital selected on the basis of pus in the pleural space, a positive Gram stain or culture, a pH of less than 7.0 or a glucose level of less than 40 mg per dL, the mean dura-

tion of pleural drainage was 21 ± 18 days, with a mortality rate of 10% (5).

HISTORY

Empyema has been recognized to be a serious problem for centuries. Around 500 B.C. Hippocrates recommended treating empyema with open drainage (6). He made the following interesting observation (6): "Those cases of empyema which are treated by incision or the cautery, if the water flows rapidly all at once certainly prove fatal. When empyema is treated, either by the incision or the cautery, if pure and white pus flows slowly from the wound, the patients recover." His observation is opposite to that which most of us would have anticipated. However, when one reflects on the observation, its validity becomes obvious. If the fluid was thin, the patient probably did not have an empyema and the lung would collapse. However, if the fluid was pus, the patient had an empyema and drainage was likely to be beneficial.

From the time of Hippocrates, the treatment of empyema remained essentially unchanged until the middle of the nineteenth century. At this time Bowditch (7) in the United States and Trousseau (8) in France popularized the use of thoracentesis and demonstrated that open drainage was not necessary in many patients. The next advance in the management of empyema came in 1876 when Hewitt (9) described a method of closed drainage of the chest in which a rubber tube was placed into the empyema cavity through a cannula. He was the first to use the water seal for chest tubes.

In the 1890s, two articles appeared that described thoracoplasty as a means of obliterating the empyema cavity (10, 11). Thoracoplasty involves resecting the ribs, intercostal muscles, and parietal pleural peel over the cavity, and covering the remaining defect by the few remaining muscles, the scapula, and the subcutaneous tissue and skin. At approximately the same time, the initial reports (12, 13) describing decortication appeared. By 1923, Eggers (14) had reported on a series of 99 patients treated by decortication at the Walter Reed Hospital, of whom two thirds subsequently healed.

Although Hippocrates had recognized before the birth of Christ that open drainage procedures were dangerous if the empyema fluid was not thick (6) and Paget (15) had emphasized in 1896 that open drainage should not be instituted for empyema before at least the 15th day of the illness, by World War I, open drainage was the accepted treatment for all cases of empyema. During World War I, there was a high incidence of postpneumonic empyema in American soldiers and the treatment of all such patients with open drainage had disastrous results. In a survey in 1919, the United States Surgeon General found an average mortality rate of 30.2% in the armed forces for individuals with pleural infections, with a range of up to 70% in some hospitals (16). The primary reason for this very high mortality rate was that many cases of parapneumonic effusions in military recruits were due to *Streptococcus hemolyticus,* which is associated with a large pleural effusion but without loculation of the pleural space (17). When an open procedure is performed on such patients, there is a high likelihood that the lung will collapse. In 1918, Graham (18) reported that when chest tubes were inserted early in dogs with experimental empyemas, the mortality rate was higher and the dogs died sooner. The Empyema Commission headed by Dr. Evarts Graham soon made the following recommendations, which really form the basis for the treatment of empyema today: (1) The pleural fluid should be drained, but one must avoid an open pneumothorax in the acute exudative phase; (2) care should be taken to avoid

a chronic empyema by rapid sterilization and obliteration of the infected cavity; and (3) careful attention should be paid to the nutrition of the patient. When these guidelines were observed, the mortality rate from streptococcal empyema secondary to influenza fell to 4.3% (19, 20).

The next advance in the treatment of parapneumonic effusion came about 1950, when Tillett and Sherry proposed enzymatic debridement with a combination of streptokinase and streptodornase for postpneumonic empyema (21). Then in the 1950s and 1960s, the pleural fluid glucose was proposed as an indicator for tube thoracostomy (22). Then in 1972, Light et al. (23) suggested that a low pleural fluid pH was an indicator for tube thoracostomy, and in 1980, the same group suggested that a high pleural fluid lactic dehydrogenase (LDH) level was an indicator for a poor prognosis (2). In the last decade, the use of video-assisted thoracoscopy (VATS) has become widespread in the treatment of loculated parapneumonic effusions (24).

DEFINITIONS

Any pleural effusion associated with bacterial pneumonia, lung abscess, or bronchiectasis is a parapneumonic effusion (23). An empyema, by definition, is pus in the pleural space, but how many white blood cells need be present in pleural fluid to make it pus? Weese et al. (25) defined an empyema as pleural fluid with a specific gravity greater than 1.018, a white blood cell count (WBC) greater than 500 cells per mm^3, or a protein level greater than 2.5 g per dL. Vianna (26) defined an empyema as pleural fluid on which the bacterial cultures are positive or the WBC is greater than 15,000 per mm^3 and the protein level is above 3.0 g per dL. Because many pleural effusions meeting these criteria resolve without operative intervention (2), I prefer to reserve the term empyema for those pleural effusions with thick, purulent appearing pleural fluid. Of course, some patients with empyema have no associated pneumonic process, as shown in Table 9.1.

The main decision in managing a patient with a parapneumonic effusion is whether or not to insert chest tubes. Therefore, I use the term complicated parapneumonic effusion to refer to

TABLE 9.1. *Event or state precipitating empyema in 319 patients*

Event or State	Number	Percentage
Pulmonary infection	177	55
Following a surgical procedure	66	21
Following trauma	18	6
Esophageal perforation	15	5
Spontaneous pneumothorax	7	2
Following thoracentesis	6	2
Subdiaphragmatic infection	4	1
Septicemia	4	1
Miscellaneous or unknown	22	7
Total	319	100

Data from Yeh TJ, Hall DP, Ellison RG. Empyema thoracis: a review of 110 cases. *Am Rev Respir Dis* 1963;88:785–790; Snider GL, Saleh SS. Empyema of the thorax in adults: review of 105 cases. *Chest* 1968;54:12–17; and Smith JA, Mullerworth MH, Westlake GW, et al. Empyema thoracis: 14-year experience in a teaching center. *Ann Thorac Surg* 1991;51:39–42, with permission.

those effusions that do not resolve without tube thoracostomy. Many complicated parapneumonic effusions are empyemas, but some parapneumonic effusions with nonpurulent-appearing pleural fluid are also complicated parapneumonic effusions.

PATHOPHYSIOLOGIC FEATURES

The evolution of a parapneumonic pleural effusion can be divided into three stages, which are not sharply defined but gradually merge together (27). First is the exudative stage, characterized by the rapid outpouring of sterile pleural fluid into the pleural space. The origin of this fluid is not definitely known, but it is probably the interstitial spaces of the lung. The origin of the pleural fluid in sheep with *Pseudomonas aeruginosa* pneumonia is the interstitial spaces of the lung (28). It is possible that some of the pleural fluid originates in the capillaries in the visceral pleura owing to their increased permeability secondary to the contiguous pneumonitis. The pleural fluid in this stage is characterized by a low WBC, a low LDH level, and a normal glucose level and pH (29). If appropriate antibiotic therapy is instituted at this stage, the pleural effusion progresses no further, and the insertion of chest tubes is not necessary.

If appropriate antibiotic therapy is not instituted, in some instances, bacteria invade the pleural fluid from the contiguous pneumonic process, and the second, fibropurulent, stage evolves. This stage is characterized by the accumulation of large amounts of pleural fluid with many polymorphonuclear leukocytes, bacteria, and cellular debris. Fibrin is deposited in a continuous sheet covering both the visceral and parietal pleura in the involved area. As this stage progresses, there is a tendency toward loculation and the formation of limiting membranes. These loculi prevent extension of the empyema but make drainage of the pleural space with chest tubes increasingly difficult. As this stage progresses, the pleural fluid pH and glucose levels become progressively lower and the LDH level becomes progressively higher.

The last stage is the organization stage, in which fibroblasts grow into the exudate from both the visceral and parietal pleural surfaces and produce an inelastic membrane called the pleural peel. This inelastic pleural peel encases the lung and renders it virtually functionless. At this stage, the exudate is thick, and if the patient remains untreated, the fluid may drain spontaneously through the chest wall (empyema necessitatis) or into the lung, producing a bronchopleural fistula.

Empyemas may arise without an associated pneumonic process. When three series (30–32) totaling 319 cases of empyema are combined (Table 9.1), the majority of patients had pulmonary infections, but postsurgical empyemas were also important. A small percentage of empyemas complicate thoracentesis or tube thoracostomy for pneumothorax, hence the necessity for maintaining sterile techniques during these procedures. The pleural effusions associated with esophageal perforation are almost always infected (see Chapter 15). Patients with rheumatoid pleural effusions frequently develop empyema; the genesis of the empyema in this situation is thought to be the formation of a bronchopleural fistula through necrotic subpleural nodules (33).

EXPERIMENTAL EMPYEMA

There has been surprisingly little work done with experimental empyema. It is difficult to produce empyemas in animals. If *Staphylococcus aureus, Escherichia coli,* or *Bacteroides fragilis* are injected into the pleural space of guinea pigs, the animals either survive without developing empyema or die of overwhelming sepsis (34). In one older model of empyema, umbilical tape is placed into the pleural space in addition to the bacteria. The combination results in an empyema in some of the animals. The injection of *E. coli* produces a higher incidence of empyema with a higher mortality rate than does the injection of *S. aureus* (34). If blood is injected with the bacteria in the presence of the umbilical tape, the incidence of empyema is higher (35). The injection of *B. fragilis,* even in the presence of umbilical tape and blood, does not lead to an empyema. If 10^4 *B. fragilis* are injected along with 10^4 *S. aureus,* however, the incidence of empyema is 80%, compared with an incidence of 20% with *S. aureus* and 0% with *B. fragilis* alone. The guinea pigs who develop empyema are more likely to have underlying pneumonia (34, 35).

Over the last few years, we have developed a new animal model of empyema that we believe more closely mimics the empyema that occurs naturally. In this rabbit model, *Pasteurella multocida* cultured in agar (rather than broth) are injected into the pleural space of rabbits. The bacteria are placed in agar rather than in broth so they will remain in the pleural space longer (36). Then 24 hours following the initial injection, procaine penicillin G is administered once per day (if antibiotics are not administered, the animals die of sepsis). In this model, the rabbits do develop an empyema; 24 hours after injection, the mean pleural fluid pH is 7.01, the mean glucose is 10 mg per dL, the mean LDH is more than 30 times the upper normal limit for serum and the Gram stain and culture of the pleural fluid are positive. By 96 hours, the Gram stain and culture of the pleural fluid are usually negative, but gross pus remains in the pleural space (36). In this model, about 60% of the rabbits survive for 14 days, and at autopsy, most animals have pus in their pleural spaces and a thick pleural peel. Microscopic examination of the pleura at 14 days reveals large numbers of leukocytes with invasion of the adjacent lung and chest wall.

Using this model, we have attempted to answer several questions concerning the management of empyema. The first question addressed was whether the timing of the chest tube placement was important in the treatment of empyema (37). After the bacteria were injected into the pleural space, rabbits were randomized to receive no chest tube or a chest tube after 24, 48, or 72 hours. The rabbits that received the chest tube at 24 or 48 hours did significantly better than did the rabbits that received late chest tube placement (72 hours) or no chest tube placement (Fig. 9.1). This study demonstrates that at least in this model, a relatively short delay in initiating tube thoracostomy adversely affects the outcome.

Next we attempted to answer whether therapeutic thoracentesis was a reasonable alternative to tube thoracostomy in the management of rabbits with empyema (38). After an empyema was induced, the rabbits were randomized to undergo daily therapeutic thoracentesis starting at 48 hours, chest tube placement at 48 hours, or no thoracentesis or chest tube. The animals in the group with the chest tubes had their chest

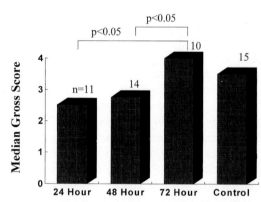

FIG. 9.1. Relationship between gross anatomical score and time of placement of chest tube. A score of 4 indicates pus in the pleural space, 3 = moderate pleural peel without gross pus, 2 = minimal pleural peel, 1 = adhesions between the visceral and parietal pleura and 0 = normal pleural space. *p < 0.05 when compared with the two other groups. (From Sasse S, Nguyen TK, Mulligan M, et al. The effects of early chest tube placement on empyema resolution. *Chest* 1997;111:1679–1683, with permission.)

tubes aspirated at 12-hour intervals. Between aspirations, the chest tubes were attached to a Heimlich valve. In this study the mortality rate in the therapeutic thoracentesis group (0 of 16) was significantly less ($p = 0.02$) than the mortality rate in the other two groups combined (9 of 33). Moreover, when the animals were sacrificed at 10 days, the gross empyema score in the therapeutic thoracentesis group (2.1 ± 0.3) was significantly lower ($p < 0.05$) than that in the chest tube group (2.8 ± 0.3) or the control group (3.5 ± 0.2). From this study, we concluded that, in our rabbit model of empyema, therapeutic thoracentesis is at least as effective as early chest tube placement (38).

The ease of penetrance of various antibiotics into the pleural space in our rabbit model was also studied (39). Antibiotic levels in samples of pleural fluid and serum were collected serially for up to 8 hours after penicillin, clindamycin, gentamicin, metronidazole, vancomycin, or ceftriaxone were administered intravenously. The degree to which the different antibiotics penetrated the infected pleural space was highly variable. Metronidazole penetrated most easily, followed by penicillin, clindamycin, vancomycin, ceftriaxone, and gentamicin (Fig. 9.2) (39). This variance in the penetrance of antibiotics into the pleural fluid should be considered when an antibiotic is selected for the treatment of patients with parapneumonic effusions.

BACTERIOLOGIC FEATURES

The bacteriologic features of culture-positive parapneumonic effusions have changed since the introduction of antibiotics. Before the antibiotic era, most empyema fluids grew *Streptococcus pneumoniae* or hemolytic streptococci (40). Then between 1955 and 1965, *S. aureus* was the bacteria most commonly isolated from pleural fluid (40). In the early 1970s, anaerobic organisms were most commonly isolated (41). However, in the 1980s and 1990s, it appears that the aerobic organisms again are responsible for the majority of empyema. Brook and Frazier (42) reviewed the microbiology of 197 patients whose pleural fluid was culture positive for bacteria in two military hospitals. In 64% of the patients, only aerobic bacteria were isolated, whereas in 13% of patients, only anaerobic organisms were isolated and, in 23% of patients, both aerobic and anaerobic organisms were isolated. Alfrageme et al. (43) reviewed the microbiology of 82 patients treated for empyema at a respiratory unit in Spain and reported results similar to those of Brook and Frazier (42). Of their patients, 62% had exclusively aerobic bacteria, whereas 12% had exclusively anaerobic bacteria and 16% had both aerobic and anaerobic organisms.

The organisms isolated from positive pleural fluid cultures in three separate series (41, 42, 44) are tabulated in Table 9.2. These series represent 342 patients, from whom 580 organisms were isolated. Aerobic organisms alone were isolated from 181 patients (53%), anaerobic organisms only were isolated from 76 patients (22%), and both aerobic and anaerobic organisms were isolated from 85 patients (25%).

Several conclusions can be made from Table 9.2. First, aerobic organisms are isolated slightly more frequently than anaerobic organisms. Second, *S. aureus* and *S. pneumoniae* account for approximately 70% of all aerobic gram-positive isolates. Third, when there is a single aerobic gram-positive organism in the pleural fluid, it almost always is *S. aureus, S. pneumoniae,* or *S. pyogenes.* Fourth, gram-positive aerobic organisms are isolated about twice as frequently as are gram-negative aerobic organisms. Fifth, although *E. coli* is the most commonly isolated gram-negative aerobic organism, it is rarely the lone pathogen isolated from pleural fluid. Sixth, *Klebsiella* sp, *Pseudomonas* sp, and *H. influenzae* are the next three most commonly isolated aerobic gram-negative organisms, and these three organisms account for approximately 75% of all aerobic gram-negative empyemas with a single organism. Seventh, *Bacteroides* sp and *Peptostreptococcus* are the two most commonly isolated anaerobic organisms from infected pleural fluid. Eighth, it is uncommon for a single anaerobic organism to be isolated from pleural fluid.

Several other points should be made concerning the bacteriology of infected pleural fluid.

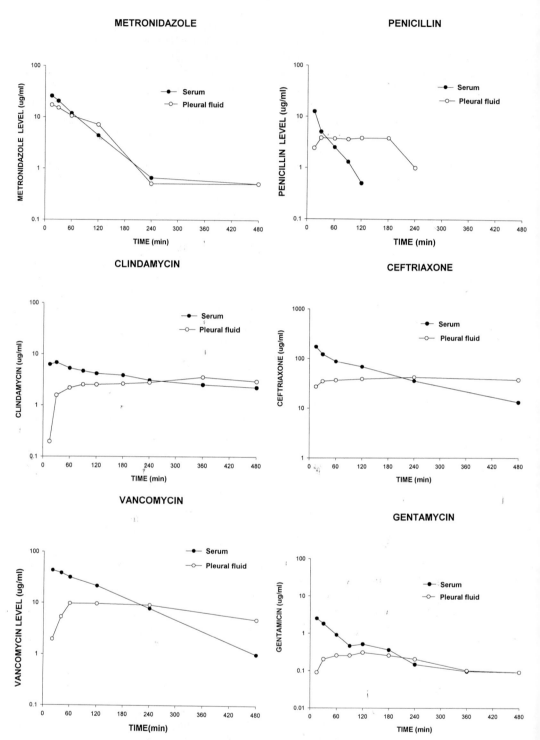

FIG. 9.2. Relationship between serum and pleural fluid antibiotic levels for six different antibiotics. (From Teixeira LR, Sasse SA, Villarino MA, et al. Antibiotic levels in empyemic pleural fluid. *Chest* 2000;117:1734–1739, with permission.)

TABLE 9.2. *Organisms isolated from infected pleural fluid in three separate series*

Organisms	Series 1974[a]	Series 1981[b]	Series 1993[c]	Total	%
Gram-Positive Organisms					
Staphylococcus aureus	17 (6)	7 (4)	58 (39)	82 (49)	36
S. epidermidis	5 (0)	0 (0)	3 (0)	8 (0)	3
Streptococcus pneumoniae	5 (2)	6 (6)	70 (33)	81 (41)	35
Enterococcus faecalis	5 (0)	4 (1)	4 (0)	13 (1)	6
Streptococcus pyogenes	4 (0)	5 (0)	9 (9)	18 (9)	8
Other streptococci	8 (0)	6 (3)	13 (0)	27 (3)	12
Total	44 (8)	28 (14)	157 (81)	229 (103)	
Gram-Negative Organisms					
Escherichia coli	11 (0)	4 (1)	17 (1)	32 (2)	30
Klebsiella species	6 (1)	1 (1)	16 (6)	23 (8)	21
Proteus species	2 (0)	1 (0)	5 (1)	8 (1)	7
Pseudomonas species	10 (2)	8 (6)	9 (3)	27 (11)	25
Enterobacter species	0 (0)	3 (3)	0 (0)	3 (3)	3
Hemophilus influenzae	1 (0)	0 (0)	12 (7)	13 (7)	12
Others	0 (0)	2 (0)	0 (0)	2 (0)	2
Total	30 (3)	19 (11)	59 (18)	108 (32)	
Anaerobic organisms					
Bacteroides species	23 (1)	13 (4)	26 (6)	62 (11)	20
Peptostreptococcus species	26 (1)	8 (1)	28 (4)	62 (6)	20
Fusobacterium species	16 (3)	7 (2)	20 (4)	43 (9)	14
Prevotella species	13 (0)	5 (1)	22 (2)	40 (3)	13
Streptococcus species	15 (5)	4 (2)	12 (0)	31 (7)	10
Clostridium species	13 (1)	5 (3)	5 (1)	23 (5)	7
Others	34 (1)	4 (2)	14 (0)	52 (4)	16
Total	140 (12)	46 (15)	127 (17)	313 (45)	

The numbers in parentheses indicate the number of isolates that were recovered in pure culture.

[a] Data from Bartlett JG, Gorbach SL, Thadepalli H, et al. Bacteriology of empyema. *Lancet* 1974;1:338–340, with permission.

[b] Data from Varkey B, Rose HD, Kutty CPK, et al. Empyema thoracis during a ten-year period. *Arch Intern Med* 1981;141:1771–1776, with permission.

[c] Data from Brook I, Frazier EH. Aerobic and anaerobic microbiology of empyema. A retrospective review in two military hospitals. *Chest* 1993;103:1502–1507, with permission.

First, to a large part, the incidence of anaerobic isolates is dependent on the care with which the pleural fluid is cultured for anaerobes. The relatively high incidence of anaerobes in the series of Bartlett et al. (41) is partially explained by the intense interest these investigators had in culturing anaerobes. Second, the organisms cultured depend somewhat on the population studied. If aspiration is responsible for the underlying pneumonia, anaerobic organisms are more likely to be responsible (42). This also explains somewhat the high incidence of anaerobes in Bartlett's series because their patient population was elderly veteran patients. In contrast, *S. pneumoniae* is more likely to be the causative factor in young ambulatory patients whereas in postthoracotomy patients, *S. aureus* is most likely to to be responsible.

The bacteriology of infected pleural fluid in children varies somewhat from that in adults in that *H. influenzae* is more common and anaerobic organisms are less common. In one study of 72 culture-positive pleural fluids (45), aerobic organisms were found in 48 (67%), anaerobic organisms were found in 17 (24%), and mixed aerobes and anaerobes were found in seven (10%). The most commonly isolated organisms in this series were *H. influenzae* (15 isolates), *Bacteroides* sp (15), *S. pneumoniae* (13), *S. aureus* (10), and anaerobic cocci (9). In another series (46) of 173 culture positive pleural fluids in children younger than 15 years of age, 38% were due to *S. aureus,* 28% were due to *S. pneumoniae,* 23% were due to *H. influenzae,* and 11% were due to other organisms. In this series, anaerobic isolates were rare (46).

INCIDENCE OF PLEURAL EFFUSIONS WITH VARIOUS BACTERIAL PNEUMONIAS

Once a patient has a bacterial pneumonia, the incidence of associated pleural effusion and the frequency with which the pleural fluid becomes infected largely depend on the infecting organism (Table 9.3). Infected pleural fluid is most common in anaerobic pneumonia. In one series of 143 patients with anaerobic infections of the lung (47), 50 (35%) had pleural effusions and, in 47 (94%), the pleural fluid cultures were positive for anaerobic organisms. Aerobic organisms were also cultured from the pleural fluid in 18 (40%) of the patients with positive anaerobic pleural fluid cultures. Some patients with anaerobic pleural infection have no concomitant parenchymal disease.

GRAM-POSITIVE BACTERIA

S. pneumoniae is still responsible for most bacterial pneumonias, and many patients have an associated pleural effusion. Taryle et al. (48) studied 53 patients with pneumococcal pneumonia and found that 57% had an associated parapneumonic effusion, whereas my colleagues and I found that 40% of 153 patients with pneumococcal pneumonia had an associated pleural effusion (2). Pleural fluid cultures are usually negative in patients with pneumococcal parapneumonic effusions. Of the 81 patients with pleural effusions in the foregoing two series, only three (4%) had pleural fluid cultures that were positive for *S. pneumoniae*. Nevertheless, as shown in Table 9.2, *S. pneumoniae* is responsible for many positive pleural fluid cultures. The explanation for this apparent paradox is the fact that such a large percentage of pneumonias are due to *S. pneumoniae*. The incidence of parapneumonic effusions is higher when patients wait 48 hours or more after the development of symptoms before seeking medical attention (48).

Pneumonia secondary to *S. aureus* is likely to have an accompanying culture-positive pleural effusion. Indeed, in one study of the causes of pleural effusion in children, staphylococcal empyema was the most frequent cause (49). Wolfe et al. (49) reviewed 98 children with pleural effusions seen at Duke University between 1952 and 1967 and reported that *S. aureus* was responsible for 35 (36%). In a series of 75 cases of staphylococcal pneumonia in infants and young children (50), more than 70% had pleural effusions, and the pleural fluid cultures were positive in nearly 80%. In adults, pleural effusions accompany staphylococcal pneumonia about 40% of the time (41), which is less frequent than in children. Pleural fluid cultures are positive in

TABLE 9.3. *Percentage of pleural effusions and of positive pleural fluid cultures with various bacterial pneumonias*

Organism	Reference	Pleural effusion (%)	Positive pleural fluid culture (%)
Anaerobic	47	35	90
Gram-Positive			
Streptococcus pneumoniae	2, 48	40–60	1–5
Staphylococcus aureus			
Adults	51	40	20
Children	50	70	80
Streptococcus pyogenes	53, 54	55–95	30–40
Bacillus anthracis	67	90–100	20
Aerobic Gram-Negative			
Escherichia coli	56	40	80
Pseudomonas	57	25–50	40–50
Klebsiella pneumoniae	52, 58	10	20
Haemophilus influenzae			
Adults	55, 61	45	20
Children	53, 54, 59, 60	75	80
Proteus species	62	20	50
Legionella species	63–647	25–60	?

about 20% of adults with pleural effusions (51). Patients who have right-sided endocarditis from *S. aureus* frequently have pleural effusions, but the cultures are positive in only a small percentage (52). In this situation, the effusions are exudates with a very high pleural fluid LDH.

Pneumonias due to *Streptococcus pyogenes* are uncommon, but they are associated with parapneumonic effusion in the majority of cases. Welch et al. (53) reported that 95% of 20 patients had an associated pleural effusion, whereas Basiliere et al. (54) reported that 57% of 95 patients with streptococcal pneumonia had a pleural effusion. The pleural fluid cultures are positive in 30% to 40% of those with pleural effusion (53, 54). The pleural effusions secondary to streptococcal pneumonia are located more commonly on the left side. Of the 73 pleural effusions in the foregoing series, nearly two thirds were on the left side. Streptococcal pneumonia occurs in epidemics, particularly among military recruits (54). In some patients, the development of the pleuritis is explosive with this organism. Patients may develop large pleural effusions with low glucose levels and pH in less than 12 hours (55).

GRAM-NEGATIVE BACTERIA

Of pneumonias due to gram-negative aerobic organisms, those caused by *E. coli* are most likely to have complicated parapneumonic effusions. In one series of 20 patients (56), 40% had pleural effusion, and in six of these eight patients, pleural fluid cultures were positive. All eight patients with pleural effusion in this series had to be treated by tube thoracostomy or open thoracotomy. Rarely, however, is *E. coli* the sole isolate from pleural fluid (Table 9.2). Patients with *Pseudomonas* pneumonia are also likely to have pleural effusions. In one series (57) of 56 patients with ventilator-associated *P. aeruginosa* pneumonia, 13 (23%) had a pleural effusion and seven (12.5%) developed empyema (57). As evident in Table 9.2, *Pseudomonas* sp and *E. coli* account for more than 50% of all aerobic gram-negative isolations from pleural fluid. Although *Klebsiella pneumoniae* is responsible for many gram-negative pneumonias, pleural effusions are

uncommon and are complicated in only a small percentage of patients (58). In recent years, *Haemophilus influenzae* has been responsible for an increasing number of pneumonias in both children (46, 59, 60) and adults (61). With *H. influenzae* pneumonia, the pleura is frequently involved, particularly in children (60). In a series of 65 cases in children (60), 49 (75%) had pleural effusions, and the cultures were positive in 36 of 46 (78%). In another series of 24 adult patients (61), 11 (45%) had pleural fluid, and cultures were positive in 2 of 11 (18%). *Proteus* sp cause a substantial proportion of gram-negative pneumonias, but associated pleural effusions are uncommon, and when they are present, they are usually small and uncomplicated (62).

Pleural effusions may also occur in 30% to 65% of patients with pneumonias due to *Legionella* sp (63, 64). In one recent series of 43 patients with Legionnaire's disease, pleural effusions were present in 10 patients (23%) on admission, whereas another 14 developed effusions during the first week after admission, and three new effusions were discovered after the first week. In some cases, the organisms can be demonstrated by direct immunofluorescence or culture of the pleural fluid (65). Usually, the pleural effusions are small and clinically unimportant, but one reported patient had a multiloculated pleural effusion due to *Legionella* and required a decortication (66).

MISCELLANEOUS PATHOGENIC ORGANISMS

Several unusual organisms should be considered in patients with pneumonia and pleural effusions. *Bacillus anthracis* is a large gram-positive, spore-forming, rod-shaped organism that may contaminate goat hair, wool, or animal hides (67). Although only one case of anthrax has been reported in the United States in the past 20 years, interest has been rekindled in this organism with the threat of anthrax germ warfare. This virulent organism causes pulmonary disease when the spores are inhaled into the alveoli, are engulfed by alveolar macrophages, and are carried to the hilar lymph nodes, where they multiply in their vegetative state. After causing flulike symptoms for several days, the bacteria are disseminated hematogenously. This dissemination is marked by the acute onset of dyspnea, cyanosis, tachycardia, fever, and shock. The characteristic radiologic findings are mediastinal widening, patchy nonsegmental pulmonary infiltrates, and unilateral or bilateral pleural effusions. Because this disease is fatal within 24 hours of hematogenous dissemination unless an appropriate antibiotic (penicillin) is administered, this diagnosis should be considered in all patients with mediastinal widening, parenchymal infiltrates, and pleural effusions (67).

Tularemia may be manifested as a pneumonia and, if so, there is frequently an accompanying pleural effusion (68). Interestingly, the pleural fluid in association with tularemia is a lymphocyte predominant exudate with a high adenosine deaminase (ADA) level (68). Clostridial pleuropulmonary infections are uncommon; by 1970, only 17 cases had been reported (69). Almost all patients with clostridial pulmonary infections have a pleural effusion that is culture positive (69). Complicated parapneumonic pleural effusions have also been reported with pneumonias due to *Haemophilus parainfluenzae* (70), *Bacillus cereus* (71), *Citrobacter diversus* (72), and *Listeria monocytogenes* (73), and can probably occur with any bacterium that is a pathogen in humans.

CLINICAL MANIFESTATIONS

The clinical manifestations of parapneumonic effusions and empyema depend to a large part on whether the patient has an aerobic or an anaerobic infection.

Aerobic Bacterial Pneumonia

The clinical presentation of patients with aerobic bacterial pneumonia and a pleural effusion is no different from that of patients with bacterial pneumonia without effusion (2, 48, 74). The patients first manifest an acute febrile illness with chest pain, sputum production, and leukocytosis. In one series (2), the incidence of pleuritic chest pain was 59% in 113 patients without effusion and 64% in 90 patients with pleural effusion. The mean peripheral WBC was 17,100 in patients without effusion and 17,800 in patients with effusion. The longer the patient has symptoms before seeking medical attention, the more likely he or she is to have a pleural effusion (48). A complicated parapneumonic effusion is suggested by the presence of fever for more than 48 hours after antibiotic therapy is instituted, but, of course, the diagnosis of parapneumonic effusion should ideally be established when the patient with pneumonia is first evaluated.

Not all patients with aerobic pneumonias and pleural effusions have acute illnesses. Sahn et al. (75) reported three cases of aerobic empyema in patients who were receiving corticosteroid therapy, and all were afebrile with minimal symptoms referable to the chest. The absence of fever or chest symptoms should not deter one from considering the diagnosis of complicated parapneumonic effusions because, in recent years, a higher percentage of such effusions has occurred in hospitalized patients, many of whom are debilitated or are receiving corticosteroids (40).

Anaerobic Bacterial Infections

In contrast to patients with aerobic bacterial pneumonias, patients with anaerobic bacterial infections involving the pleural space are usually first seen with subacute illnesses. In a series of 47 patients (47), 70% of the patients had symptoms for more than 7 days before presentation, with a median symptom duration of 10 days. In this same series of patients (47), 60% had substantial weight loss (mean 29 pounds). Many patients have a history of alcoholism, an episode of unconsciousness, or another factor that predisposes them to aspiration. The majority of patients also have poor oral hygiene. Laboratory evaluation reveals leukocytosis (median WBC 23,500 per mm^3) and mild anemia (median hematocrit 36%) in the majority of patients (47).

DIAGNOSIS

The possibility of a parapneumonic effusion should be considered during the initial evaluation of every patient with a bacterial pneumonia. At this evaluation, it is important to determine whether a complicated parapneumonic effusion is present because a delay in instituting proper pleural drainage in such patients substantially increases morbidity.

The presence of a significant amount of pleural fluid is usually suggested by the appearance of the lateral chest radiograph. If both diaphragms are visible throughout their length and the posterior costophrenic angle is not blunted, one can assume that a significant amount of pleural fluid is not present. If either of the posterior costophrenic angles is blunted or if a diaphragm is obscured by the infiltrate, however, bilateral decubitus chest radiographs should be obtained. With the suspect side down, free pleural fluid is indicated by the presence of fluid between the chest wall and the inferior part of the lung (Fig. 3.3). The view with the suspect side up is also valuable because, in this position, the free fluid gravitates toward the mediastinum and allows one to assess how much of the increased radiodensity is due to the fluid and how much is due to the parenchymal infiltrate. The amount of free pleural fluid can be semiquantitated by measuring the distance between the inside of the chest wall and the bottom of the lung. If this distance measures less than 10 mm, one can assume that the effusion is not clinically significant and, therefore, a thoracentesis is not indicated. My colleagues and I reported that 53 patients with acute bacterial pneumonia had such small effusions, and in each of the patients, the pneumonia and the pleural effusion cleared with only antibiotics and left no residual pleural disease (2).

If the thickness of the fluid is greater than 10 mm on the decubitus radiograph, a therapeutic thoracentesis should be performed immediately because it is impossible to separate complicated from uncomplicated effusions without a thoracentesis. The pleural fluid is examined grossly for color, turbidity, and odor. Aliquots are sent for determination of the pleural fluid glucose, LDH, and protein levels, pH (must be analyzed with a blood gas machine), and differential and total WBC. Samples of pleural fluid are also sent for bacterial cultures, both aerobic and anaerobic, and for Gram's stain, as well as for cytologic studies and mycobacterial and fungal smears and cultures, if clinically indicated.

Not all patients with an acute illness, parenchymal infiltrates, and pleural effusion have an acute bacterial pneumonia; pulmonary embolization, acute pancreatitis, tuberculosis, Dressler's syndrome, and other diseases can produce identical pictures. The possibility of pulmonary embolization should always be considered if the patient does not have purulent sputum or a peripheral leukocytosis above 15,000 per mm^3. Most patients with acute tuberculous pleuritis have no infiltrate on the decubitus film with the involved side superior.

The pleural fluid with parapneumonic effusions varies from a clear, yellow exudate to thick, foul-smelling pus. If the odor of the pleural fluid is feculent, the patient is likely to have an anaerobic pleural infection (47, 76). Although Sullivan et al. (76) reported that 11% of aerobic empyemas were described as foul smelling, it is probable that these represented mixed aerobic and anaerobic pleural infections in that sophisticated anaerobic culture techniques were not used in this study. Only about 60% of anaerobic empyemas have a foul odor (47, 76). If frank pus is obtained with the diagnostic thoracentesis, a pleural fluid pH determination should not be obtained. When thick, purulent material is processed through blood gas machines, it is likely to plug up the machine or damage the membranes. Once laboratory personnel have this experience with one pleural fluid, they are hesitant to process additional pleural fluids. The differential WBC on the pleural fluid usually reveals predominantly polymorphonuclear leukocytes. If many small lymphocytes, mesothelial cells, or macrophages are seen, alternate diagnoses should be considered. If food particles are seen in the pleural fluid, the patient has an esophageal pleural fistula (77).

Not all patients with parapneumonic effusions have an acute illness, so the possibility of a parapneumonic effusion should be considered in all patients with pleural effusion. Anaerobic pleural infections are particularly likely to produce subacute or chronic illness (47, 78), and many patients with anaerobic pleural infections do not have associated parenchymal infiltrates (78).

Accordingly, aerobic and anaerobic bacterial cultures should be obtained on all exudative pleural effusions.

INDICATORS OF POOR PROGNOSIS FROM PLEURAL FLUID ANALYSIS

Pleural fluid characteristics associated with a need for pleural fluid drainage are tabulated in Table 9.4. If the pleural fluid is thick pus, the patient has an empyema and drainage of the pleural space is indicated. No other tests are needed for confirmation of the need for drainage. The odor of the fluid should be noted because a feculant odor is an indication for anaerobic antibiotic coverage.

If the fluid is not thick pus, then much information on the prognosis of the patient can be obtained from the Gram stain and culture of the pleural fluid, as well as the levels of glucose, pH, and LDH in the pleural fluid. If the Gram stain is positive, there is a large bacterial burden in the pleural space and the fluid needs to be drained. If the Gram stain is negative but the culture is positive, it is likely that the patient will have difficulty with their pleural infection and the pleural space should be drained.

The pleural fluid chemistries are also useful in identifying which patients have complicated parapneumonic effusions. Patients with complicated parapneumonic effusions have a lower pleural fluid glucose and pH, and a higher pleural fluid LDH than those with uncomplicated parapneumonic effusions (Fig. 9.3). If the pleural fluid pH is higher than 7.20, the pleural fluid glucose is higher than 40 mg per dL, and the pleural fluid LDH is below three times the upper normal limit

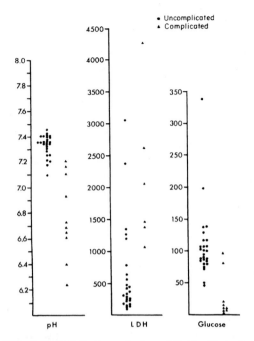

FIG. 9.3. Distribution of pleural fluid pH, lactic dehydrogenase (LDH), and glucose levels in uncomplicated and complicated parapneumonic effusions. (From Light RW, Girard WM, Jenkinson SG, et al. Parapneumonic effusions. *Am J Med* 1980;69:507–511, with permission.)

for serum, the parapneumonic effusion is a Class 3 parapneumonic effusion (Table 9.5), and no further diagnostic or therapeutic maneuvers need be directed toward the pleural effusion.

A pleural fluid pH less than 7.00 or a glucose level less than 40 mg per dL are also bad prognostic indicators in patients with parapneumonic effusions. It is important to understand that the pleural fluid pH and glucose levels should be used as indicators for pleural fluid drainage only in patients with parapneumonic effusions; patients with pleural effusions of other etiologies, including those secondary to rheumatoid disease, malignant tumors, and tuberculosis (23), may also have a low pH or a low glucose level and need not always be treated by tube thoracostomy. If one uses the pleural fluid pH as a guide for the placement of chest tubes, it must be measured with a blood gas machine. If the pleural fluid pH is measured with a pH meter or with pH indicator strip paper, the results are not sufficiently

---

TABLE 9.4. *Bad prognostic factors for parapneumonic effusions and empyema[a]*

Pus present in pleural space
Gram stain of pleural fluid positive
Pleural fluid glucose below 40 mg/dL
Pleural fluid culture positive
Pleural fluid pH < 7.0
Pleural fluid LDH > 3 × upper normal limit for serum
Pleural fluid loculated

LDH, lactic dehydrogenase.
[a] Listed in order of decreasing importance.

TABLE 9.5. *A classification and treatment scheme for parapneumonic effusions and empyema*

Class 1 Nonsignificant pleural effusion	Small Less than 10 mm thick on decubitus x-ray study No thoracentesis indicated
Class 2 Typical parapneumonic pleural effusion	More than 10 mm thick Glucose >40 mg/dL, pH > 7.2 LDH <3 × upper limit normal for serum Gram's stain and culture negative Antibiotics alone
Class 3 Borderline complicated pleural effusion	7.0 < pH < 7.20 and/or LDH >3 × upper limit normal and glucose >40 mg/dL Gram's stain and culture negative Antibiotics plus serial thoracentesis
Class 4 Simple complicated pleural effusion	pH < 7.0 or glucose <40 mg/dL or Gram's stain or culture positive Not loculated not frank pus Tube thoracostomy plus antibiotics
Class 5 Complex complicated pleural effusion	pH < 7.0 and/or glucose <40 mg/dL or Gram's stain or culture positive Multiloculated Tube thoracostomy plus fibrinolytics (Rarely require thoracoscopy or decortication)
Class 6 Simple empyema	Frank pus present Single locule or free flowing Tube thoracostomy ± decortication
Class 7 Complex empyema	Frank pus present Multiple locules Tube thoracostomy ± fibrinolytics Often require thoracoscopy or decortication

LDH, lactic dehydrogenase.

accurate (79). Moreover, because the pleural fluid pH is influenced by the arterial pH (23), the arterial pH should be measured before the pleural fluid is drained if it is to be drained solely on the basis of the pleural fluid pH. To serve as a definite indication for tube thoracostomy, the pleural fluid pH should be at least 0.30 units less than the arterial pH.

The one situation in which the pleural fluid pH is not reduced in complicated parapneumonic effusion is when the offending organism is of the *Proteus* sp. These organisms produce ammonia by their urea splitting ability, which can lead to an elevated pleural fluid pH. Pine and Hollman (80) reported three cases of complicated parapneumonic effusions due to *Proteus* organisms in which the pleural fluid pH exceeded 7.8.

In the natural evolution of a parapneumonic effusion, the pleural fluid pH falls before the glucose level falls (23, 81) and, therefore, the pH is a more sensitive indicator of complicated parapneumonic effusion than the pleural fluid glucose level. The lowered pH with complicated parapneumonic effusions appears to be caused by the metabolism of glucose by the leukocytes in the pleural fluid, resulting in increased levels of lactate and carbon dioxide in the pleural fluid (81). When some loculi are infected and others are sterile in patients with loculated pleural effusions, the carbon dioxide probably equilibrates across the fibrin membranes, separating the different loculi, more readily than does the glucose. Accordingly, pleural fluid acidosis is present in all loculi, even though some loculi may contain nearly normal glucose levels (82).

It should be mentioned that there is not universal agreement concerning the usefulness of using the pleural fluid glucose and pH as indicators for pleural fluid drainage. Berger and Morganroth (83) reviewed the clinical courses of 26 patients who had a pH of less than 7.20, a positive Gram stain, or a positive culture. Sixteen patients were initially treated with intravenous antibiotics alone without tube thoracostomy, whereas the remaining 10 were treated with tube thoracostomy plus intravenous antibiotics. Only two of the 16 patients treated with antibiotics alone subsequently required tube thoracostomy. Three of the four patients with pleural fluid pH less than 7.00 never required tube thoracostomy. The mean duration of hospitalization was longer in the group that received a chest tube immediately. Poe et al. (84) reviewed 91 patients with parapneumonic effusions and concluded that measurement of the pleural fluid glucose, pH, and LDH has limited usefulness in predicting the need for eventual chest tube drainage or decortication, or both. However, if their data is examined closely (85), this conclusion is not supported. When patients with frank empyemas are excluded, 10 of 18 patients (56%) who had a pleural fluid pH value below 7.00 or a pleural fluid glucose below 40 mg per dL received chest tubes. In contrast, only eight of 52 patients (15%) who did not meet these criteria received tube thoracostomy ($p < 0.005$).

Heffner et al. (86) performed a meta-analysis regarding the ability of the pleural fluid levels of pH (n = 251), LDH (n = 114), and glucose (n = 135) to identify those parapneumonic effusions that need drainage. In general, they found that those effusions that were drained had a lower glucose, a lower pH, and a higher LDH than did those that were not drained, but that there was much overlap (86). In general, the pleural fluid pH was a little better at making the differentiation than was the pleural fluid glucose or LDH, but there was much overlap in the values for all three measurements between those patients who received drainage and those who did not. Overall one encounters several problems when trying to assess the value of these measurements. First, the individual who made the decision to institute pleural drainage knew the results of the biochemical tests. Second, the upper limit of LDH may have varied from institution to institution. Third, some of the pleural fluid pHs may have not been measured with a blood gas machine (substantial number of pleural fluid pH's above 7.50).

In view of the above-mentioned factors, there is no doubt that some patients with parapneumonic effusions who have a pleural fluid pH below 7.00, a pleural fluid glucose below 40 mg per dL, a positive Gram stain or a positive pleural fluid culture can be cured with antibiotics alone. Nevertheless, it is recommended that the pleural fluid be drained in patients with parapneumonic effusions who have a pleural fluid pH below 7.00, a pleural fluid glucose below 40 mg per dL, or a positive pleural fluid Gram stain (85), because these are indicators that it is likely that the parapneumonic process will not resolve with antibiotics alone. The risk of more severe morbidity associated with delayed tube thoracostomy justifies the placement of a few extra chest tubes.

LOCULATED PLEURAL EFFUSIONS

Pleural effusions are already loculated in some patients with pneumonia and pleural effusion when they are first evaluated. Although small amounts of freely moving fluid can be demonstrated in most patients with loculated pleural effusion, such is not invariably the case. Loculated pleural effusions manifest as pleural-based masses without air bronchograms on the standard chest radiograph (Fig. 3.5). Frequently, it is difficult to distinguish pleural fluid loculi from peripheral parenchymal infiltrates on standard chest radiographs. Ultrasonic techniques are effective in distinguishing pleural fluid loculi from parenchymal infiltrates (87, 88). As little as 5 mL of loculated pleural fluid can be identified by ultrasound. Therefore, if a loculated pleural effusion is suspected, ultrasonic examination of the pleural space should be performed.

Loculated pleural effusion should also be suspected in patients with pneumonia who do not respond clinically to appropriate antibiotic therapy within 48 hours. If one pleural fluid loculation is identified with ultrasound, it is important to examine the entire pleural space ultrasonically because multiple loculi are often present. If pleural fluid is identified by ultrasound, thoracentesis should be performed immediately because if the skin is marked and the patient is sent back to his room, the relationship between the skin and the underlying pleural fluid may be altered with the patient in a different position. If more than one pleural fluid loculation is discovered, all should be diagnostically aspirated because the character of the pleural fluid may vary from one loculus to another (47).

The presence of loculated pleural fluid by itself is not an indication for tube thoracostomy. The presence of loculi does indicate that there is or has been an intense inflammatory response in the pleural space. Parapneumonic effusions that are loculated tend to have a lower pH and glucose level, and a higher LDH level than do nonloculated parapneumonic pleural effusions (89). Tube thoracostomy with loculated pleural effusions is indicated only if the pleural fluid has one or more poor prognostic factors (Table 9.4). The pleural fluid analysis from the majority of patients with loculated parapneumonic pleural effusions indicates that tube thoracostomy should be performed.

HYDROPNEUMOTHORAX VERSUS LUNG ABSCESS

Frequently, on the standard chest radiographs, it is difficult to distinguish a loculated hydropneumothorax with a bronchopleural fistula from a peripheral lung abscess. This differentiation is important because the loculated hydropneumothorax with the bronchopleural fistula needs to be treated with chest tubes immediately in order to prevent discharge of the infected pleural fluid throughout the remainder of the lung. In contrast, usually only antibiotic therapy is necessary for the peripheral lung abscess. If any doubt exists as to whether the air–fluid level is in the pleural space or the lung parenchyma, ultrasound (87) or CT studies (90) should be obtained to make this differentiation (see Chapter 3).

CLASSIFICATION OF COMPLICATED PARAPNEUMONIC EFFUSIONS

It is important to realize that there is a wide range in parapneumonic effusions and empyemas (91). A patient with a very small effusion will do well regardless of treatment, as long as appropriate antibiotics are given. In contrast, a patient with multiloculated pus in the pleural space will probably require a decortication. The classification in Table 9.5 was developed to assist the practicing physician in the initial care of patients with parapneumonic effusions. This classification, however, is probably most useful for stratifying patients with parapneumonic effusions who are research subjects. Much of the literature on parapneumonic effusions and empyema is confusing because the characteristics of the patients being reported is not adequately described. The classification in Table 9.5 is based on the amount of fluid, the gross characteristics of the pleural fluid, the biochemical characteristics of the pleural fluid, and whether or not the pleural fluid is loculated. As one proceeds farther down Table 9.5, the treatment of the parapneumonic

effusion becomes more difficult and increasingly invasive procedures are required.

Class 1: Nonsignificant Parapneumonic Effusion

Patients with Class 1 parapneumonic effusions have free-flowing fluid that is less than 10 mm thick on the decubitus chest radiograph. Individuals with Class 1 effusions should not be subjected to thoracentesis because if they are treated with appropriate antibiotics, the effusion almost always resolves (2). In addition, a thoracentesis is more difficult in patients with a small amount of pleural fluid. If a patient with a Class 1 effusion subsequently develops a larger pleural effusion, a diagnostic thoracentesis should be performed.

Class 2: Typical Parapneumonic Effusion

Patients with Class 2 parapneumonic effusion have pleural fluid that is free flowing, with a thickness of greater than 10 mm on the decubitus radiograph. In addition the pleural fluid glucose is above 40 mg per dL, the pleural fluid pH is above 7.20, the pleural fluid LDH is below three times the upper limit of normal for serum, and the bacterial smears and cultures are negative. Patients with Class 2 parapneumonic effusions require no invasive procedure other than the initial thoracentesis to delineate the characteristics of the pleural effusion (3). If a Class 2 effusion rapidly enlarges in size or if the patient remains toxic with significant pleural fluid, then a repeat thoracentesis should be performed.

Class 3: Borderline Complicated Parapneumonic Effusion

Patients with Class 3 parapneumonic effusions have negative bacterial smears and cultures, and a glucose level above 40 mg per dL, but the pH is between 7.00 and 7.20, the LDH is above $3\times$ the upper limit of normal, or the pleural fluid is loculated. The relatively low pH, the relatively high LDH, and the loculus all indicate a high level of inflammation in the pleural space. Some Class 3 pleural effusions resolve with no invasive procedure, whereas others do not.

Class 4: Simple Complicated Parapneumonic Effusion

Patients with Class 4 parapneumonic effusions have a pleural fluid pH less than 7.00, a pleural fluid glucose level less than 40 mg per dL or a positive Gram stain or culture. The pleural fluid does not look like pus and it is not loculated. Patients with Class 4 parapneumonic effusions should be treated with some form of invasive therapy because many will not resolve solely with antibiotics.

Class 5: Complex Complicated Parapneumonic Effusion

Patients with Class 5 parapneumonic effusion meet the criteria for Class 4 parapneumonic effusions, but, in addition, the fluid is loculated. These patients require fibrinolytics or thoracoscopy to break down the adhesions, and some of the patients require thoracotomy with decortication.

Class 6: Simple Empyema

Patients with Class 6 parapneumonic effusions have pleural fluid that is frank pus that is either free flowing or confined to a single loculus. These patients should be treated with a relatively large (~28 to 36F) chest tube because the thick pus is likely to obstruct a smaller tube. Patients who have Class 6 parapneumonic effusions frequently have a thick peel over the visceral pleura that prevents the underlying lung from expanding. If a sizable empyema cavity remains after several days of chest tube drainage, consideration should be given to performing a decortication in order to eradicate the empyema cavity.

Class 7: Complex Empyema

Patients with Class 7 parapneumonic effusions have frank pus in their pleural space that is multiloculated. Although these patients should initially be treated with large chest tubes and attempts can be made to facilitate drainage with fibrinolytics, more invasive measures such as thoracoscopy with the breakdown of adhesions or racoscopy with the breakdown of adhesions or thoracotomy with decortication are necessary in the majority.

MANAGEMENT

The management of parapneumonic effusions and empyemas involves two separate areas—selection of an appropriate antibiotic and management of the pleural fluid.

Antibiotic Selection

All patients with parapneumonic effusions or empyema should be treated with antibiotics. If the Gram stain of the pleural fluid is positive, it should guide the selection of an antibiotic. The initial antibiotic selection is usually based on whether the pneumonia is a community-acquired pneumonia or a hospital-acquired pneumonia and how sick the patient is. The initial antibiotic selection and the dose are influenced somewhat by whether or not a pleural effusion is present because some antibiotics, for example, aminoglycosides, do not penetrate pleural fluid easily (39). No reason exists to increase the dose of antibiotics merely because a pleural effusion is present. For patients hospitalized with community-acquired pneumonias that are not severe, the recommended agents are a fluoroquinolone alone, such as levofloxacin, sparfloxacin, or grepafloxacin, or a β-lactam-β-lactamase inhibitor (ampicillin/sulbactam, ticarcillin/clavulanate, or piperacillin/tazobactam) with or without a macrolide such as erythomycin, azithromycin, or clarithromycin (92). For patients with severe community-acquired pneumonia, the recommended agents are erythromycin, azithromycin or a fluoroquinolone plus cefotaxime, ceftriaxone, or a β-lactam-β-lactamase inhibitor (92). If an anaerobic infection is suspected, a fluoroquinolone plus either clindamycin or metronidazole or a β-lactam-β-lactamase inhibitor are recommended (92).

Pneumonia acquired in institutions such as nursing homes or hospitals is frequently caused by enteric gram-negative bacilli, *P. aeruginosa,* or *S. aureus* with or without oral anaerobes. If *S. aureus* is suspected, the patient should be treated with nafcillin or vancomycin. If a gram-negative infection is suspected, the patient should be treated with a third generation cephalosporin or a β-lactam-β-lactamase inhibitor plus an aminoglycoside.

There are no useful studies of duration of therapy for bacterial pleural space infections, and the current standard of practice is to continue antibiotics for several weeks (93).

Intrapleural Antibiotics

Intrapleural antibiotics were first used to treat an infected pneumonectomy space by Clagett and Geraci (94) in 1963. Since that time, there have been several reports (95–99) regarding the use of intrapleural antibiotics in the treatment of empyema complicating pneumonia. All of these reports have reported positive results, but in none was there a randomized control group. Until such controlled studies documenting the efficacy of intrapleural antibiotics are completed, they are not recommended for patients with parapneumonic effusions.

Options for Management of Pleural Fluid

There are several treatment options available for the management of the pleural fluid in patients with parapneumonic effusion and these include observation, therapeutic thoracentesis, tube thoracostomy, intrapleural instillation of fibrinolytics, thoracoscopy with the breakdown of adhesions, thoracotomy with decortication and the breakdown of adhesions, and open drainage.

Observation

In general, observation is not an acceptable option because the pleural fluid from patients with parapneumonic effusions should be sampled as soon as it is identified. This sampling is important because examination of the fluid is necessary to determine if drainage of the fluid is indicated (2) (Table 9.4). Although only about 10% of patients with parapneumonic effusions require drainage of their effusion, it is important not to delay drainage in those who require it because

an effusion that is free flowing and easy to drain can become loculated and difficult to drain over a period of 12 to 24 hours (47,100). Observation is the appropriate course if the patient has a Class 1 parapneumonic effusion, that is, the effusion is less than 10 mm in thickness on the decubitus chest radiograph.

Therapeutic Thoracentesis

Therapeutic thoracentesis was first proposed as a treatment modality for parapneumonic effusions in the middle of the nineteenth century (6, 7). In 1962, the American Thoracic Society recommended repeated thoracentesis for nontuberculous empyemas that were in the early exudative phase (27). In 1968, Snider and Saleh recommended that patients with empyema could be managed with two therapeutic thoracenteses, but if fluid accumulated after that time, then tube thoracostomy should be performed (30). Recently, however, therapeutic thoracentesis as a treatment for parapneumonic effusions has received relatively little consideration.

As discussed earlier in this chapter, studies in our rabbit model of empyema have shown that daily therapeutic thoracentesis starting 48 hours after empyema induction is at least as effective as tube thoracostomy initiated at the same time (38). In addition, there have been some recent studies that have suggested that there is a role for therapeutic thoracentesis in this situation. Storm et al. (99) reported that 48 of 51 patients (94%) with empyema (e.g., purulent pleural fluid or positive microbiologic studies on the pleural fluid) were successfully treated with daily thoracentesis. Simmers et al. (101) treated 29 patients with complicated parapneumonic effusions with daily ultrasound-guided thoracenteses and reported that 24 (86%) were successfully treated. The drawback to this study was that the patients underwent an average of 7.7 ± 3.5 thoracenteses and the average hospitalization was 31 days (101). Ferguson and colleagues (102) reported that 19 of 46 patients (41%) with empyema (e.g., opaque fluid in the pleural space with the cloudiness due to neutrophils or organisms) were treated successfully with repeated thoracentesis. There have been no controlled studies comparing therapeutic thoracentesis with small tube thoracostomy in the treatment of patients with complicated nonloculated parapneumonic effusions.

Tube Thoracostomy

For the past several decades, the initial drainage modality for most patients with complicated parapneumonic effusions has been tube thoracostomy. The chest tube should be positioned in a dependent part of the pleural effusion. Initially, the chest tube should be connected to an underwater-seal drainage system. If the visceral pleura is covered with a fibrinous peel, the application of negative pressure to the chest tube may help expand the underlying lung and hasten the obliteration of the empyema cavity. The management of patients with chest tubes is discussed in Chapter 26.

What size chest tubes should be used to treat complicated parapneumonic effusions? In the past, relatively large (28 to 36F) tubes have been recommended owing to the belief that smaller tubes would become obstructed with the thick fluid. Indeed, in a recent edition of the major thoracic surgical text (103), large-bore (36F or larger) tubes were recommended. There is, however, some data to suggest that such large tubes are unnecessary. In one recent study, 8 to 12F pigtail or 10 to 14F Malecot catheters were placed using the Seldinger technique to treat 103 patients with empyema (104). These small catheters served as the definitive treatment in 80 of the patients (78%). These results are certainly as good as those reported in recent surgical series (105, 106) in which much larger tubes were used, but the parapneumonic effusions in the surgical series may have been in a higher class. The advantage of the smaller tube is that it is easier to insert and is less painful to the patient. The percutaneous catheters in the two studies referenced were placed by interventional radiologists, and it is quite likely that the excellent results are due to accurate catheter placement.

Successful closed-tube drainage of complicated parapneumonic effusions is evidenced by improvement in the clinical and radiologic status within 24 hours. If the patient has not demonstrated significant improvement within 24 hours of initiating tube thoracostomy, either the pleural drainage is unsatisfactory or the patient is receiving the wrong antibiotic. In such patients, the culture results should be reviewed. Unsatisfactory pleural drainage is frequently due to positioning the tube in the wrong location (107). Failure can also be due to loculi of the pleural fluid that prevent complete pleural drainage, or the failure may be due to fibrinous tissues coating the visceral pleura that prevent the underlying lung from expanding. If drainage is inadequate, a chest CT scan should be obtained to delineate which of the above-mentioned factors is responsible. If multiple loculi of pleural fluid are demonstrated, consideration should be given to administering a fibrinolytic agent or performing thoracoscopy with the lysis of adhesions.

If the patient responds clinically and radiologically to closed-tube drainage of the pleural space, how long should the chest tubes be left in place? In general, chest tubes should be left in place until the volume of the pleural drainage is under 50 mL for 24 hours and until the draining fluid becomes clear yellow. If the chest tube ceases to function (no spontaneous fluctuation with respiratory efforts), it should be removed because it serves no useful purpose and can be a conduit for pleural superinfection.

At times, a patient responds clinically and radiologically to closed-tube drainage, but purulent drainage continues from the chest tube. In this situation, the decision to take a more aggressive approach, e.g., decortication, can be aided by the injection of contrast material through the chest tube into the pleural space (108). When only a tube tract remains, the chest tube is gradually withdrawn over a few days, and the cavity is allowed to fill in with granulation tissue. When a larger cavity (greater than 50 mL) is demonstrated, empyemectomy with decortication or an open drainage procedure should be performed.

Intrapleural Fibrinolytics

Difficulties arise in the drainage of complicated parapneumonic effusions as a result of pleural fluid loculi. Many years ago, Tillett et al. (21)

reported that the intrapleural injection of streptokinase and streptodornase facilitated pleural drainage in patients with empyemas by eliminating the pleural loculi. Subsequently, the use of intrapleural streptokinase and streptodornase was largely abandoned because its intrapleural injection was associated with systemic side effects, including febrile reactions, general malaise, and leukocytosis (109). In the late 1970s, Bergh et al. (110) reported the results with the intrapleural injection of streptokinase alone in 12 patients with empyema. They reported radiologic improvement in 10 of their 12 patients.

In the last few years, there have been at least five uncontrolled studies (111–115), each with more than 20 patients, that concluded that fibrinolytics are useful in the management of patients with loculated parapneumonic effusions. Success has been reported with both streptokinase (111–114) and urokinase (111, 114, 115). Each agent is administered intrapleurally in a total volume of 50 to 100 mL as long as it appears to be facilitating pleural drainage. The usual dose of urokinase is 100,000 IU, whereas that for streptokinase is 250,000 IU. One vial of urokinase that contains 250,000 IU costs $490, whereas one vial of streptokinase containing 250,000 IU costs $127. One possible advantage for urokinase in comparison to streptokinase is that streptokinase (which is a bacterial protein) forms a complex with plasminogen, which produces an antibody response. Accordingly, if a patient is treated with streptokinase for a loculated effusion, the subsequent administration of the agent might produce an allergic reaction (116). Similar antibodies are not produced with urokinase. At the present time, however, urokinase is unavailable because of difficulties with viral contamination. The intrapleural injection of fibrinolytics has no effect on the systemic coagulation parameters (117).

In the past few years, there have been three controlled studies on the use of fibrinolytics for loculated parapneumonic effusions (118–120). The first study was not randomized or blinded in that the patients received no fibrinolytics for the first part of the study and then received streptokinase for the latter part of the study (118). This study, which included 52 patients, concluded that there was no significant difference in the need for more invasive surgery or the mortality rate in the two groups (118). In a second study, 24 patients were randomized to receive streptokinase 250,000 IU per day, or saline flushes as controls for up to 3 days (119). The streptokinase group had a significantly greater reduction in the size of the pleural fluid collection and greater improvement in the chest radiograph (119). In a third study, 31 patients were randomly assigned to receive either intrapleural urokinase or normal saline for 3 days. Pleural fluid drainage was complete in 13 (86.5%) patients in the group taking urokinase but in only four (25%) in the control group. Subsequently, eight patients in whom saline had failed were given streptokinase for 3 days, but six still required additional surgery. This study supports the contention that fibrinolytic agents are more likely to be effective if they are administered early in the course of the parapneumonic effusion, before fibrosis has developed.

From the above-mentioned studies, one can conclude that the intrapleural administration of fibrinolytics does obviate the need for subsequent surgery in some but not all patients with loculated parapneumonic effusions. The results that can be expected from the management of patients with parapneumonic effusions with bad prognostic factors are exemplified by a recent study from Singapore. Lim and Chin (121) studied 82 patients with parapneumonic effusions and at least one of the following: (a) distinctly purulent pleural fluid, (b) positive bacterial culture or Gram's stain of the pleural fluid, (c) pleural fluid pH < 7.00, or pleural fluid LDH level < 1,000 U per L. These patients were managed in a sequential fashion—initially a chest tube was placed, then intrapleural fibrinolytics were administered if the chest tube was ineffective, and then surgical drainage (thoracoscopy or thoracotomy) was performed if the fibrinolytic was ineffective. They found that 29 patients (35%) were managed with tube thoracostomy alone, 23 patients (28%) were managed successfully with tube thoracostomy plus fibrinolytics, and 30 (37%) required surgical drainage.

The original articles on enzymatic debridement for loculated parapneumonic effusions used Varidase, which consists of a fibrinolytic (streptokinase) and a DNAse (streptodornase). It is unclear how much the DNAse contributed to the efficacy of the preparation. We have shown that when thick empyemic material from rabbits is incubated with either streptokinase or urokinase, there is no significant liquefaction of the fluid (109). In contrast, when the fluid is incubated with Varidase, the fluid becomes completely liquefied over 4 hours. Although Varidase is currently not available in the United States, recombinant human DNAse (Pulmozyme, Genentech, San Francisco, CA) is available. Simpson et al. (122) have recently demonstrated that recombinant DNAase by itself is very effective at reducing the viscosity of human empyema fluid. The usefulness of DNAase with or without a fibrinolytic in the treatment of complicated parapneumonic effusions or empyema needs to be evaluated.

Thoracoscopy with Lysis of Adhesions

One option for the patient with an incompletely drained parapneumonic effusion is thoracoscopy. A chest CT scan should be obtained before thoracoscopy to provide anatomic information about the size and extent of the empyema cavity (123). With thoracoscopy, the loculi in the pleural space can be disrupted, the pleural space can be completely drained, and the chest tube can be optimally placed (123). In addition, the pleural surfaces can be inspected to determine the necessity for further intervention such as decortication. If at thoracoscopy, the patient is found to have a very thick pleural peel with a large amount of debris and entrapment of the lung, the thoracoscopy incision can be enlarged to allow for decortication (123).

Thoracoscopy is very effective at treating incompletely drained parapneumonic effusions. Since the last edition of this book, there have been at least four articles that reported the results of thoracoscopy in this situation (124–127). When these four studies with a total of 232 patients are combined, thoracoscopy was the definitive procedure in 178 of the patients (77%). The overall mortality rate was 3%, and the median time for chest tube drainage after the procedure ranged from 3.3 to 7.1 days. The median hospital stay after thoracoscopy ranged from 5.3 to 12.3 days (124–127). There was one small study that randomized 20 patients with either a loculated pleural effusion or a pleural fluid pH < 7.20 to receive either chest tube drainage plus streptokinase or thoracoscopy (128). In this study, thoracoscopy was the definitive procedure in 10 of 11 patients (91%), whereas streptokinase was definitive in 4 of 9 patients (44%) (128). The authors of this study concluded that in patients with loculated parapneumonic effusions, a primary treatment strategy of thoracoscopy is associated with a higher efficacy, shorter hospital duration, and less cost than a treatment strategy that uses catheter-directed fibrinolytic therapy (128).

Decortication

With decortication, a full thoracotomy is performed and all the fibrous tissue is removed from the visceral pleura and parietal pleura, and all pus is evacuated from the pleural space (129). Decortication eliminates the pleural sepsis and allows the underlying lung to expand. Decortication is a major thoracic operation requiring a full thoracotomy incision and, therefore, should not be performed on patients who are markedly debilitated.

Even though decortication is a major procedure, the postsurgical hospitalization is not long. In a recent study (130), the median postoperative stay after decortication in 71 patients was 7 days. The mortality rate in this latter series was 10%, but all the patients who died had other serious medical problems (130). It should be noted that postprocedure times for chest tube drainage and hospitalization are longer after decortication than after thoracoscopy with the lysis of adhesions (131).

When managing patients with pleural infections in the acute stages, decortication should only be considered for the control of pleural infection. Decortication should not be performed just to remove thickened pleura because such thickening usually resolves spontaneously over several months (132). If after 6 months the pleura remains thickened and the patient's pulmonary function is sufficiently reduced to limit activities, decortication should be considered.

Open Drainage

Chronic drainage of the pleural space can be achieved with open drainage procedures. Two different types of procedures can be performed. The simplest procedure involves resecting segments of one to three ribs overlying the lower part of the empyema cavity and inserting one or more short, large-bore tubes into the empyema cavity. Following this procedure, the tubes are irrigated daily with a mild antiseptic solution. The drainage from the tubes can be collected in a colostomy bag placed over the tubes. The advantage of this method over closed-tube drainage is that drainage is more complete and the patient is freed from his attachment to the chest-tube bottles.

A similar but more complicated procedure is open-flap drainage, in which a skin and muscle flap is positioned so it lines the tract between the pleural space and the surface of the chest (133, 134) after two or more overlying ribs are resected. The advantage of this open flap (Eloesser flap) is that it creates a skin-lined fistula that provides drainage without tubes. Therefore, it can be more easily managed by the patient at home and permits gradual obliteration of the empyema space.

It is important not to convert to an open drainage procedure too early in the course of a complicated parapneumonic effusion. With an open drainage procedure, the pleural space is exposed to atmospheric pressure. If the visceral and parietal pleura adjacent to the empyema cavity have not been fused by the inflammatory process, exposure of the pleural space to atmospheric pressure will result in a pneumothorax. Before open drainage procedures, this possibility can be evaluated by leaving the chest tube exposed to atmospheric pressure for a short period and determining radiologically whether the lung has collapsed. If the lung does collapse in this situation, an open drainage procedure can still be performed by creating an airtight seal and connecting the large tube to a water-seal drainage apparatus (134). The high rate of mortality in patients with parapneumonic effusions during World War I has been attributed to performing open drainage procedures too early (19).

A patient treated with an open procedure can expect to have an open chest wound for a prolonged period. In one series of 33 patients treated by open drainage procedures (47), the median time for healing the drainage site was 142 days. With decortication, the period of convalescence is much shorter (133), but decortication is a major surgical procedure that cannot be tolerated by markedly debilitated patients.

Recommended Management of Parapneumonic Effusions

When a patient with a pneumonia is initially evaluated, one should ask if the patient has a parapneumonic effusion. If the diaphragms are not visible throughout their entire length on the lateral radiographs, decubitus radiographs should be obtained to determine whether free pleural fluid is present. If free pleural fluid is present and the distance between the inside of the chest wall and the outside of the lung is more than 10 mm, the pleural fluid needs to be sampled. If there is doubt as to how much of the density in a hemithorax is parenchymal and how much is pleural, a CT scan of the chest should be obtained. If more than minimal fluid is demonstrated on the CT, the pleural fluid should be sampled. The reason for sampling the pleural fluid in these situations is to determine whether any bad prognostic factors are present (Table 9.4).

The options for the invasive treatment of complicated parapneumonic effusions are listed in Table 9.6. In general, one moves from the less invasive treatments to the more invasive treatments. It is important to abandon a treatment within 1 or 2 days if it is ineffective. Not every treatment needs to be used. If a patient is going to need a decortication, it should be performed

TABLE 9.6. *Treatment option for complicated parapneumonic effusions*[a]

Therapeutic thoracentesis
Tube thoracostomy
Tube thoracostomy with the intrapleural administration of fibrinolytics
Thoracoscopy with the breakdown of adhesions
Thoracotomy with decortication

[a] Listed in order of increasing invasiveness.

within 10 days of the initial identification of the parapneumonic effusion.

If a patient has sufficient pleural fluid to warrant a thoracentesis, a therapeutic rather than a diagnostic thoracentesis should be performed initially (Fig 9.4). The reasoning behind this recommendation is as follows. If no fluid reaccumulates after the initial therapeutic thoracentesis, one need not worry about the parapneumonic effusion. If the pleural fluid reaccumulates and there were no bad prognostic factors at the time of the initial thoracentesis, no additional therapy is indicated as long as the patient is doing well.

If the fluid reaccumulates and there were bad prognostic factors present at the time of the initial thoracentesis, a second therapeutic thoracentesis should be performed. If the fluid reaccumulates a second time, a tube thoracostomy should be performed if any of the bad prognostic factors were present at the time of the second therapeutic thoracentesis.

Performance of the therapeutic thoracentesis also delineates whether the pleural fluid is loculated. If the pleural fluid is loculated, and if any of the other bad prognostic factors listed in Table 9.4 are present, then more aggressive therapy should

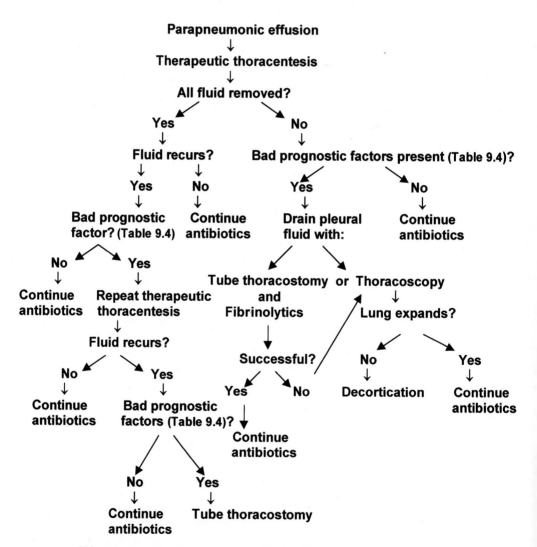

FIG. 9.4. Algorithm for managing patients with parapneumonic effusions.

be initiated. The two primary options at this time are tube thoracostomy with the instillation of fibrinolytics or thoracoscopy with the lysis of adhesions. The choice between these two options is dictated somewhat by local circumstances. If thoracoscopy is unavailable, the obvious choice is fibrinolytics. If both are available, one may want to try tube thoracostomy with fibrinolytics initially. However, if complete drainage is not obtained with one or two administrations of the fibrinolytics, one should move to thoracoscopy or thoracotomy with decortication without delay. Along the same lines, if thoracoscopy is not successful, thoracotomy with decortication should be performed without delay. If thoracoscopy is unavailable and fibrinolytics are ineffective after one to three treatments, the patient should be subjected to decortication or transferred to a facility where thoracoscopy is available.

SPECIAL SITUATIONS WITH EMPYEMA

Empyema in Children

As mentioned earlier in this chapter, the bacteriology of empyema in children varies somewhat from that in adults. In children the incidence of anaerobic infection is lower, whereas that of *H. influenzae* is higher. Another difference between children and adults is that the complicated parapneumonic effusions can lead to scoliosis in the children. Hoff et al. (135) reported that scoliosis of 5 degrees or more was noted in 27 of 61 pediatric patients (44%). They also found that 80% of children presenting with more than 10 degrees of scoliosis required decortication (135).

The criteria for tube thoracostomy, namely a low pleural fluid pH or a low pleural fluid glucose, appear to be appropriate for children as well as for adults (135). Additional indicators of a poor outcome in children were significant scoliosis, evidence of parenchymal entrapment, and anaerobic infection. Tube thoracostomy, thoracoscopy, or decortication should be instituted if the patient has two or more of these indicators of a poor prognosis.

In general, the management of children with empyema is very similar to that for adults. The children are usually healthy, so there is very little if any role for open drainage procedures. If the pleural fluid is loculated, fibrinolytic agents can be administered intrapleurally (136) or the patient can be taken directly to thoracoscopy (137). If the sepsis is still not controlled, then the patient should be subjected to decortication (135, 137). Doski et al. (137) recommend that VATS be the primary means of therapy for pediatric patients. In a series of 41 patients, all were cured with thoracoscopy and the median length of stay was only 7 days.

Empyema Associated with Bronchopleural Fistula

When an empyema is complicated by the presence of a bronchopleural fistula, adequate pleural drainage is crucial (Fig. 9.5). Pleural fluid that is not drained exteriorly with chest tubes is likely to drain interiorly into the lung. The bacteria then are spread throughout the bronchopulmonary tree and an overwhelming pneumonia can result. It should be emphasized that the presence of a bronchopleural fistula in conjunction with infected pleural fluid is a medical emergency. Drainage should be instituted immediately to prevent the possibility of contaminating the entire respiratory system by the infected pleural fluid (Fig. 9.5).

The presence of a bronchopleural fistula should be suspected when a patient with a pleural fluid collection raises more sputum than would be expected from the associated pulmonary disease. If the patient raises large amounts of sputum only when lying in one position, a bronchopleural fistula is strongly suggested. Radiologically, a bronchopleural fistula is manifested by the presence of an air–fluid level in the pleural space when the radiograph is obtained with the patient in the upright position (Fig. 9.5). It is sometimes difficult to determine whether the air–fluid levels are in the lung parenchyma or the pleural space. The utility of ultrasound and CT studies in making this differentiation is discussed in Chapter 3.

Empyema Distal to an Obstructed Bronchus

One contraindication to the placement of chest tubes in patients with complicated parapneumonic effusions is the presence of a malignant tumor obstructing a lobar or main stem bronchus.

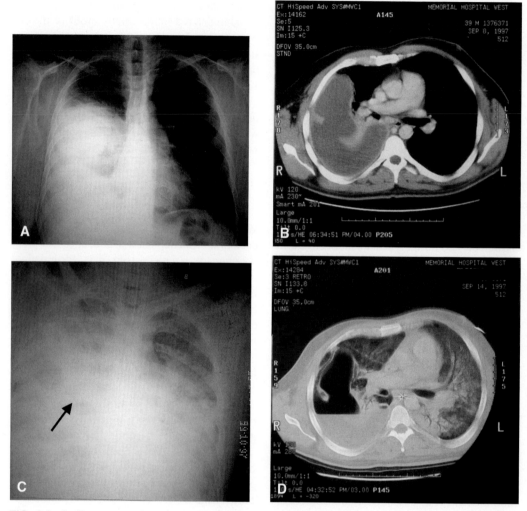

FIG. 9.5. A: Posteroanterior chest radiograph of a 44-year-old male who had pleuritic chest pain, fever, and leukocytosis for 1 week. **B:** CT scan demonstrating that most of the opacity in the right lung field in the PA chest radiograph is pleural fluid. **C:** Anteroposterior chest radiograph 2 days later demonstrating extensive infiltrates throughout both lungs in addition to pleural effusion. Note lucent area (arrow) in right midlung field indicating area in the pleural space that had drained. The infiltrates are a result of the pleural pus entering the tracheobronchial tree. **D:** CT scan from 1 day after the AP chest radiograph demonstrating extensive bilateral pulmonary infiltrate. Note that there is no chest tube in place so that the pus in the pleural space continues to drain through the tracheobronchial tree.

If chest tubes are placed in such patients, the bronchial obstruction will prevent expansion of the lung underlying the pleural effusion and the unfortunate patient will be saddled with a chest tube or an open chest wound for the remainder of his life. When a patient is discovered to have a complicated parapneumonic effusion distal to an obstructed bronchus, appropriate antibiotics should be administered in conjunction with therapy for the obstructed bronchus, which could include radiotherapy, an endobronchial stent, or laser therapy. Tube thoracostomy can be instituted if the obstruction is relieved with the therapy. If the obstruction persists, the patient can be sent home with a prescription of appropriate oral antibiotics. In my experience, the continuous administration of oral antibiotics to patients with pleural sepsis and bronchial obstruction allows them to live in symbiosis with their pleural infection without excessive systemic toxicity.

Postpneumonectomy Empyema

Empyemas following thoracic surgical procedures account for approximately 25% of all empyemas (25, 30, 44), and the procedure is usually a pneumonectomy. After a pneumonectomy, there is a characteristic evolution of radiologic findings, and deviations from this pattern suggest the possibility of postpneumonectomy empyema. Immediately after pneumonectomy, the ipsilateral pleural space contains air, the mediastinum is shifted to the ipsilateral side, and the hemidiaphragm is elevated (Fig. 9.6A). The postpneumonectomy space then begins to fill with serosanguineous fluid at a rate of approximately two rib spaces a day. In the majority of

patients, the pleural space becomes 80% to 90% filled with fluid within 2 weeks and completely filled within 2 to 4 months (138). During this period, the mediastinum progressively shifts ipsilaterally (Fig. 9.6B). Failure of the mediastinum to shift in the postoperative period indicates an abnormality in the postpneumonectomy space (138). Similarly, the most sensitive indicator of late complications in the pneumonectomy space is the return to the midline of a previously shifted mediastinum or a shift of the mediastinum to the contralateral side (Fig. 9.7) (138).

The postoperative occurrence of empyema is a dreaded complication of pneumonectomy. The complication is particularly serious because it is impossible to eliminate the space containing the infection, and, consequently, it is difficult to sterilize the space. Approximately 80% of patients with postpneumonectomy empyema have a bronchopleural or an esophagopleural fistula as a complication (139, 140). Therefore, all patients with this type of empyema should have a barium swallow and a bronchoscopic examination (140).

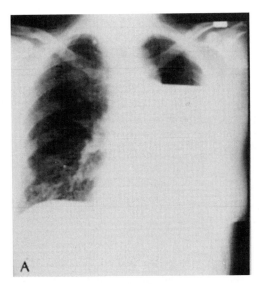
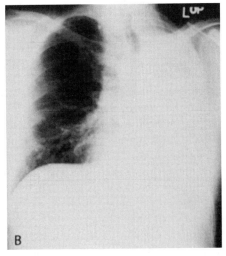

FIG. 9.6. Appearance of chest radiograph after pneumonectomy. **A:** Posteroanterior chest radiograph from a patient 1 week after pneumonectomy. Note that the postpneumonectomy space contains an air–fluid level and that the mediastinum is shifted toward the side of the pneumonectomy. **B:** Posteroanterior chest radiograph from the same patient 1 year after pneumonectomy. The mediastinum has shifted more toward the side with the pneumonectomy, and the hemithorax is completely opacified.

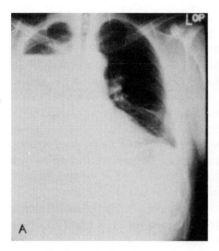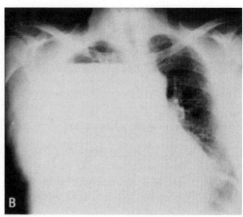

FIG. 9.7. A: Posteroanterior chest radiograph from a patient who had undergone a right pneumonectomy 2 weeks previously. **B:** Posteroanterior chest radiograph from the same patient a week later. Note the marked interval shift in the mediastinum. This patient had a *Staphylococcus aureus* infection of his pneumonectomy space.

The incidence of empyema following pneumonectomy is about 5% (139, 140), and the mortality rate from postpneumonectomy empyema is about 12% (139). The administration of antibiotics prophylactically starting before surgery and continuing until the pleural drains are removed resulted in a significant reduction in postpneumonectomy empyema in one study (141). An infected pneumonectomy space usually becomes manifest in one of four ways: (a) a febrile illness with signs of systemic toxicity; (b) expectoration of large amounts of pleural fluid; (c) an air–fluid level in the pneumonectomy space; or (d) the drainage of purulent material from the surgical incision. The time from pneumonectomy to the development of an empyema ranges from 2 days to 7 years, with most infections evident within 4 weeks (142, 143). The diagnosis should be suspected in any patient who, following this operation, becomes febrile, starts expectorating large amounts of pleural fluid, has purulent drainage from his thoracotomy wound, or has a mediastinum that is midline or shifted to the contralateral side (Fig. 9.7). The diagnosis is established by a thoracentesis demonstrating bacteria on the Gram stain of the pleural fluid. If more than several weeks have passed since the patient's pneumonectomy, ultrasound examination of the pleural space should be performed to identify the appropriate location for the thoracentesis. *S. aureus* is the bacterium responsible for the majority of postpneumonectomy empyemas (142, 144, 145), but gram-negative organisms such as *E. coli, Pseudomonas* sp, and *Proteus* sp, as well as fungi are at times responsible.

All patients with postpneumonectomy empyema should be treated with a chest tube and appropriate antibiotics. Placement of a chest tube more than 1 week following the pneumonectomy may be difficult, because the evacuated hemithorax rapidly loses volume by apposition of ribs and shift of the mediastinum. Therefore, a chest CT scan is useful to assess the size and location of the residual space, and to determine the optimal line of approach. Placement of the tube in the 4th or 5th intercostal space in the anterior axillary line is usually appropriate (140). In the first few weeks following pneumonectomy, the mediastinum is not stable. Therefore, suction should not be applied to the chest tube and an open drainage procedure should not be performed.

After the initial drainage, the treatment is largely dependent on whether the patient has a bronchopleural fistula. If the patient does not have a bronchopleural fistula, then the treatment of choice is closed-tube drainage of the pleural space in conjunction with antibiotic irrigation (139, 144, 146). A chest tube is inserted into the most dependent portion of the patient's empyema cavity and is connected to an underwater-seal drainage apparatus. The antibiotics to which the offending organisms are susceptible can be instilled by this tube, if a double-lumen tube is used (146), or through a separate, smaller tube inserted into the second or third intercostal space at the midclavicular line. The antibiotics can be infused through the pleural space continuously. Alternatively, with the drainage tube clamped, several hundred milliliters of antibiotic solution can be instilled into the pleural space and allowed to remain for several hours. The pleural fluid is then drained, and the sequence is repeated. When the drained fluid becomes clear, the irrigation fluid is changed to normal saline solution for 24 hours. If the culture of this drainage is sterile, 100 mL of concentrated irrigation fluid is left in the pleural space, and the chest tubes are removed. Hollaus et al. recommend thoracoscopic debridement shortly after the initial chest tube is placed (147). The debridement facilitates sterilization of the postpneumonectomy space.

Antibiotic irrigation of the pneumonectomy space is also effective in patients in whom the bronchopleural fistula is repaired surgically. Gharagozloo et al. (139) reported that this approach was successful in all 22 patients in whom they had repaired the bronchopleural fistula primarily. At the time that the bronchopleural fistula was repaired, the pleural space was meticulously debrided. In 20 patients, the Gram stain pleural fluid was negative on day 8 of the irrigation, and in the remaining two patients, Gram's stain of the pleural fluid was negative on day 16 of the operation.

An alternate approach to postpneumonectomy empyema involves the creation of a large opening in the chest by resecting several inches of the rib inferior to the thoracotomy incision and one or more ribs superior to it. The procedure is called the Clagett procedure after the surgeon who first described it (94). The superficial fascia is sutured down to the periosteum of the resected ribs to leave a large window in the thoracic wall. Each day, the empyema cavity is irrigated with a mildly antiseptic solution such as half-strength Dakin's solution or chlorhexidine (Hibitane) (145). These irrigations are continued for several weeks until the drainage is no longer purulent and the empyema cavity appears to be well debrided. At this time, the opening in the chest wall is closed, and a 0.25% solution of neomycin is placed in the cavity.

Goldstraw (145) treated 29 patients with postpneumonectomy empyemas in the foregoing manner and attempted closure in 22 of the patients. In 17 of these 22 patients (77%), closure was successful in that no evidence was seen of a recurrence of the empyema from 5 weeks to 9 years after closure. The five patients in whom closure failed initially were subjected to a second fenestration, and a successful closure was eventually obtained in two of these patients. Other workers have reported much poorer results with the Clagett procedure. Shamji and colleagues (148) achieved successful closure in only two of 31 patients (6%) managed in this manner, whereas Bayes et al. (149) reported success in 10 of 28 patients (36%). This treatment is time-consuming, with a mean interval between fenestration and closure of 40 days (145) (range 21 to 74 days), and patients usually have to remain hospitalized for the entire period. The closed irrigation method is the procedure of choice in my opinion.

If a bronchopleural fistula is present, several different procedures can be used to attempt to close the fistula. On occasion, the bronchopleural fistula will close with continuous irrigation of the infected pleural space, but usually more extensive procedures must be done. If the bronchopleural fistula develops within the first few weeks of surgery, attempts can be made to close the bronchopleural fistula directly. Recently, Gharagozloo et al. (139) reported the successful primary repair of all 22 bronchopleural fistulas. None of the patients had a bronchial stump opening that was more than 25% of the diameter of the bronchus. Attempts can be made to close the bronchopleural fistula with fibrin glue endoscopically. In one study, 8 of 36 patients had their bronchopleural fistula successfully treated using fibrin sealant and decalcified spongy calf bone (147). Pairolero et al. (150) advocate the intrathoracic transposition of extrathoracic skeletal muscle to facilitate closure of the fistula. They attempted this procedure in 28 patients following open drainage and reported success in 24. The median number of operations was 5, with a range of 1 to 19. The median hospitalization time was 34 days, with a range of 4 to 137. A related method closes the fistula with an omentopexy (151, 152).

Posttraumatic Empyema

Empyema remains a distressing complication after thoracic injury. In one recent study, the incidence of empyema requiring decortication was 4% in 584 patients who were treated with tube thoracostomy (153), whereas in another series, the incidence was 1.8% of 5,474 patients (154). Factors that predicted the development of an empyema were retained hemothorax (odds ratio, 12:5), pulmonary contusion (odds ratio, 6:3), and multiple chest tube placement (odds ratio, 2:5). Factors that did not predict empyema were severity of injury, mechanism of injury, setting in which tube thoracostomy was performed, number of days chest tubes were in place, and antibiotics at the time of tube thoracostomy (153). Aguilar et al. (153) recommend the early drainage of the pleural space with the VATS technique in posttrauma patients with fluid collections in the pleural space. In general, the management of posttraumatic empyema is the same as that of parapneumonic empyema.

REFERENCES

1. Neiderman MS, Bass JB, Campbell GD, et al. Guidelines for the initial management of adults with community-acquired pneumonia: diagnosis, assessment of severity, and initial antimicrobial therapy. *Am Rev Respir Dis* 1993;148:1418–1426.
2. Light RW, Girard WM, Jenkinson SG, et al. Parapneumonic effusions. *Am J Med* 1980;69:507–511.
3. Hasley PB, Albaum MN, Li Y-H, et al. Do pulmonary radiographic findings at presentation predict mortality in patients with community-acquired pneumonia? *Arch Intern Med* 1996;156:2206–2212.
4. Fine MJ, Auble TE, Yealy DM, et al. A prediction rule to identify low-risk patients with community-acquired pneumonia. *JAMA* 1996;275:134–141.
5. Broaddus VC. Infections in the pleural space. An update on pathogenesis and management. *Semin Respir Crit Care Med* 1995;16:303–314.
6. Adams F. *The genuine works of Hippocrates.* New York: William Wood, 1948:266.
7. Bowditch HI. Paracentesis thoracic: an analysis of 25 cases of pleuritic effusion. *Am Med Monthly* 1853:3–45.
8. Trousseau A. *Lectures on clinical medicine delivered at the Hotel-Dieu Paris,* Vol 3. JR McCormick (trans). London: The New Sydenham Society, 1987;3:198.
9. Hewitt C. Drainage for empyema. *Br Med J* 1876;1:317.
10. Estlander JA. Sur le resection des côté dans l'empyème chronique. *Rev Mens* 1897;8:885.
11. Schede M. Die Behandlung der empyeme. *Verh Innere Med Weisbaden* 1890;9:41.
12. Fowler GR. A case of thoracoplasty for the removal of a large cicatricial fibrous growth from the interior of the chest, the result of an old empyema. *Med Rec* 1893;44:938.
13. Beck C. Thoracoplasty in America and visceral pleurectomy with report of a case. *JAMA* 1897;28:58.
14. Eggers C. Radical operation for empyema. *Ann Surg* 1923;77:327.
15. Paget S. *The surgery of the chest.* Bristol: John Wright & Co., 1896:204–206.
16. Graham EA. *Some fundamental considerations in the treatment of empyema thoracis.* St. Louis: C.V. Mosby Co, 1925:14.
17. Olch PD. Evarts A. Graham in World War I: the Empyema Commission and Service in the American Expeditionary Forces. *J Hist Med Allied Sci* 1989;44:430–446.
18. Graham EA, Bell RD. Open pneumothorax: its relations to the treatment of empyema. *Am J Med Sci* 1918;156:839–871.
19. Empyema Commission. Cases of empyema at Camp Lee, Virginia. *JAMA* 1918;71:366–373.
20. Stone WJ. The management of postpneumonic empyema based on 310 cases. *Am J Med Sci* 1919;158:1–29.
21. Tillett WS, Sherry S, Read CT. The use of streptokinase-streptodornase in the treatment of postpneumonic empyema. *J Thorac Surg* 1951;21:275–297.
22. Glenert J. Sugar levels in pleural effusions of different etiologies. *Acta Tuberc Scand* 1962;42:222–227.
23. Light RW, MacGregor MI, Ball WC Jr, et al. Diagnostic significance of pleural fluid pH and Pco_2. *Chest* 1973;64:591–596.
24. Ferguson MK. Thoracoscopy for empyema, bronchopleural fistula, and chylothorax. *Ann Thorac Surg* 1993;56:644–645.
25. Weese WC, Shindler ER, Smith IM, et al. Empyema of the thorax then and now. *Arch Intern Med* 1973;131:516–520.
26. Vianna NJ. Nontuberculous bacterial empyema in patients with and without underlying diseases. *JAMA* 1971;215:69–75.
27. Andrews NC, Parker EF, Shaw RR, et al. Management of nontuberculous empyema. *Am Rev Respir Dis* 1962;85:935–936.
28. Wiener-Kronish JP, Sakuma T, Kudoh I, et al. Alveolar epithelial injury and pleural empyema in acute *P. aeruginosa* pneumonia in anesthetized rabbits. *J Appl Physiol* 1993;75:1661–1669.
29. Light RW. Management of parapneumonic effusions. *Arch Intern Med* 1981;141:1339–1341.
30. Snider GL, Saleh SS. Empyema of the thorax in adults: review of 105 cases. *Chest* 1968;54:12–17.

31. Yeh TJ, Hall DP, Ellison RG. Empyema thoracis: a review of 110 cases. *Am Rev Respir Dis* 1963;88:785–790.
32. Smith JA, Mullerworth MH, Westlake GW, et al. Empyema thoracis: 14-year experience in a teaching center. *Ann Thorac Surg* 1991;51:39–42.
33. Jones FL, Blodgett RC. Empyema in rheumatoid pleuropulmonary disease. *Ann Intern Med* 1971;74:665–671.
34. Mavroudis C, Ganzel BL, Katzmark S, et al. Effect of hemothorax on experimental empyema thoracis in the guinea pig. *J Thorac Cardiovasc Surg* 1985;89:42–49.
35. Mavroudis C, Ganzel BL, Cox SK, et al. Experimental aerobic-anaerobic thoracic empyema in the guinea pig. *Ann Thorac Surg* 1987;43:295–297.
36. Sasse SA, Causing LA, Mulligan ME, et al. Serial pleural fluid analysis in a new experimental model of empyema. *Chest* 1996;109:1043–1048.
37. Sasse S, Nguyen TK, Mulligan M, et al. The effects of early chest tube placement on empyema resolution. *Chest* 1997;111:1679–1683.
38. Sasse S, Nguyen T, Teixeira LR, et al. The utility of daily therapeutic thoracentesis for the treatment of early empyema. *Chest* 1999;116:1703–1708.
39. Teixeira LR, Sasse SA, Villarino MA, et al. Antibiotic levels in empyemic pleural fluid. *Chest* 2000;117:1734–1739.
40. Finland M, Barnes MW. Changing ecology of acute bacterial empyema: occurrence and mortality at Boston City Hospital during 12 selected years from 1935 to 1972. *J Infect Dis* 1978;137:274–291.
41. Bartlett JG, Gorbach SL, Thadepalli H, et al. Bacteriology of empyema. *Lancet* 1974;1:338–340.
42. Brook I, Frazier EH. Aerobic and anaerobic microbiology of empyema. A retrospective review in two military hospitals. *Chest* 1993;103:1502–1507.
43. Alfageme I, Munoz F, Pena N, et al. Empyema of the thorax in adults. Etiology, microbiologic findings, and management. *Chest* 1993;103:839–843.
44. Varkey B, Rose HD, Kutty CPK, et al. Empyema thoracis during a ten-year period. *Arch Intern Med* 1981;141:1771–1776.
45. Brook I. Microbiology of empyema in children and adolescents. *Pediatrics* 1990;85:722–726.
46. Freij BJ, Kusmiesz H, Nelson JD, et al. Parapneumonic effusions and empyema in hospitalized children: a retrospective review of 227 cases. *Pediatr Infect Dis* 1984;3:578–591.
47. Bartlett JG, Finegold SM. Anaerobic infections of the lung and pleural space. *Am Rev Respir Dis* 1974;110:56–77.
48. Taryle DA, Potts DE, Sahn SA. The incidence and clinical correlates of parapneumonic effusions in pneumococcal pneumonia. *Chest* 1978;74:170–173.
49. Wolfe WG, Spock A, Bradford WD. Pleural fluid in infants and children. *Am Rev Respir Dis* 1968;98:1027–1032.
50. Hendren WH III, Haggerty RJ. Staphylococcic pneumonia in infancy and childhood. *JAMA* 1958;168:6–16.
51. Kaye MG, Fox MJ, Bartlett JG, et al. The clinical spectrum of *Staphylococcus aureus* pulmonary infection. *Chest* 1990;97:788–792.
52. Sexauer WP, Quezado Z, Lippmann ML, et al. Pleural effusions in right-sided endocarditis: characteristics and pathophysiology. *South Med J* 1992;85:1176–1180.
53. Welch CC, Tombridge TL, Baker WJ, et al. Beta-hemolytic streptococcal pneumonia: report of an outbreak in a military population. *Am J Med Sci* 1961;242:157–165.
54. Basiliere JL, Bistrong HW, Spence WF. Streptococcal pneumonia: recent outbreaks in military recruit populations. *Am J Med* 1968;44:580–589.
55. Braman SS, Donat WE. Explosive pleuritis. Manifestation of Group A beta-hemolytic streptococcal infection. *Am J Med* 1986;81:723–726.
56. Tillotson JR, Lerner AM. Characteristics of pneumonias caused by *Escherichia coli*. *N Engl J Med* 1967;277:115–122.
57. Winer-Muram HT, Jennings SG, Wunderink RG, et al. Ventilator-associated *Pseudomonas aeruginosa* pneumonia: radiographic findings. *Radiology* 1995;195:247–252.
58. Holmes RB. Friedlander's pneumonia. *AJR Am J Roentgenol* 1956;75:728–747.
59. Asmar BI, Slovis TL, Reed JO, et al. *Hemophilus influenzae* type b pneumonia in 43 children. *J Pediatr* 1978;93:389–393.
60. Ginsburg CM, Howard JB, Nelson JD. Report of 65 cases of *Haemophilus influenzae* b pneumonia. *Pediatrics* 1979;64:283–286.
61. Levin DC, Schwarz MI, Matthay RA, et al. Bacteremic *Haemophilus influenzae* pneumonia in adults: a report of 24 cases and a review of the literature. *Am J Med* 1977;62:219–223.
62. Tillotson JR, Lerner AM. Characteristics of pneumonias caused by *Bacillus proteus*. *Ann Intern Med* 1968;68:287–294.
63. Evans AF, Oakley RH, Whitehouse GH. Analysis of the chest radiograph in Legionnaires' disease. *Clin Radiol* 1981;32:361–365.
64. Tan MJ, Tan JS, Hamor RH, et al. The radiologic manifestations of Legionnaire's disease. *Chest* 2000;117:398–403.
65. Kroboth FJ, Yu VL, Reddy SC, et al. Clinicoradiographic correlation with extent of Legionnaire disease. *AJR Am J Roentgenol* 1983;141:263–268.
66. Randolph KA, Beekman JF. Legionnaires' disease presenting with empyema. *Chest* 1979;75:404–406.
67. Shafazand S, Doyle R, Ruoss S, et al. Inhalational anthrax: epidemiology, diagnosis, and management. *Chest* 1999;116:1369–1376.
68. Pettersson T, Nyberg P, Nordstrom D, et al. Similar pleural fluid findings in pleuropulmonary tularemia and tuberculous pleurisy. *Chest* 1996;109:572–575.
69. Patel SB, Mahler R. Clostridial pleuropulmonary infections: case report and review of the literature. *J Infect* 1990;21:81–85.
70. Cooney TG, Harwood BR, Meisner DJ. *Haemophilus parainfluenzae* thoracic empyema. *Arch Intern Med* 1981;141:940–941.
71. Bekemeyer WB, Zimmerman GA. Life-threatening complications associated with *Bacillus cereus* pneumonia. *Am Rev Respir Dis* 1985;131:466–469.
72. Madrazo A, Henderson MD, Baker L, et al. Massive empyema due to *Citrobacter diversus*. *Chest* 1975;68:104–106.
73. Mazzulli T, Salit IE. Pleural fluid infection caused by *Listeria monocytogenes:* case report and review. *Rev Infect Dis* 1991;13:564–570.
74. Van De Water JM. The treatment of pleural effusion complicating pneumonia. *Chest* 1970;57:259–262.

75. Sahn SA, Lakshminarayan S, Char DC. "Silent" empyema in patients receiving corticosteroids. *Am Rev Respir Dis* 1973;107:873–876.

76. Sullivan KM, O'Toole RD, Fisher RH, et al. Anaerobic empyema thoracis. *Arch Intern Med* 1973;131:521–527.

77. Massard G, Wihlm JM; Early complications. Esophagopleural fistula. *Chest Surg Clin N Am* 1999;9:617–631.

78. Landay MJ, Christensen EE, Bynum LJ, et al. Anaerobic pleural and pulmonary infections. *AJR Am J Roentgenol* 1980;134:233–240.

79. Cheng D-S, Rodriguez RM, Rogers J, et al. Comparison of pleural fluid pH values obtained using blood gas machine, pH meter, and pH indicator strip. *Chest* 1998;114:1368–1372.

80. Pine JR, Hollman JL. Elevated pleural fluid pH in *Proteus mirabilis* empyema. *Chest* 1983;84:109–111.

81. Sahn SA, Taryle DA, Good JT Jr. Experimental empyema: time course and pathogenesis of pleural fluid acidosis and low pleural fluid glucose. *Am Rev Respir Dis* 1979;120:355–361.

82. Light RW, Moller DJ Jr, George RB. Low pleural fluid pH in parapneumonic effusion. *Chest* 1975;68:273–274.

83. Berger HA, Morganroth ML. Immediate drainage is not required for all patients with complicated parapneumonic effusions. *Chest* 1990;97:731–735.

84. Poe RH, Matthew GM, Israel RH, et al. Utility of pleural fluid analysis in predicting tube thoracostomy/decortication in parapneumonic effusions. *Chest* 1991;100:963–967.

85. Light RW. Management of parapneumonic effusions. *Chest* 1991;100:892–893.

86. Heffner JE, Brown LK, Barbieri C, et al. Pleural fluid chemical analysis in parapneumonic effusions. A meta-analysis. *Am J Respir Crit Care Med* 1995;151:1700–1708.

87. McLoud TC, Flower CD. Imaging the pleura: sonography, CT, and MR imaging. *AJR Am J Roentgenol* 1991;156:1145–1153.

88. Yang PC, Luh KT, Chang DB, et al. Value of sonography in determining the nature of pleural effusion: analysis of 320 cases. *AJR Am J Roentgenol* 1992;159:29–33.

89. Himelman RB, Callen PW. The prognostic value of loculations in parapneumonic pleural effusions. *Chest* 1986;90:852–856.

90. Stark DD, Federle MP, Goodman PC, et al. Differentiating lung abscess and empyema: radiography and computed tomography. *AJR Am J Roentgenol* 1983;141:163–167.

91. Light RW. A new classification of parapneumonic effusions and empyema. *Chest* 1995;108:299–301.

92. Bartlett JG, Breiman RF, Mandell LA, et al. Community-acquired pneumonia in adults: guidelines for management. *Clin Infect Dis* 1998:26:811–838.

93. Everts RJ, Reller LB. Pleural space infections: microbiology and antimicrobial therapy. *Semin Respir Infect* 1999;14:18–30.

94. Clagett OT, Geraci JE. A procedure for the management of postpneumonectomy empyema. *J Thorac Cardiovasc Surg* 1963;45:141–145.

95. Dieter RA Jr, Pifarre R, Neville WE, et al. Empyema treated with neomycin irrigation and closed-chest drainage. *J Thorac Cardiovasc Surg* 1970;59:496–500.

96. Rosenfeldt FL, McGibney D, Braimbridge MV, et al. Comparison between irrigation and conventional treatment for empyema and pneumonectomy space infection. *Thorax* 1981;36:272–277.

97. Hutter JA, Harari D, Braimbridge MV. The management of empyema thoracis by thoracoscopy and irrigation. *Ann Thorac Surg* 1985;39:517–520.

98. Hakim M, Milstein BB. Empyema thoracis and infected pneumonectomy space: case for cyclical irrigation. *Ann Thorac Surg* 1986;41:85–88.

99. Storm HKR, Krasnik M, Bang K, et al. Treatment of pleural empyema secondary to pneumonia: thoracocentesis regimen versus tube drainage. *Thorax* 1992;47:821–824.

100. Cham CW, Haq SM, Rahamim J. Empyema thoracis: a problem with late referral? *Thorax* 1993;48:925–927.

101. Simmers TA, Jie C, Sie B. Minimally invasive treatment of thoracic empyema. *Thorac Cardiovasc Surg* 1999;47:77–81.

102. Ferguson AD, Prescott RJ, Selkon JB, et al. The clinical course and management of thoracic empyema. *QJM* 1996;89:285–289.

103. McLaughlin JS, Krasna MJ. Parapneumonic empyema. In: Shields TW, ed: *General thoracic surgery,* 5th ed. Baltimore: Williams & Wilkins, 2000:699–708.

104. Shankar S, Gulati M, Kang M, et al. Image-guided percutaneous drainage of thoracic empyema: can sonography predict the outcome? *Eur Radiol* 2000;10:495–499.

105. Ali I, Unruh H. Management of empyema thoracis. *Ann Thorac Surg* 1990;50:355–359.

106. Ashbaugh DG. Empyema thoracis. Factors influencing morbidity and mortality. *Chest* 1991;99:1162–1165.

107. Kerr A, Vasudevan VP, Powell S, et al. Percutaneous catheter drainage for acute empyema. Improved cure rate using CAT scan, fluoroscopy, and pigtail drainage catheters. *NY State J Med* 1991;91:4–7.

108. Sherman MM, Subramanian V, Berger RL. Management of thoracic empyema. *Am J Surg* 1977;133:474–479.

109. Light RW. Nguyen T, Mulligan ME, et al. The in vitro efficacy of varidase versus streptokinase or urokinase for liquefying thick purulent exudative material from loculated empyema. *Lung* 2000;178:13–18.

110. Bergh NP, Ekroth R, Larsson S, et al. Intrapleural streptokinase in the treatment of haemothorax and empyema. *Scand J Thorac Cardiovasc Surg* 1977;11:265–268.

111. Bouros D, Schiza S, Patsourakis G, et al. Intrapleural streptokinase versus urokinase in the treatment of complicated parapneumonic effusions: a prospective, double-blind study. *Am J Respir Crit Care Med* 1997;155:291–295.

112. Jerjes-Sanchez C, Ramirez-Rivera A, Elizalde JJ, et al. Intrapleural fibrinolysis with streptokinase as an adjunctive treatment in hemothorax and empyema: a multicenter trial. *Chest* 1996;109:1514–1519.

113. Laisaar T, Puttsepp E, Laisaar V. Early administration of intrapleural streptokinase in the treatment of multiloculated pleural effusions and pleural empyemas. *Thorac Cardiovasc Surg* 1996;44:252–256.

114. Temes RT, Follis F, Kessler RM, et al. Intrapleural fibrinolytics in management of empyema thoracis. *Chest* 1996;110:102–106.

115. Moulton JS, Benkert RE, Weisiger KH, et al. Treatment of complicated pleural fluid collections with

image-guided drainage and intracavitary urokinase. *Chest* 1995;108:1252–1259.

116. Light RW. Pleural disease. *Dis Mon* 1992;38:265–331.

117. Berglin E, Ekroth R, Teger-Nilsson AL, et al. Intrapleural instillation of streptokinase. Effects on systemic fibrinolysis. *Thorac Cardiovasc Surg* 1981;29:124–126.

118. Chin NK, Lim TK. Controlled trial of intrapleural streptokinase in the treatment of pleural empyema and complicated parapneumonic effusions. *Chest* 1997;111:275–279.

119. Davies RJO, Traill ZC, Gleeson FV. Randomised controlled trial of intrapleural streptokinase in community acquired pleural infection. *Thorax* 1997;52:416–421.

120. Bouros D, Schiza S, Tzanakis N, et al. Intrapleural urokinase versus normal saline in the treatment of complicated parapneumonic effusions and empyema. A randomized, double-blind study. *Am J Respir Crit Care Med* 1999;159:37–42.

121. Lim TK, Chin NK. Empirical treatment with fibrinolysis and early surgery reduces the duration of hospitalization in pleural sepsis. *Eur Respir J* 1999;13:514–518.

122. Simpson G, Roomes D, Heron M. Effects of streptokinase and deoxyribonuclease on viscosity of human surgical and empyema pus. *Chest* 2000;117:1728–1733.

123. Silen ML, Naunheim KS. Thoracoscopic approach to the management of empyema thoracis. Indications and results. *Chest Surg Clin N Am* 1996;6:491–469.

124. Landreneau RJ, Keenan RJ, Hazelrigg SR, et al. Thoracoscopy for empyema and hemothorax. *Chest* 1995;109:18–24.

125. Cassina PC, Hauser M, Hillejan L, et al. Video-assisted thoracoscopy in the treatment of pleural empyema: stage-based management and outcome. *J Thorac Cardiovasc Surg* 1999;117:234–238.

126. Lawrence DR, Ohri SK, Moxon RE, et al. Thoracoscopic debridement of empyema thoracis. *Ann Thorac Surg* 1997;64:1448–1450.

127. Striffeler H, Gugger M, Im Hof V, et al. Video-assisted thoracoscopic surgery for fibrinopurulent pleural empyema in 67 patients. *Ann Thorac Surg* 1998;65:319–323.

128. Wait MA, Sharma S, Hohn J, et al. A randomized trial of empyema therapy. *Chest* 1997;111:1548–1551.

129. Thurer RJ. Decortication in thoracic empyema. Indications and surgical technique. *Chest Surg Clin N Am* 1996;6:461–490.

130. Pothula V, Krellenstein DJ. Early aggressive surgical management of parapneumonic empyemas. *Chest* 1994;105:832–836.

131. Angelillo Mackinlay TA, Lyons GA, Chimondeguy DJ, et al. VATS debridement versus thoracotomy in the treatment of loculated postpneumonia empyema. *Ann Thorac Surg* 1996;61:1626–1630.

132. Neff CC, van Sonnenberg E, Lawson DW, et al. CT follow-up of empyemas: pleural peels resolve after percutaneous catheter drainage. *Radiology* 1990;176:195–197.

133. Morin JE, Munro DD, MacLean LD. Early thoracotomy for empyema. *J Thorac Cardiovasc Surg* 1972;64:530–536.

134. Samson PC. Empyema thoracis: essentials of present-day management. *Ann Thorac Surg* 1971;11:210–220.

135. Hoff SJ, Neblett WW, Edwards KM, et al. Parapneumonic empyema in children: decortication hastens

recovery in patients with severe pleural infections. *Pediatr Infect Dis J* 1991;10:194–199.

136. Rosen H, Nadkarni V, Theroux M, et al. Intrapleural streptokinase as adjunctive treatment for persistent empyema in pediatric patients. *Chest* 1993;103:1190–1193.

137. Doski JJ, Lou D, Hicks BA, et al. Management of parapneumonic collections in infants and children. *J Pediatr Surg* 2000;35:265–270.

138. Fraser RS, Muller NL, Colman N, et al. *Diagnosis of diseases of the chest*, 4th ed. Philadelphia: W.B. Saunders, 2000:2659–2695.

139. Gharagozloo F, Trachiotis G, Wolfe A, et al. Pleural space irrigation and modified Clagett procedure for the treatment of early postpneumonectomy empyema. *J Thorac Cardiovasc Surg* 1998;116:943–948.

140. Wain JC. Management of late postpneumonectomy empyema and bronchopleural fistula. *Chest Surg Clin N Am* 1996;6:529–541.

141. Ratto GB, Fantino G, Tassara E, et al. Long-term antimicrobial prophylaxis in lung cancer surgery: correlation between microbiological findings and empyema development. *Lung Cancer* 1994;11:345–352.

142. Virkkula L, Eerola S. Treatment of postpneumonectomy empyema. *Scand J Thorac Cardiovasc Surg* 1974;8:133–137.

143. Ueda H, Shibata K, Kusano T. Postoperative pyothorax. *Surg Today* 1992;22:115–119.

144. Karkola P, Kairaluoma MI, Larmi TKI. Postpneumonectomy empyema in pulmonary carcinoma patients. *J Thorac Cardiovasc Surg* 1976;72:319–322.

145. Goldstraw P. Treatment of postpneumonectomy empyema: the case for fenestration. *Thorax* 1979;34:740–745.

146. Rosenfeldt FL, McGibney D, Braimbridge MV, et al. Comparison between irrigation and conventional treatment for empyema and pneumonectomy space infection. *Thorax* 1981;36:272–277.

147. Hollaus PH, Lax F, Wurnig PN, et al. Videothoracoscopic treatment of postpneumonectomy empyema. *J Thorac Cardiovasc Surg* 1999;117:397–398.

148. Shamji FM, Ginsberg RJ, Cooper JD, et al. Open window thoracostomy in the management of postpneumonectomy empyema with or without bronchopleural fistula. *J Thorac Cardiovasc Surg* 1983;86:818–822.

149. Bayes AJ, Wilson JA, Chiu RC, et al. Clagett open-window thoracostomy in patients with empyema who had and had not undergone pneumonectomy. *Can J Surg* 1987;30:329–331.

150. Pairolero PC, Arnold PG, Trastek VF, et al. Postpneumonectomy empyema. The role of intrathoracic muscle transposition. *J Thorac Cardiovasc Surg* 1990;99:958–968.

151. Saito H, Tatsuzawa T, Kikkawa H, et al. Transpericardial bronchial closure with omentopexy for postpneumonectomy bronchopleural fistula. *Ann Thorac Surg* 1989;47:312–313.

152. Shirakusa T, Ueda H, Takata S, et al. Use of pedicled omental flap in treatment of empyema. *Ann Thorac Surg* 1990;50:420–424.

153. Aguilar MM, Battistella FD, Owings JT, et al. Post-traumatic empyema. Risk factor analysis. *Arch Surg* 1997;132:647–650.

154. Mandal AK, Thadepalli H, Mandal AK, et al. Post-traumatic empyema thoracis: a 24-year experience at a major trauma center. *J Trauma* 1997;43:764–771.

10

Tuberculous Pleural Effusions

The diagnosis of tuberculous pleuritis should be considered in any patient with an exudative pleural effusion. A pleural effusion as an isolated manifestation of tuberculosis has been likened to a primary chancre as a manifestation of syphilis. Both are self-limited and of little immediate concern, but both may lead to serious disease many years later.

PATHOGENESIS AND PATHOPHYSIOLOGIC FEATURES

When a tuberculous pleural effusion occurs in the absence of radiologically apparent tuberculosis, it may be the sequel to a primary infection 6 to 12 weeks previously or it may represent reactivation tuberculosis (1). In industrialized countries, more pleural effusions may be due to reactivation than are due to postprimary infection (1). The tuberculous pleural effusion is thought to result from rupture of a subpleural caseous focus in the lung into the pleural space (2). Supporting evidence comes from the operative findings of Stead et al. (3), who reported that they could demonstrate a caseous tuberculous focus in the lung contiguous with the diseased pleura in 12 of 15 patients with tuberculous pleuritis. The remaining three patients in this series were found to have parenchymal tuberculosis, although these patients did not have caseous foci adjacent to the pleura.

It appears that delayed hypersensitivity plays a large role in the pathogenesis of tuberculous pleural effusion. Several workers (4–7) have reported that when guinea pigs or mice are immunized to tuberculous protein by injecting Freund's adjuvant containing dead tubercle bacilli into their footpads, an intrapleural injection of purified protein derivative of tuberculin (PPD) 3 to 5 weeks later causes the rapid appearance (over 12 to 48 hours) of an exudative pleural effusion. The development of the pleural effusion is suppressed when the animals are given antilymphocyte serum (6).

The neutrophil appears to play a key role in the development of experimental tuberculous pleuritis. When bacillus Calmette-Guérin (BCG)–sensitized rabbits are given BCG intrapleurally, the resulting pleural fluid contains predominantly neutrophils for the first 24 hours (8). If the animals are made neutropenic, the accumulation of pleural fluid and inflammatory cells, particularly macrophages, is decreased. The intrapleural injection of neutrophils in the neutropenic animals restores the response to control levels. The neutrophils in the pleural space appear to secrete a monocyte chemotaxin that recruits monocytes to the pleural space and thereby contributes to the formation of granulomas (8).

In this BCG model of experimental tuberculous pleuritis, macrophages predominate in the pleural fluid from day 2 to day 5 (8). It has been shown that mesothelial cells stimulated with BCG or interferon-gamma produce macrophage inflammatory protein and monocyte chemotactic peptide (9). These two proteins account for more than 75% of the mononuclear chemotactic factor in tuberculous pleural fluid (9). After this period, lymphocytes are the predominant cell in the pleural fluid (10). When the lymphocytes first appear in the pleural fluid on approximately day 3, they do not respond to PPD. From day 5 onward, however, reactivity to PPD is found in most cases (11). The reactivity of the lymphocytes in the peripheral blood parallels that of the pleural lymphocytes (11).

It is probable that delayed hypersensitivity also plays a large role in the development of tuberculous pleural effusions in humans. The pleural fluid mycobacterial cultures from the majority of patients with tuberculous pleural effusions are negative (2, 12, 13). T lymphocytes specifically sensitized to tuberculous protein are present in the pleural fluid (14). In one report, approximately one in 2,000 of the lymphocytes in the pleural fluid was specifically sensitized to tuberculous protein (14). In the same report, only one in 15,000 of the lymphocytes in the peripheral blood was specifically sensitized to the tuberculous protein. It is unknown whether the increased percentage of specifically sensitized lymphocytes in the pleural fluid is due to their clonal expansion in the pleural fluid or is due to the migratory loss of PPD-responding T lymphocytes from the blood to the pleural space. When pleural lymphocytes from patients with tuberculous pleural effusions are cocultured with PPD, lymphokines are produced (15). The level of lymphokine production is much greater with pleural lymphocytes than with peripheral blood lymphocytes (15).

Rupture of a subpleural caseous focus into the pleural space allows tuberculous protein to enter the pleural space and to generate the hypersensitivity reaction responsible for most of the clinical manifestations.

Although delayed hypersensitivity to tuberculous protein is probably responsible for most clinical manifestations of tuberculous pleuritis, many patients when first evaluated have a negative PPD skin test. The explanation for this paradox may be a combination of two factors. First, in some (16), but not in all (17), patients with tuberculous pleuritis, a circulating mononuclear adherent cell suppresses the specifically sensitized circulating T lymphocytes in the peripheral blood. Second, there may be sequestration of PPD-reactive T lymphocytes in the pleural space involving both Leu-2 (suppressor/cytotoxic) and Leu-3 (helper) positive T cells (17).

Tuberculous pleural effusions are enriched with many potentially immunoreactive cells and substances that comprise the vigorous local cell-mediated immune response (18). Compared with peripheral blood, pleural fluid is enriched with T lymphocytes. The CD4 (helper-inducer) to CD8 (suppressor/cytotoxic) ratio is 3:4 in pleural fluid, compared with 1:7 in blood (18). Pleural fluid lymphocytes from patients with tuberculous pleuritis show greater responsiveness to PPD than do peripheral blood lymphocytes (19).

The obvious explanation for the development of the tuberculous pleural effusion is that the delayed hypersensitivity reaction increases the permeability of the pleural capillaries to protein, and the increased protein levels in the pleural fluid result in a much higher rate of pleural fluid formation and accordingly result in the accumulation of pleural fluid. However, this does not appear to be the mechanism for the pleural fluid formation. Allen and Apicella (5) were unable to demonstrate any striking increase in the inflow of protein into the pleural space in their experimental model of delayed-hypersensitivity tuberculous pleuritis. They did, however, demonstrate a dramatic decrease in the clearance of protein from the pleural space (5). Leckie and Tothill (20) reported that the pleural lymphatic flow from patients with tuberculosis was approximately 50% that of patients with congestive heart failure. It is probable that the intense inflammatory reaction in the parietal pleura impedes the lymphatic drainage from the pleural space (see Chapter 2) and leads to the accumulation of pleural fluid.

INCIDENCE

In many areas of the world, tuberculosis remains the most common cause of pleural effusions in the absence of demonstrable pulmonary disease. For example, in a recent series of 642 pleural effusions from northern Spain, tuberculosis was the most common etiology of pleural effusion, accounting for 25% of all pleural effusions (21). A recent study from Saudi Arabia demonstrated that tuberculosis was also the most common cause of pleural effusions in that country, accounting for 37% of all pleural effusions (22).

In the United States, the annual incidence of tuberculous pleuritis has been estimated to be about 1,000 cases, and it is said that approximately one in 30 patients with tuberculosis will have tuberculous pleuritis (23). It is likely that both of these numbers are low. Patients with tuberculous pleuritis tend to be under reported because their mycobacterial cultures are frequently negative. Between 1988 and 1994, there were 2,817 cases of tuberculosis in patients without the acquired immunodeficiency syndrome (AIDS) who were reported to the South Carolina state tuberculosis registry; 6% of these patients had pleural effusions (24). However, in Burundi, pleural effusions occur in more than 25% of non-AIDS patients with new-onset intrathoracic tuberculosis (25), whereas a 20% incidence has been reported in South Africa in non-AIDS patients (26).

One might anticipate that the incidence of tuberculous pleuritis would be relatively low in patients with AIDS and tuberculosis because the patient with AIDS has a compromised immunologic system, and pleural tuberculosis is thought to be due to hypersensitivity. However, overall it appears that the incidence of pleural effusions is higher in patients with AIDS. Although in the series referenced above from Burundi, a slightly smaller percentage of human immunodeficiency virus (HIV)–positive patients (24%) than HIV-negative patients (28%) had pleural effusions (25), other series have shown that pleural effusions are more common in HIV-negative patients. The percentage of patients with thoracic tuberculosis who had a pleural effusion with thoracic tuberculosis was higher in HIV-positive patients than in HIV-negative patients in series from South Africa (38% versus 20%) (26), Uganga (23% versus 11%) (27), and Zimbabwe (27% versus 13%) (28).

CLINICAL MANIFESTATIONS

Although tuberculosis is usually considered a chronic illness, tuberculous pleuritis most commonly manifests as an acute illness. In one series of 71 patients, 25 (31%) had initial symptoms of less than a week in duration, whereas 50 (62%) had been symptomatic for less than a month (29). In another series, 31 of 49 patients (62%) had an acute illness that most commonly mimicked acute bacterial pneumonia (2). Most patients (~70%) have a cough, usually nonproductive, and most (~75%) have chest pain, usually pleuritic in nature (1, 2, 30). If both cough and pleuritic chest pain are present, the pain usually precedes the cough. Most patients are febrile, but a normal temperature does not rule out the diagnosis. In one series, 7 of 49 patients (14%) were afebrile (2). Occasionally, the onset of tuberculosis is less acute, with only mild chest pain, perhaps with a low-grade fever and a nonproductive cough, weight loss, and easy fatigability.

In general, patients with tuberculous pleuritis are younger than patients with parenchymal tuberculosis. In one series, the mean age of patients with tuberculous pleuritis was 28 years, whereas the mean age of patients with parenchymal tuberculosis was 54 years (31). In the United States, tuberculous pleuritis is increasingly becoming a disease of the older individual. In 1987, Epstein et al. (32) reported that the median age of their 26 patients with tuberculous pleuritis was 54 years, and one third of the patients were older than 60 years of age. Patients with pleural effusions secondary to reactivation tend to be older than those with postprimary pleural effusion (1).

Pleural effusions secondary to tuberculous pleuritis are usually unilateral and can be of any size. In one series, the effusions occupied more than two thirds the hemithorax in 18%, between one third and two thirds of the hemothorax in 47%, and less than one third of the hemithorax in 34% (33). In another series of 46 patients with massive pleural effusions (34), 4% of the effusions were due to tuberculosis. In about 20% of patients with pleural effusions secondary to tuberculosis (33), coexisting parenchymal disease is radiologically visible. In such patients, the pleural effusion is almost always on the side of the parenchymal infiltrate and invariably indicates active parenchymal disease.

Clinical Manifestations in Human Immunodeficiency Virus–Positive Patients

The clinical manifestations of pleural tuberculosis tend to be somewhat different in the HIV-positive patient. Patients with HIV tend to have a longer duration of illness and a lower incidence of chest pain (35). Systemic signs and symptoms such as night sweats, fatigue, diarrhea, hepatomegaly, splenomegaly, and lymphadenopathy are significantly more common in HIV-infected patients (30). Their pleural fluid is more likely to be smear positive for acid-fast bacilli (AFB) and culture positive for AFB (35). If the CD4 count is less than 100, nearly 50% have a positive smear for AFB on their pleural fluid (35).

NATURAL HISTORY OF UNTREATED TUBERCULOUS PLEURITIS

Without treatment, tuberculous pleuritis usually resolves spontaneously, only to return as active tuberculosis at a later date. Patiala (36) followed for at least 7 years all 2,816 members of the Finnish Armed Forces who developed pleural effusions between 1939 and 1945. They reported that 43% of this large group of young men developed tuberculosis during the follow-up period. Even in the 1-year observation period 5 years following the initial episode, 5% of the total population studied developed active tuberculosis. Confirmatory evidence for this large series comes from the series of Roper and Waring (37) in the United States, who followed 141 military personnel first seen from 1940 to 1944 with a pleural effusion and a positive PPD test. In most patients, the effusions resolved and all the other symptoms disappeared within 2 to 4 months.

Nevertheless, 92 of the 141 individuals (65%) subsequently developed some form of active tuberculosis. Manifest tuberculosis did not develop in the lung or elsewhere in any of the patients within 8 months of the onset of the original pleurisy. The incidence of subsequent tuberculosis was 60% in those with initially negative pleural fluid cultures for tuberculosis and 65% in those with initially positive pleural fluid cultures. In addition, the size of the original effusions and the presence or the absence of small radiologic residual pleural disease were not correlated with the subsequent appearance of active tuberculosis (37). The foregoing series emphasize the importance of making the diagnosis of tuberculous pleuritis.

Because the administration of antituberculous chemotherapy reduces the incidence of subsequent tuberculosis (2, 38), it is important to establish the diagnosis of tuberculous pleuritis and initiate proper treatment. Moreover, patients in whom the diagnosis cannot be established but in whom the diagnosis is considered likely should also be treated.

DIAGNOSIS

The diagnosis of tuberculous pleuritis depends on the demonstration of tubercle bacilli in the sputum, pleural fluid, or pleural biopsy specimen, or the demonstration of granulomas in the pleura. The diagnosis can also be established with reasonable certainty by demonstrating elevated levels of adenosine deaminase (ADA) or interferon-gamma in the pleural fluid (39). Study of the peripheral blood is not useful; most patients do not have leukocytosis (2). The chest radiograph usually demonstrates only the pleural fluid, but as previously mentioned, about 20% of the patients also have a parenchymal infiltrate due to tuberculosis (33). The observations of Stead et al. (3) that most patients with tuberculous pleuritis have concomitant parenchymal disease that is subclinical radiologically, raises the possibility that computed tomographic (CT) studies might be useful in demonstrating such parenchymal disease. However, in one study, CT scans were obtained in 66 patients with pleural tuberculosis, and parenchymal abnormalities were demonstrated in less than 40% (40). Interestingly, 39% of the patients in the series had hilar or mediastinal lymphadenopathy (40).

Tuberculin Skin Testing

In the past, the tuberculin skin test was an important diagnostic aid in patients suspected of having tuberculous pleuritis. However, a negative skin test does not rule out the diagnosis of tuberculous pleuritis. In one recent series from Spain, the PPD was positive in only 66.5% of 254 patients with tuberculous pleuritis (33). In another recent series from Hong Kong, more than one half the patients tested had a negative PPD (13). The factors responsible for the negative skin test in patients with tuberculous pleuritis are discussed earlier in this chapter. If the patient with a negative tuberculin skin test and tuberculous pleuritis is skin tested more than 8 weeks after the development of symptoms, the skin test will almost always be positive. Therefore, in patients with an undiagnosed exudative pleural effusion, a negative tuberculin skin test performed 8 weeks after the development of symptoms can be used to exclude the diagnosis of tuberculous pleuritis. However, if the patient is markedly immunosuppressed with HIV infection or is severely malnourished, the PPD may remain negative.

Pleural Fluid Analysis

Pleural fluid analysis is useful in the diagnosis of tuberculous pleuritis. The fluid is invariably an exudate. Frequently, the pleural fluid protein level is above 5.0 g per dL, and this finding suggests tuberculous pleuritis. In most patients, the pleural fluid differential white blood cell count (WBC) reveals more than 50% small lymphocytes (2, 33, 41–43). In one series of 254 patients with tuberculous pleuritis (33), only 17 (6.7%) had fewer than 50% lymphocytes in the pleural fluid. In patients with symptoms of less than 2 weeks' duration, the pleural fluid differential WBC may reveal predominantly polymorphonuclear leukocytes (29). If serial thoracenteses are performed, the differential WBC reveals a change to predominantly small lymphocytes (2). The separation of the lymphocytes into T lymphocytes and B lymphocytes is not useful diagnostically (see Chapter 4). If eosinophils are found in the pleural fluid in significant numbers (>10%), one can virtually exclude the diagnosis of tuberculous pleuritis, unless the patient has a pneumothorax or has had a previous thoracentesis (see Chapter 4).

A useful study for ruling out tuberculous pleuritis is analysis of the pleural fluid for mesothelial cells (Fig. 4.1A). Four separate series have confirmed that pleural fluid from patients with tuberculosis rarely contains more than 5% mesothelial cells (41, 42, 44, 45). Unfortunately, the absence of mesothelial cells is not diagnostic of tuberculosis because in any condition in which the pleural surfaces are extensively involved by an inflammatory process, mesothelial cells are not found in the pleural fluid. It has been suggested that HIV-infected patients with tuberculous pleuritis may have significant numbers of

mesothelial cells in their pleural fluid (46). In one report (46), three HIV-infected patients with tuberculous pleuritis all had significant numbers of mesothelial cells in their pleural fluid. Each of the patients had CD4 counts of less than 100 per mm^3 in their peripheral blood.

Adenosine Deaminase

Demonstration of an elevated pleural fluid ADA level is useful in establishing the diagnosis of tuberculous pleuritis. ADA is the enzyme that catalyzes the conversion of adenosine to inosine. ADA is a predominant T lymphocyte enzyme, and its plasma activity is high in diseases in which cellular immunity is stimulated. In an early study, Ocana et al. (47) measured the pleural fluid ADA levels in 221 pleural or peritoneal effusions (Fig. 10.1). All patients with a pleural fluid ADA level above 70 U per L had tuberculosis, whereas no patient with a pleural fluid ADA level below 40 U per L had tuberculous pleuritis. Subsequent

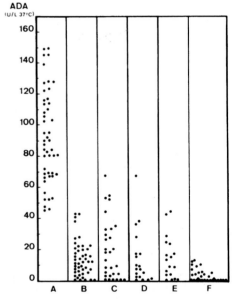

FIG. 10.1. Levels of adenosine deaminase (ADA) activity in pleuroperitoneal effusions. Tuberculosis **(A)**; malignancies **(B)**; pleuropneumonia **(C)**; miscellaneous **(D)**; unknown origin **(E)**; transudates **(F)**. (From Ocana I, Martinez-Vazquez JM, Segura RM, et al. Adenosine deaminase in pleural fluids. *Chest* 1983;84:51–53, with permission.)

studies of larger numbers of patients with tuberculous pleural effusions have demonstrated that the pleural fluid ADA level is higher in patients with tuberculous pleuritis than in patients with other types of pleural effusions (48–51). Different authors have used various cutoff levels for the pleural fluid ADA between 33 and 50 U per L for the diagnosis of pleural tuberculosis. The higher the pleural fluid ADA level, the more likely the patient is to have tuberculous pleuritis.

In general, the main two diseases other than tuberculous pleuritis that are associated with a high pleural fluid ADA are empyema and rheumatoid pleuritis. However, it should be easy to differentiate these two diseases from tuberculous pleuritis by the clinical picture and the fact that these latter two diseases do not have pleural fluid lymphocytosis. Indeed, if the diagnostic criteria for tuberculous pleuritis includes a pleural fluid lymphocyte-to-neutrophil ratio of 0:75 or more, the specificity of the test is increased (52). This increase in specificity is due to excluding the cases with rheumatoid pleuritis or empyema. An occasional patient with a lymphoma and patients with Q fever and pleural effusions have a lymphocytic pleural effusion with a high ADA.

Almost all patients with tuberculous pleuritis have an ADA level above 40 U per L. The levels of ADA in patients with and without AIDS are comparable (51). The pleural fluid ADA level can be used to exclude the diagnosis of tuberculous pleural effusions in patients with undiagnosed pleural effusions.

Ferrer et al. (53) followed 40 patients with undiagnosed pleural effusions and a pleural fluid ADA level below 43 U per L for a mean of 5 years and reported that none of the patients developed tuberculosis.

There are two molecular forms of ADA—ADA1 and ADA2. ADA1 is found in all cells, but has its greatest activity in lymphocytes and monocytes (54). ADA2 is found only in monocytes, and the majority of ADA in tuberculous pleural fluid is ADA2, whereas the majority of ADA in other pleural fluids is ADA1 (54). Although the use of a ratio of the ADA1 to ADA total of less than 0:42 will slightly increase the sensitivity and specificity of the ADA in diagnosing tuberculous pleuritis, the separation of ADA

into its isoenzymes is not necessary in the vast majority of cases (54, 55).

In the United States, one of the most common causes of an exudate with predominantly lymphocytes is the postcoronary artery bypass graft (CAGB) surgery pleural effusion (see Chapter 16) (56). On rare occasions, patients post-CABG can develop a tuberculous pleural effusion (57). However, it has recently been shown that the lymphocytic predominant pleural effusion post-CABG has a pleural fluid ADA level below 40 U/L (58).

Interferon-Gamma

Another test that is useful in the diagnosis of tuberculous pleuritis is the level of interferon-gamma in the pleural fluid (48, 59–62). Interferon-gamma is produced by the $CD4^+$ lymphocytes from patients with tuberculous pleuritis (61). In one report, 33 of 35 patients with tuberculous pleuritis had interferon-gamma levels above 140 pg per mL, whereas only 9 of 110 other pleural fluids had levels that exceeded this (Fig. 4.5) (48). Excluding empyemas, there was only one nontuberculous pleural fluid that had a interferon-gamma level above 200 pg per mL (48). Comparable results have been reported in other series (59, 60–62), but comparison of the series is difficult because the units have differed from one study to another. In general, measurement of the pleural fluid ADA level is preferred to measurement of the pleural fluid interferon-gamma level in evaluating patients suspected of having pleural tuberculosis because the ADA measurement is less expensive.

Polymerase Chain Reaction

In the field of infectious diseases, the polymerase chain reaction (PCR) tests have been quite useful in establishing the diagnosis and pathogenesis of viral diseases. Therefore, it was hypothesized that PCR would be useful in diagnosing tuberculous pleuritis. It appears, however, that PCR is certainly not superior to either the pleural fluid ADA or interferon-gamma levels in establishing the diagnosis of tuberculous pleuritis. The best results with PCR came from a report by

Querol et al. (63) who performed PCR on the pleural fluid from 21 patients with pleural tuberculosis and 86 controls. They reported that the sensitivity and specificity of PCR for the diagnosis of tuberculous pleuritis were 81% and 100%, respectively. In the same patients, the sensitivity and specificity for an ADA level of 45 U per L was nearly identical (86% and 98%, respectively) (63). The PCR has been much less accurate in other studies. For example Villena et al. (64) reported that the PCR was positive in only 42% of patients with tuberculous pleuritis. The PCR of the pleural fluid should be considered to be an investigative test until there is more data regarding its sensitivity and specificity.

Pleural Fluid Tuberculous Proteins or Antibodies

In recent years, the possibility of establishing the diagnosis of tuberculous pleuritis by the demonstration of tuberculous antigens or specific antibodies against tuberculous proteins in the pleural fluid has been investigated. None of these tests have proven to be of use in the diagnosis of tuberculous pleuritis. The presence of antituberculous antibodies in the pleural space appears to result from their passive diffusion from the serum rather than local antibody production (65). Therefore, it is unlikely that measurement of such antibodies in the pleural fluid will ever be diagnostically useful.

Other Chemical Tests

Other chemical analyses of the pleural fluid are of limited value in establishing the diagnosis of tuberculous pleuritis. Although in the past it was believed that the pleural fluid glucose level was reduced in most cases of tuberculous pleuritis (66), more recent studies show that the majority of patients with tuberculous pleuritis have a pleural fluid glucose level above 60 mg per dL (2, 32, 35). A low pleural fluid pH was once thought to be suggestive of tuberculous pleuritis (67), and I concluded that tuberculous pleural effusions had a lower pleural fluid pH than malignant pleural effusions in the first article my

colleagues and I wrote on pleural fluid pH (68). Subsequent articles (69, 70), however, and my own observations indicate that the pleural fluid pH has about the same distribution in malignant as in tuberculous pleural effusions.

The levels of lysozyme in the pleural fluid have been proposed to be useful diagnostically (71, 72), and there is no doubt that the mean level of lysozyme in the pleural fluid from patients with tuberculous pleuritis is higher than it is in other exudative pleural fluids. A value of 1.2:1 for the ratio of the pleural fluid to the serum lysozyme has been proposed as a good test for diagnosing tuberculous pleuritis (72). When the utility of this ratio is compared with that of the pleural fluid ADA or interferon-gamma level, the lysozyme ratio is distinctly inferior (48). For this reason, the measurement of the lysozyme ratio is not recommended (48).

Pleural Fluid Stains and Cultures

For nonimmunosuppresed patients, routine smears of the pleural fluid for mycobacteria are not indicated because they are usually negative, unless the patient has a tuberculous empyema (12, 33). Cultures for mycobacteria should be obtained, however. If the patient is HIV positive, the smears may be positive in more than 20% (35). Both pleural fluid and sputum should be cultured for mycobacteria when tuberculous pleuritis is suspected. In most series of patients with tuberculous pleuritis, the pleural fluid cultures are positive for mycobacteria in fewer than 40% (2, 33). For mycobacterial cultures, use of a BACTEC system with bedside inoculation provides higher yields and faster results than do conventional methods. In one study, the median time for the BACTEC cultures to become positive was 18 days (range 3 to 40 days), whereas the median time for conventional cultures was 33.5 days (range 21 to 48 days) (73).

Pleural Biopsy

For the past 40 years, the diagnosis of tuberculous pleuritis has been most commonly made with needle biopsy of the pleura. The demonstration of granuloma in the parietal pleura suggests tuberculous pleuritis; caseous necrosis and AFB need not be demonstrated. Although other disorders including fungal diseases, sarcoidosis, tularemia (74), and rheumatoid pleuritis may produce granulomatous pleuritis, more than 95% of patients with granulomatous pleuritis have tuberculosis. Even when granulomas are not demonstrated in the pleural biopsy, the biopsy specimen should be examined for AFB because organisms are occasionally demonstrated when no granulomas are present in the biopsy. In a recent study of 248 patients undergoing needle biopsy of the pleura, the biopsy showed granulomas in 198 patients (80%), the acid-fast stain of the biopsy was positive in 64 (25.8%), the culture of the biopsy tissue was positive in 140 (56%), and at least one of the above three tests was positive in 227 (91%) (33).

In recent years, the availability of tests on the pleural fluid, such as the ADA, which are at least as sensitive in diagnosing tuberculous pleuritis as is needle biopsy of the pleura, have resulted in a decreased use of needle biopsy of the pleura (75). A possible criticism of relying on the pleural fluid tests rather than the pleural biopsy is that with, for example, the pleural fluid ADA, no culture results are obtained. Accordingly, the sensitivities of the organisms cannot be determined. It should be noted that although the cultures of the biopsy are positive in about 55%, cultures of the fluid itself are positive in 35%. Therefore, the culture of the biopsy itself provides additional positive cultures in only 20% of the patients.

Recommended Diagnostic Approach in Patients with Undiagnosed Exudative Pleural Effusion

When a patient is seen with a pleural effusion, the diagnosis of tuberculous pleuritis should always be considered. When the initial thoracentesis is performed, the pleural fluid should be analyzed for the ADA level and differential cell count, and the fluid should be cultured for mycobacteria. If the pleural fluid ADA is above 70 U per L and the pleural fluid has a lymphocyte-to-neutrophil ratio of more than 0.75, the diagnosis of tuberculosis is virtually established. If the pleural fluid

ADA level is between 40 and 70 U per L and the patient has a lymphocyte-to-neutrophil ratio of more than 0.75, a presumptive diagnosis of tuberculosis can be made. In this situation, consideration can be given to further studies (thoracoscopy or needle biopsy of the pleura) if the patient's clinical picture is not typical for tuberculous. If the patient's pleural fluid ADA is below 40, the diagnosis of tuberculosis is unlikely. However, if the patient has a clinical picture typical for tuberculosis and, particularly, if the pleural fluid has a high percentage of lymphocytes, the possibility of tuberculosis can be further evaluated with thoracoscopy or needle biopsy of the pleura.

TREATMENT

The treatment of tuberculous pleuritis has three goals: (a) to prevent the subsequent development of active tuberculosis, (b) to relieve the patient's symptoms, and (c) to prevent the development of a fibrothorax.

Chemotherapy

The recommendations by the American Thoracic Society for the treatment of all pulmonary and extrapulmonary tuberculosis are as follows (76). The initial phase of a 6-month regimen should consist of a 2-month period of isoniazid, rifampin, and pyrazinamide. Ethambutol should be included in the initial regimen until the results of drug susceptibility studies are available, unless there is little possibility of drug resistance. The second phase of the treatment should be isoniazid and rifampin given for 4 months. Directly observed therapy (DOT) is recommended. Nine-month regimens using isoniazid and rifampin are also effective when the organisms are fully susceptible to the drug.

The above-mentioned recommendations may be somewhat too intensive for isolated tuberculous pleuritis. Less intensive regimens appear to be effective. In one study, Canete et al. (77) treated 130 patients with 5 mg per kg of isoniazid and 10 mg per kg of rifampin daily for 6 months and reported no treatment failures. In a second study, Dutt et al. (78) administered 300 mg of INH plus 600 mg of rifampin daily for 1 month, followed by 900 mg of INH plus 600 mg of rifampin twice a week for the next 5 months to 198 patients. This regimen failed only one patient (78).

The patient with isolated tuberculous pleuritis appears to have a small bacterial burden because many of the symptoms are due to delayed hypersensitivity. In the series of Patiala and Mattila (38), the administration of chemotherapy decreased the subsequent incidence of tuberculosis from 28% to 9%, even though the majority of their patients received only one drug for less than 6 months. Falk and Stead (79) reported that antituberculous therapy reduced the incidence of subsequent tuberculosis from 19% to 4%, and, again, many of their patients did not receive two drugs for even 6 months. From the foregoing studies, it appears that 6 months of isoniazid and rifampin administration are sufficient if the patient does not have resistant organisms.

With treatment, the patient's symptoms and radiologic abnormalities gradually abate. The average patient becomes afebrile within 2 weeks, but temperature elevations may persist for as long as 2 months (80). If a therapeutic thoracentesis is performed at the time that antituberculous therapy is initiated, most patients become afebrile within 5 days (81, 82). The mean duration for complete resorption of the pleural fluid is about 6 weeks, but it can be as long as 12 weeks (80).

The incidence of pleural thickening at 6 to 12 months after beginning treatment is approximately 50% (83). The incidence of residual pleural thickening is not related to the initial pleural fluid findings; patients with a low glucose or a high pleural fluid LDH are not any more likely to have residual pleural thickening (83).

No reason exists to keep the patient in bed (2), and patients need be isolated only if their sputum tests are positive for mycobacteria.

An occasional patient will develop paradoxical worsening of their disease after antituberculous therapy is initiated. Al-Majed (84) serially studied 61 patients with tuberculous pleural effusion who were started on a standard regimen of rifampin, isoniazid, pyrazinamide, and ethambutol for the first 2 months. He reported that the size of the effusion worsened in 10 of the 61 patients (17%) after the initiation of antituberculous

therapy. Six of the patients developed increasing dyspnea and were treated with pleural aspiration and oral prednisolone with complete resolution of the pleural effusion. A second report suggested that such paradoxical responses might be due to isoniazid-induced lupus pleuritis (85).

Corticosteroids

The role of oral corticosteroids in the treatment of tuberculous pleurisy is controversial. There were no benefits with systemic corticosteroids in two recent controlled studies (81, 82) in which therapeutic thoracentesis was also performed. In a third study, however, the duration of fever and the time required for fluid resorption were decreased, but in this study, no therapeutic thoracentesis was performed (86). In none of the three reports did the administration of corticosteroids influence the degree of residual pleural thickening at 6 or 12 months after therapy was initiated.

In view of the above-mentioned factors, if the patient is more than mildly symptomatic with tuberculous pleuritis, a therapeutic thoracentesis is recommended. It should be noted, however, that although the studies outlined earlier suggested a beneficial effect of therapeutic thoracentesis, an older study by Large and Levick (87) was unable to demonstrate any difference in the clinical courses of 33 patients who had serial therapeutic thoracenteses and those of 19 patients who had only a single diagnostic thoracentesis. If the patient continues to have severe systemic symptoms (fever, malaise, pleuritic chest pain) after a therapeutic thoracentesis, and a definite diagnosis has been established, the administration of 80 mg of prednisone every other day until the acute symptoms have subsided is recommended. Thereafter, the corticosteroids are rapidly tapered.

Surgical Procedures

If the patient is dyspneic from a large pleural effusion, a therapeutic thoracentesis should be performed. Surgery should not be performed early for pleural thickening. Although the pleura may be thickened when the patient's disorder is first diagnosed, the thickening decreases with treatment, so decortication should not be considered until the patient has undergone treatment for at least 6 months. After this period of observation, decortication is rarely necessary.

TUBERCULOUS BRONCHOPLEURAL FISTULA

Tuberculous bronchopleural fistulas are uncommon today because most cases of tuberculosis are easily controlled with modern antituberculous chemotherapy. These fistulas are usually seen in patients with old, healed tuberculosis, and especially in patients with a previous therapeutic pneumothorax who were never treated with chemotherapy (88–90). When such patients develop a bronchopleural fistula, their sputum production usually increases in variable amounts, and superinfection of the pleural space by bacteria sometimes results (88). The diagnosis is suggested by the presence of an air–fluid level in the pleural space, particularly if the level fluctuates with serial chest radiographs (88). The fistula can be confirmed by the injection of methylene blue or a radiopaque dye into the pleural space.

A tuberculous bronchopleural fistula is dangerous to the patient for three reasons. First, the communication between the bronchus and the pleural space allows bacteria to gain access to the pleural space and to cause pleural infection with its attendant toxicity. Second, once the pleural space becomes superinfected, the patient is at risk for a fulminant pneumonia caused by entrance of the infected material from the pleural space into the remainder of the tracheobronchial tree. Third, the tuberculous bacilli in the pleural space are likely to become resistant to antituberculous drugs (88).

The initial treatment of tuberculous bronchopleural fistulas should be the institution of appropriate antituberculous chemotherapy in addition to the insertion of chest tubes into the lower part of the pleural cavity, because a tuberculous bronchopleural fistula does not heal spontaneously (88). Insertion of the chest tubes eliminates the danger of contamination of the contralateral lung by the infected pleural fluid and controls the systemic toxicity from the bacterial infection. Before a definitive surgical procedure is attempted, the patient should be given antituberculous chemotherapy for 90 to 120 days, or until sputum tests become negative for AFB.

Definitive surgical treatment consists of decortication, which sometimes must be combined with thoracoplasty because the underlying lung has usually been damaged by the tuberculosis to such an extent that it cannot expand to fill the pleural space (88, 90). This is a major operation and is dangerous to the patient with severely damaged lungs. In Jensen's series (89) of 15 patients with tuberculous bronchopleural fistulas, three were cured with conservative treatment, two were deemed unfit to undergo definitive surgical treatment and died within a year, and 10 were operated on with an operative mortality rate of 20%.

TUBERCULOUS EMPYEMA

Tuberculous empyema is a rare entity characterized by purulent pleural fluid that is loaded with tuberculous organisms on AFB stains (91). It usually develops in fibrous scar tissue resulting from pleurisy, artificial pneumothorax, or thoracoplasty (92). In one recent series of 12 patients from Italy, nine patients had received artificial pneumothorax therapy, one had received a thoracoplasty, and two had received inadequate antimycobacterial therapy (92). The mean duration between the therapy with the artificial pneumothoraces and the development of the empyema was over 40 years (92). Frequently, the underlying pleura is heavily calcified. The patient usually has a subacute or chronic illness characterized by fatigue, low-grade fever, and weight loss. Radiographically, there may be an obvious pleural effusion, but frequently the chest radiograph only shows pleural thickening. The chest CT scan usually demonstrates a thick, calcific pleural rind and rib thickening surrounding loculated pleural fluid. The diagnosis is established with diagnostic thoracentesis, which yields thick pus on which the AFB smear is markedly positive. Treatment is difficult, and decortication, extrapleural pneumonectomy, and thoracoplasty have all been recommended. All of these procedures have substantial morbidity and some mortality at least in part because of the compromised pulmonary status of the patient. Because intensive chemotherapy coupled with serial thoracentesis can be curative at times (93), this approach should be attempted initially. It is important to use a multiple (three or more) drug regimen and to employ agents at their maximal tolerated dosages, because these patients have a strong tendency to develop resistant organisms. This is probably because the antituberculous drugs frequently do not reach their normal levels in the pleural space owing to the thick, fibrous, and often calcified pleura (94).

The entity of bacterial empyema complicating collapse therapy for pulmonary tuberculosis, which is sometimes confused with tuberculous empyema, is discussed in Chapter 9.

ATYPICAL MYCOBACTERIA

Pleural effusions due to atypical mycobacteria are rare. Pleural effusions without parenchymal disease analogous to the postprimary pleural effusion with *Mycobacterium tuberculosis* do not occur. However, approximately 5% of patients with parenchymal disease due to either *M. kansasii* or *M. intracellulare* have an associated small pleural effusion, an incidence similar to that seen with parenchymal disease due to *M. tuberculosis* (95). About 15% of patients with parenchymal disease due to *M. intracellulare* have marked pleural thickening (>2 cm), as compared with fewer than 3% of patients with disease due to *M. tuberculosis* or *M. kansasii* (95).

If the cultures of the pleural fluid yield a nontuberculous mycobacterium, one must be cautious in attributing the pleural effusion to that organism. Gribetz et al. (96) reviewed the case records of 22 patients whose pleural fluid grew nontuberculous mycobacterium. In 16 of the patients, there was another explanation for the pleural effusion, and in only three did the nontuberculous mycobacterium appear to be responsible for the pleural effusion. All three patients had nontuberculous mycobacterial infection of other tissues. These authors concluded that nontuberculous mycobacteria isolated from pleural fluid should not be considered etiologic, unless there is evidence of the same organism infecting other tissues (96).

Before the AIDS epidemic, disseminated nontuberculous mycobacterial infections were very uncommon. However, disseminated disease due to *M. intracellulare* or *M. avium* (collectively referred to as the *Myobacterium avium* complex [MAC]) is an important cause of infection in patients with AIDS (97). Some autopsy studies have shown that more than 50% of patients who die with AIDS have disseminated disease due to MAC (97). Pleural effusions do occur in some patients with disseminated disease due to MAC (97), and pleural fluid cultures are sometimes positive for MAC. Nevertheless, it is unclear whether the atypical mycobacteria are responsible for the effusion (97). Overall, disease due to MAC accounts for at most only a small percentage of the pleural effusions in patients with AIDS.

REFERENCES

1. Moudgil H, Sridhar G, Leitch AG. Reactivation disease: the commonest form of tuberculous pleural effusion in Edinburgh, 1980–1991. *Respir Med* 1994;88:301–304.
2. Berger HW, Mejia E. Tuberculous pleurisy. *Chest* 1973;63:88–92.
3. Stead WW, Eichenholz A, Stauss H-K. Operative and pathologic findings in twenty-four patients with syndrome of idiopathic pleurisy with effusion, presumably tuberculous. *Am Rev Respir Dis* 1955;71:473–502.
4. Allen JC, Apicella MA. Experimental pleural effusion as a manifestation of delayed hypersensitivity to tuberculin PPD. *J Immunol* 1968;101:481–487.
5. Apicella MA, Allen JC. A physiologic differentiation between delayed and immediate hypersensitivity. *J Clin Invest* 1969;48:250–259.
6. Leibowitz S, Kennedy L, Lessof MH. The tuberculin reaction in the pleural cavity and its suppression by antilymphocyte serum. *Br J Exp Pathol* 1973;54:152–162.
7. Yamamoto S, Dunn CJ, Willoughby DA. Studies on delayed hypersensitivity pleural exudates in guinea pigs: II. The interrelationship of monocytic and lymphocytic cells with respect to migration activity. *Immunology* 1976;30:513–519.
8. Antony VB, Sahn SA, Antony AC, et al. Bacillus Calmette-Guerin–stimulated neutrophils release chemotaxins for monocytes in rabbit pleural space in vitro. *J Clin Invest* 1985;76:1514–1521.
9. Mohammed KA, Nasreen N, Ward MJ, et al. Mycobacterium-mediated chemokine expression in pleural mesothelial cells: role of C-C chemokines in tuberculous pleurisy. *J Infect Dis* 1998;178:1450–1456.
10. Widstrom O, Nilsson BS. Pleurisy induced by intrapleural BCG in immunized guinea pigs. *Eur J Respir Dis* 1982;63:425–434.
11. Widstrom O, Nilsson BS. Low in vitro response to PPD and PHA in lymphocytes from BCG-induced pleurisy in guinea pigs. *Eur J Respir Dis* 1982;63:435–441.

12. Bueno CE, Clemente G, Castro BC, et al. Cytologic and bacteriologic analysis of fluid and pleural biopsy specimens with Cope's needle. *Arch Intern Med* 1990;150:1190–1194.

13. Chan CH, Arnold M, Chan CY, et al. Clinical and pathological features of tuberculous pleural effusion and its long-term consequences. *Respiration* 1991;58: 171–175.

14. Fujiwara H, Tsuyuguchi I. Frequency of tuberculin-reactive T-lymphocytes in pleural fluid and blood from patients with tuberculous pleurisy. *Chest* 1986;89: 530–532.

15. Shimokata K, Kawachi H, Kishimoto H, et al. Local cellular immunity in tuberculous pleurisy. *Am Rev Respir Dis* 1982;128:822–824.

16. Ellner JJ. Pleural fluid and peripheral blood lymphocyte function in tuberculosis. *Ann Intern Med* 1978;89: 932–933.

17. Rossi GA, Balbi B, Manca F. Tuberculous pleural effusions: evidence for selective presence of PPD-specific T-lymphocytes at site of inflammation in the early phase of the infection. *Am Rev Respir Dis* 1987;136: 575–579.

18. Ellner JJ, Barnes PF, Wallis RS, et al. The immunology of tuberculous pleurisy. *Semin Respir Infect* 1988;3: 335–342.

19. Mehra V, Gong JH, Iyer D, et al. Immune response to recombinant mycobacterial proteins in patients with tuberculosis infection and disease. *J Infect Dis* 1996;174: 431–434.

20. Leckie WJH, Tothill P. Albumin turnover in pleural effusions. *Clin Sci* 1965;29:339–352.

21. Valdes L, Alvarez D, Valle JM, et al. The etiology of pleural effusions in an area with high incidence of tuberculosis. *Chest* 1996;109:158–162.

22. al-Qorain A, Larbi EB, al-Muhanna F, et al. Pattern of pleural effusion in Eastern Province of Saudi Arabia: a prospective study. *East Afr Med J* 1994;71:246–249.

23. Mehta JB, Dutt A, Harvill L, et al. Epidemiology of extrapulmonary tuberculosis. *Chest* 1991;99:1134–1138.

24. Frye MD, Pozsik CJ, Sahn SA. Tuberculous pleurisy is more common in AIDS than in non-AIDS patients with tuberculosis. *Chest* 1997;112:393–397.

25. Mlika-Cabanne N, Brauner M, Kamanfu G, et al. Radiographic abnormalities in tuberculosis and risk of coexisting human immunodeficiency virus infection. *Am J Respir Crit Care Med* 1995;152:794–799.

26. Saks AM, Posner R. Tuberculosis in HIV positive patients in South Africa: a comparative radiological study with HIV negative patients. *Clin Radiol* 1992;46: 387–390.

27. Awil PO, Bowlin SJ, Daniel TM. Radiology of pulmonary tuberculosis and human immunodeficiency virus infection in Gulu, Uganda. *Eur Respir J* 1997;10: 615–618.

28. Pozniak AL, MacLeod GA, Ndlovu D, et al. Clinical and chest radiographic features of tuberculosis associated with human immunodeficiency virus in Zimbabwe. *Am J Respir Crit Care Med* 1995;152:1558–1561.

29. Levine H, Szanto PB, Cugell DW. Tuberculous pleurisy: an acute illness. *Arch Intern Med* 1968;122:329–332.

30. Richter C, Perenboom R, Mtoni I, et al. Clinical features of HIV-seropositive and HIV-seronegative patients with tuberculous pleural effusion in Dar es Salaam, Tanzania. *Chest* 1994;106:1471–1475.

31. Aho K, Brander E, Patiala J. Studies for primary drug resistance in tuberculous pleurisy. *Scand J Respir Dis* 1968; 63[Suppl]:111–114.

32. Epstein DM, Kline LR, Albelda SM, et al. Tuberculous pleural effusions. *Chest* 1987;91:106–109.

33. Valdes L, Alvarez D, San Jose E, et al. Tuberculous pleurisy: a study of 254 patients. *Arch Intern Med* 1998;158:2017–2021.

34. Maher GG, Berger HW. Massive pleural effusion: malignant and non-malignant causes in 46 patients. *Am Rev Respir Dis* 1972;105:458–460.

35. Heyderman RS, Makunike R, Muza T, et al. Pleural tuberculosis in Harare, Zimbabwe: the relationship between human immunodeficiency virus, CD4 lymphocyte count, granuloma formation and disseminated disease. *Trop Med Int Health* 1998;3:14–20.

36. Patiala J. Initial tuberculous pleuritis in the Finnish Armed Forces in 1939–1945 with special reference to eventual post pleuritic tuberculosis. *Acta Tuberc Scand* 1954;36[Suppl]:1–57.

37. Roper WH, Waring JJ. Primary serofibrinous pleural effusion in military personnel. *Am Rev Respir Dis* 1955;71:616–634.

38. Patiala J, Mattila M. Effect of chemotherapy of exudative tuberculous pleurisy on the incidence of post pleuritic tuberculosis. *Acta Tuberc Scand* 1964;44:290–296.

39. Light RW. Establishing the diagnosis of tuberculous pleuritis. *Arch Intern Med* 1998;158:1967–1968.

40. Yilmaz MU, Kumcuoglu Z, Utkaner G, et al. Computed tomography findings of tuberculous pleurisy. *Int J Tuberc Lung Dis* 1998;2:164–167.

41. Yam LT. Diagnostic significance of lymphocytes in pleural effusions. *Ann Intern Med* 1967;66:972–982.

42. Light RW, Erozan YS, Ball WC. Cells in pleural fluid: their value in differential diagnosis. *Arch Intern Med* 1973;132:854–860.

43. De Oliveira HG, Rossatto ER, Prolla JC. Pleural fluid adenosine deaminase and lymphocyte proportion: clinical usefulness in the diagnosis of tuberculosis. *Cytopathology* 1994;5:27–32.

44. Spriggs AI, Boddington MM. *The cytology of effusions,* 2nd ed. New York: Grune & Stratton, 1968.

45. Hurwitz S, Leiman G, Shapiro C. Mesothelial cells in pleural fluid: TB or not TB? *S Afr Med J* 1980;57: 937–939.

46. Jones D, Lieb T, Narita M, et al. Mesothelial cells in tuberculous pleural effusions of HIV-infected patients. *Chest* 2000;117:289–291.

47. Ocana I, Martinez-Vazquez JM, Segura RM, et al. Adenosine deaminase in pleural fluids: test for diagnosis of tuberculous pleural effusion. *Chest* 1983;84: 51–53.

48. Valdes L, San Jose E, Alvarez D, et al. Diagnosis of tuberculous pleurisy using the biologic parameters adenosine deaminase, lysozyme, and interferon gamma. *Chest* 1993;103:458–465.

49. Burgess LJ, Maritz FJ, Le Roux I, et al. Use of adenosine deaminase as a diagnostic tool for tuberculous pleurisy. *Thorax* 1995;50:672–674.

50. Valdes L, Alvarez D, San Jose E, et al. Value of adenosine deaminase in the diagnosis of tuberculous pleural effusions in young patients in a region of high prevalence of tuberculosis. *Thorax* 1995;50:600–603.

51. Riantawan P, Chaowalit P, Wongsangiem M, et al. Diagnostic value of pleural fluid adenosine deaminase in

tuberculous pleuritis with reference to HIV coinfection and a Bayesian analysis. *Chest* 1999;116:97–103.

52. Burgess LJ, Maritz FJ, Le Roux I, et al. Combined use of pleural adenosine deaminase with lymphocyte/neutrophil ratio. Increased specificity for the diagnosis of tuberculous pleuritis. *Chest* 1996;109: 414–419.

53. Ferrer JS, Munoz XG, Orriols RM, et al. Evolution of idiopathic pleural effusion. A prospective, long-term follow-up study. *Chest* 1996;109:1508–1513.

54. Perez-Rodriguez E, Castro DJ. The use of ADA and ADA isoenzymes in the diagnosis of tuberculous pleuritis. *Curr Opin* 2000;6:259–266.

55. Valdes L, San Jose E, Alvarez D, et al. Adenosine deaminase (ADA) isoenzyme analysis in pleural effusions: diagnostic role, and relevance to the origin of increased ADA in tuberculous pleurisy. *Eur Respir J* 1996;9:747–751.

56. Sadikot RT, Rogers JT, Cheng D-S, et al. Pleural fluid characteristics of patients with symptomatic pleural effusion post coronary artery bypass surgery. *Arch Intern Med* 2000;160:2665–2668.

57. Meysman M, Schoors DF, Noppen M, et al. Tuberculous pleural effusion following coronary artery bypass graft. *Acta Clin Belg* 1995;50:305–309.

58. Lee YC, Rogers JT, Rodriguez RM, et al. Adenosine deaminase (ADA) levels in non-tuberculous lymphocytic pleural effusions. *Chest* 2000;118:1315.

59. Shimokata K, Saka H, Murate T, et al. Cytokine content in pleural effusion. *Chest* 1991;99:1103–1107.

60. Ribera E, Ocana I, Martinez-Vazquez JM, et al. High level of interferon gamma in tuberculous pleural effusion. *Chest* 1988;93:308–311.

61. Barnes PF, Mistry SD, Cooper CL, et al. Compartmentalization of a CD4+ T lymphocyte subpopulation in tuberculous pleuritis. *J Immunol* 1989;142:1114–1119.

62. Villena V, Lopez-Encuentra A, Echave-Sustaeta J, et al. Interferon-gamma in 388 immunocompromised and immunocompetent patients for diagnosing pleural tuberculosis. *Eur Respir J* 1996;9:2635–2639.

63. Querol JM, Minguez J, Garcia-Sanchez E, et al. Rapid diagnosis of pleural tuberculosis by polymerase chain reaction. *Am J Respir Crit Care Med* 1995;152; 1977–1981.

64. Villena V, Rebollo MJ, Aguado JM, et al. Polymerase chain reaction for the diagnosis of pleural tuberculosis in immunocompromised and immunocompetent patients. *Clin Infect Dis* 1998;26:212–214.

65. Levy H, Wayne LG, Anderson BE, et al. Antimycobacterial antibody levels in pleural fluid reflect passive diffusion from serum. *Chest* 1990;97: 1144–1147.

66. Barber LM, Mazzadi L, Deakins DD, et al. Glucose level in pleural fluid as a diagnostic aid. *Dis Chest* 1957;31:680–681.

67. Holton K. Diagnostic value of some biochemical pleural fluid examinations. *Scand J Respir Dis* 1968;63(Suppl):121–125.

68. Light RW, MacGregor MI, Ball WC Jr, et al. Diagnostic significance of pleural fluid pH and Pco_2. *Chest* 1973;64:591–596.

69. Chavalittamrong B, Angsusingha K, Tuchinda M, et al. Diagnostic significance of pH, lactic acid dehydrogenase, lactate and glucose in pleural fluid. *Respiration* 1979;38:112–120.

70. Good JT Jr, Taryle DA, Maulitz RM, et al. The diagnostic value of pleural fluid pH. *Chest* 1980;78:55–59.

71. Fontan Bueso J, Verea Hernando H, Garcia-Buela JP, et al. Diagnostic value of simultaneous determination of pleural adenosine deaminase and pleural lysozyme/serum lysozyme ratio in pleural effusion. *Chest* 1988;93:303–307.

72. Verea Hernando HR, Masa Jimenez JF, Dominguez Juncal L, et al. Meaning and diagnostic value of determining the lysozyme level of pleural fluid. *Chest* 1987;91: 342–345.

73. Maartens G, Bateman ED. Tuberculous pleural effusions: increased culture yield with bedside inoculation of pleural fluid and poor diagnostic value of adenosine deaminase. *Thorax* 1991;46:96–99.

74. Schmid GP, Catino D, Suffin SC, et al. Granulomatous pleuritis caused by *Francisella tularensis:* possible confusion with tuberculous pleuritis. *Am Rev Respir Dis* 1983;128:314–316.

75. Light RW. Closed needle biopsy of the pleura is a valuable diagnostic procedure. Con closed needle biopsy. *J Bronchol* 1998;5:332–336.

76. Bass JB Jr, Farer LS, Hopewell PC, et al. Treatment of tuberculosis and tuberculosis infection in adults and children. *Am J Respir Crit Care Med* 1994;149: 1359–1374.

77. Canete C, Galarza I, Granados A, et al. Tuberculous pleural effusion: experience with six months of treatment with isoniazid and rifampicin. *Thorax* 1994;49: 1160–1161.

78. Dutt AK, Moers D, Stead WW. Tuberculous pleural effusion: 6-month therapy with isoniazid and rifampin. *Am Rev Respir Dis* 1992;145:1429–1432.

79. Falk A, Stead WW. US Veterans Administration Armed Forces cooperative studies of tuberculosis: V. Antimicrobial theory in treatment of primary tuberculous pleurisy with effusion: the effect upon the incidence of subsequent tuberculous relapse. *Am Rev Tuberc Pulmon Dis* 1956;74:897–902.

80. Tani P, Poppius H, Makipaja J. Cortisone therapy for exudative tuberculous pleurisy in the light of the follow-up study. *Acta Tuberc Scand* 1964;44:303–309.

81. Galarza I, Canete C, Granados A, et al. Randomised trial of corticosteroids in the treatment of tuberculous pleurisy. *Thorax* 1995;50:1305–1307.

82. Wyser C, Walzl G, Smedema JP, et al. Corticosteroids in the treatment of tuberculous pleurisy. A double-blind, placebo-controlled, randomized study. *Chest* 1996;110:333–338.

83. Barbas CSV, Cukier A, de Varvalho CRR, et al. The relationship between pleural fluid findings and the development of pleural thickening in patients with pleural tuberculosis. *Chest* 1991;100:1264–1267.

84. Al-Majed SA. Study of paradoxical response to chemotherapy in tuberculous pleural effusion. *Resp Med* 1996;90:211–214.

85. Hiraoka K, Nagata N, Kawajiri T, et al. Paradoxical pleural response to antituberculous chemotherapy and isoniazid-induced lupus. Review and report of two cases. *Respiration* 1998;65:152–155.

86. Lee CH, Wang WJ, Lan RS, et al. Corticosteroids in the treatment of tuberculous pleurisy: a double-blind, placebo-controlled, randomized study. *Chest* 1988;94:1256-1259.

87. Large SE, Levick RK. Aspiration in the treatment

of primary tuberculous pleural effusion. *Br Med J* 1958;1:1512–1514.

88. Johnson TM, McCann W, Davey WN. Tuberculous bronchopleural fistula. *Am Rev Respir Dis* 1973;107: 30–41.

89. Jenssen AD. Chronic calcified pleural empyema. *Scand J Respir Dis* 1969;50:19–27.

90. Mouroux J, Maalouf J, Padovani B, et al. Surgical management of pleuropulmonary tuberculosis. *J Thorac Cardiovasc Surg* 1996;111:662–670.

91. Sahn SA, Iseman MD. Tuberculous empyema. *Semin Respir Infect* 1999;14:82–87.

92. Mancini P, Mazzei L, Zarzana A, et al. Post-tuberculosis chronic empyema of the "forty years after." *Eur Rev Med Pharmacol Sci* 1998;2:25–29.

93. Neihart RE, Hof DG. Successful nonsurgical treatment of tuberculous empyema in an irreducible pleural space. *Chest* 1985;88:792–794.

94. Iseman MD, Madsen LA. Chronic tuberculous empyema with bronchopleural fistula resulting in treatment failure and progressive drug resistance. *Chest* 1991;100: 124–127.

95. Christensen EE, Dietz GW, Ahn CH, et al. Initial roentgenographic manifestations of pulmonary *Mycobacterium tuberculosis, M. kansasii,* and *M. intracellularis* infections. *Chest* 1981;80:132–136.

96. Gribetz AR, Damsker B, Marchevsky A, et al. Nontuberculous mycobacteria in pleural fluid: assessment of clinical significance. *Chest* 1985;87:495–498.

97. Aronchick JM, Miller WT. Disseminated nontuberculous mycobacterial infections in immunosuppressed patients. *Semin Roentgenol* 1993;8:150–157.

11

Pleural Effusion Secondary to Fungal Infections, Actinomycosis, and Nocardiosis

In this chapter, pleural disease resulting from fungal infections is discussed. Although fungal diseases account for less than 1% of all pleural effusions, it is important to identify correctly patients with fungal disease of the pleura because effective treatment is available. Actinomycosis and nocardiosis are also included in this chapter because they produce a chronic disease similar to that caused by the fungi even though they actually are bacteria.

ASPERGILLOSIS

Occasionally, the pleural space becomes infected with the *Aspergillus* species of fungus. The usual infecting organism is *Aspergillus fumigatus* (1), but other species such as *Aspergillus niger* may also be responsible (2). Pleural aspergillosis is uncommon, but 13 cases were observed at one institution during a recent 5-year period (3).

Clinical Manifestations

Pleural aspergillosis usually occurs in one of two settings. Most commonly, it occurs in patients who were treated in the past with artificial pneumothorax therapy for tuberculosis (2–4). Such patients have signs and symptoms of a chronic infection, including weight loss, malaise, a low-grade fever, and a chronic, productive cough (1). The chest radiograph reveals increasing degrees of pleural thickening and usually an air–fluid level in the pleural space indicating the presence of a bronchopleural fistula (1). Fungus balls,

although uncommon, may be evident radiographically either in the lungs or the pleural space (1, 5).

The second situation in which pleural aspergillosis occurs is postoperatively after lobectomy or pneumonectomy for lung cancer or tuberculosis (3, 4). A bronchopleural fistula is almost invariably present. The clinical picture is similar to that with a pleural bacterial infection after lung resection (see Chapter 9). On rare occasions, the pleural fluid becomes infected with aspergillus in the immunosuppressed patient with systemic aspergillosis (6). One report cited two patients with pleural effusion complicating allergic bronchopulmonary aspergillosis (7), but the relationship between the pleural effusion and the allergic aspergillosis was not convincing.

Diagnosis

The diagnosis of pleural aspergillosis should be suspected in any patient with a history of artificial pneumothorax therapy for tuberculosis who has a chronic pleural infection, particularly when a bronchopleural fistula is present. Similarly, the diagnosis should be suspected in any patient with a pleural infection after lung resection. The diagnosis is confirmed by the demonstration of aspergillus on fungal cultures of the pleural fluid. The presence of brown clumps containing fungal hyphae in the pleural fluid suggests the diagnosis (4). Patients with pleural aspergillosis almost always have positive precipitin blood tests for antibodies against aspergillus (1, 4). Aspergillus antigens can also be demonstrated in the pleural fluid by radioimmunoassay (8). The presence of calcium oxalate crystals in the pleural fluid suggests an infection due to *A. niger* (2). The presence of the black-pigmented spores of *A. niger* can impart a black color to the pleural fluid (9).

Treatment

The optimal treatment for pleural aspergillosis is early excision of the involved pleura with resection of the upper lobe or the entire ipsilateral lung, if necessary (1). When this definitive surgical treatment is undertaken, itraconazole or amphotericin B should be administered systemically before and after the operation because the incidence of postoperative pleural infection with aspergillus is high if systemic antifungal drugs are not administered (1, 10). The reason for performing this extensive operation is that the infection is likely to invade and destroy the underlying lung. The longer the surgical procedure is postponed, the more severe the damage to the underlying lung and the more debilitated the patient becomes (1). The bronchopleural fistulas are often difficult to manage and frequently require muscle transpositions or omentoplasty (3). Even if there is no bronchopleural fistula, muscle transpositions are sometimes necessary because the pleural space cannot be obliterated with just the damaged underlying lung (3).

Some patients with pleural aspergillosis are too debilitated to undergo a surgical procedure, or their pleural aspergillosis is a complication of pulmonary resection. In such patients, a chest tube should be inserted, and the pleural space should be irrigated daily with amphotericin B or nystatin (4, 5, 11). The usual dose of amphotericin B is 25 mg, and the usual dose of nystatin is 75,000 U (5). After instillation of the antifungal agents, the chest tube is clamped for an hour. An open-drainage procedure (see Chapter 9) can be performed for the patient's comfort (5). Although this treatment takes many months, it is successful in most patients (4, 5, 11).

BLASTOMYCOSIS

Infection with *Blastomyces dermatitidis* frequently is associated with pleural disease. In one series of 118 patients with pulmonary blastomycosis, four (3%) had pleural effusions (12). In a more recent study of 63 cases with proven pulmonary blastomycosis, 13 of the patients (21%) had a pleural effusion. The effusions in this series were small and caused only mild to moderate blunting of the costophrenic sulci (13). However, an occasional patient with pleural blastomycosis has an effusion that occupies more than 50% of a hemithorax (14).

Patients with pleural blastomycosis have signs and symptoms similar to those with tuberculous pleuritis (see Chapter 10). In addition to the pleural effusion, there may be an associated parenchymal infiltrate (15, 16). With pleural blastomycosis, the pleural fluid is an exudate containing predominantly lymphocytes or polymorphonuclear leukocytes (14–16). The pleural fluid glucose level is normal, and the LDH is usually not higher than the upper limits of normal for serum (14). Microscopic examination of the pleural fluid at times reveals the budding yeasts typical of *B. dermatitidis* (14). Pleural biopsy may reveal noncaseating granulomas (15–16). Therefore, one should consider the diagnosis of blastomycosis in patients with a clinical picture suggestive of tuberculous pleuritis, and one should obtain fungal cultures of the pleural fluid in all such patients. The complement-fixation test is the most widely used test for the serologic diagnosis of blastomycosis; however, its clinical value is limited because fewer than 25% of culture-proven cases are detected using this method (17). There is no commercially available skin test for blastomycosis.

Patients with pleural blastomycosis should be treated with itraconazole 400 mg qd for 6 months, ketoconazole 400 to 800 mg per day for 6 months, or amphotericin B with a total dose of 2 g. It appears that the treatment of choice is itraconazole (10), which cures virtually all immunocompetent individuals with pulmonary blastomycosis. Amphotericin B remains the drug of choice for all forms of blastomycosis in the immunosuppressed host (10).

COCCIDIOIDOMYCOSIS

Coccidioides immitis is an infectious fungus endemic to the southwestern United States, particularly the San Joaquin Valley in California. The disease is acquired by inhaling the light, fluffy, and infectious arthrospores produced by the mycelial form growing in appropriate soil. Once inhaled, the arthrospores develop into the yeast form that produces disease in humans. Pleural disease of two types occurs in association with coccidioidomycosis (18). The first type is associated with the primary benign infection and may or may not have concomitant parenchymal involvement. The second type occurs when a coccidioidal cavity adjacent to the pleura ruptures to produce a hydropneumothorax with a bronchopleural fistula.

Primary Infection

The pleura is frequently involved in primary infections with *Coccidioides immitis*. As many as 70% of patients have pleuritic chest pain, and about 20% have blunting of the costophrenic angles radiologically (19). Approximately 7% of all symptomatic patients with primary coccidioidomycosis have pleural effusions (19). Patients with pleural effusions secondary to coccidioidomycosis are almost always febrile, and over 80% have pleuritic chest pain (19). Nearly 50% of patients have either erythema nodosum or erythema multiforme (19). The chest radiograph reveals parenchymal infiltrates in addition to the pleural effusion in about 50% of patients. The pleural effusion varies in size, but it often occupies more than 50% of the hemithorax (19, 20). In one series of 28 patients, all pleural effusions were unilateral (19).

Pleural fluid analysis reveals an exudate that usually contains predominantly small lymphocytes (19). Although nearly 50% of patients have peripheral eosinophilia, pleural fluid eosinophilia is uncommon and occurred in only one of 15 patients in one series (19). The pleural fluid glucose level is almost always above 60 mg per dL (19). The pleural fluid cultures are positive for *Coccidioides immitis* in about 20% of patients, but cultures of pleural biopsy specimens are positive in almost all patients (19). In one series, eight of eight pleural biopsy cultures were positive, and cocci spherules were identified in six of eight specimens (19). The pleural biopsy may

reveal caseating or noncaseating granulomas (19, 20). The cocci skin tests are usually positive, and the mean complement fixation (CF) titer 6 weeks after the onset of symptoms is 1:32 (19).

Most patients with primary coccidioidomycosis and pleural effusion require no systemic antifungal therapy (19). In a series of 28 such patients, 23 (82%) recovered completely without specific therapy. Two patients with disseminated disease died within a short period, whereas the other three patients had minor complications and were treated with amphotericin B. Even though the CF titers are high in patients with pleural coccidioidomycosis (19) and high (>1:16) CF titers are used by some as an indication of dissemination (21), patients with pleural coccidioidomycosis and high CF titers should be treated only if their skin tests are negative or if other evidence of dissemination exists. The treatment of choice is either itraconazole or amphotericin B (10).

Rupture of Coccidioidal Cavity

The second situation in which pleural disease occurs with coccidioidomycosis is when a coccidioidal cavity adjacent to the pleura ruptures into the pleural space to produce a bronchopleural fistula and a hydropneumothorax. Hydropneumothoraces develop in 1% to 5% of patients with chronic cavitary coccidioidomycosis and occasionally occur without a prior cavitation (18). Many patients who experience rupture of a coccidioidal cavity have no history of coccidioidomycosis (22). Accordingly, in endemic areas, all patients with spontaneous hydropneumothoraces should be evaluated for the possibility of coccidioidomycosis.

When a coccidioidal cavity ruptures into the pleural space, the patient usually becomes acutely ill, with systemic signs of toxicity. The pleural fluid cultures are usually positive for *Coccidioides immitis* and the CF tests are almost always positive (22). A patient with a hydropneumothorax should have a chest tube inserted immediately to drain the air and the fluid from the pleural space. They should also be given itraconazole or amphotericin B systemically. The majority require additional surgery such as a partial lobectomy for control of the cavity. In one series of

23 patients, all but two required surgical treatment in addition to the tube thoracostomy (22). In view of this factor, it is recommended that patients who have a persistent bronchopleural fistula for more than 7 days be subjected to surgery.

CRYPTOCOCCOSIS

Cryptococcus neoformans, a fungus distributed worldwide, lives in soil, particularly that contaminated by pigeon excreta. On rare occasions, infection with *C. neoformans* produces a pleural effusion. Until 1980, only 30 cryptococcal pleural effusions had been reported (23). With the advent of the acquired immunodeficiency syndrome (AIDS) epidemic, pleural effusions secondary to cryptococcosis have become much more frequent. In one series of 12 patients with pulmonary cryptococcal involvement proven by culture, three (25%) had a pleural effusion (24). In another series of 75 patients with AIDS and pleural effusion from Paris, four (5%) had pleural cryptococcosis (25). Pleural cryptococcosis appears to result from an extension of a primary subpleural cryptococcal nodule into the pleural space (26).

In patients with pleural cryptococcosis, the disease is localized to the hemithorax in about 50% and is disseminated in the remaining 50% (23). Over half the patients have serious underlying disease, most commonly leukemia, lymphoma, or AIDS (23, 27). In 27 of the 30 cases reported up to 1980, the pleural effusion was unilateral (23) and most of the effusions associated with AIDS are also unilateral. The size of the pleural effusion ranges from massive to minimal (23). Most patients also have an accompanying parenchymal lesion in the form of a nodule, a mass, or an interstitial infiltrate (23). The pleural fluid is an exudate, usually with a predominance of small lymphocytes. One case report cited an effusion in which the pleural fluid contained 15% eosinophils (28). Cultures of the pleural fluid were positive in 11 of 26 patients in the 1980 series (23). In the remaining patients, the diagnosis was made by histologic study or by culture of lung tissue obtained at operation or autopsy (23). Patients with cryptococcal pleural effusion have high titers of cryptococcal antigen in their pleural fluid and serum (23).

It is not clear whether treatment with systemic antifungal agents is necessary for all patients with pleural cryptococcosis. Several patients have recovered without any specific therapy (23, 29, 30). Therefore, it is recommended that blood and cerebral spinal fluid be studied for cryptococcal antigen. If cryptococcal antigen is detected in either of these fluids, amphotericin B or 5-fluorocytosine, or both, should be administered. Immunosuppressed patients, such as those with AIDS, leukemia, lymphoma, diabetes mellitus, or sarcoidosis, and patients receiving corticosteroids or immunosuppressant agents should also be treated. If none of the foregoing conditions are met, it is recommended that the patient be treated with 400 mg per day of fluconazole for 6 months. On rare occasions in immunosuppressed individuals, the pleural infection is so overwhelming that tube thoracostomy is indicated (31).

HISTOPLASMOSIS

Histoplasma capsulatum is a fungus that lives in the mycelial form in soil and is distributed throughout the temperate zones of the world but is most heavily endemic in the central United States (32). Infection with *H. capsulatum* only rarely produces pleural effusions. Although it has been estimated that 500,000 persons are infected annually in the United States (32), fewer than 20 pleural effusions secondary to histoplasmosis have been reported. In a review of the radiographic manifestations of pulmonary histoplasmosis, only one patient of 259 with abnormal chest radiographs had a pleural effusion (33).

Patients with pleural effusions secondary to histoplasmosis usually have a subacute illness characterized by a low-grade fever and pleuritic chest pain. The chest radiograph usually reveals an infiltrate or a subpleural nodule in addition to the pleural effusion (34–37). Pleural fluid analysis reveals an exudate containing predominantly lymphocytes. In two of the reported cases (34, 36), pleural fluid eosinophilia was present. The pleural biopsy may reveal noncaseating granulomas. The diagnosis is made by culturing *H. capsulatum* from the pleural fluid, sputum, or biopsy material by routine fungal cultures or by demonstrating the organism in biopsy material with appropriate stains. A presumptive diagnosis can sometimes be established by demonstrating a high histoplasmosis CF titer or an H band on counterimmunoelectrophoresis. It appears that treatment is not necessary for pleural effusions secondary to histoplasmosis (35, 37, 38). The pleural effusion usually resolves spontaneously over several weeks (34, 35, 39). On rare occasions, however, a patient develops a fibrosing pleuritis for which a decortication should be considered if the patient is symptomatic (35, 40).

An isolated pleural effusion due to infection with *H. capsulatum* has been reported in a patient with AIDS (41). This particular patient presented with fever and bilateral small pleural effusions. Thoracentesis revealed an exudate, and many organisms typical of *H. capsulatum* were seen on the Wright-Giemsa stain of the pleural fluid. This patient appeared to respond to therapy with amphotericin B (41). Pleural effusions can also occur in patients with AIDS and disseminated histoplasmosis (42), but pleural involvement is not a prominent part of the disease picture.

On rare occasions, patients with parenchymal histoplastmosis may develop a bronchopleural fistula with the subsequent development of a loculated fungal empyema (43). Such patients should be treated with drainage and decortication.

ACTINOMYCOSIS

Actinomyces israelii, an anaerobic or microaerophilic gram-positive bacterium, is a normal inhabitant of the mouth and oropharynx. Although this organism and *Nocardia asteroides* are actually bacteria, they are usually grouped with fungi because they cause chronic illness.

Clinical Manifestations

Actinomycosis is characterized by the formation of abscesses and multiple sinus tracts (44). The infection arises from endogenous sources such as infected gums, infected tonsils, or carious teeth (44). The pleura is involved in over 50% of patients with thoracic actinomycosis. In one series of 15 cases of this disorder, six patients had pleural effusions, and an additional six patients had marked pleural thickening (45). The pleura is particularly likely to be thickened in areas where parenchymal actinomycosis has extended through the chest wall to produce a chest wall abscess or a draining sinus. In a more recent series using computed tomography (CT) scans, pleural effusions were present in five of eight patients (62.5%) with actinomycosis, although there was only enough pleural fluid for thoracentesis in three (46). Pleural thickening was demonstrated with CT scans in all eight of the patients in this latter series (46).

The pleural fluid with actinomycosis may be either frank pus with predominantly polymorphonuclear leukocytes (47) or serous fluid with predominantly lymphocytes (48). I have seen a patient with thoracic actinomycosis in which the associated pleural effusion was serous and contained more than 50% eosinophils.

Diagnosis

The diagnosis of thoracic actinomycosis should be suspected in any patient with a chronic infiltrative pulmonary disease, particularly when the parenchymal disease crosses lung fissures. The presence of chest wall abscesses or draining sinus tracts suggests the diagnosis, as do bone changes consisting of periosteal proliferation or bone destruction (45). Thoracic actinomycosis sometimes becomes disseminated and produces peripheral abscesses in the skin, subcutaneous tissues, or muscles (49). The diagnosis is suggested by the presence of sulfur granules in the draining exudate or the pleural fluid. These granules are 1 to 2 mm in diameter and consist of clumps of thin bacterial filaments that possess peripheral radiations with or without clubbing at their ends. Sulfur granules may be associated with cutaneous nocardiosis, but their presence in viscera only occurs in actinomycosis.

Gram's stains of the exudate should be carefully examined for the presence of the slender, gram-positive, long-branching filaments characteristic of actinomycosis (49). The definitive diagnosis is established with the demonstration of *Actinomyces israelii* by anaerobic cultures. The diagnosis of thoracic actinomycosis cannot be established from cultures of expectorated sputum or bronchoscopic washings because *A. israelii* can frequently be cultured from such specimens in the absence of invasive disease. Bacterial culture of the pleural fluid frequently reveals organisms in addition to *A. israelii* (47, 49). The organism most commonly isolated is *Actinobacillus actinomycetemcomitans,* a gram-negative aerobic coccobacillus (49). It has been suggested that the aerobic actinobacillus reduces the oxygen level in the lesion to facilitate the growth of *Actinomyces israelii* (49).

Treatment

The cornerstone of treatment of actinomycosis is the administration of high doses of antibiotics for prolonged periods. Penicillin is the antibiotic of choice, and a dose of 10 million units per day for 4 to 6 weeks is recommended, followed by 12 to 18 months of therapy with oral penicillin phenoxymethyl potassium (49). Tetracycline, erythromycin, lincomycin, and clindamycin have been used successfully in the treatment of patients with actinomycosis and a history of penicillin hypersensitivity. The management of the pleural effusion in patients with actinomycosis is similar to that of patients with any other type of bacterial pneumonia (see Chapter 9). If the pleural fluid is serous and contains predominantly lymphocytes or eosinophils, a tube thoracostomy procedure is not necessary. Alternately, if the pleural fluid is frank pus, tube thoracostomy should be performed (50). Decortication is sometimes necessary for resolution of the process (47).

NOCARDIOSIS

Nocardia asteroides is an aerobic, gram-positive, filamentous bacterium that has a worldwide distribution and can be cultured from the soil (51).

Clinical Manifestations

The disease produced by this organism is similar to actinomycosis, but there is less abscess and sinus tract formation and more hematogenous dissemination with nocardiosis (44). Nocardiosis also has a greater propensity to occur in patients with AIDS and other immunosuppressed patients than does actinomycosis. Because most patients who develop nocardiosis are immunosuppressed (52), the incidence of nocardiosis is increasing because there are more immunosuppressed patients due to AIDS, organ transplantation, and chemotherapy. The lung is involved in about 75% of patients with nocardiosis (53), and as many as 50% of patients with pulmonary nocardiosis have a pleural effusion (52, 54, 55). Patients with pleural effusions secondary to nocardiosis usually have associated parenchymal infiltrates (52, 54, 56). The pleural fluid is an exudate, which can range from serous fluid to frank pus. Pleural fluid cultures may or may not be positive for *N. asteroides.*

Diagnosis

The diagnosis of nocardiosis should be suspected in patients with subacute or chronic pulmonary infiltrates and pleural effusion, particularly if the patient is immunosuppressed. Support for the diagnosis is obtained from a Gram stain of sputum, bronchoscopic washings, or pleural fluid revealing the typical gram-positive, branching, filamentous bacteria or from an acid-fast stain revealing variably acid-fast, filamentous bacteria (51). The definitive diagnosis is made by the demonstration of *N. asteroides* with aerobic bacterial cultures of the sputum, bronchoscopic washings, or pleural fluid. Because *N. asteroides* is a slow-growing organism, when nocardiosis is suspected, the bacterial cultures must be flagged so that they can be maintained for at least 2 weeks (56). Not all patients with positive sputum cultures for *N. asteroides* have nocardiosis. In a series of 20 patients with positive sputum cultures for *N. asteroides,* nine of the patients (45%) did not have radiographic abnormalities (57).

Treatment

The cornerstone of treatment for nocardiosis is the administration of sulfonamides. Sulfamethoxazole (1 g t.i.d.), sulfisoxazole (1 to 2 g q.i.d.), or sulfadiazine (6 to 12 g qd) are all efficacious. The medications are continued for at least 6 weeks after the disease is completely cleared, and lifelong therapy has been recommended by some (53). The recommended management of the pleural effusion with nocardiosis is the same as the management of the pleural effusion with actinomycosis (see the previous section of this chapter on actinomycosis).

REFERENCES

1. Hillerdal G. Pulmonary aspergillus infection invading the pleura. *Thorax* 1981;36:745–751.
2. Reyes CV, Kathuria S, MacGlashan A. Diagnostic value of calcium oxalate crystals in respiratory and pleural fluid cytology: a case report. *Acta Cytol* 1979;23:65–68.
3. Wex P, Utta E, Drozdz W. Surgical treatment of pulmonary and pleuro-pulmonary *Aspergillus* disease. *Thorac Cardiovasc Surg* 1993;41:64–70.
4. Krakowka P, Rowinska E, Halweg H. Infection of the pleura by *Aspergillus fumigatus*. *Thorax* 1970;25:245–253.
5. Colp CR, Cook WA. Successful treatment of pleural aspergillosis and bronchopleural fistula. *Chest* 1975;68:96–98.
6. Walsh TJ, Bulkley BH. *Aspergillus* pericarditis: clinical and pathologic features in the immunocompromised patient. *Cancer* 1982;49:48–54.
7. Murphy D, Lane DJ. Pleural effusion in allergic bronchopulmonary aspergillosis: two case reports. *Br J Dis Chest* 1981;75:91–95.
8. Weiner MH. Antigenemia detected by radioimmunoassay in systemic aspergillosis. *Ann Intern Med* 1980;92:793–796.
9. Metzger JB, Garagusi VF, Kerwin DM. Pulmonary oxalosis caused by *Aspergillus niger*. *Am Rev Respir Dis* 1984;129:501–502.
10. Klein NC, Cunha BA. New antifungal drugs for pulmonary mycoses. *Chest* 1996;110:525–532.
11. Shirakusa T, Ueda H, Saito T, et al. Surgical treatment of pulmonary aspergilloma and *Aspergillus* empyema. *Ann Thorac Surg* 1989;48:779–782.
12. Blastomycosis Cooperative Study of the Veterans Administration. Blastomycosis. A review of 198 collected cases in Veterans Administration hospitals. *Am Rev Respir Dis* 1964;89:659–672.
13. Sheflin JR, Campbell JA, Thompson GP. Pulmonary blastomycosis: findings on chest radiographs in 63 patients. *AJR Am J Roentgenol* 1990;154:1177–1180.
14. Faila PJ, Cerise FP, Karam GH, et al. Blastomycosis: pulmonary and pleural manifestations. *South Med J* 1995;88:405–410.
15. Kinasewitz GT, Penn RL, George RB. The spectrum and significance of pleural disease in blastomycosis. *Chest* 1984;86:580–584.
16. Nelson O, Light RW. Granulomatous pleuritis secondary to blastomycosis. *Chest* 1977;71:433–434.
17. Sarosi GA, Armstrong D, Davies SF, et al. Laboratory diagnosis of mycotic and specific fungal infections. *Am Rev Respir Dis* 1985;132:1373–1380.
18. Drutz DJ, Catanzaro A. Coccidioidomycosis. *Am Rev Respir Dis* 1978;117:727–771.
19. Lonky SA, Catanzaro A, Moser KM, et al. Acute coccidioidal pleural effusion. *Am Rev Respir Dis* 1976;114:681–688.
20. Pinckney L, Parker BR. Primary coccidioidomycosis in children presenting with massive pleural effusion. *AJR Am J Roentgenol* 1978;130:247–249.
21. Sarosi GA, Armstrong D, Barbee RA, et al. Treatment of fungal diseases. *Am Rev Respir Dis* 1979;120:1393–1397.
22. Cunningham RT, Einstein H. Coccidioidal pulmonary cavities with rupture. *J Thorac Cardiovasc Surg* 1982;84:172–177.
23. Young EJ, Hirsh DD, Fainstein V, et al. Pleural effusions due to *Cryptococcus neoformans:* a review of the literature and report of two cases with cryptococcal antigen determinations. *Am Rev Respir Dis* 1980;121:743–747.
24. Chechani V, Kamholz SL. Pulmonary manifestations of disseminated cryptococcosis in patients with AIDS. *Chest* 1990;98:1060–1065.
25. Cadranel JL, Chouaid C, Denis M, et al. Causes of pleural effusion in 75 HIV-infected patients. *Chest* 1993;104:655.
26. Salyer WR, Salyer DC. Pleural involvement in cryptococcosis. *Chest* 1974;66:139–140.
27. Wasser L, Talavera W. Pulmonary cryptococcosis in AIDS. *Chest* 1987;92:692–695.
28. Epstein R, Cole R, Hunt KK Jr. Pleural effusion secondary to pulmonary cryptococcosis. *Chest* 1972;61:296–298.
29. Duperval R, Hermans PE, Brewer NS, et al. Cryptococcosis, with emphasis on the significance of isolation of *Cryptococcus neoformans* from the respiratory tract. *Chest* 1977;72:13–19.
30. Warr W, Bates JH, Stone A. The spectrum of pulmonary cryptococcosis. *Ann Intern Med* 1968;69:1109–1116.
31. Tenholder MF, Ewald FW Jr, Khankhanian NK, et al. Complex cryptococcal empyema. *Chest* 1992;101:586–588.
32. Goodwin RA Jr, Des Prez RM. Histoplasmosis. *Am Rev Respir Dis* 1978;117:929–956.
33. Connell JV Jr, Muhm JR. Radiographic manifestations of pulmonary histoplasmosis: a 10-year review. *Radiology* 1976;121:281–285.
34. Brewer PL, Himmelwright JP. Pleural effusion due to infection with *Histoplasma capsulatum*. *Chest* 1970;58:76–79.
35. Schub HM, Spivey CG Jr, Baird GD. Pleural involvement in histoplasmosis. *Am Rev Respir Dis* 1966;94:225–232.
36. Campbell GD, Webb WR. Eosinophilic pleural effusion. *Am Rev Respir Dis* 1964;90:194–201.
37. Weissbluth M. Pleural effusion in histoplasmosis. *J Pediatr* 1976;88:894–895.
38. Quasney MW, Leggiadro RJ. Pleural effusion associated with histoplasmosis. *Pediatr Infect Dis J* 1993;12:415–418.
39. Ericsson CD, Pickering LK, Salmon GW. Pleural effusion in histoplasmosis. *J Pediatr* 1977;90:326–327.
40. Kilburn CD, McKinsey DS. Recurrent massive pleural effusion due to pleural, pericardial, and epicardial fibrosis in histoplasmosis. *Chest* 1991;100:1715–1717.
41. Marshall BC, Cox JK Jr, Carroll KC, et al. Histoplasmosis as a cause of pleural effusion in the acquired immunodeficiency syndrome. *Am J Med Sci* 1990;300:98–101.
42. Ankobiah WA, Vaidya K, Powell S, et al. Disseminated

histoplasmosis in AIDS. Clinicopathologic features in seven patients from a non-endemic area. *NY State J Med* 1990;90:234–238.

43. Richardson JV, George RB. Bronchopleural fistula and lymphocytic empyema due to *Histoplasma capsulatum. Chest* 1997;112:1130–1132.

44. Peabody JW Jr, Seabury JH. Actinomycosis and nocardiosis: a review of basic differences in therapy. *Am J Med* 1960;28:99–115.

45. Flynn MW, Felson B. The roentgen manifestations of thoracic actinomycosis. *AJR Am J Roentgenol* 1970;110:707–716.

46. Kwong JS, Muller NL, Godwin JD, et al. Thoracic actinomycosis: CT findings in eight patients. *Radiology* 1992;183:189–192.

47. Karetzky MS, Garvey JW. Empyema due to *Actinomyces naeslundii. Chest* 1974;65:229–230.

48. Barker CS. Thoracic actinomycosis. *Can Med Assoc J* 1954;71:332–334.

49. Varkey B, Landis FB, Tang TT, et al. Thoracic actinomycosis: dissemination to skin, subcutaneous tissue and muscle. *Arch Intern Med* 1974;134:689–693.

50. McQuarrie DG, Hall WH. Actinomycosis of the lung and chest wall. *Surgery* 1968;64:905–911.

51. Neu HC, Silva M, Hazen E, et al. Necrotizing nocardial pneumonitis. *Ann Intern Med* 1967;66:274–284.

52. Feigin DS. Nocardiosis of the lung: chest radiographic findings in 21 cases. *Radiology* 1986;159:9–14.

53. Uttamchandani RB, Daikos GL, Reyes RR, et al. Nocardiosis in 30 patients with advanced human immunodeficiency virus infection: clinical features and outcome. *Clin Infect Dis* 1994;18:348–353.

54. Rubin E, Shin MS. Pleural and extrapleural disease in nocardia infections. *Can Assoc Radiol J* 1984;35: 189–191.

55. Kramer MR, Uttamchandani RB. The radiographic appearance of pulmonary nocardiosis associated with AIDS. *Chest* 1990;98:382–385.

56. Palmer DL, Harvey RL, Wheeler JK. Diagnostic and therapeutic considerations in *Nocardia asteroides* infection. *Medicine* 1974;53:391–401.

57. Frazier AR, Rosenow EC III, Roberts GD. Nocardiosis: a review of 25 cases occurring during 24 months. *Mayo Clin Proc* 1975;50:657–663.

12

Pleural Effusion Due to
Parasitic Infection

Pleural effusions secondary to parasitic infections are uncommon in the United States, but in some countries, they account for a sizable percentage of all pleural effusions. With worldwide travel more prevalent, one can anticipate that the incidence of pleural effusions secondary to parasitic disease will gradually increase in the United States.

AMEBIASIS

Amebiasis, the disease caused by *Entamoeba histolytica*, occurs throughout the world. Humans acquire the disease by ingesting the cyst, which is the infectious form of the organism. After ingestion by the host, eight daughter trophozoites develop and colonize the proximal large intestine. The trophozoites, which can proliferate, are the potentially invasive form. These trophozoites may migrate through the portal system to the liver, where the liberation of cytolytic enzymes gives rise to liver abscesses. The trophozoite can also revert to a cyst. When the cyst is passed in the stool, it can be ingested by another individual, to complete the parasite's life cycle. Trophozoites can also be passed in the stool but are not infectious (1).

The prevalence of amebiasis is most dependent on the level of sanitation in the community, as would be expected from the life cycle of this parasite. About 5% of the population in the United States are carriers. Amebiasis is most prevalent in the southeastern United States, but the condition is reported with low frequency from every state. Amebic abscess is not unusual in the

United States. For example, there were 30 patients seen with hepatic amebiasis at the Santa Clara Valley Medical Center in San Jose, California, during the period of 1981 to 1988. None of the patients, however, were born in the United States (2).

Pathogenesis

Pleural effusions arise by two mechanisms in association with amebic liver abscess. The first occurs when an amebic abscess produces diaphragmatic irritation and a sympathetic pleural effusion in a manner analogous to that seen with pyogenic liver abscesses (3, 4) (see Chapter 15). Amebic liver abscesses also produce pleural effusions when the abscess ruptures through the diaphragm into the pleural space (3, 4). In this situation, the pleural fluid is described as "chocolate sauce" or "anchovy paste" (1). Such pleural fluid does not contain purulent material but is rather a mixture of blood, cytolyzed liver tissue, and small solid particles of liver parenchyma that have resisted dissolution.

Clinical Manifestations and Diagnosis

The sympathetic effusion seen with amebic liver abscess is more common than rupture of an abscess through the diaphragm into the pleural space (2, 3). Approximately 20% to 35% of patients with an amebic liver abscess will have a sympathetic pleural effusion (2). Patients with the sympathetic effusion frequently experience pleuritic chest pain referred to the tip of the scapula or the shoulder. Most patients have a tender enlarged liver (5). Eosinophilia is not associated with extraintestinal amebiasis. The level of alkaline phosphatase is elevated in more than 75% of patients, whereas the levels of transaminases are elevated in 50% (1). The chest radiograph reveals a pleural effusion of small to moderate size, often with a concomitant elevation of the hemidiaphragm and platelike atelectasis at the base (2–4). The pleural fluid in this situation has not been well characterized, but is an exudate (2).

The diagnosis of amebiasis should be considered in all patients with right-sided pleural effusions for which no other explanation is obvious. Ultrasonic studies and computed tomography (CT) scanning can demonstrate the hepatic abscess but cannot differentiate pyogenic from amebic abscesses (6). The diagnosis is aided with the use of serologic tests. The gel-diffusion test is positive in more than 95% of patients with acute invasive disease and reverts to negative after 6 to 12 months. With the indirect hemagglutination tests, an antibody titer of 1:128 or more is seen in 95% of cases, but the titer remains elevated for up to 10 years (7).

Treatment

The treatment of choice is metronidazole, 750 mg t.i.d. orally, for 10 days (7). If the patient is dyspneic from the pleural effusion, a single therapeutic thoracentesis is usually sufficient to control the symptoms. More than 90% of patients can be cured with the foregoing regimen. Catheter drainage adds no significant benefit to amebicidal therapy alone (1).

TRANSDIAPHRAGMATIC RUPTURE OF LIVER ABSCESS

The transdiaphragmatic rupture of an amebic liver abscess is usually signaled by an abrupt exacerbation of pain in the right upper quadrant and may be accompanied by a tearing sensation (3). These symptoms are followed by the development of rapidly progressive respiratory distress and sepsis, occasionally with shock (3). The pleural effusion is frequently massive, with opacification of the entire hemithorax and shift of the mediastinum to the contralateral side (3). The rupture is into the right pleural space in more than 90% of patients. The symptoms are sometimes subacute or chronic in nature (8). The diagnosis of amebic abscess with transdiaphragmatic rupture is suggested by the discovery of anchovy paste or chocolate sauce pleural fluid on diagnostic thoracentesis. Amebas can be demonstrated in the pleural fluid in fewer than 10% of patients. Concomitant rupture into the airways occurs in about 30% of patients (3), and this complication is usually manifested by the expectoration of chocolate sauce sputum that may be confused with hemoptysis by the patient and the physician.

The diagnosis is established by the characteristic appearance of the pleural fluid and can be confirmed by serologic tests for amebiasis. Ultrasound or CT scanning of the abdomen can delineate the extent of the intrahepatic disease and the presence or absence of a subphrenic abscess. Patients with transdiaphragmatic rupture should be treated with the same drugs as patients with sympathetic pleural effusions due to amebic hepatic abscess. Patients with transdiaphragmatic rupture should also undergo percutaneous drainage of both the liver abscess and the collection of material in the pleural space. The drainage can be accomplished with small tubes (12 to 14F) (9). The combination of the drugs and the percutaneous drainage tubes results in clinical cure in almost all patients (9).

About a third of patients with transhepatic rupture also have a bacterial infection of their pleural space (4, 8). Such patients should be treated with the appropriate antibiotics. In addition, an open-drainage procedure or decortication is frequently necessary, indications for which are outlined in Chapter 9. In patients who undergo decortication, the visceral pleura is found to be covered with a thick membrane (8), but this membrane can easily be stripped off the visceral pleura (8). Even when no bacterial superinfection is present, decortication should be performed if the lung has not fully expanded in 10 days (8). The prognosis with transdiaphragmatic rupture is excellent if the patient is not too debilitated initially or if the diagnosis is not delayed (3, 4, 8).

ECHINOCOCCOSIS (HYDATID DISEASE)

Echinococcosis is caused by the tapeworm *Echinococcus granulosus.* The definitive host for this small tapeworm is the dog or wolf. When dog feces containing the parasite's eggs are ingested by humans, larvae emerge in the duodenum, enter the blood, and usually lodge in either the liver or the lung. In these tissues, the parasite gradually grows, and years may pass before symptoms appear. It takes about 6 months for the cyst to reach a diameter if 1 cm and thereafter it increases in size by 2 to 3 cm per year (10). The dog becomes infected by eating meat containing the larvae. Echinococcosis is seen in most sheep- and cattle-raising areas of the world including Australia, New Zealand, Argentina, Uruguay, Chile, parts of Africa, Eastern Europe, and the Middle East. The disease is particularly common in Lebanon and Greece.

Pathogenesis

Pleural involvement with hydatid disease can occur in one of four situations (11, 12): (a) a hepatic hydatid cyst or, on rare occasions, a splenic cyst may rupture through the diaphragm into the pleural space; (b) a pulmonary hydatid cyst may rupture into the pleural space; (c) on rare occasions, the pleura may be primarily involved by the slowly enlarging cyst (11); or (d) a pulmonary or hepatic hydatid cyst may be accompanied by a pleural effusion (13, 14). The incidence of pulmonary and hepatic cyst rupture into the pleural space is equivalent (11). Fewer than 5% of hepatic or pulmonary hydatid cysts are complicated by intrapleural rupture (11, 12, 15). Approximately 5% of patients with a hepatic or a pulmonary hydatid cyst have a pleural effusion (13). The characteristics of the pleural fluid in this situation have not been characterized.

Clinical Manifestations and Diagnosis

When a hepatic cyst ruptures into the pleural space, the patient usually becomes acutely ill, with sudden tearing chest pain, dyspnea, and shock from the antigenic challenge to the body (16). In about 50% of patients with rupture into the pleural space, simultaneous rupture into the tracheobronchial tree occurs (16). Such patients may cough up large quantities of pus and membranes of the cyst. When a pulmonary cyst ruptures into the pleural space, similar symptoms are frequently present. In addition, a bronchopleural fistula often produces a hydropneumothorax that may become secondarily infected.

The diagnosis of pleural echinococcosis is established by the demonstration of echinococcal scolices with hooklets in the pleural fluid (17). A CT scan demonstrating multiple round cysts is very suggestive of the diagnosis (18). Eosinophils are frequently present in the pleural fluid unless it becomes secondarily infected (12, 17, 19). The Casoni skin test is positive in about 75% of patients (16), and the Weinberg complement-fixation (CF) test is positive in a higher percentage.

Treatment

Attempts should be made to remove the cyst in patients with hydatid disease. In the past, all thoracic cysts have been removed through thoracotomy. However, it appears that the cysts can be removed by percutaneous catheter drainage (20) or thoracoscopy (21).

An immediate thoracotomy is recommended for patients who have rupture of a hepatic cyst into the pleural space (16). When a hepatic cyst has ruptured, the objectives of surgical treatment are to remove the parasite, to drain the hepatic cavity, and to reexpand the lung immediately (16). If the surgical procedure is delayed, a decortication may also be required (16). An exploratory thoracotomy should also be performed when a pulmonary hydatid cyst ruptures into the pleural space, to remove the parasite, to excise the original cyst, and to close the bronchopleural fistula. Patients with hydatid cysts should be treated with antiprotozoal therapy if all the cysts cannot be removed or when rupture of a cyst has occurred. The treatment of choice is albendazole, 400 mg b.i.d. over 28 days (22).

PARAGONIMIASIS

Paragonimiasis is caused by the lung flukes *Paragonimus westermani* and *P. miyazakii* (23), which have a fascinating life cycle. Humans acquire the disease by eating raw or undercooked crabs or crayfish containing the larvae of these parasites (24, 25). Once ingested, the larvae bore through the intestinal wall and enter the peritoneal cavity. They then migrate upward in the peritoneal cavity to the diaphragm, bore through the diaphragm, and then, after traversing the pleural space, bore through the visceral pleura and enter the lung (24, 25). In the lung, the larvae lodge near small bronchi and mature into the adult lung fluke, persisting in the lungs for years while producing about 10,000 eggs daily. The eggs produced by the mature flukes are expectorated or are swallowed and excreted in the feces. Once in water, the eggs develop into ciliated miracidia that infect freshwater snails. Another larval form develops in the snails and is eventually liberated as cercariae that penetrate crayfish and crabs, to complete the cycle (24, 25).

Pathogenesis and Incidence

The pleural disease associated with paragonimiasis is thought to arise when the parasites traverse the pleural space and penetrate the visceral pleura. Pleural disease is common with paragonimiasis (26, 27). In a series of 71 cases of pleuropulmonary paragonimiasis from Korea (27), 43 patients (61%) had pleural disease. Of the 43 patients with pleural disease, 28 had unilateral pleural effusions, six had bilateral pleural effusions, six had unilateral hydropneumothorax, six had bilateral hydropneumothorax, and five had pleural thickening (27). In another series from Japan, nine of 13 patients (69%) had a pleural effusion (26).

Although paragonimiasis is confined mainly to residents of the Far East, there was an increased incidence of this disease in the United States in the 1980s with the influx of refugees from Southeast Asia (24, 28). Johnson and Johnson reported a series of 25 cases of paragonimiasis that occurred in Indochinese refugees between March 1980 and December 1982. Seventeen cases occurred in Minneapolis, whereas eight cases occurred in Seattle (28). Twelve of the patients (48%) had pleural effusions. The effusions were bilateral in three individuals and were massive in six. Non-Asian individuals in the United States have developed paragonimiasis from ingesting infected crayfish (29) or crabs (30).

Diagnosis

The diagnosis of pleural paragonimiasis should be suspected in Asian patients or in patients with a pleural effusion who have recently traveled to the Orient. The diagnosis of paragonimiasis is made either by detecting eggs in sputum, stool, fluid from bronchoscopic lavage, or biopsy specimens, or by a positive anti-Paragonimus antibody test (27). Enzyme-linked immunosorbent assay (ELISA) is highly sensitive and specific in detecting antibodies, whereas eggs are demonstrable in less than 50% of cases (27).

The characteristics of the pleural fluid are virtually pathognomonic for paragonimiasis. The pleural fluid with paragonimiasis is an exudate with a low glucose level (<10 mg per dL), a low pH (<7.10), and a high lactic dehydrogenase (LDH) level (>1,000 IU per L) (24, 28). Cholesterol crystals are usually present in the pleural fluid. Most patients with pleural paragonimiasis have significant eosinophilia in their pleural fluid (23, 24, 28). The only other disease that produces an eosinophilic exudate with a low glucose level and a low pH is the Churg-Strauss syndrome (31).

Yokogawa et al. (23) reported that pleural fluid IgE levels are elevated and are higher than the simultaneous serum IgE levels in patients with pleural paragonimiasis. Subsequently Ikeda et al. (32) used ELISA to measure *P. westermani*–specific IgE and IgG in seven patients. They reported that the levels of parasite-specific IgE and IgG were significantly higher in the pleural effusion than in the serum in all patients (32). This latter study suggests that measurement of parasite-specific IgE and IgG is useful diagnostically and indicates that these antibodies are produced in the pleural space.

Treatment

The treatment of choice is praziquantel, 25 mg per kg body weight three times a day for 3 days. Bithionol, 35 to 50 mg/kg on alternate days for 10 to 15 doses, is also effective, but its toxic gastrointestinal effects can be troublesome (32). If pleural disease has been present for such a prolonged period that the pleural surfaces are abnormally thickened, penetration of the drugs into the pleural space is insufficient to eradicate the infection, and thoracotomy with decortication may be necessary (24, 33).

OTHER PARASITIC INFECTIONS

Pleural disease due to other parasites is uncommon. A rare patient with *Pneumocystis carinii* pneumonia has a pleural effusion, but the effusion hardly ever dominates the clinical picture. Because *P. carinii* infection usually occurs in patients with acquired immunodeficiency syndrome, this entity is discussed in Chapter 13. Patients who die from malaria frequently have pleural effusions (5). The pleural effusions in this circumstance are probably secondary to the pulmonary edema and have little, if any, clinical significance (5). There have been case reports of pleural effusions due to *Strongyloides sterocoralis* (34), Trichomonas (35), *Toxocara canis* (36), loiasis (37), and sporotrichosis (38).

REFERENCES

1. Lyche KD, Jensen WA. Pleuropulmonary amebiasis. *Semin Respir Infect* 1997;12:106–112.
2. Lyche KD, Jensen WA, Kirsch CM, et al. Pleuropulmonary manifestations of hepatic amebiasis. *West J Med* 1990;153:275–278.
3. Ibarra-Perez C. Thoracic complications of amebic abscess of the liver. *Chest* 1981;79:672–676.
4. Cameron EWJ. The treatment of pleuropulmonary amebiasis with metronidazole. *Chest* 1978;73:647–650.
5. Sharma OP, Maheshwari A. Lung diseases in the tropics. Part 2: Common tropical lung diseases: diagnosis and management. *Tuber Lung Dis* 1993;74:359–370.
6. Boultbee JE, Simjee AE, Rooknoodeen F, et al. Experiences with grey scale ultrasonography in hepatic amoebiasis. *Clin Radiol* 1979;30:683–689.
7. Petersen C, Mills J. Parasitic infections. In: Murray JF, Nadel JA, eds. *Textbook of respiratory medicine*, 2nd ed. Philadelphia: WB Saunders, 1994:1201–1243.
8. Rasaretnam R, Paul ATS, Yoganathan M. Pleural

empyema due to ruptured amoebic liver abscess. *Br J Surg* 1974;61:713–715.
9. Baijal SS, Agarwal DK, Roy S, et al. Complex ruptured amebic liver abscesses: the role of percutaneous catheter drainage. *Eur J Radiol* 1995;20:65–67.
10. von Sinner WN. Ultrasound, CT and MRI of ruptured and disseminated hydatid cysts. *Eur J Radiol* 1990; 11:31–37.
11. Rakower J, Milwidsky H. Hydatid pleural disease. *Am Rev Respir Dis* 1964;90:623–631.
12. Barzilai A, Pollack S, Kaftori JK, et al. Splenic echinococcal cyst burrowing into left pleural space. *Chest* 1977;72:543–545.
13. Jerray M, Benzarti M, Garrouche A, et al. Hydatid disease of the lung. *Am Rev Respir Dis* 1992;146:185–189.
14. von Sinner W. Pleural complications of hydatid disease (*Echinococcus granulosus*). *Rofo Fortschr Geb Rontgenstr Nuklearmedizin* 1990;152:718–722.
15. Balikian JP, Mudarris, FF. Hydatid disease of the lungs: a roentgenologic study of 50 cases. *AJR Am J Roentgenol* 1974;122:692–707.
16. Xanthakis DS, Katsaras E, Efthimiadis M, et al. Hydatid cyst of the liver with intrathoracic rupture. *Thorax* 1981;36:497–501.
17. Jacobson ES. A case of secondary echinococcosis diagnosed by cytologic examination of pleural fluid and needle biopsy of pleura. *Acta Cytol* 1973;17:76–79.
18. Gouliamos AD, Kalovidouris A, Papailiou J, et al. CT appearance of pulmonary hydatid disease. *Chest* 1991;100:1578–1581.
19. Yacoubian HD. Thoracic problems associated with hydatid cyst of the dome of the liver. *Surgery* 1976;79:544–548.
20. Men S, Hekimoglu B, Yucesoy C, et al. Percutaneous treatment of hepatic hydatid cysts: an alternative to surgery. *AJR Am J Roentgenol* 1999;172:83–89.
21. Paterson HS, Blyth DF. Thoracoscopic evacuation of dead hydatid cyst. *J Thorac Cardiovasc Surg* 1996;111:1280–1281.
22. Drugs for parasitic infections. *The Medical Letter* 1998;40:1–7.
23. Yokogawa M, Kojima S, Araki K, et al. Immunoglobulin E: raised levels in sera and pleural exudates of patients with paragonimiasis. *Am J Trop Med Hyg* 1976;25:581–586.
24. Minh V-D, Engle P, Greenwood JR, et al. Pleural paragonimiasis in a southeast Asian refugee. *Am Rev Respir Dis* 1981;124:186–188.
25. Eikas J, Kim PK. Clinical investigation of paragonimiasis. *Acta Tuberc Scand* 1960;39:140–147.
26. Nawa Y. Recent trends of paragonimiasis westermani in Miyazaki Prefecture, Japan. *Southeast Asian J Trop Med Public Health* 1991;22[Suppl]:342–344.
27. Im JG, Whang HY, Kim WS, et al. Pleuropulmonary paragonimiasis: radiologic findings in 71 patients. *AJR Am J Roentgenol* 1992;159:39–43.
28. Johnson RJ, Johnson JR. Paragonimiasis in Indochinese refugees: roentgenographic findings with clinical correlations. *Am Rev Respir Dis* 1983;128:534–538.
29. Pachucki CT, Levandowski RA, Brown VA, et al. American paragonimiasis treated with praziquantel. *N Engl J Med* 1984;311:582–584.
30. Sharma OP. The man who loved drunken crabs: a case of pulmonary paragonimiasis. *Chest* 1989;95:670–672.

31. Erzurum SE, Underwood GA, Hamilos DL, et al. Pleural effusion in Churg-Strauss syndrome. *Chest* 1989;95:1357–1359.
32. Ikeda T, Oikawa Y, Owhashi M, et al. Parasite-specific IgE and IgG levels in the serum and pleural effusion of *paragonimiasis westermani* patients. *Am J Trop Med Hyg* 1992;47:104–107.
33. Dietrick RB, Sade RM, Pak JS. Results of decortication in chronic empyema with special reference to paragonimiasis. *J Thorac Cardiovasc Surg* 1981;82:58–62.
34. Emad A. Exudative eosinophilic pleural effusion due to *Strongyloides stercoralis* in a diabetic man. *South Med J* 1999;92:58–60.
35. Walzer PD, Rutherford I, East R. Empyema with *Trichomonas* species. *Am Rev Respir Dis* 1978;118:415–418.
36. Jeanfaivre T, Cimon B, Tolstuchow N, et al. Pleural effusion and toxocariasis. *Thorax* 1996;51:106–107.
37. Klion AD, Eisenstein EM, Smirniotopoulos TT, et al. Pulmonary involvement in loiasis. *Am Rev Respir Dis* 1992;145:961–963.
38. Morrissey R, Caso R. Pleural sporotrichosis. *Chest* 1983;84:507.

13

Pleural Effusion Due to the Acquired Immunodeficiency Syndrome, Other Viruses, *Mycoplasma pneumoniae*, and Rickettsiae

Over the past decade, the acquired immunodeficiency syndrome (AIDS) epidemic has had a profound impact on the practice of medicine. Accordingly, the first part of this chapter deals with pleural effusions in patients with AIDS. Because the organism responsible for AIDS is a virus, we have also included pleural diseases due to viruses in this chapter. Additionally, we have included the pleural effusions resulting from infection with *Mycoplasma pneumoniae*, ehrlichia, and the rickettsial diseases, Q fever, and Rocky Mountain spotted fever. Diseases secondary to mycoplasma, ehrlichia, and rickettsiae are discussed in this chapter because they produce clinical pictures simulating viral pneumonias.

sions in patients with AIDS varies widely from series to series. In the series of 160 patients from Jacksonville, the five leading causes of pleural effusions were pneumonia and empyema (33%), renal failure (9%), hypoalbuminemia (8%), tuberculosis (6%) and pancreatitis (4%) (1). In a second, older series of 61 patients from Paris, 52% of the effusions were due to Kaposi's sarcoma (2), 18% had aerobic bacteria, 15% had tuberculosis, 10% had opportunistic infections, and 5% had effusions due to other malignancies (2). In a third series from Rwanda (3), tuberculosis was responsible for the pleural effusion in 82 of 91 (90%) of patients who were HIV positive and had a pleural effusion.

PLEURAL EFFUSIONS IN PATIENTS WITH THE ACQUIRED IMMUNODEFICIENCY SYNDROME

Pleural effusions are not uncommon in patients with AIDS. In a recent series of 1,225 consecutive hospital admissions of patients with AIDS in Jacksonville, FL, the incidence of pleural effusion was 14.6% (1). In an older series from Metropolitan Hospital Center in New York, the incidence was 1.7% in a large series of 4,511 human immunodeficiency virus (HIV)–positive patients who were hospitalized (1). The distribution of the diseases responsible for pleural effu-

Kaposi's Sarcoma

Kaposi's sarcoma (KS) is one of the more common causes of a pleural effusion in patients with AIDS. KS occurs almost exclusively in male homosexual patients with AIDS (4). The explanation for the occurrence of KS primarily in homosexual men is the observation that almost all individuals with KS are infected with the Kaposi's sarcoma–associated herpes virus (KSHV) (5). It is thought that KSHV is particularly likely to be spread by male homosexual contacts. In the past, KS occurred in 20% to 25% of individuals with AIDS (4). In recent years, there has been a precipitous decline in the prevalence of KS (6). For example, in the state of Washington, the prevalence of KS in the homosexual HIV-positive population was 6% in 1990, but the prevalence had fallen to 2% by 1997 and apparently has fallen more in the past 3 years (6). It is likely that the decrease in the prevalence of KS is, at least in part, related to the introduction of the highly active antiretroviral therapy (HAART) (6).

Cutaneous violaceous plaques are the most common presentation of KS. At autopsy, 50% to 75% of patients with cutaneous KS have pulmonary involvement (6), but clinically apparent pulmonary involvement is less common during life (6). Most patients with pleuropulmonary KS present with progressive shortness of breath, nonproductive cough, and fever. Patients with pulmonary KS generally have abnormal chest roentgenograms characterized by bilateral infiltrates (4). The incidence of pleural effusion with pulmonary KS is approximately 50% (4). Most patients with a pleural effusion due to KS also have bilateral parenchymal infiltrates (4). The pleural effusions may be unilateral or bilateral. The computed tomography (CT) scans are somewhat characteristic with KS. In a review of 53 patients with pulmonary KS, 42 patients (79%) had nodules, 35 (66%) had bronchovascular bundle thickening, 28 (53%) had tumoral masses, and 29 (55%) had pleural effusions (7). The effusions were bilateral in 40 (76%) and were usually at least medium sized (7). Autopsy studies demonstrate multiple cherry red to purple lesions on the visceral surface but not on the parietal pleural surface (4).

The pathogenesis of the pleural effusions in KS is not conclusively defined. Approximately 20% of the pleural effusions with KS are chylothoraces, and, in these instances, the pleural effusion is probably due to involvement of the thoracic duct by the sarcoma (4). In the remaining patients, lymphatic blockade is probably not the responsible mechanism because the lymphatic drainage of the pleura is through the parietal pleura and KS does not involve the parietal pleura. It has been hypothesized that the effusion is due to the elaboration of vascular endothelial growth factor (VEGF) by the tumor (8). VEGF increases the permeability of the microvessels and is present in large quantities in AIDS-KS cell–derived conditioned media (9).

The diagnosis of pulmonary KS is usually established at bronchoscopy, which demonstrates erythematous or violaceous macules or papules in the respiratory tree (10). It is important to remember that many patients with pulmonary KS have a coexisting opportunistic infection (6). If the CT scan reveals ground-glass opacities or mediastinal adenopathy, alternative diagnoses must be sought (7). The definitive diagnosis of pleural KS is not easy and is virtually one of exclusion. The pleural fluid is an exudate that is usually serosanguineous or hemorrhagic. The differential cell count shows a mononuclear cell—predominant pattern (4). In one series of 10 patients, the pleural fluid glucose and pH levels were normal in nine patients but were reduced to 63 mg per dL and 7.02, respectively, in one patient (4). Cytologic examination of the pleural fluid is not helpful because the diagnosis requires a characteristic architectural appearance and not a particular neoplastic cell type (11). Needle biopsy of the pleura does not establish the diagnosis of KS because the parietal pleura is not involved (4). It is probable that the diagnosis could be established with thoracoscopy given the characteristic appearance of the KS lesions on the visceral pleura (4).

The prognosis of a patient with pleuropulmonary KS is poor. In one study, the average interval from diagnosis of pulmonary KS to death was 4 ± 3 months (4). The presence of the pleural effusion is a significant problem for many patients with pleuropulmonary KS. In one series, recurrent, massive, progressive effusions dominated the final days of a substantial percentage of patients and contributed significantly to their death in about 50% (4).

The treatment of the pleural effusion associated with KS is difficult. Tube thoracostomy with the instillation of tetracycline is usually not successful (4). If the diagnosis is made with thoracoscopy, pleural abrasion or parietal pleurectomy is probably the treatment of choice. Otherwise, the best alternatives are probably the insertion of a pleuroperitoneal shunt or an indwelling catheter (e.g., Pleurx).

Primary Effusion Lymphoma

This rare lymphoma occurs almost exclusively in patients with HIV infection and is discussed in Chapter 8.

Parapneumonic Effusion and Empyema and Acquired Immunodeficiency Syndrome

Community-acquired bacterial pneumonia occurs frequently in patients with AIDS. It appears that patients with AIDS are probably more likely to develop pleural complications with their pneumonias than are other patients (12) because they are more likely to have bacteremia with their pneumonia (12). In one series of 81 cases of community-acquired pneumonia, pleural effusion occurred in 21 (26%) patients (12). The pleural fluid was culture positive in 11 of these 21 (52%) patients. The distribution of organisms responsible for community-acquired bacterial pneumonia in AIDS is very similar to that of patients without AIDS (12). The management of the patient with AIDS and a parapneumonic effusion or an empyema is the same as that for any patient with a parapneumonic effusion.

Pneumocystis carinii Pneumonia and Acquired Immunodeficiency Syndrome

Although pleural effusions due to *Pneumocystis carinii* account for only a small percentage of pleural effusions in patients with AIDS, they do occur. By 1993 a total of seven cases of pleural effusion due to *P. carinii* infection had been reported (13, 14). In most cases, the diagnosis was established by visualization of *Pneumocystis* in pleural fluid stained with Gomori methenamine silver. All seven of the reported patients were receiving aerosolized pentamidine, and five of the seven had documented underlying *P. carinii* pneumonia. Two patients presented with primary pleural infection with *Pneumocystis*. It appears that *Pneumocystis* pleural disease is an anatomic extension of smoldering subpleural *Pneumocystis* pneumonia, and the prognosis is not worse than with pneumonia alone. Four of the seven

patients with pleural *Pneumocystis* also had a bronchopleural fistula (13).

The pleural fluid is an exudate with pleural *Pneumocystis*. The pleural fluid lactate dehydrogenase (LDH) has been higher than 400 IU, and the ratio of the pleural fluid to serum LDH has exceeded 1:0. Interestingly, the pleural fluid protein level has been below 3.0 g per dL, and the ratio of the pleural fluid to the serum protein has been below 0:50 in all patients. The pleural fluid glucose and pH are not reduced, and the differential cell count can reveal either neutrophils or mononuclear cells (13). The treatment of pleural *Pneumocystis* is the same as the treatment of pulmonary *Pneumocystis*.

Tuberculous Pleural Effusions and Acquired Immunodeficiency Syndrome

In some series, tuberculosis is the most common etiology for pleural effusions associated with AIDS (3). The clinical picture of tuberculous pleuritis in patients with and without AIDS is similar, but there are some differences. In patients with tuberculosis, some reports have demonstrated that a higher percentage of patients with AIDS have a pleural effusion (15), whereas others report a similar incidence (16). The percentage of tuberculosis cases that have pleural effusions in patients with AIDS is higher in patients with $CD4^+$ counts above 200 than in those with $CD4^+$ counts below 200 per mm^3 (17).

The purified protein derivative (PPD) skin test is less frequently positive in patients with AIDS who have tuberculous pleuritis. In one series of patients with tuberculous pleuritis, the PPD was positive in 76% of patients without AIDS but in only 41% of patients with AIDS (18). The lower the $CD4^+$ count, the less likely the PPD is to be positive. In patients without AIDS, the pleural fluid acid-fast bacilli (AFB) stain is only rarely positive ($\sim$1%), but in one series, the AFB pleural fluid smear was positive in 15% of patients with AIDS (18). In another series the pleural fluid smear was positive in 37% of patients with AIDS and a $CD4^+$ count under 200 per mm^3 (19). The granuloma on pleural biopsy are less well formed in some patients with AIDS, and there are numerous AFB (20). Patients with the poorly defined granuloma appear to respond less well to antituberculous therapy (20). The incidence of granuloma on pleural biopsy is comparable in patients with and without AIDS (18). Cultures of the pleural biopsy specimen are positive more frequently (~50%) than are cultures of the pleural fluid (~10%).

Miscellaneous Pleural Effusion in Patients with Acquired Immunodeficiency Syndrome

Other opportunistic diseases such as cryptococcosis (21), histoplasmosis (22), nocardiosis (23), and atypical mycobacteria (24) at times are responsible for a pleural effusion in patients with AIDS. In their terminal stages, some patients with AIDS develop hypoproteinemia and this may lead to a transudative pleural effusion (25). Patients with AIDS may also develop hypervolemia owing to heart failure or renal failure, which can lead to a pleural effusion (26). In one series, pancreatitis was the fifth leading cause of pleural effusion in patients with AIDS (1). The diagnosis and management of pleural effusions due to these different entities are described in the appropriate chapters in this book.

Approach to the Patient with Acquired Immunodeficiency Syndrome and Pleural Effusion

AIDS patients with a pleural effusion should have a diagnostic thoracentesis. Studies on the fluid should include smears and cultures for bacteria, mycobacteria, and fungi; cytology with special consideration for primary effusion lymphoma; and either a interferon-gamma or an adenosine deaminase measurement for pleural tuberculosis. If the patient has a positive PPD (<5 mm) or if there are no mesothelial cells in the pleural fluid, chemotherapy with isoniazid and rifampin for 9 months is recommended. If the patient is receiving aerosolized pentamidine, silver stains of the pleural fluid should be obtained to rule out *Pneumocystis*.

If the diagnosis is not apparent after the thoracentesis and the patient has an exudative pleural effusion, what should be the next diagnostic procedure? Possible courses of action include a needle biopsy of the pleura, thoracoscopy, bronchoscopy, or observation. In general, a thoracoscopy is recommended, if any procedure is going to be done. With thoracoscopy one can establish the diagnosis of KS, other intrathoracic malignancies, tuberculous pleuritis, or other opportunistic pleural infections. In addition, a pleural abrasion can be performed to prevent reaccumulation of the pleural fluid.

VIRUSES

Viral infections probably account for a larger percentage of pleural effusions than is generally realized. The diagnosis usually depends on isolation of the virus or the demonstration of a significant increase in the antibodies to the virus. Because most pleural effusions secondary to viruses are self-limiting, paired sera from patients in the acute and convalescent phases of disease are not usually obtained for diagnosis. Moreover, most hospitals are not equipped to culture viruses.

The most interesting epidemic of pleural effusions attributed to viral infection occurred in Turkey in 1955, when 559 individuals at a military base developed a pleural effusion in conjunction with an acute illness characterized by fever, cough, malaise, anorexia, and shortness of breath (27). None of the patients had parenchymal infiltrates, but about 30% had an enlarged hilar shadow. The peripheral white blood cell count (WBC) was normal or reduced, with an increased percentage of lymphocytes. The differential WBC on the pleural fluid revealed mostly mononuclear cells. The disease was self-limited, and almost all patients recovered completely within 90 days. Because all bacterial cultures were negative, as were serologic tests for Q fever, and because the patients recovered without any specific therapy, it was concluded that the disease was due to a viral infection (27). This report is important because it documents that viral infections can cause pleural effusions and in large numbers. One wonders what fraction of undiagnosed pleural effusions is due to viral infections.

Small pleural effusions frequently accompany primary atypical pneumonia. Fine et al. (28) prospectively studied 59 patients with atypical pneumonia that satisfied serologic criteria for association with either a mycoplasma, viral, or cold-agglutinin–positive pneumonia. Twelve of these patients (20%) had small pleural effusions, which in four patients, could only be demonstrated on lateral decubitus radiographs. This finding compares with a 45% incidence of pleural effusions in patients with acute bacterial pneumonia (29). In the series of Fine et al., six of 29 (21%) patients with *Mycoplasma* pneumonia, one of seven (14%) with adenoviral pneumonia, one of four (25%) with influenza pneumonia, and four of 19 (21%) with only increased titers of cold agglutinins had pleural effusions (28).

In patients with viral infections, the pleural effusions are usually small (27, 28), but occasionally may be large (30). The pleural fluid is an exudate (28), and usually mononuclear cells are predominant on the pleural fluid differential WBC (27, 31). I have seen a patient with a viral pneumonia, however, in whom the initial thoracentesis revealed predominantly polymorphonuclear leukocytes, but a subsequent thoracentesis 48 hours later revealed predominantly mononuclear cells. The diagnosis of pleural effusions secondary to viral infections is established by documenting increasing titers with the specific serologic tests or by culturing viruses from the pleural fluid (31, 32). At times, with pleural effusions secondary to herpes infections or cytomegalovirus, the cytologic findings in the pleural fluid, consisting of intranuclear inclusions and multinuclear giant cells with gelatinous nuclear changes, suggest the diagnosis (33, 34).

Hantavirus Infections

The hantavirus pulmonary syndrome is a recently described entity that is due to infection with a previously unknown hantavirus species now called Sin Nombre virus. As of May 31, 1996, 139 cases had been confirmed from 24 states, representing all regions of the United States, with a mortality rate of 49.6%. An additional 12 cases had been reported from Canada (35). The majority of cases have occurred in the Four Corners Region, where New Mexico, Arizona, Colorado, and Utah meet. The deer mouse, *Peromyscus maniculatus*, has been identified as the likely principal reservoir of the Sin Nombre virus (36, 37). There are several other hantaviruses that can produce a similar syndrome including the New York virus, which produces disease in New York State; the Bayou virus, which produces disease in Louisiana; and the Black Creek Canal virus, which produces disease in Florida and the southeastern United States (38). Hantaviruses have also been recognized in several locations in South America (38).

The hantavirus pulmonary syndrome is characterized by a brief prodromal illness, followed by rapidly progressive, noncardiogenic pulmonary edema (36, 37). The median age of infected individuals is about 30 years, and 50% of the patients have been Native American Indians (36). Most patients present with fever or chills, and gastrointestinal complaints such as nausea or vomiting, abdominal pain, or diarrhea. Most patients report myalgias and cough. Dyspnea tends to be a late-developing symptom, occurring just before respiratory decompensation.

Patients who present with the hantavirus pulmonary syndrome have many abnormal laboratory tests. They characteristically have the triad of thrombocytopenia, a left shift in the myeloid series, and large immunoblastoid lymphocytes. The PaO_2/FiO_2 is usually severely reduced, and 50% of the patients require mechanical ventilation. The chest radiograph of patients who progress to respiratory failure initially shows bibasilar infiltrates, which rapidly spread to include all four quadrants of the lung. The heart size is normal. Patients with the hantavirus pulmonary syndrome tend to decompensate rapidly with refractory hypoxemia and hypotension. The mean duration of hospitalization before death is only about 3 days.

Pleural effusions were common in the 23 patients seen at the University of New Mexico Hospital (35). At the time of admission, 21 of the 23 patients had pleural effusions. Effusions of similar size were present bilaterally in most patients. The maximum size of the effusion was achieved within 24 to 48 hours of admission. Three of the patients had effusions of sufficient size that chest tubes were inserted. A thoracentesis was performed in four of the patients. Although none of the fluids was very inflammatory, all four met exudative criteria with a pleural fluid LDH greater than two thirds the upper normal serum limit. However, the pleural fluid protein level was below 2.5 g per dL in three of the four patients, and the pleural fluid WBC was below 200 per mm^3 in all patients (35). At autopsy, patients dying of the hantavirus pulmonary syndrome have large serous effusions with severe edema of the lungs. It is probable that the pleural effusion results from interstitial fluid traversing the visceral pleura to the pleural space.

It is important to make the diagnosis of the hantavirus pulmonary syndrome early, because antiviral therapy requires time to be beneficial. The diagnosis can be established by serologic tests for immunoglobulin M (IgM) and immunoglobulin G (IgG) antibody, which are usually demonstrated by enzyme-linked immunosorbent assay (ELISA) (38). The broad-spectrum antiviral agent ribavirin is active against hantavirus *in vitro*, but an open-label trial of intravenous ribavirin in patients with the hantavirus syndrome was inconclusive (38).

Adenovirus Pneumonia

After *Mycoplasma pneumoniae*, adenoviruses are the second leading cause of primary atypical pneumonia. Pleural effusions occur in 15% to 62% of patients with adenoviral pneumonia (39, 40). The pleural effusions are usually bilateral, and most are moderate to large in size. When adenovirus infection results in a pleural effusion, a concomitant parenchymal infiltrate is usually present (39, 40).

Infectious Hepatitis

Pleural effusions occasionally occur in conjunction with infectious hepatitis and at times precede the development of icterus (31, 41–45). In a review of 2,500 patients with viral hepatitis (41), four patients (0.16%) had pleural effusions. In another prospective study of 156 patients with hepatitis (45), however, 70% of the patients had at least a small pleural effusion. Patients with pleural effusions secondary to viral hepatitis do not have parenchymal infiltrates. The pleural fluid is an exudate with predominantly mononuclear cells (31, 46). The pleural effusion frequently resolves before the hepatitis (42). One must be careful in handling pleural fluid when infectious hepatitis is suspected because the infectious hepatitis B e antigen has been demonstrated in pleural fluid secondary to hepatitis (44, 46).

Infectious Mononucleosis

Pleural effusions occasionally occur in the course of infectious mononucleosis (47–49). Lander and Palayew reviewed the chest radiographs of 59 patients with infectious mononucleosis and reported that three (5%) had pleural effusions (47). Two of the patients had bilateral interstitial infiltrates and small bilateral pleural effusions, whereas the third patient had a moderate-sized, left-sided pleural effusion without any parenchymal infiltrates (47). The pleural effusions are exudates and usually take several months to resolve (48, 49).

Dengue Hemorrhagic Fever

Dengue fever is caused by four antigenically distinct dengue viruses, and the disease is transmitted to human beings by mosquitoes. Classic dengue fever is not uncommon among travelers to tropical areas but dengue hemorrhagic fever is rare. The characteristics of dengue hemorrhagic fever are increased capillary permeability with leakage of plasma and abnormal hemostasis (50). Pleural effusions are common with dengue hemorrhagic fever and are usually exudates (51) but can be transudates (50). In one study of 40 adults with severe dengue hemorrhagic fever, 21 (53%) had pleural effusions (52). In another study, pleural effusions were found in 95% of patients with severe dengue hemorrhagic fever. The effusions are usually bilateral but sometimes are right sided only, and rarely, if ever, left sided only (53). The effusions are small in most instances. It appears that the pathogenesis of the effusions is similar to than with the hantavirus syndrome, namely, a systemic increase in the permeability of capillaries induced by cytokines. In one study, the interleukin 8 (IL-8) levels in the pleural fluid were very high (51).

Other Viral Infections

Pleural effusions have also been reported to result from infection with respiratory syncytial virus

(54), influenza viruses (28), measles after the administration of inactivated virus vaccine (55), herpes simplex virus (56), and Lassa fever virus (30). Pleural effusions probably result from infection by many other viruses as well.

MYCOPLASMA PNEUMONIAE

This organism is actually a small bacterium rather than a virus. It is included in this chapter because the disease it produces more closely resembles a viral than a bacterial disease. Pleural effusions occur in 5% to 20% of patients with pneumonias due to *Mycoplasma pneumoniae* (28, 57). The effusions are usually small (28) but can be large (57–59). The diagnosis, suggested by increased titers of cold agglutinins, is established by increasing specific antibody titers. It may take several weeks for a fourfold rise in specific antibody titer to become evident. In an occasional patient, the diagnosis can be established by isolating *M. pneumoniae* from the pleural fluid (60). The treatment of choice is tetracycline or erythromycin administration. No specific treatment need be directed toward the pleural effusion, but a diagnostic thoracentesis should be performed to ensure that a complicated parapneumonic effusion is not present.

RICKETTSIAE

Q Fever

The causative agent for Q fever is the rickettsial agent *Coxiella burnetii*. This disease is sometimes manifested as a primary atypical pneumonia. Q fever is acquired by the inhalation of contaminated dust particles or by drinking infected, unpasteurized milk. Because the infection is prevalent among livestock in the United States, farmers and stockyard workers are particularly likely to contract the disease. Patients with Q fever pneumonia present with the clinical picture of primary atypical pneumonia, with a high fever, cough, headache, and myalgias. Nearly half of the patients have no respiratory symptoms, although one third have pleuritic chest pain (61). Pleural involvement is relatively common with Q fever pneumonia. In one series of 164 cases

from the Basque country of Spain, 12% had a pleural effusion (61). In another review, five of 25 patients (20%) with chest radiographic abnormalities due to Q fever had a pleural effusion, and in one of these patients the effusion was large (62). The pleural fluid is an exudate, and the differential reveals predominantly mononuclear cells (63) or eosinophils (64). In one report, the pleural fluid adenosine deaminase level was increased to 64 IU per L with Q fever (63). The diagnosis is usually established by demonstrating a fourfold increase in the antibody titers in the patient's serum. This increase becomes apparent in most patients within 2 weeks of the onset of the illness. The treatment of choice is tetracycline or doxycycline, which appear to be superior to erythromycin (61).

Rocky Mountain Spotted Fever

Rocky Mountain spotted fever is due to *Rickettsia rickettsii*, and humans acquire the infection after a tick bite. Most infections occur in the southeastern and coastal Atlantic states. Classically, Rocky Mountain spotted fever is manifested by the triad of fever, rash, and a history of tick exposure. The usual onset of illness is 5 to 7 days after the tick bite. Fever, malaise, frontal headache, myalgia, and vomiting are common. A pleural effusion is present in 10% to 36% and a pulmonary infiltrate is present in a comparable percentage (65). The infiltrates are probably due to vasculitis with increased permeability of the blood vessels. At times, fluid overload in conjunction with myocardial vasculitis can lead to increased left atrial pressures and transudative pleural effusions. The characteristics of the pleural fluid have not been well-defined. The treatment of choice is doxycycline 200 mg a day in two divided doses.

EHRLICHIOSIS

Ehrlichiae are obligate intracellular bacteria that grow within membrane-bound vacuoles in leukocytes. Humans acquire ehrlichiosis through a tick bite. The two most important human ehrlichial diseases are human monocytic ehrlichiosis (HME), which is caused by *Ehrlichia chaffeensis*, and human granulocytic ehrlichiosis (HGE), which is caused by a species currently known as the *human granulocytic ehrlichia*. Ehrlichiosis is not uncommon; at Saint Thomas Hospital in Nashville, TN, there have been more than 20 confirmed cases within the past 5 years. Clinical illness begins approximately 7 days after a tick bite and is characterized by high fever with headache. Frequently, there is also malaise, myalgia, nausea, vomiting, and anorexia. Pulmonary infiltrates develop in approximately 50% of patients (65) and at least some patients develop a pleural effusion (66). Frequently the chest radiograph is normal initially, but the condition then progresses rapidly with the development of bilateral pulmonary infiltrates and pleural effusions. It is probable that the infiltrates represent noncardiogenic pulmonary edema with a pathogenesis similar to those with hantavirus syndrome or Rocky Mountain spotted fever. The treatment of choice for ehrlichiosis is doxycycline.

REFERENCES

1. Afessa B. Pleural effusion and pneumothorax in hospitalized patients with HIV infection: The Pulmonary Complications, ICU Support, and Prognostic Factors of Hospitalized Patients With HIV (PIP) Study. *Chest* 2000;117:1031–1037.
2. Cadranel JL, Chouaid C, Denis M, et al. Causes of pleural effusion in 75 HIV-infected patients (Letter). *Chest* 1993;104:655.
3. Batungwanayo J, Taelman H, Allen S, et al. Pleural effusion, tuberculosis and HIV-1 infection in Kigali, Rwanda. *AIDS* 1993;7:73–79.
4. O'Brien RF, Cohn DL. Serosanguineous pleural effusions in AIDS-associated Kaposi's sarcoma. *Chest* 1989;96:460–466.
5. Cesarman E, Knowles DM. Kaposi's sarcoma–associated herpesvirus: a lymphotropic human herpesvirus associated with Kaposi's sarcoma, primary effusion lymphoma, and multicentric Castleman's disease. *Semin Diagn Pathol* 1997;14:54–66.
6. Aboulafia DM. The epidemiologic, pathologic, and clinical features of AIDS-associated pulmonary Kaposi's sarcoma. *Chest* 2000;117:1128–1145.
7. Khalil AM, Carette MF, Cadranel JL, et al. Intrathoracic Kaposi's sarcoma. CT findings. *Chest* 1995;108:1622–1626.
8. Light RW, Hamm H. Pleural disease and the acquired immune deficiency syndrome. *Eur Respir J* 1997;10:2638–2643.
9. Nakamura S, Murakami-Mori K, Rao N, et al. Vascular endothelial growth factor is a potent angiogenic factor in AIDS-associated Kaposi's sarcoma–derived spindle cells. *J Immunol* 1997;158:4992–5001.
10. Huang L, Schnapp LM, Gruden JF, et al. Presentation of AIDS-related pulmonary Kaposi's sarcoma di-

agnosed by bronchoscopy. *Am J Respir Crit Care Med* 1996;153:1385–1390.
11. Ognibene FP, Shelhamer JH. Kaposi's sarcoma. *Clin Chest Med* 1988;9:459–463.
12. Suay V, Cordero PJ, Martinez E, et al. Parapneumonic effusions secondary to community-acquired bacterial pneumonia in human immunodeficiency virus–infected patients. *Eur Respir J* 1995;8:1934–1939.
13. Horowitz ML, Schiff M, Samuels J, et al. *Pneumocystis carinii* pleural effusion. Pathogenesis and pleural fluid analysis. *Am Rev Respir Dis* 1993;148:232–234.
14. Jayes RL, Kamerow HN, Hasselquist SM, et al. Disseminated pneumocystosis presenting as a pleural effusion. *Chest* 1993;103:306–308.
15. Frye MD, Pozsik CJ, Sahn SA. Tuberculous pleurisy is more common in AIDS than in non-AIDS patients with tuberculosis. *Chest* 1997;112:393–397.
16. Cordero PJ, Gil Suay V, Greses JV, et al. The clinical characteristics of pleural tuberculosis in patients with and without human immunodeficiency virus infection. [Translated from Spanish.] *Arch Bronconeumol* 1995;31:512–518.
17. Jones BE, Young SMM, Antoniskis D, et al. Relationship of the manifestations of tuberculosis to CD4 cell counts in patients with human immunodeficiency virus infection. *Am Rev Respir Dis* 1993;148:1292–1297.
18. Relkin F, Aranda CP, Garay SM, et al. Pleural tuberculosis and HIV infection. *Chest* 1994;105:1338–1341.
19. Heyderman RS, Makunike R, Muza T, et al. Pleural tuberculosis in Harare, Zimbabwe: the relationship between human immunodeficiency virus, CD4 lymphocyte count, granuloma formation and disseminated disease. *Trop Med Int Health* 1998;3:14–20.
20. Kitinya JN, Richter C, Perenboom R, et al. Influence of HIV status on pathological changes in tuberculous pleuritis. *Tuberc Lung Dis* 1994;75:195–198.
21. Newman TG, Soni A, Acaron S, et al. Pleural cryptococcosis in the acquired immune deficiency syndrome. *Chest* 1987;91:459–460.
22. Ankobiah WA, Vaidya K, Powell S, et al. Disseminated histoplasmosis in AIDS. Clinicopathologic features in seven patients from a non-endemic area. *NY State J Med* 1990;90:234–288.
23. Uttamchandani RB, Daikos GL, Reyes RR, et al. Nocardiosis in 30 patients with advanced human immunodeficiency virus infection: clinical features and outcome. *Clin Infect Dis* 1994;18:348–353.
24. Aronchick JM, Miller WT. Disseminated nontuberculous mycobacterial infections in immunosuppressed patients. *Semin Roentgenol* 1993;28:150–157.
25. Joseph J, Strange C, Sahn SA. Pleural effusions in hospitalized patients with AIDS. *Ann Intern Med* 1993;118:856–869.
26. Lababidi HMS, Gupta K, Newman T, et al. A retrospective analysis of pleural effusion in human immunodeficiency virus infected patients. *Chest* 1994;106:86S.
27. Alptekin F. An epidemic of pleurisy with effusion in Bitlis, Turkey: study of 559 cases. *US Armed Forces Med J* 1958;9:1–11.
28. Fine NL, Smith LR, Sheedy PF. Frequency of pleural effusions in mycoplasma and viral pneumonias. *N Engl J Med* 1970;283:790–793.
29. Light RW, Girard WM, Jenkinson SG, et al. Parapneumonic effusions. *Am J Med* 1980;69:507–511.

30. Monath TP, Maher M, Casals J, et al. Lassa fever in the Eastern Province of Sierra Leone, 1970–1972. II. Clinical observations and virological studies on selected hospital cases. *Am J Trop Med Hyg* 1974;23: 1140–1149.

31. Gross PA, Gerding DN. Pleural effusion associated with viral hepatitis. *Gastroenterology* 1971;60: 898–902.

32. Cho CT, Hiatt WO, Behbehami AM. Pneumonia and massive pleural effusion associated with adenovirus type 7. *Am J Dis Child* 1973;126:92–94.

33. Goodman ZD, Gupta PK, Frost JK, et al. Cytodiagnosis of viral infections in body cavity fluids. *Acta Cytol* 1979;23:204–208.

34. Charles RE, Katz RL, Ordonez NG, et al. Varicella-zoster infection with pleural involvement. *Am J Clin Pathol* 1986;85:522–526.

35. Bustamante EA, Levy H, Simpson SQ. Pleural fluid characteristics in hantavirus pulmonary syndrome. *Chest* 1997;112:1133–1136.

36. Levy H, Simpson SQ. Hantavirus pulmonary syndrome. *Am J Respir Crit Care Med* 1994;149:1710–1713.

37. Duchin JS, Koster FT, Peters CJ, et al. Hantavirus pulmonary syndrome: a clinical description of 17 patients with a newly recognized disease. The Hantavirus Study Group. *N Engl J Med* 1994;330:949–955.

38. Treanor JJ, Hayden FG. Viral infections. In: Murray JF, Nadel JA, eds. *Textbook of respiratory medicine,* 3rd ed. Philadelphia: WB Saunders, 2000:929–984.

39. Simila S, Ylikorkala O, Wasz-Hockert O. Type 7 adenovirus pneumonia. *J Pediatr* 1971;79:605–611.

40. Han BK, Son JA, Yoon HK, et al. Epidemic adenoviral lower respiratory tract infection in pediatric patients: radiographic and clinical characteristics. *AJR Am J Roentgenol* 1998;170:1077–1080.

41. Katsilabros L, Triandafillou G, Kontoyiannis P, et al. Pleural effusion and hepatitis. *Gastroenterology* 1972; 63:718.

42. Cocchi P, Silenzi M. Pleural effusion in HBsAG-positive hepatitis. *J Pediatr* 1976;89:329–330.

43. Owen RL, Shapiro H. Pleural effusion, rash, and anergy in icteric hepatitis. *N Engl J Med* 1974;291: 963–964.

44. Tabor E, Russell RP, Gerety RJ, et al. Hepatitis B surface antigen and e antigen in pleural effusion: a case report. *Gastroenterology* 1977;73:1157–1159.

45. Sposito M, Petroni VA, Valeri L. Importanza diagnostica dei piccoli versamenti pleurici nella virus epatite. *Epatologia* 1966;12:228–231.

46. Lee HS, Yang PM, Liu BF, et al. Pleural effusion coinciding with acute exacerbations in a patient with chronic hepatitis B. *Gastroenterology* 1989;96:1604–1606.

47. Lander P, Palayew MJ. Infectious mononucleosis: a review of chest roentgenographic manifestations. *J Can Assoc Radiol* 1974;25:303–306.

48. Fermaglich DR. Pulmonary involvement in infectious mononucleosis. *J Pediatr* 1975;86:93–95.

49. Sarkar TK. Infectious mononucleosis with pleural effusion. *Chest* 1969;56:359–360.

50. Laferi H. Pleural effusion and ascites on return from Pakistan. *Lancet* 1997;350:1072.

51. Avirutnan P, Malasit P, Seliger B, et al. Dengue virus infection of human endothelial cells leads to chemokine production, complement activation, and apoptosis. *J Immunol* 1998;161:6338–6346.

52. Thulkar S, Sharma S, Srivastava DN, et al. Sonographic findings in grade III dengue hemorrhagic fever in adults. *J Clin Ultrasound* 2000;28:34–37.

53. Setiawan MW, Samsi TK, Wulur H, et al. Dengue haemorrhagic fever: ultrasound as an aid to predict the severity of the disease. *Pediatr Radiol* 1998;28:1–4.

54. Milder JE, McDearmon SC, Walzer PD. Presumed respiratory syncytial virus pneumonia in an adolescent compromised host. *South Med J* 1979;72:1195–1198.

55. Fulginiti VA, Eller JJ, Downie AW, et al. Altered reactivity to measles virus. *JAMA* 1967;202:1075–1080.

56. Trudo FJ, Gopez EV, Gupta PK, et al. Pleural effusion due to herpes simplex type II infection in an immunocompromised host. *Am J Respir Crit Care Med* 1997;155:371– 373.

57. Mansel JK, Rosenow EC III, Smith TF, et al. *Mycoplasma pneumoniae* pneumonia. *Chest* 1989;95:639– 646.

58. Decancq HG Jr, Lee FA. *Mycoplasma pneumoniae* pneumonia. *JAMA* 1965;194;1010–1011.

59. Grix A, Giammona ST. Pneumonitis with pleural effusion in children due to *Mycoplasma pneumoniae*. *Am Rev Respir Dis* 1974;109:665–671.

60. Nagayama Y, Sakurai N, Tamai K, et al. Isolation of *Mycoplasma pneumoniae* from pleural fluid and/or cerebrospinal fluid: report of four cases. *Scand J Infect Dis* 1987;19:521–524.

61. Sobradillo V, Ansola P, Baranda F, et al. Q fever pneumonia: a review of 164 community-acquired cases in the Basque country. *Eur Respir J* 1989;2:263–266.

62. Gordon JK, MacKeen AD, Marrie TJ, et al. The radiographic features of epidemic and sporadic Q fever pneumonia. *J Can Assoc Radiol* 1984;35:293–296.

63. Esteban C, Oribe M, Fernandez A, et al. Increased adenosine deaminase activity in Q fever pneumonia with pleural effusion. *Chest* 1994;105:648.

64. Murphy PP, Richardson SG. Q fever pneumonia presenting as an eosinophilic pleural effusion. *Thorax* 1989;44:228–229.

65. Byrd RP Jr, Vasquez J, Roy TM. Respiratory manifestations of tick-borne diseases in the Southeastern United States. *South Med J* 1997;90:1–4.

66. Fordham LA, Chung CJ, Specter BB, et al. Ehrlichiosis: findings on chest radiographs in three pediatric patients. *AJR Am J Roentgenol* 1998;171:1421–1424.

14

Pleural Effusion Due to Pulmonary Embolization

The disorder most commonly overlooked in the workup of a patient with pleural effusion is pulmonary embolization. The possibility of pulmonary embolization should be excluded in every patient with a pleural effusion of uncertain origin.

INCIDENCE

It is estimated that at least 500,000 persons have a pulmonary embolic event each year in this country (1). Because pleural effusions occur in 30% to 50% of patients with pulmonary emboli (2–4), over 150,000–250,000 pleural effusions secondary to pulmonary emboli should occur annually. Therefore, one should expect to see more cases of pleural effusions secondary to pulmonary embolization than to bronchogenic carcinoma. Nevertheless, in most large series, pulmonary embolization accounts for fewer than 5% of the pleural effusions. This discrepancy probably occurs because the diagnosis is frequently not considered in patients with undiagnosed pleural effusions. Indeed, in a recent epidemiologic study from the Czech Republic, pulmonary embolism was the fourth leading cause of pleural effusion (5).

It is likely that pulmonary embolism is responsible for a substantial fraction of undiagnosed pleural effusions. Gunnels (6) followed 27 patients with exudative pleural effusions in whom no diagnosis was established after an initial workup, including pleural biopsy. Of the 19 patients who did not have malignant disease, two subsequently died, and both had pulmonary emboli at autopsy. One wonders how many of the remaining 17 patients might have had pulmonary emboli if this diagnosis had been considered. Along the same lines, Storey et al. (7) reported on a series of 133 patients with pleural effusions in which only three were due to pulmonary emboli, but causes were not determined in 25 patients. Because these authors do not mention any evaluation of their patients for pulmonary emboli, one wonders how many of the 25 patients would have been switched from the undetermined category to the pulmonary embolus category if the possibility of pulmonary embolus had been explored.

PATHOPHYSIOLOGIC MECHANISMS

Pulmonary embolization appears to produce a pleural effusion by two distinct mechanisms. First, the obstruction of the pulmonary vasculature can lead to the development of right-sided heart failure and increased pressures in the capillaries in the parietal pleura. This increased pressure increases pleural fluid formation (see Chapter 2) and can lead to pleural fluid accumulation (8). The pleural fluid is a transudate with this mechanism. In the series of 29 patients with pleural effusions secondary to pulmonary embolization reported by Bynum and Wilson (9), seven (24%) had transudative pleural effusions.

The second mechanism by which pulmonary emboli can produce pleural effusion is by increasing the permeability of the capillaries in the lung. The interstitial fluid that results from this increased permeability traverses the visceral pleura and leads to the accumulation of pleural fluid. In the experimental situation, it has been shown (10) that more than 20% of the fluid formed in the lung with increased permeability pulmonary edema is cleared through the pleural space. It is probable that ischemia of the capillaries in the visceral pleura plays at most a minor role because these capillaries are supplied by the bronchial circulation (11). Leckie and Tothill (12) have demonstrated that patients with exudative pleural effusion secondary to pulmonary emboli have a large amount of protein entering and leaving the pleural space. The main factor responsible for the increased permeability of the pulmonary capillaries is probably the release of inflammatory mediators from the platelet-rich thrombi. It is possible that vascular endothelial growth factor (VEGF) may play a role in the formation of pleural fluid in at least some patients, because the pleural fluid VEGF level was very high in one patient with pulmonary embolism (13). The release of such mediators can increase the permeability of the capillaries in either the visceral pleura or the lung. Ischemia of the capillaries distal to the embolus may also contribute to the increased permeability.

CLINICAL MANIFESTATIONS

Symptoms and Signs

There are three symptom complexes associated with pulmonary emboli: (a) pleuritic pain or hemoptysis, (b) isolated dyspnea, and (c) circulatory collapse. In the Prospective Investigation of Pulmonary Embolism Diagnosis (PIOPED) study, 56% of the 119 patients with pleuritic chest pain or hemoptysis had pleural effusion, 26% of those with isolated dyspnea had pleural effusion, and none with circulatory collapse had pleural effusion (14). More than 75% of patients with pleural effusions secondary to pulmonary emboli have pleuritic chest pain (15), which is almost invariably on the side of the effusion (2). Indeed, the presence of pleuritic chest pain in a patient with pleural effusion is suggestive of pulmonary embolus. In one series, pulmonary emboli were present in 12 of 22 patients (55%) younger than the age of 40 who presented as outpatients with pleural effusion and pleuritic chest pain (16).

Dyspnea, also present in more than 70% of patients (15, 17), is usually out of proportion to the size of the pleural effusion. Cough and apprehension are present in approximately 50% of patients (15, 17). Nearly 50% of these patients are febrile (17) but less than 10% have temperatures above 38.5°C (15, 17). Approximately 15% have hemoptysis (15). Most patients have a respiratory rate above 20 per min, and tachycardia above 100 per min occurs in about 30% (15). In the PIOPED study, 113 of 117 patients (97%) with no preexisting cardiac or pulmonary disease had dyspnea or tachypnea or pleuritic chest pain (15).

Chest Radiograph

When a pleural effusion is secondary to pulmonary emboli, an associated parenchymal infiltrate may or may not be present. In one series of 62 patients with pleural effusions secondary to pulmonary embolism, 28 (45%) had no associated infiltrate (2), but in another series of 20 patients (18), only 1 (5%) did not have an associated infiltrate. In a third series of 10 patients with pulmonary emboli and bilateral pleural effusions, only three (30%) had parenchymal infiltrates (19). Infiltrates are usually in the lower lobes, are pleura based, and are convex toward the hilum. Patients with an embolic occlusion of segmental pulmonary arteries are more likely to have infiltrates than those with an embolic occlusion of the central arteries (18).

The pleural effusions secondary to pulmonary emboli are small, with the mean size equal to about 15% of the hemithorax (2). In the PIOPED study, 48 of the 56 effusions (86%) were manifest only as blunting of the costophrenic angle and in no patient did the pleural effusion occupy more than one third of a hemithorax (15). If parenchymal infiltrates are present, the pleural effusions are larger. In one series, the pleural effusion occupied greater than 15% of the hemithorax in 74% of the patients with parenchymal infiltrates but in only 21% of those without parenchymal infiltrates (2). The pleural effusions are usually unilateral, but in a recent series, chest computed tomography (CT) demonstrated bilateral pleural fluid in six of 13 patients with pulmonary embolization (20).

Pleural Fluid Findings

In patients with pulmonary emboli, analysis of the pleural fluid is not helpful in establishing the diagnosis because the pleural fluid associated with pulmonary emboli can vary widely. Nevertheless, a thoracentesis should be performed in patients suspected of having pulmonary emboli to exclude other causes of pleural effusion such as tuberculosis, malignant disease, or pneumonia with a parapneumonic effusion.

As mentioned previously, the pleural fluid may be either a transudate or an exudate, depending on the mechanism of its production. The pleural fluid is not always blood tinged or bloody. The pleural fluid red blood cell count (RBC) is below 10,000 per mm^3 in about 30% of effusions secondary to pulmonary emboli, whether they are transudates or exudates. The pleural fluid RBC exceeds 100,000 per mm^3 in fewer than 20% of such effusions (9). The pleural fluid white blood cell count (WBC) ranges from under 100 to over 50,000 cells per mm^3 (9). The differential WBC may reveal predominantly polymorphonuclear leukocytes or lymphocytes (9). Spriggs and Boddington (21) have reported that pleural effusions secondary to pulmonary emboli frequently have large numbers of mesothelial cells or eosinophils.

DIAGNOSIS

The diagnosis of pulmonary embolization should be considered in every patient with a pleural effusion. Because the patient may or may not have fever, chest pain, or a parenchymal infiltrate, and because the pleural fluid may be either a transudate or an exudate, all patients who have a pleural effusion with no clear-cut etiology should be evaluated for pulmonary emboli. Even patients with pleural effusions and obvious congestive heart failure may have pulmonary emboli. In an autopsy series of 290 patients with congestive heart failure and pleural effusions, 60 (21%) had pulmonary emboli (22). The possibility of pulmonary embolization should be considered in patients with heart failure in whom the effusions are unilateral or bilateral but greatly disparate in size.

In the past, the perfusion lung scan was the procedure of choice as the initial screening procedure for pulmonary emboli. More recently, contrast-enhanced CT using spiral or electron-beam technique has become the method of choice in many centers (23). For the reasons detailed later, spiral CT scan appears to be the initial procedure of choice for the patient with an undiagnosed pleural effusion. In some instances, particularly if a perfusion lung scan is used as the initial test, a pulmonary arteriogram will have to be performed. The pulmonary arteriogram remains the gold standard for the diagnosis of pulmonary embolism.

Lung Scans

In general, the perfusion lung scan has significant limitations in the diagnosis of pulmonary embolism. If the perfusion lung scan is negative, a pulmonary embolus is virtually ruled out. If the perfusion lung scan is a high-probability lung scan, 87% of the patients will have pulmonary emboli, and when coupled with a high clinical probability of embolism, the positive predicted value increases to 96% (1). However, the patients most likely to have a pleural effusion are those with pleuritic pain or hemoptysis, and less than one third of these patients will have a high-probability lung scan (14).

If a pleural effusion is present, the perfusion lung scan is even more difficult to interpret (Fig. 14.1). A large effusion severely restricts the ability of the lung to expand and causes a shift of perfusion to the contralateral lung (24). Small, mobile effusions of any origin may gravitate to different regions of the pleural space, depending on the position of the patient at the time of the examination. For example, fluid may enter the major fissures when the patient lies down and produce a perfusion defect on the lung scan, when no comparable defect is seen on the erect chest radiograph. Similarly, mismatching of the ventilation and perfusion lung scans can be produced by the pleural fluid itself when the scans are obtained in different positions (Fig. 14.1) (24). For these reasons, a therapeutic thoracentesis (see Chapter 25) should be performed before obtaining the lung scan whenever feasible.

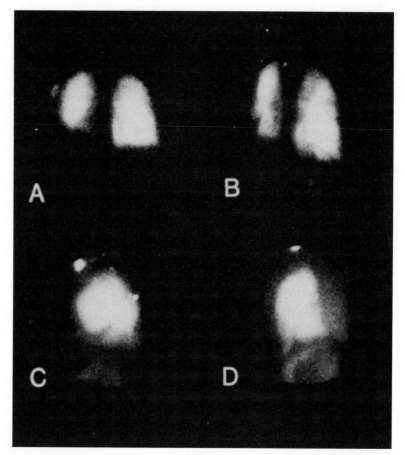

FIG. 14.1. Influence of pleural fluid on lung scans. Posterior perfusion lung scans with the patient upright **(A)** and in the left lateral decubitus **(B)** position from a patient with a left pleural effusion. Note the marked difference in the configuration of the left lung as the patient's position is changed, owing to shifts in the pleural fluid. Left lateral scans with the same patient upright **(C)** and supine **(D)**. The perfusion defect seen posteriorly with the patient upright disappears when the patient is supine. (Courtesy of Norah Milne, M.D.)

Spiral (Helical) Computed Tomography

In many centers, the spiral CT scan is being used rather than the perfusion scan as the initial screening test for pulmonary emboli. The diagnosis of pulmonary embolism is based on the presence of partial or complete filling defects on the contrast-enhanced CT (Fig. 14.2). In general, the spiral CT detects between 75% and 100% of emboli and the specificity of the test exceeds 90%. Spiral CT has its greatest sensitivity for detecting emboli in the main, lobar, or segmental pulmonary arteries (25). This should not be too much of a problem because in the PIOPED study, only 6%

of the patients with pulmonary emboli had isolated subsegmental emboli (26). A big advantage of the spiral CT over the perfusion lung scan is the information it provides regarding pleural thickening, parenchymal abnormalities, lymphadenopathy, and concomitant pericardial disease.

Impedance Plethysmogram and Venogram

Another approach for establishing the diagnosis of pulmonary emboli is to study the veins in the legs. The basis for this approach is that over 90% of pulmonary emboli originate from

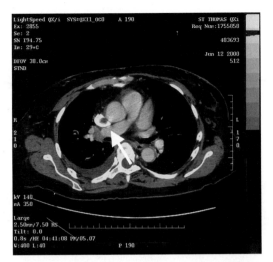

FIG. 14.2. Spiral CT showing a small right pleural effusion, a peripheral infiltrate in the right lower lobe, and a dark area in the artery to the right lower lobe *(arrow)* that represents the pulmonary embolus.

the deep venous system in the legs. Therefore, if the deep venous system of the legs is normal, the patient probably does not have a pulmonary embolus. Electrical impedance plethysmography (IPG) has been extensively evaluated during the last decade for its utility as a screening test for pulmonary embolism. It does not appear sufficiently sensitive to serve as a good screening test for pulmonary emboli. In one series of 83 patients with pulmonary emboli demonstrated angiographically, only 36 (43%) had a positive IPG (27). Similarly, in another series of 41 patients with pulmonary emboli, only 71% had positive venograms of the lower extremities (27). Accordingly, it appears that neither IPG nor lower extremity venograms are good screening tests for patients suspected of having pulmonary emboli.

TREATMENT

The treatment of the patient with pleural effusion secondary to pulmonary embolization is the same as that for any patient with pulmonary emboli. Since the last edition of this book in 1995, low-molecular-weight heparins (LMWHs) have become the initial drugs of choice for the treatment of pulmonary embolism (28). The advantages of LMWHs compared with unfractionated heparin include the following: (a) improved bioavailability and a longer half-life; (b) a more predictable dose-response curve so that laboratory monitoring is rarely needed; (c) less frequent heparin-induced thrombocytopenia; and (d) less heparin-associated osteopenia. After the initial administration of LMWHs, the patient should be treated with oral anticoagulants. With treatment, pleural effusions gradually resolve, particularly if no infiltrates are present. In one series, the effusions had cleared completely after 7 days of therapy in 18 of 28 patients (64%) without parenchymal infiltrates, but in none of 30 patients with parenchymal infiltrates (2).

The presence of bloody pleural fluid is not a contraindication to the administration of LMWHs. Bynum and Wilson (9) treated three patients who had pleural fluid RBC greater than 100,000 per mm^3 with intravenous heparin, and in none did the effusion increase in size.

If the pleural effusion increases in size with anticoagulant therapy or if a contralateral pleural effusion develops, the patient probably has recurrent emboli or another complication. In one series, two patients developed an enlarged ipsilateral effusion and one had recurrent pulmonary emboli, whereas the other had developed infected pleural fluid (2). Two other patients developed contralateral pleural effusions, and both had recurrent emboli.

On rare occasions, the administration of anticoagulants to patients with pulmonary emboli can lead to the development of a hemothorax. Rostan et al. (29) reviewed 11 such cases and reported that the clotting studies were within an acceptable range when the hemothorax occurred in seven of the patients. Hemothorax developed within the first week of anticoagulation in nine of the 11 reported cases and developed on the side of the embolus in each of these patients. In two patients, the hemothorax developed while they were receiving long-term anticoagulation. When a pleural effusion increases in size in a patient with pulmonary emboli, a diagnostic thoracentesis should be performed to rule out a complicated parapneumonic effusion or a hemothorax. If bloody pleural fluid is obtained, the hematocrit of the pleural fluid should be determined. If the hematocrit on the pleural fluid is greater than 50% of that of the peripheral blood, anticoagulation should be discontinued and chest tubes should be inserted (see Chapter 22).

PLEURAL EFFUSIONS WITH RIGHT-SIDED ENDOCARDITIS AND SEPTIC EMBOLI

Patients who have right-sided endocarditis may have septic pulmonary emboli and pleural effusions (30). The incidence of pleural effusion with right-sided endocarditis is about 25% (30). The pleural fluid is an exudate, and the cultures are usually negative. The differential cell count can reveal neutrophils, lymphocytes, or mono-mesothelial cells (30). The pleural fluid lactate dehydrogenase (LDH) is usually greater than the serum LDH and may be elevated to 10 times or more the upper limit for serum.

PLEURAL EFFUSIONS WITH LEMIERRE'S SYNDROME

Lemierre's syndrome is a rare life-threatening septic thrombophlebitis of a jugular vein with anaerobic septicemia (31). The most common pathogen associated with the syndrome is *Fusobacterium necrophorum.* Patients with Lemierre's syndrome frequently have septic pulmonary emboli and may develop pleural effusions and empyema. Lemierre's syndrome should be suspected in febrile patients with painful thrombophlebitis of the jugular vein. The treatment for the syndrome is high doses of intravenous antibiotics with anaerobic activity. If the pleural effusion is infected, tube thoracostomy or thoracoscopy with the breakdown of adhesions may be necessary.

PLEURAL EFFUSIONS WITH SICKLE CELL ANEMIA

There is a high incidence of pleural effusions in patients with sickle cell anemia who develop the acute chest syndrome. In one recent series of 107 episodes of the acute chest syndrome in 77 adults, unilateral pleural effusions were present in 35%, whereas bilateral pleural effusions were present in 14% (32). The pathogenesis of these effusions is not definitely known but is believed to be either *in situ* thrombosis of the pulmonary arteries or fat embolization (32). The characteristics of the pleural fluid associated with the acute chest syndrome with sickle cell anemia are not known.

REFERENCES

1. Fedullo PF. Pulmonary thromboembolism. In: Murray JF, Nadel JA, eds. *Textbook of respiratory medicine*, 3rd ed. Philadelphia: WB Saunders, 2000:1503–1531.
2. Bynum LJ, Wilson JE III. Radiographic features of pleural effusions in pulmonary embolism. *Am Rev Respir Dis* 1978;117:829–834.
3. Worsley DF, Alavi A, Aronchick JM, et al. Chest radiographic findings in patients with acute pulmonary embolism: observations from the PIOPED study. *Radiology* 1993;189:133–136.
4. Stein PD, Athanasoulis C, Greenspan RH, et al. Relation of plain chest radiographic findings to pulmonary arterial pressure and arterial blood oxygen levels in patients with acute pulmonary embolism. *Am J Cardiol* 1992;69:394–396.
5. Marel M, Arustova M, Stasny B, et al. Incidence of pleural effusion in a well-defined region: epidemiologic study in central Bohemia. *Chest* 1993;104:1486–1489.
6. Gunnels JJ. Perplexing pleural effusion. *Chest* 1978;74:390–393.
7. Storey DD, Dines DE, Coles DT. Pleural effusion: a diagnostic dilemma. *JAMA* 1976;236:2183–2186.
8. Mellins RB, Levine OR, Fishman AP. Effect of systemic and pulmonary venous hypertension on pleural and pericardial fluid accumulation. *J Appl Physiol* 1970;29:564–569.
9. Bynum LJ, Wilson JE III. Characteristics of pleural effusions associated with pulmonary embolism. *Arch Intern Med* 1976;136:159–162.
10. Wiener-Kronish JP, Broaddus VC, Albertine KH, et al. Relationship of pleural effusions to increased permeability pulmonary edema in anesthetized sheep. *J Clin Invest* 1988;82:1422–1429.
11. Albertine KH, Wiener-Kronish JP, Roos PJ, et al. Structure, blood supply, and lymphatic vessels of the sheep's visceral pleura. *Am J Anat* 1982;165:277–294.
12. Leckie WJH, Tothill P. Albumin turnover in pleural effusions. *Clin Sci* 1965;29:339–352.
13. Cheng C-S, Rodriguez RM, Perkett EA, et al. Vascular endothelial growth factor in pleural fluid. *Chest* 1999;115:760–765.
14. Stein PD, Henry JW. Clinical characteristics of patients with acute pulmonary embolism stratified according to their presenting syndromes. *Chest* 1997;112:974–979.
15. Stein PD, Terrin ML, Hales CA, et al. Clinical, laboratory, roentgenographic, and electrocardiographic findings in patients with acute pulmonary embolism and no pre-existing cardiac or pulmonary disease. *Chest* 1991;100:598–603.
16. Branch WR, McNeil BJ. Analysis of the differential

diagnosis and assessment of pleuritic chest pain in young adults. *Am J Med* 1983;75:671–679.

17. Bell WR, Simon TL, DeMets DL. The clinical features of submassive and massive pulmonary emboli. *Am J Med* 1977;62:355–360.

18. Dalen JE, Haffajee CI, Alpert JS III, et al. Pulmonary embolism, pulmonary hemorrhage and pulmonary infarction. *N Engl J Med* 1977;296:1431–1435.

19. Rabin CB, Blackman NS. Bilateral pleural effusion: its significance in association with a heart of normal size. *J Mt Sinai Hosp* 1957;24:45–63.

20. Coche EE, Muller NL, Kim KI, et al. Acute pulmonary embolism: ancillary findings at spiral CT. *Radiology* 1998;207:753–758.

21. Spriggs AI, Boddington MM. *The cytology of effusions*, 2nd ed. New York: Grune & Stratton, 1968.

22. Race GA, Scheifley CH, Edward JE. Hydrothorax in congestive heart failure. *Am J Med* 1957;22:83–89.

23. Fraser RS, Muller NL, Colman N, et al. *Diagnosis of diseases of the chest*, 4th ed. Philadelphia: WB Saunders, 2000:2659–2695.

24. Baum S, Vincent NR, Lyons KP, et al. *Atlas of nuclear medicine imaging*. New York: Appleton-Century-Crofts, 1981.

25. Clinical Practice Guideline. The diagnostic approach to acute venous thromboembolism. *Am J Respir Crit Care Med* 1999;160:1043–1066.

26. The PIOPED Investigators. Value of the ventilation/perfusion scan in acute pulmonary embolism. *JAMA* 1990;263:2753–2759.

27. Hull RD, Hirsh J, Carter CJ, et al. Pulmonary angiography, ventilation lung scanning, and venography for clinically suspected pulmonary embolism with abnormal perfusion lung scan. *Ann Intern Med* 1983;98:891–899.

28. Aguilar D, Goldhaber SZ. Clinical uses of low-molecular-weight heparins. *Chest* 1999;115:1418–1423.

29. Rostand RA, Feldman RL, Block ER. Massive hemothorax complicating heparin anticoagulation for pulmonary embolus. *South Med J* 1977;70:1128–1130.

30. Sexauer WP, Quezado Z, Lippmann ML, et al. Pleural effusions in right-sided endocarditis: characteristics and pathophysiology. *South Med J* 1992;85:1176–1180.

31. Alifano M, Venissac N, Guillot F, et al. Lemierre's syndrome with bilateral empyema thoracis. *Ann Thorac Surg* 2000;69:930–931.

32. Maitre B, Habibi A, Roudot-Thoraval F, et al. Acute chest syndrome in adults with sickle cell disease. *Chest* 2000;117:1386–1392.

15

Pleural Effusion Secondary to Diseases of the Gastrointestinal Tract

Diseases of the gastrointestinal tract are sometimes associated with pleural effusion. In this chapter, the exudative pleural effusions resulting from pancreatic disease, intraabdominal abscesses, esophageal perforation, abdominal operations, diaphragmatic hernia, variceal sclerotherapy, hepatic transplantation, and disease of the biliary tract are discussed. The transudative pleural effusion that occurs with cirrhosis and ascites is discussed in Chapter 6.

PANCREATIC DISEASE

Four different types of nonmalignant pancreatic disease can have an accompanying pleural effusion: acute pancreatitis, pancreatic abscess, chronic pancreatitis with pseudocyst, and pancreatic ascites.

Acute Pancreatitis

In older reports, the incidence of pleural effusion with acute pancreatitis was relatively low (3% to 17%) (1, 2). More recent reports, however, have documented a much higher incidence of pleural effusion. Lankisch et al. (3) obtained computed tomography (CT) scans of the chest within 72 hours of admission in 133 consecutive patients with their first attack of acute pancreatitis and reported that 50% of the patients had a pleural effusion. The effusions were bilateral in 77%, left sided in 16%, and right sided in 8%. The thickness of the fluid on the CT scan was less than 10 mm in 32 patients, 1 to 2 cm in 18 patients, and greater than 2 cm in 16 patients with the CT scans (3).

The presence of a pleural effusion in patients with acute pancreatitis is an indication of more severe pancreatitis (4). In one series, the incidence of pleural effusion was 84% in 19 patients with severe pancreatitis but only 8.6% in 116 patients with mild pancreatitis (4). The presence of a pleural effusion is also associated with the development of a pseudocyst. In the series of Lankisch et al. (3), 29% of 66 patients with pleural effusions had pancreatic pseudocysts compared with 6% of 67 patients without pleural effusions.

The exudative pleural effusion accompanying acute pancreatitis results primarily from the transdiaphragmatic transfer of the exudative fluid arising from acute pancreatic inflammation and from diaphragmatic inflammation (2). Numerous lymphatic networks join the peritoneal and pleural aspects of the diaphragm (1). Anatomically, the tail of the pancreas is in direct contact with the diaphragm. Hence, the exudate resulting from acute pancreatic inflammation, which is rich in pancreatic enzymes, enters the lymphatic vessels on the peritoneal side of the diaphragm and is conveyed to the pleural side of the diaphragm. Because this fluid contains high levels of pancreatic enzymes, the permeability of the lymphatic vessels is increased, and fluid leaks from the pleural lymphatic vessels into the pleural space. The high enzymatic content of the pancreatic exudate may also cause partial or complete obstruction of the pleural lymphatic vessels that leads to more pleural fluid formation (1). Of course, the diaphragm itself may be inflamed from the adjacent inflammatory process, and this inflammation may increase the permeability of the capillaries in the diaphragmatic pleura. This mechanism cannot be entirely responsible for the pleural fluid accumulation, because the pleural fluid amylase concentration is almost always higher than the simultaneous serum amylase.

In the patient with acute pancreatitis, the clinical picture is usually dominated by abdominal symptoms including pain, nausea, and vomiting. At times, however, respiratory symptoms consisting of pleuritic chest pain and dyspnea may dominate the clinical picture. The chest radiograph may reveal, in addition to the small- to moderate-sized pleural effusion, an elevated diaphragm and basilar infiltrates (5). In addition, on ultrasound or fluoroscopy, the diaphragm is sluggish or immobile. The clinical picture may look much like that of pneumonia or pulmonary embolism complicated by pleural effusion.

The diagnosis is usually established by demonstrating an elevated serum amylase or lipase level in a patient with abdominal symptoms. In a patient with the typical clinical picture for pancreatitis, a thoracentesis need not be performed. If the patient has a large pleural effusion and the patient is dyspneic, a therapeutic thoracentesis should be performed to relieve the dyspnea. If the patient is persistently febrile, a thoracentesis should be performed to rule out an empyema.

In patients with acute pancreatitis, the pleural fluid amylase level is usually elevated (1). Ball and I reported on five patients with pleural effusions secondary to pancreatic disease (6), and in one of the patients, the pleural fluid amylase was originally within normal limits for serum, but subsequent pleural fluid amylase levels were elevated. The pleural fluid amylase level is usually higher than the serum amylase (1, 6) and remains elevated longer than the serum amylase. The pleural fluid amylase level in patients with acute pancreatitis and pleural effusion tends to be lower than that in patients with chronic pancreatic disease (2). Levels of phospholipase A2 are also elevated in patients with acute pancreatitis (7).

Other characteristics of the pleural fluid with pancreatic disease are as follows. The pleural fluid is an exudate with high protein and lactate dehydrogenase (LDH) levels. Frequently, the pleural fluid is serosanguineous, and it can be bloody. The pleural fluid glucose level is comparable to that of the serum (6). The pleural fluid differential white blood cell count (WBC) usually reveals predominantly polymorphonuclear leukocytes, and the pleural fluid WBC can vary from 1,000 to 50,000 cells per mm^3 (6).

In the patient with acute pancreatitis, the pleural effusion usually resolves as the pancreatic inflammation subsides. If the pleural effusion does not resolve within 2 weeks of treatment of the pancreatic disease, the possibility of a pancreatic abscess or a pancreatic pseudocyst must be considered.

Pancreatic Abscess

Pancreatic abscess usually follows an episode of acute pancreatitis. Typically, the acute pancreatitis initially responds to therapy, but 10 to 21 days later, the patient becomes febrile with abdominal pain and leukocytosis (8). The diagnosis is also suggested if a patient with acute pancreatitis does not respond to the usual therapy within several days (8). It is important to establish the diagnosis because the mortality rate approaches 100% if the abscess is not drained surgically (8). Both ultrasound (8) and abdominal CT scanning (9) are useful in establishing the diagnosis of pancreatic abscess preoperatively. Pleural effusion occurs commonly in patients with pancreatic abscess. In one series of 63 patients, 38% had pleural effusions (8). Although pleural fluid findings were not described in this series, another patient with a pleural effusion associated with pancreatic abscess had a high pleural fluid amylase level (10). The other complication that can cause a pleural effusion to persist in patients with acute pancreatitis is a pancreatic pseudocyst.

Pancreatic Pseudocyst and Chronic Pancreatic Pleural Effusion

A pancreatic pseudocyst is not a true cyst but rather a collection of fluid and debris rich in pancreatic enzymes near or within the pancreas. The walls consist of granulation tissue without an epithelial lining (11). About 10% of patients with acute pancreatitis have a clinically significant pseudocyst (12). Approximately 5% of patients with a pancreatic pseudocyst have a pleural effusion (12). Pleural effusions due to pancreatic pseudocysts are relatively uncommon. By 1990, only 96 cases had been reported in the English literature (12). Between 1983 and 1989, there were only seven cases at the Moffitt-Long and San Francisco General Hospitals (12).

The mechanism responsible for the pleural effusion in patients with a chronic pseudocyst is the development of a direct sinus tract between the pancreas and the pleural space (10, 13). When the pancreatic ductal system is disrupted, the extruded pancreatic fluid sometimes passes through the aortic or esophageal hiatus into the mediastinum. Once in the mediastinum, the process either can be contained, to form a mediastinal pseudocyst, or it may decompress into one or both pleural spaces. Once fluid enters the pleural space, the pancreaticopleural fistula is likely to result in a massive chronic pleural effusion.

Most patients with chronic pancreatic pleural effusion are men. In more than 90% of male patients, the pancreatic disease is a result of alcoholism (12, 14). Chest symptoms usually dominate the clinical picture of the patient with chronic pancreatic disease and a pleural effusion (14). These patients report chest pain and shortness of breath. In one series of 101 patients from Japan, 42 complained of dyspnea and 29 complained of chest and back pain, whereas only 23 complained of upper abdominal pain (14). The explanation for the lack of abdominal symptoms is that the pancreaticopleural fistula decompresses the pseudocyst. Weight loss is common in patients with chronic pancreatic pleural effusions (12). The pleural effusion is usually large, sometimes occupying the entire hemithorax. In the majority of cases the effusion is unilateral and left sided, but about 20% are unilateral and right sided. Fifteen percent are bilateral (12, 14). If a therapeutic thoracentesis is performed, the pleural effusion reaccumulates rapidly. In one patient, over 13 L of pleural fluid were removed during three separate thoracenteses over a short period (15). Because chest symptoms dominate the clinical picture and some patients have no history of prior pancreatic disease, the diagnosis is easily missed unless the pleural fluid amylase is measured.

The diagnosis of a chronic pancreatic pleural effusion should be suspected in any individual with a large pleural effusion who appears to be chronically ill or has a history of pancreatic disease or abdominal trauma (16). Many patients have no history of pancreatic disease (12). The best screening test for chronic pancreatic pleural effusion is to measure the pleural fluid amylase. The pleural fluid amylase is usually markedly elevated ($>1,000$ U per L) (16), whereas the serum amylase may be normal or mildly elevated (16). An elevated pleural fluid amylase level is not diagnostic of pancreatic disease, as discussed in Chapter 4.

The other main diagnosis to consider in a patient with a chronic pleural effusion with a high amylase level is malignant disease. Approximately 10% of patients with a malignant pleural effusion have an elevated pleural fluid amylase level (6). With malignancy, the cytology is frequently positive. In addition, it is uncommon to have a malignant pleural effusion with an amylase above 1,000 U per L. If there is difficulty in distinguishing between these two entities, the differentiation can be made by obtaining amylase isoenzymes on the pleural fluid. With malignant effusions, the amylase is of the salivary rather than the pancreatic type (17).

The diagnosis can usually be established by CT of the chest and abdomen, which frequently shows both the pseudocyst and the sinus tract (12). Endoscopic retrograde cholangiopancreatography (ERCP) also plays an important role in the evaluation and management of patients with pancreaticopleural fistula. ERCP is useful in delineating the ductal structure, the pseudocyst, and the fistulous connection to the pleura through the sinus tract (12). The greatest utility for ERCP is in defining the precise anatomic relationship preoperatively so that a direct and expeditious surgical procedure can be planned. Recently, some patients have been successfully treated by placing stents in the pancreatic duct at the time the ERCP is performed (18).

The initial therapy of a patient with a pancreatic pseudocyst and a pleural effusion should probably be nonoperative. The theory behind conservative therapy is that if pancreatic secretions are minimized, the pseudocyst will regress and the sinus tract will close. Accordingly, a nasogastric tube is inserted and the patient is given intravenous hyperalimentation. It is probable that the patients are benefited if they are given somatostatin or octreotide, a synthetic analog of somatostatin (19). Somatostatin has numerous inhibitory actions on gastrointestinal functions, one of which is its inhibitory effect on pancreatic exocrine secretion (12). It has been shown that somatostatin decreases the output from an external pancreatic fistula by more than 80% (20). Some authors recommend serial thoracentesis and subsequent tube thoracostomy if the effusions recur, but there in no evidence that such procedures are beneficial.

If after 2 weeks, the patient remains symptomatic and the pleural fluid continues to accumulate, surgical intervention should be considered. Approximately 50% of patients require surgery. Surgery is more likely to be required in patients with more severe pancreatic disease (19). Before surgery, an endoscopic retrograde pancreatogram and an abdominal CT scan should be performed to aid in planning the surgical procedure (21). For example, if a leak from the duct or pseudocyst is demonstrated in the distal portion of the gland, distal pancreatectomy will be curative. If a direct pancreatic duct leak is found in the more proximal portion of the gland, without a pseudocyst, a direct anastomosis between the leak and a Roux-en-Y jejunal loop or a Whipple resection should be considered. Conversely, if a large cyst is present within the body of the gland, internal drainage should be performed either into the stomach or with a Roux-en-Y jejunal loop. Procedures that do not focus on removal of the disrupted portion of the gland or on drainage of the pseudocyst usually fail. If the preoperative ERCP is unsuccessful, pancreatography may be performed at the time of surgery (12).

An alternative approach to the patient with a pancreatic pseudocyst is to drain the pseudocyst percutaneously. Under CT guidance, a catheter is introduced through the anterior abdominal wall, and then through the anterior and then the posterior wall of the stomach into the pseudocyst cavity. Side holes are cut into the part of the catheter that lies in the pseudocyst and that which lies in the stomach. Maintenance of this drainage for 15 to 20 days is thought to create a fistulous tract between the pseudocyst and stomach akin to surgical marsupialization. In one series, 20 of 26 patients (77%) were cured by this procedure (22). To my knowledge, there are no randomized studies comparing the results with surgery and with percutaneous drainage of pseudocysts.

The prognosis of patients with pancreaticopleural fistula appears to be favorable (12). In the series of 96 patients reviewed by Rockey and Cello (12), the overall mortality rate was 5%, and three patients died of unrelated illnesses during their follow-up period. Both patients who died as a direct result of the pancreatic process were managed conservatively and died of sepsis.

In patients with chronic pleural effusions secondary to pancreatic disease, the pleural surfaces may become thickened, and in several patients, decortications have been performed (23). However, because the pleural thickening gradually improves spontaneously, decortication should be delayed for at least 6 months following definitive treatment of the pancreatic disease in order to ascertain whether the pleural disease will resolve spontaneously.

One rare complication of pancreatic pleural effusion is the development of a bronchopleural fistula. Kaye (1) reported one such patient in whom the development of the bronchopleural fistula was heralded by the expectoration of copious quantities of clear yellow fluid. In this situation, chest tubes should be inserted immediately to drain the pleural space and to protect the lung from the fluid with its high enzymatic content.

Pancreatic Ascites

Some patients with pancreatic disease develop ascites characterized by high amylase and protein levels (19, 24). The genesis of the ascites is leakage of fluid from a pseudocyst directly into the peritoneal cavity or a sinus tract from the pseudocyst into the peritoneal cavity. If such a patient should happen to have a defect in his diaphragm, he will develop a large pleural effusion as a result of the flow of fluid from the peritoneal to the pleural cavity in the same way that pleural effusions develop secondary to ascites from cirrhosis (see Chapter 6). Approximately 20% of patients with pancreatic ascites have a pleural effusion (24).

Most patients with pancreatic ascites and pleural effusion are initially thought to have cirrhosis and ascites. The diagnosis is easily established if amylase determinations are made on the peritoneal and pleural fluid in such patients (24). Most patients have a protein level above 3.0 g per dL in their ascitic fluid. The treatment for pancreatic ascites is the same as for pancreatic pleural effusion, except serial paracenteses rather than serial thoracenteses are performed (24).

SUBPHRENIC ABSCESS

Subphrenic abscess continues to be a significant clinical problem despite the development of potent antibiotics.

Incidence

In most large medical centers, between six and 15 subphrenic abscesses are seen each year (25–27). Subphrenic abscesses are discussed in this chapter because a pleural effusion is present in approximately 80% of cases.

Pathogenesis

Approximately 80% of subphrenic abscesses follow intraabdominal surgical procedures (28, 29). Splenectomy is likely to be complicated by a left subphrenic abscess (29), as is gastrectomy. Deck and Berne (30) noted a high incidence of subphrenic abscess after exploratory laparotomy for trauma; in their study, 59% of subphrenic abscesses occurred after such an operation. Overall, about 1% of abdominal operations are complicated by subphrenic abscess (27). Sanders (27) reviewed the incidence of subphrenic abscesses following 1,566 abdominal surgical procedures at the Radcliffe Infirmary in 1965 and found 15 patients with subphrenic abscess. Sanders also reviewed the cases of 23 patients with pleural effusion following intraabdominal surgical procedures during the same period. He found that 12 of the 23 patients had definite subphrenic

abscesses, and he believed that another five patients possibly had subphrenic abscesses.

Subphrenic abscess may also occur without antecedent abdominal surgical procedures. It may result from processes such as gastric, duodenal, or appendiceal perforation; diverticulitis; cholecystitis; pancreatitis; or trauma (28). In such patients, the diagnosis of subphrenic abscess is frequently not considered. In one series of 22 patients in whom abscesses occurred without antecedent abdominal operations, the diagnosis was established before the patient's death in only 41% (28).

The pathogenesis of the pleural effusion associated with subphrenic abscess is probably related to inflammation of the diaphragm. Although Carter and Brewer (25) proposed that the pleural effusion arose from the transdiaphragmatic transfer of abscess material by the lymphatic vessels, this hypothesis is unlikely because fluid from these pleural effusions is only rarely culture-positive. If the pleural effusion arose from the transdiaphragmatic transport of abscess material, bacteria as well as leukocytes should be transported. The diaphragmatic inflammation resulting from the adjacent abscess probably increases the permeability of the capillaries in the diaphragmatic pleura and causes pleural fluid to accumulate.

Clinical Manifestations

The clinical picture of a patient with subphrenic abscess can be dominated by either chest or abdominal symptoms. In the series of 125 cases of Carter and Brewer (25), chest findings dominated the clinical picture in 44% of patients. The main chest symptom is pleuritic chest pain. Radiographic abnormalities include pleural effusion, basal pneumonitis, compression atelectasis, and an elevated diaphragm on the affected side. Pleural effusions occur in 60% to 80% of patients (25, 26, 29–31), and are usually small to moderate in size, but may be large, occupying more than 50% of the hemithorax.

Most patients with postoperative subphrenic abscesses have fever, leukocytosis, and abdominal pain (25, 26, 30), but frequently no localizing signs or symptoms are present. The symptoms and signs of subphrenic abscess are variable. In a series of 60 patients, 37% had no abdominal pain, 21% had no abdominal tenderness, 15% had no temperature elevation greater than 39°C, and 8% had no leukocytosis above 10,000 per mm^3 (26). The interval between the surgical procedure and the development of the subphrenic abscess is usually 1 to 3 weeks but can be as long as 5 months (28, 29).

Examination of the pleural fluid from patients with subphrenic abscesses usually reveals an exudate with predominantly polymorphonuclear leukocytes. Although the pleural fluid WBC may approach or may even exceed 50,000 per mm^3, the pleural fluid pH and glucose level remain above 7.20 and 60 mg per dL, respectively. It is distinctly uncommon for the pleural fluid to become infected (25). However, empyemas have resulted from contamination of the pleural space when the abscesses were drained percutaneously (32).

Diagnosis

The diagnosis of subphrenic abscess should be suspected in any patient who develops a pleural effusion several days or more after an abdominal surgical procedure or in any other patient who has an undiagnosed exudative pleural effusion containing predominantly polymorphonuclear leukocytes. The chest radiographs from such a patient are shown in Fig. 15.1. This patient had left-sided chest pain and a low-grade fever without any abdominal symptoms. Thoracentesis revealed an exudate with a WBC of 29,000, an LDH level of 340 IU per L, a glucose level of 117 mg per dL, and a pH of 7.36. He was treated with parenteral antibiotics for a presumed parapneumonic effusion but had little clinical response. Two subsequent thoracenteses revealed similar pleural fluid findings. Two weeks after admission, a gallium scan revealed increased uptake of the gallium in the left upper quadrant (Fig. 15.2). At laparotomy, this patient was found to have a left subphrenic abscess resulting from a colonic perforation secondary to a colonic carcinoma. At no time did this patient have more than mild left upper quadrant tenderness.

Routine chest or abdominal radiographs frequently establish the diagnosis of subphrenic

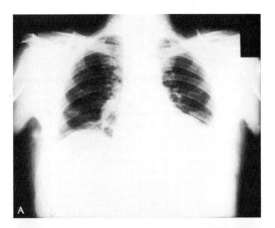
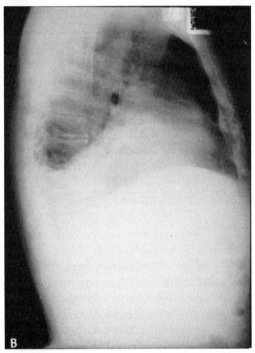

FIG. 15.1. Posteroanterior chest radiograph **(A)** and left lateral radiograph **(B)**, demonstrating elevated left diaphragm and blunting of the left diaphragm posteriorly.

abscess. A pathognomonic radiologic finding is an air–fluid level below the diaphragm outside the gastrointestinal tract. These air–fluid levels are best demonstrated with heavily exposed abdominal films that include the diaphragm, with the patient upright and in the lateral decubitus position (29). In one series of 82 patients, these

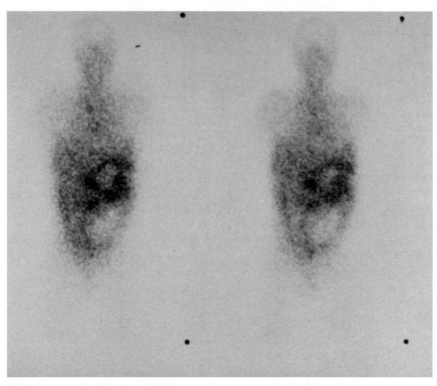

FIG. 15.2. Gallium scan from the patient whose radiographs are shown in Fig. 15.1. Note the increased activity in the left upper abdominal quadrant with the "cold" spot in the center of the area with the increased uptake.

routine radiographs demonstrated air within the abscess in 70% (29). In over 25% of the patients with air in the abscess, the air had been overlooked on the initial radiologic interpretation (29). A second radiographic sign sometimes seen on routinely obtained radiographs is displacement of intraabdominal viscera. Contrast studies including upper gastrointestinal series and barium enemas are helpful in demonstrating the extraluminal location of gas, leakage, and deformity or displacement of normal structures. Some investigators have recommended water-soluble contrast material for these studies because of the possibility of perforation or leakage and because retained barium can make subsequent CT scans and ultrasound studies more difficult.

In recent years, CT scans, ultrasound studies, and gallium scans have proved useful in diagnosing subphrenic abscesses. As demonstrated in Fig. 15.2, gallium scans can be helpful in establishing the diagnosis. Gallium scans are not always positive when subphrenic abscesses are present. In one series, four of 11 patients (36%) with subphrenic abscesses had negative gallium scans (30). Abdominal CT scans are probably the best means by which to establish the diagnosis of subphrenic abscess (33). One advantage of CT scans over gallium scans is that, with CT scans, the precise anatomic location and extent of the abscess can be defined (29). Ultrasonic examination effectively demonstrates fluid-filled abscess cavities, but ultrasound is technically difficult in the left subphrenic region because of overlying lung, ribs, and gas in the gastrointestinal tract (29). In one series, ultrasonic examinations were negative in 41% of 22 patients with subphrenic abscesses (30).

Treatment and Prognosis

The two main aspects of treatment are the administration of appropriate antibiotics and drainage.

Sepsis is an ever-present threat to the patient with a subphrenic abscess. In a series of 125 cases, 29 patients (23%) developed positive blood cultures, and the mortality rate in these 29 patients was 93% (25). Most subphrenic abscesses contain more than a single organism; *Escherichia coli, Staphylococcus aureus*, and anaerobic organisms are most commonly isolated (34). Broad-spectrum antibiotics with anaerobic coverage should be instituted before any drainage procedure is attempted to prevent bacteremia during this procedure.

Drainage of the subphrenic abscess can be accomplished either percutaneously or with surgery. Because the results seem comparable with the two procedures (35), it is recommended that percutaneous drainage be used in most cases, although posterior subphrenic abscesses are best approached surgically (36). The results with percutaneous drainage by experienced individuals are excellent. Voros et al. (36) reported that 92% of 185 patients with intraabdominal abscesses were successfully treated with percutaneous drainage. These investigators inserted the catheters under CT guidance and left the catheters in place for a mean of 6 days (36).

Mortality rates among patients with subphrenic abscesses remain high, ranging from 20% to 45% (25, 26, 28, 31). Because much of the mortality is due to delayed diagnosis or lack of a diagnosis before autopsy, the possibility of a subphrenic abscess must be considered in every patient with an exudative pleural effusion containing predominantly polymorphonuclear leukocytes. In such patients, heavily penetrated abdominal radiographs should be examined for extravisceral gas, and one should consider obtaining an abdominal CT scan.

INTRAHEPATIC ABSCESS

Pleural effusions accompany intrahepatic abscesses in about 20% of patients (37). The pathogenesis of the pleural fluid and the pleural fluid findings with intrahepatic abscess are similar to those for subphrenic abscess, as previously discussed. Because the mortality rate of patients with untreated liver abscesses approaches 100% (38), the diagnosis of intrahepatic abscess should

be considered in every patient with a right-sided exudative pleural effusion with predominantly polymorphonuclear leukocytes on the pleural fluid differential. Amebic liver abscesses are discussed in Chapter 12.

Clinical Manifestations

Most patients with pyogenic intrahepatic abscesses have fever and anorexia (38), and approximately 50% give a history of shaking chills. About 50% of patients with hepatic abscesses have hepatobiliary disease, most commonly hepatolithiasis, whereas 50% have no illness that predisposes them to liver abscess (39). Abdominal pain is common, but it frequently is not localized to the right upper quadrant. Most patients have an enlarged, tender liver. Laboratory tests usually reveal leukocytosis, anemia, elevated alkaline phosphatase levels, and hyperbilirubinemia. However, because none of these findings are invariably present in patients with pyogenic liver abscesses, this diagnosis should be pursued in all patients with right-sided exudative pleural effusions containing polymorphonuclear leukocytes.

Diagnosis

The best way to establish the diagnosis of pyogenic liver abscess is by abdominal CT scan (40). With CT scanning, abscesses with diameters as small as 0.5 cm can be readily appreciated. Abdominal ultrasound studies can also identify fluid-filled intrahepatic lesions (41), but because CT scanning provides more precise anatomic information, it is the procedure of choice. Not all fluid-filled intrahepatic lesions are pyogenic abscesses; cysts, hematomas, hemangiomas, and amebic abscesses can produce identical findings on ultrasound studies and CT scans. The definitive diagnosis can be established by percutaneous aspiration guided by CT scanning or ultrasound.

Treatment

The treatment of a pyogenic liver abscess consists of the administration of appropriate parenteral antibiotics and drainage of the abscess. The preferred method of drainage is image-guided aspiration with or without catheter drainage (39). Emergency laparotomy is indicated when there are signs of peritonitis, ongoing deterioration of the patient's condition despite aspiration or catheter drainage, or CT evidence of persistent abscess (39).

INTRASPLENIC ABSCESS

Splenic abscess is an unusual entity. In the 30 years between 1950 and 1980, there were only 11 cases diagnosed at Johns Hopkins Hospital (42). In a more recent series from the University of California at Davis Medical Center (43), nine patients were seen between 1980 and 1990. In this latter series, all patients had an associated pleural effusion, but in prior series only 20% to 50% of patients with splenic abscess had a left-sided pleural effusion (42, 44). In most patients, the splenic suppuration arises from primary hematogenous seeding such as with endocarditis. Splenic abscess appears to be more common in individuals with diseases producing splenic abnormalities, such as chronic hemolytic anemia or sickle cell anemia (42).

Most but not all patients with a splenic abscess have localized pain in the left upper quadrant. One combination that is particularly suggestive of the diagnosis is a left pleural effusion plus thrombocytosis. In the series of Ho and Wisner (43), seven of nine patients (78%) had this combination. The diagnosis can be made presumptively with ultrasonography or CT and can be confirmed by fine needle aspiration (45). Although most patients are treated with splenectomy plus antibiotics (43), some patients have been cured with catheter drainage (45).

ESOPHAGEAL PERFORATION

Esophageal rupture should always be considered in the differential diagnosis of pleural effusions, because if this entity is not rapidly treated, the mortality rate approaches 100%.

Incidence

Esophageal perforation is uncommon. Michel et al. (46) reported only 85 cases at the Massa-chusetts General Hospital over a 21-year period, whereas Reeder et al. (47) found 41 cases at The University of Chicago Hospitals over a 14-year period.

Pathogenesis and Pathophysiologic Mechanisms

Esophageal perforation most commonly arises as a complication of esophagoscopic examination. In one series of 108 cases, 67% occurred as a complication of esophagoscopy (48). Esophageal perforation is particularly common with esophagoscopy when one has attempted to remove a foreign body or to dilate an esophageal stricture (48). Overall, between 0.15% and 0.70% of all esophagoscopic examinations are complicated by esophageal perforation (46). The insertion of a Blakemore tube for esophageal varices can also be complicated by esophageal rupture; this mechanism accounted for 11% of all esophageal perforations in one series (46). Frequently, the diagnosis of esophageal perforation is missed in patients with Blakemore tubes because they are so ill with multiple problems (46).

Esophageal perforations may also arise from foreign bodies themselves, carcinomas, gastric intubation, chest trauma, and chest operations. Finally, esophageal rupture may occur as a complication of vomiting (Boerhaave's syndrome). Spontaneous rupture almost always involves the lower esophagus, just above the diaphragm.

The clinical symptoms of esophageal perforation are due to contamination of the mediastinum by oropharyngeal contents that produces an acute mediastinitis. When the mediastinal pleura ruptures, a pleural effusion develops, frequently complicated by a pneumothorax. Most of the morbidity from esophageal perforation is due to the infection of the mediastinum and the pleural space by the oropharyngeal bacterial flora (49).

Clinical Manifestations

With esophageal perforation secondary to esophagoscopic examination, the endoscopist usually does not realize that the esophagus has been perforated (50). Because, however, such patients usually report persistent chest or epigastric pain within several hours of the procedure (51), such complaints should serve as indications for an emergency contrast study of the esophagus.

Patients with spontaneous rupture of the esophagus usually have a history of vomiting, followed by chest pain (52), and they frequently describe a sensation of tearing or bursting in the lower part of the chest or the epigastrium. The chest pain is characteristically excruciating and is often unrelieved by opiates. Small amounts of hematemesis are present in more than 50% of these patients (52). Dyspnea is frequently a prominent symptom. The presence of subcutaneous emphysema that first appears in the suprasternal notch suggests esophageal perforation, but this appears late in the course of perforation. In Abbott et al.'s series of 47 patients, only four (9%) had subcutaneous emphysema within the first 4 hours (52). The clinical picture may be much less dramatic than that described. Chandrasekhara and Levitan described a patient with a ruptured esophagus and symptoms present for 5 days who had only mild distress (53).

In patients with esophageal perforation, the chest radiograph reveals a pleural effusion in about 60% and a pneumothorax in about 25% (46). Most patients with spontaneous rupture have a pleural effusion (54). The pleural effusion is usually left sided, but it may be right sided or bilateral. Other radiographic findings may include widening of the mediastinum and visible air within the mediastinal compartments.

Diagnosis

Because the mortality rate approaches 60% (54) when treatment is delayed for more than 24 hours, the diagnosis of esophageal rupture should be entertained any time one sees a patient with an exudative pleural effusion, particularly when the patient appears acutely ill. Examination of the pleural fluid is helpful in suggesting the diagnosis of esophageal perforation because it is characterized by (a) a high amylase level, (b) a low pH, (c) the presence of squamous epithelial cells, and sometimes (d) ingested food particles.

An elevated pleural fluid amylase level appears to be the best indication of esophageal rupture. In the experimental model, the pleural fluid amylase level is elevated within 2 hours of esophageal rupture (43). In one clinical series, all seven patients with esophageal rupture had elevated pleural fluid amylase levels (52). The origin of the amylase is salivary rather than pancreatic because the saliva, with its high amylase content, enters the pleural space through the defect in the esophagus (55). To my knowledge, in only two reported cases have pleural fluid amylase levels been within normal limits with esophageal perforation and pleural effusion (56, 57). One of these patients (57) had Sjögren's syndrome and essentially no production of saliva. The other (56) had a chronic perforation due to esophageal carcinoma.

The pleural fluid pH is usually decreased with esophageal rupture (58, 59). In fact, Dye and Laforet (59) concluded that a pleural fluid pH below 6.0 was highly suggestive of esophageal rupture and attributed the low pleural fluid pH to the leakage of acidic gastric juice through the esophageal tear. Both of these conclusions appear to be wrong. Patients with severe infections of the pleural space and an intact esophagus frequently have a pleural fluid pH below 6.0.

Good et al. (60) demonstrated, in an experimental model, that the pleural fluid pH falls just as rapidly after esophageal perforation when the esophagogastric junction is ligated. These authors concluded that leukocyte metabolism was the major contributor to the low pleural fluid pH with esophageal rupture. Nevertheless, the presence of a pleural fluid pH below 7.00 increases the likelihood that the patient has a ruptured esophagus.

Another useful test in diagnosing esophageal perforation is examination of the Wright stain of the pleural fluid for squamous epithelial cells (61). Eriksen demonstrated the presence of squamous epithelial cells in the pleural fluid from all 14 patients with esophageal perforation. Again, as with amylase, the squamous epithelial cells enter the pleural space through the esophageal perforation. Obviously, the demonstration of food particles in pleural fluid is diagnostic of esophageal perforation.

The diagnosis of esophageal perforation is established when esophageal disruption is confirmed by contrast studies of the esophagus.

The contrast agent of choice is probably meg-lumine and ioxaglate sodium (Hexabrix, 320 mg per mL) (62). Barium has a greater radiographic density, better mucosal adherence, and minimal irritation to the tracheobronchial tree, but it is not absorbed once it leaks into the mediastinum or pleura and produces a marked inflammatory re-action in the pleura. When water-soluble agents, such as Hexabrix or meglumine and diatrizoate sodium (Gastrografin), are injected in the pleural space, they are almost completely absorbed af-ter 24 hours (62) and neither create much of an inflammatory response. Hexabrix is considered the agent of choice because Gastrografin creates marked bronchospasm when it is aspirated and Hexabrix does not create such a reaction (62). The contrast studies are positive in about 85% of patients (46). If the perforation is small or has already closed spontaneously, the esophagogram may not be diagnostic. It has been suggested that contrast studies of the esophagus when perfora-tion is suspected be done in the decubitus position (63). In this position, the contrast material fills the whole length of the esophagus and thereby allows the actual site of the perforation and its inter-connecting cavities to be demonstrated in almost all patients (63).

If the esophageal perforation is not demon-strated by the contrast study of the esophagus, chest CT scan may facilitate the diagnosis (64). White et al. (64) performed chest CT scans on 12 patients with esophageal perforation. They found esophageal thickening in nine patients, perieso-phageal fluid in 11 patients, extraluminal air in 11 patients, and pleural effusion in nine. The site of the perforation was visible on CT scan in two patients. The finding that most commonly pointed to esophageal rupture was extraluminal air (64).

Treatment

The treatment of choice for esophageal rupture is exploration of the mediastinum with primary repair of the esophageal tear and drainage of the pleural space and mediastinum (47, 65, 66). Par-enteral antibiotics should be given to treat the me-diastinitis and pleural infection. Although con-servative treatment consisting of antibiotics and nasogastric suction is adequate in some patients with esophageal perforation (66), in patients with pleural effusion or pneumothorax complicating esophageal perforation, mediastinal exploration should be performed. It is important to perform the mediastinal exploration as soon as possible after the diagnosis is established, because a de-lay of even 12 hours increases the mortality rate (54). If primary repair is not possible because the damaged tissue cannot hold the sutures, the pa-tient can be managed with T tube intubation of the esophageal defect (67).

ABDOMINAL SURGICAL PROCEDURES

The incidence of small pleural effusions after ab-dominal operations is high. George and I reported a series of 200 patients who had bilateral decu-bitus chest radiographs 48 to 72 hours following abdominal surgical procedures (68). Pleural ef-fusions were identified in 97 patients (49%). In a more recent series, Nielsen et al. (69) reported that 89 of 128 patients (69%) undergoing upper abdominal surgery had pleural effusions in the first 4 days postoperatively. Most of the pleural effusions are small; only 21 patients (22%) in our series had pleural fluid that measured more than 10 mm in thickness on the decubitus films (68). Larger left-sided pleural effusions are particu-larly common after splenectomy. Postoperative pleural effusions are more common in patients undergoing upper abdominal surgical procedures (68), in patients with postoperative atelectasis (68, 69), and in those with free abdominal fluid at the time of operation (68). In our series (68), a thoracentesis was performed on 20 patients, and in 16 of these, the pleural fluid was an exudate (68). The pleural effusions in all but a single pa-tient, who had a staphylococcal pleural infection, resolved spontaneously without any specific ther-apy. In summary, pleural effusions frequently oc-cur after abdominal surgical procedures and are usually related to diaphragmatic irritation or at-electasis. If the pleural effusion measures more than 10 mm in thickness on the decubitus film, a diagnostic thoracentesis should be performed to rule out pleural infection. Although pulmonary embolization and subphrenic abscess can cause pleural effusion postoperatively, most effusions occurring within the first 72 hours after abdominal surgery are not due to these factors and resolve spontaneously.

DIAPHRAGMATIC HERNIA

Hernias through the diaphragm are important in the differential diagnosis of pleural effusions from two viewpoints. First, they may mimic a pleural effusion. Second, pleural effusions are usually present in patients with a strangulated diaphragmatic hernia.

Diaphragmatic hernia should be considered whenever an apparent pleural effusion has an atypical shape or location (Fig. 15.3). Air in the herniated intestine usually is the clue to this diagnosis. Occasionally, an upper gastrointestinal series and a small bowel follow-through study in conjunction with a barium enema are necessary for accurate diagnosis.

The possibility of a strangulated diaphragmatic hernia should always be considered in patients

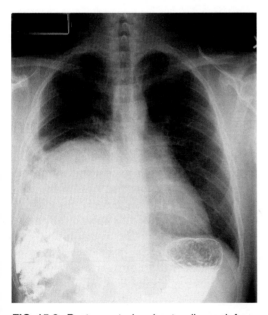

FIG. 15.3. Posteroanterior chest radiograph from a 31-year-old man who presented with increasing dyspnea. He was in an automobile accident 15 years previously and was told that he injured his right diaphragm. Note the collections of air in the upper part of the apparent mass. At surgery, both the liver and colon had herniated through the diaphragm.

with a left pleural effusion and signs of an acute abdominal catastrophe (70, 71). At least 90% of strangulated diaphragmatic hernias are traumatic in origin, and at least 95% are on the left side because the liver protects the right diaphragm. Strangulation can occur months to years after the original injury, which is usually an automobile accident. Strangulation typically occurs suddenly and progresses rapidly. Left shoulder pain is generally present from diaphragmatic irritation. Serosanguineous exudative pleural fluid with predominantly polymorphonuclear leukocytes is almost always present. The diagnosis is usually suggested by air–fluid levels in the viscera strangulated in the left pleural space. Contrast studies of the gastrointestinal tract are sometimes necessary to make the diagnosis. Immediate surgical treatment is imperative to prevent gangrene of the strangulated viscera (70, 71).

ENDOSCOPIC VARICEAL SCLEROTHERAPY

Over the past 20 years, endoscopic variceal sclerotherapy (EVS) has become one of the principal forms of therapy for patients who have bled from ruptured esophageal varices. Frequently, EVS is followed by the development of a pleural effusion. Saks et al. (72) reviewed the chest radiographs following 38 different EVS procedures and reported that 50% of the procedures were followed by the development of a pleural effusion, whereas Bacon et al. (73) reported pleural effusions following 48% of 65 procedures. The sclerosant used in both of the above-mentioned series was 5% sodium morrhuate. Parikh et al. (74) reported that the incidence of pleural effusion was only 19% in 31 patients in whom absolute alcohol was used as the sclerosant. Left, right, and bilateral effusions occur with approximately equal frequency (75). Most of the effusions are small.

In the Bacon study, 11 pleural fluids were analyzed and all were exudates, primarily by the LDH criteria (73). There is no relationship between the incidence of fever, the patient's fluid status, or the presence of ascites and the occurrence of postsclerotherapy effusions (73). Patients who develop pleural effusion are more likely to experience chest pain requiring medication after the procedure (73). It is hypothesized that the development of the pleural effusion is related to extravasation of the sclerosant into the esophageal mucosa, which results in an intense inflammatory reaction in the mediastinum and pleura (73). No treatment is necessary for the pleural effusion secondary to EVS. However, if the effusion persists for more than 24 to 48 hours and is accompanied by fever or if the effusion occupies more than 25% of the hemithorax, a thoracentesis should be performed to rule out an infection or an esophagopleural fistula (75). The latter diagnosis is suggested by a high pleural fluid amylase level.

BILIOUS PLEURAL EFFUSIONS

Bilious pleural effusions are a rare complication of biliary tract disorders. With all cases of bilious pleural effusions, there is a fistula from the biliary tree to the pleural space. Historically, the most common cause has been thoracoabdominal trauma (76); other causes have included parasitic liver disease, suppurative complications of biliary tract obstruction, and postoperative strictures of bile ducts (77). Bilious pleural effusions have also been reported to occur after percutaneous biliary drainage (78) or after an internal stent was placed for an obstructed biliary system (79). In two cases with spontaneous biliary pleural fistula, the tract was large enough to allow the passage of gallstones into the pleural space (77, 80).

When bile is instilled into the pleural space of rabbits, an inflammatory reaction is produced. The influx of fluid plus the rapid reabsorption of the bile results in the pleural fluid having a much lower bilirubin than one would anticipate (78). In one patient who developed a pleural effusion as a complication of percutaneous biliary drainage, the pleural fluid bilirubin was only 2.1 mg per dL (78). However, the pleural fluid bilirubin has exceeded 25 mg per dL in some patients (78).

The diagnosis of a bilious pleural effusion should be suspected in any patient with an obstructed biliary system. It is important to remember that the pleural fluid may not appear to be bile, although the ratio of the pleural fluid to serum bilirubin is greater than 1.0 (78). The appropriate treatment for this condition is the reestablishment of the biliary drainage. Most patients who have a bilious pleural effusion after trauma require decortication and diaphragmatic repair (76). The incidence of empyema with bilious pleural effusions approaches 50%, and one should constantly be aware of this complication.

PLEURAL EFFUSIONS AFTER LIVER TRANSPLANTATION

Almost all patients who undergo an orthotopic liver transplantation develop a pleural effusion postoperatively. Spizarny et al. (81) reviewed the chest radiographs of 42 patients undergoing liver transplantation and found that 40 of 42 patients (95%) developed a right-sided pleural effusion within 72 hours of transplantation. One of the remaining two patients had a left-sided effusion. Afessa et al. (82) reported that pleural effusions were present postoperatively in 77% of their 44 patients undergoing liver transplantation. The pleural effusions are bilateral in about one third of patients, but the amount of fluid on the right side is greater than that on the left side (82).

The pleural effusion after liver transplantation may be large. In one series of liver transplants in 48 children, effusions that were large enough to cause clinically detectable respiratory compromise occurred in 23 (19 right sided and four left sided) (83). Fifteen of the patients in this latter series were treated with chest tubes (83).

The pathogenesis of the pleural effusions after liver transplantation is not definitely known. It has been suggested that the effusion is due to injury or irritation of the right hemidiaphragm caused by the extensive right upper quadrant dissection and retraction. The natural history of a pleural effusion after transplantation is that it increases in size over the first three postoperative days and then gradually resolves over a period ranging from several weeks to several months (81). In one series, the effusion increased in size in the period after the first 3 days in 10 patients. Seven of the 10 patients had subdiaphragmatic pathology, including four with hematomas, one with a biloma, and two with abscesses. Accordingly, patients with enlarging pleural effusions after liver transplantation should be evaluated for subdiaphragmatic pathology.

To my knowledge, there has been no systematic analysis of the pleural fluid in these patients. In the series referenced earlier, there was no mention of the findings with thoracentesis.

The pleural effusion that occurs after liver transplantation can be largely prevented if a fibrin sealant is sprayed on the undersurface of the diaphragm around the insertion of the liver ligaments at the time of transplantation. When Uetsuji et al. (84) used the fibrin sealant in 25 liver transplant patients, none developed a pleural effusion postoperatively.

REFERENCES

1. Kaye MD. Pleuropulmonary complications of pancreatitis. *Thorax* 1968;23:297–306.
2. Gumaste V, Singh V, Dave P. Significance of pleural effusion in patients with acute pancreatitis. *Am J Gastroenterol* 1992;87:871–874.
3. Lankisch PG, Groge M, Becher R. Pleural effusions: a new negative prognostic parameter for acute pancreatitis. *Am J Gastroenterol* 1994;89:1849–1851.
4. Heller SJ, Noordhoek E, Tenner SM, et al. Pleural effusion as a predictor of severity in acute pancreatitis. *Pancreas* 1997;15:222–225.
5. Roseman DM, Kowlessar OD, Sleisenger MH. Pulmonary manifestations of pancreatitis. *N Engl J Med* 1960;263:294–296.
6. Light RW, Ball WC. Glucose and amylase in pleural effusions. *JAMA* 1973;225:257–260.
7. Makela A, Kuusi T, Nuutinen P, et al. Phospholipase A2 activity in body fluids and pancreatic tissue in patients with acute necrotising pancreatitis. *Eur J Surg* 1999;165:35–42.
8. Miller TA, Lindenauer SM, Frey CF, et al. Pancreatic abscess. *Arch Surg* 1974;108:545–551.
9. Kolmannskog F, Kolbenstvedt A, Aakhus T. Computed tomography in inflammatory mass lesions following acute pancreatitis. *J Comput Assist Tomogr* 1981;5:169–172.
10. Tombroff M, Loicq A, De Koster J-P, et al. Pleural effusion with pancreaticopleural fistula. *Br Med J* 1973;1:330–331.
11. Shetty AN. Pseudocysts of the pancreas: an overview. *South Med J* 1980;73:1239–1242.
12. Rockey DC, Cello JP. Pancreaticopleural fistula. Report of 7 patients and review of the literature. *Medicine* 1990;69:332–344.
13. Anderson WJ, Skinner DB, Zuidema GD, et al. Chronic pancreatic pleural effusions. *Surg Gynecol Obstet* 1973;137:827–830.
14. Uchiyama T, Suzuki T, Adachi A, et al. Pancreatic pleural effusion: case report and review of 113 cases in Japan. *Am J Gastroenterol* 1992;87:387–391.
15. Miridjianian A, Ambruoso VN, Derby BM, et al. Massive bilateral hemorrhagic pleural effusions in chronic relapsing pancreatitis. *Arch Surg* 1969;98:62–66.
16. Pottmeyer EW III, Frey CF, Matsuno S. Pancreaticopleural fistulas. *Arch Surg* 1987;122:648–654.
17. Kramer MR, Saidana MJ, Cepero RJ, et al. High amylase levels in neoplasm-related pleural effusion. *Ann Intern Med* 1989;110:567–569.
18. Safadi BY, Marks JM. Pancreatic-pleural fistula: the role of ERCP in diagnosis and treatment. *Gastrointest Endosc* 2000;51:213–215.
19. Parekh D, Segal I. Pancreatic ascites and effusion. Risk factors for failure of conservative therapy and the role of octreotide. *Arch Surg* 1992;127:707–712.
20. Pederzoli P, Bassi C, Falconi M, et al. Conservative treatment of external pancreatic fistulae with parenteral nutrition along or in combination with continuous intravenous infusion of somatostatin, glucagon or calcitonin. *Surg Gynecol Obstet* 1986;163:428–432.
21. Krasnow AZ, Collier BD, Isitman AT, et al. The value of preoperative imaging techniques in patients with chronic pancreatic pleural effusions. *Int J Pancreatol* 1987;2:269–276.
22. Lang EK, Paolini RM, Pottmeyer A. The efficacy of palliative and definitive percutaneous versus surgical drainage of pancreatic abscesses and pseudocysts: a prospective study of 85 patients. *South Med J* 1991;84:55–64.
23. Shapiro DH, Anagnostopoulos CE, Dineen JP. Decortication and pleurectomy for the pleuropulmonary complications of pancreatitis. *Ann Thorac Surg* 1970;9:76–80.
24. Lipsett PA, Cameron JL. Internal pancreatic fistula. *Am J Surg* 1992;163:216–220.
25. Carter R, Brewer LA. Subphrenic abscess: a thoracoabdominal clinical complex. *Am J Surg* 1964;108:165–174.
26. DeCosse JJ, Poulin TL, Fox PS, et al. Subphrenic abscess. *Surg Gynecol Obstet* 1974;138:841–846.
27. Sanders RC. Post-operative pleural effusion and subphrenic abscess. *Clin Radiol* 1970;21:308–312.
28. Sherman NJ, Davis JR, Jesseph JE. Subphrenic abscess: a continuing hazard. *Am J Surg* 1969;117:117–123.
29. Connell TR, Stephens DH, Carlson HC, et al. Upper abdominal abscess: a continuing and deadly problem. *AJR Am J Roentgenol* 1980;134:759–765.
30. Deck KB, Berne TV. Selective management of subphrenic abscesses. *Arch Surg* 1979;114:1165–1168.
31. van der Sluis RF. Subphrenic abscess. *Surg Gynecol Obstet* 1984;158:427–435.
32. Samelson SL, Ferguson MK. Empyema following percutaneous catheter drainage of upper abdominal abscess. *Chest* 1992;102:1612–1614.
33. Alexander ES, Proto AV, Clark RA. CT differentiation of subphrenic abscess and pleural effusion. *AJR Am J Roentgenol* 1983;145:47–51.
34. Brook I, Frazier EH. Microbiology of subphrenic abscesses: a 14-year experience. *Am Surg* 1999;65:1049–1053.
35. Bufalari A, Giustozzi G, Moggi L. Postoperative intraabdominal abscesses: percutaneous versus surgical treatment. *Acta Chir Belg* 1996;96:197–200.
36. Voros D, Gouliamos A, Kotoulas G, et al. Percutaneous drainage of intraabdominal abscesses using large lumen tubes under computed tomographic control. *Eur J Surg* 1996;162:895–898.
37. Rubin RH, Swartz MN, Malt R. Hepatic abscess: changes in clinical, bacteriologic and therapeutic aspects. *Am J Med* 1974;57:601–610.
38. Perera MR, Kirk A, Noone P. Presentation, diagnosis and management of liver abscess. *Lancet* 1980;3:629–632.
39. Chu K-M, Fan S-T, Lai ECS, et al. Pyogenic liver abscess. *Arch Surg* 1996;131:148–153.

40. Buchman TG, Zuidema GD. The role of computerized tomographic scanning in the surgical management of pyogenic hepatic abscess. *Surg Gynecol Obstet* 1981;153:1–9.

41. Newlin N, Silver TM, Stuck KJ, et al. Ultrasonic features of pyogenic liver abscesses. *Radiology* 1981;139:155–159.

42. Sarr MG, Zuidema GD. Splenic abscess: presentation, diagnosis and treatment. *Surgery* 1982;92:480–485.

43. Ho HS, Wisner DH. Splenic abscess in the intensive care unit. *Arch Surg* 1993;128:842–848.

44. Johnson JF, Raff MJ, Barnwell PA, et al. Splenic abscess complicating infectious endocarditis. *Arch Intern Med* 1983;143:905–912.

45. Tikkakoski T, Siniluoto T, Paivansalo M, et al. Splenic abscess. Imaging and intervention. *Acta Radiol* 1992;33:561–565.

46. Michel L, Grillo HC, Malt RA. Operative and nonoperative management of esophageal perforations. *Ann Surg* 1981;194:57–63.

47. Reeder LB, DeFilippi VJ, Ferguson MK. Current results of therapy for esophageal perforation. *Am J Surg* 1995;169:615–617.

48. Keszler P, Buzna E. Surgical and conservative management of esophageal perforation. *Chest* 1981;80:158–162.

49. Maulitz RM, Good JT Jr, Kaplan RL, et al. The pleuropulmonary consequences of esophageal rupture: an experimental model. *Am Rev Respir Dis* 1979;120:363–367.

50. Quintana R, Bartley TD, Wheat MW Jr. Esophageal perforation: analysis of 10 cases. *Ann Thorac Surg* 1970;10:45–53.

51. Skinner DB, Little AG, DeMeester TR. Management of esophageal perforation. *Am J Surg* 1980;139:760–764.

52. Abbott OA, Mansour KA, Logan WD, et al. Atraumatic so-called "spontaneous" rupture of the esophagus. *J Thorac Cardiovasc Surg* 1970;59:67–83.

53. Chandrasekhara R, Levitan R. Spontaneous rupture of the esophagus. *Arch Intern Med* 1970;126:1008–1009.

54. Finley RJ, Pearson FG, Weisel RD, et al. The management of non-malignant intrathoracic esophageal perforations. *Ann Thorac Surg* 1980;30:575–581.

55. Sherr HP, Light RW, Merson MH, et al. Origin of pleural fluid amylase in esophageal rupture. *Ann Intern Med* 1972;76:985–986.

56. Faling LJ, Pugatch RD, Robbins AH. Case report: the diagnosis of unsuspected esophageal perforation by computed tomography. *Am J Med Sci* 1981;281:31–34.

57. Rudin JS, Ellrodt AG, Phillips EH. Low pleural fluid amylase associated with spontaneous rupture of the esophagus. *Arch Intern Med* 1983;143:1034–1035.

58. Good JT Jr, Taryle DA, Maulitz RM, et al. The diagnostic value of pleural fluid pH. *Chest* 1980;78:55–59.

59. Dye RA, Laforet EG. Esophageal rupture: diagnosis by pleural fluid pH. *Chest* 1974;66:454–456.

60. Good JT Jr, Antony VB, Reller LB, et al. The pathogenesis of the low pleural fluid pH in esophageal rupture. *Am Rev Respir Dis* 1983;127:702–704.

61. Eriksen KR. Oesophagopleural fistula diagnosed by microscopic examination of pleural fluid. *Acta Chir Scand* 1964;128:771–777.

62. Ginai AZ. Experimental evaluation of various available contrast agents for use in the gastrointestinal tract in case of suspected leakage: effects on pleura. *Br J Radiol* 1986;59:887–894.

63. Demeester TR. Perforation of the esophagus. *Ann Thorac Surg* 1986;42:231–232.

64. White CS, Templeton PA, Attar S. Esophageal perforation: CT findings. *AJR Am J Roentgenol* 1993;160:767–770.

65. Lawrence DR, Ohri SK, Moxon RE, et al. Primary esophageal repair for Boerhaave's syndrome. *Ann Thorac Surg* 1999;67:818–820.

66. Bufkin BL, Miller JI Jr, Mansour KA. Esophageal perforation: emphasis on management. *Ann Thorac Surg* 1996;61:1447–1451.

67. Naylor AR, Walker WS, Dark J, et al. T tube intubation in the management of seriously ill patients with oesophagopleural fistulae. *Br J Surg* 1990;77:40–42.

68. Light RW, George RB. Incidence and significance of pleural effusion after abdominal surgery. *Chest* 1976;69:621–626.

69. Nielsen PH, Jensen SB, Olsen AD. Postoperative pleural effusion following upper abdominal surgery. *Chest* 1989;96:1133–1135.

70. Keshishian JM, Cox SA. Diagnosis and management of strangulated diaphragmatic hernias. *Surg Gynecol Obstet* 1962;115:626–632.

71. Aronchick JM, Epstein DM, Gefter WB, et al. Chronic traumatic diaphragmatic hernia: the significance of pleural effusion. *Radiology* 1988;168:675–678.

72. Saks BJ, Kilby AE, Dietrich PA, et al. Pleural and mediastinal changes following endoscopic injection sclerotherapy of esophageal varices. *Radiology* 1983;149:639–642.

73. Bacon BR, Bailey-Newton RS, Connors AF Jr. Pleural effusions after endoscopic variceal sclerotherapy. *Gastroenterology* 1985;88:1910–1914.

74. Parikh SS, Amarapurkar DN, Dhawan PS, et al. Development of pleural effusion after sclerotherapy with absolute alcohol. *Gastrointest Endovasc* 1993;39:404–405.

75. Edling JE, Bacon BR. Pleuropulmonary complications of endoscopic variceal sclerotherapy. *Chest* 1991;99:1252–1257.

76. Ivatury RR, O'Shea J, Rohman M. Post-traumatic thoracobiliary fistula. *J Trauma* 1984;24:438–441.

77. Delco F, Domenigheti G, Kauzlaric D, et al. Spontaneous biliothorax (thoracobilia) following cholecystopleural fistula presenting as an acute respiratory insufficiency. *Chest* 1994;106:961–963.

78. Strange C, Allen ML, Freedland PN, et al. Biliopleural fistula as a complication of percutaneous biliary drainage: experimental evidence for pleural inflammation. *Am Rev Respir Dis* 1988;137:959–961.

79. Dasmahapatra HK, Pepper JR. Bronchopleurobiliary fistula: a complication of intrahepatic biliary stent migration. *Chest* 1988;94:874–875.

80. Cunningham LW, Grobman M, Paz HL, et al. Cholecystopleural fistula with cholelithiasis presenting as a right pleural effusion. *Chest* 1990;97:751–752.

81. Spizarny DL, Gross BH, McLoud T. Enlarging pleural effusion after liver transplantation. *J Thorac Imaging* 1993;8:85–87.

82. Afessa B, Gay PC, Plevak DJ, et al. Pulmonary complications of orthotopic liver transplantation. *Mayo Clin Proc* 1993;68:427–434.

83. Bilik R, Yellen M, Superina RA. Surgical complications in children after liver transplantation. *Pediatr Surg* 1992;27:1371–1375.

84. Uetsuji S, Komada Y, Kwon AH, et al. Prevention of pleural effusion after hepatectomy using fibrin sealant. *Int Surg* 1994;79:135–137.

16

Pleural Effusion Secondary
to Diseases of the Heart

In this chapter, the pleural effusions that occur after coronary artery bypass graft surgery (CABG), those that occur after cardiac injury (Dressler's syndrome), and those that occur concomitantly with pericardial disease are discussed.

POST CORONARY ARTERY BYPASS SURGERY

Over 500,000 CABG procedures are now performed annually in the United States (1). Because pleural effusions complicate many of these procedures, pleural effusions after CABG are one of the most common types of effusions.

Incidence

In the period immediately following CABG, there is a very high incidence of pleural effusions. In one study of 152 patients who had undergone CABG surgery, the incidence of pleural effusion on routine chest radiographs 7 days postoperatively was 42% (2). In a subsequent study (3), patients underwent chest ultrasound on the 7th, 14th, and 30th postoperative day. In this latter study, the incidence of pleural effusion was 89.4% on the 7th postoperative day, 76.6% on the 14th postoperative day, and 57.4% on the 30th postoperative day (3).

In patients who have undergone CABG, there is a substantial incidence of large pleural effusions 30 days after CABG (4). In a recent study of 421 patients at our institution, the incidence of pleural effusion that occupied more than 25% of the hemithorax 30 days after CABG was

8.3% (4). In this study, more than 60% of the patients had some pleural fluid detectable on posteroanterior and lateral chest radiographs (5). Hurlbut et al. (6) reported that 4% of 100 patients who had undergone CABG developed moderate to large effusions. If 8% of all the patients undergoing CABG develop a moderate to large pleural effusion, then the exudative pleural effusion following CABG will be one of the most common types of exudative pleural effusion.

Pathogenesis and Pathologic Features

The etiology of the large early pleural effusion after CABG surgery is probably related to trauma to the pleura during surgery (3). Patients undergoing internal mammary artery (IMA) grafting are more likely to have a pleural effusion than those undergoing only saphenous vein grafting (SVG) (3). Patients undergoing bilateral (IMA) bypasses are more likely to have a pleural effusion than those undergoing unilateral IMA bypasses (7). Patients with a pericardial effusion postoperatively are more likely to have a pleural effusion, but it is likely that both are a result of trauma rather than being responsible for the other (3). The effusions occurring early in the postoperative period are frequently bloody. In one series, the mean pleural fluid red blood cell count in 45 patients with large pleural effusions within the first 30 days of surgery exceeded 2,000,000 per mm^3 (8), which is equivalent to a hematocrit of 20%.

The etiology of the effusions that occur more than 30 days after CABG is not known. The fluid is an exudate with predominantly lymphocytes (8). Because the fluid is an exudate, the effusion is probably not due to congestive heart failure. The presence of the lymphocytes suggests an immunologic basis. Pleural biopsies obtained within the first few months of surgery demonstrate an intense lymphocytic pleuritis (9). Immunohistochemical staining demonstrates that the lymphocytes in the pleural tissue are both T lymphocytes and B lymphocytes with a predominance of B lymphocytes (9). The effusions have been attributed to the post pericardiectomy syndrome (10). This explanation, however, is unsatisfactory because patients with the post pericardiectomy syndrome usually have fever, chest pain, pericarditis, and pneumonitis besides the pleural effusion. Patients with the late pleural effusions after CABG do not have fever, chest pain, pericarditis, or pneumonitis (4). Possibly, the pleural effusion after CABG is a variant of or a limited variety of the post pericardiectomy syndrome (8).

Clinical Manifestations

Dyspnea is the only symptom that most patients with pleural effusions experience after CABG (4). Pleuritic chest pain, chest wall tenderness, fever, pneumonitis, and pericarditis are all unusual. In one study, seven of 32 patients (22%) who had a pleural effusion that occupied more than 25% of their hemithorax were asymptomatic.

The pleural effusions that occur after CABG surgery tend to be unilateral on the left side. In the study using ultrasound (3) in which 42 of 47 patients had pleural effusion on the 7th postoperative day, 17 (40%) of the effusions were unilateral on the left, 24 (57%) were bilateral, and one (2%) was unilateral on the right. By the 30th postoperative day, there were 27 patients with effusions, and 18 (67%) of these were unilateral left sided, 8 (30%) were bilateral, and one (4%) was unilateral right sided (3).

In studies of patients that have larger pleural effusions, the effusions are usually left sided, or if they are bilateral, they are larger on the left. In the study by Sadikot et al. (8) of 71 patients with post CABG pleural effusions who underwent thoracentesis, 42 of the effusions (59%) were unilateral left sided, 18 (27%) were bilateral and usually larger on the left, and 11 (15%) were unilateral on the right.

In general, the larger pleural effusions that occur after CABG can be divided into those that occur within the first 30 days of the surgery and those that occur more than 30 days after surgery (8, 11). The late effusions do not appear to evolve from the early effusions. The characteristics of the pleural fluid in the two situations are quite different. The pleural fluid with the early effusions is bloody, with a mean red blood cell count of approximately 2,000,000 per mm^3 (8, 11). The pleural fluid is frequently eosinophilic, with a mean eosinophil percentage of greater than 40% (8). The pleural fluid eosinophilia is probably due to the blood in the pleural space. The mean pleural fluid lactate dehydrogenase (LDH) with the bloody effusions is approximately twice the upper limit of normal for serum (8). It is likely that much of the pleural fluid LDH is LDH-1, which is the LDH from the red blood cells. The pleural fluid protein is in the exudative range, and the pleural fluid glucose is not reduced (8).

In contrast to the bloody exudates seen early, the pleural fluid that occurs more than 30 days after CABG is a clear yellow lymphocyte-predominant exudate. The mean lymphocyte count for 26 late effusions in one series was 61%, whereas the mean eosinophil count was only 2% (8). The pleural fluid LDH tends to be lower with the late effusions than with the early effusions and averages about the upper limit of normal for serum (8). As with the early effusions, the pleural fluid protein is in the exudative range and the pleural fluid glucose is not reduced (8).

Diagnosis

The diagnosis of pleural effusion secondary to CABG is one of exclusion. In the days immediately after CABG, the main diagnoses to exclude are congestive heart failure, pulmonary embolus, parapneumonic effusion, and chylothorax. Congestive heart failure is excluded if the patient has an exudative pleural effusion. Chylothorax is excluded if the fluid is clear yellow or it if is very bloody. Pulmonary embolus is more difficult to exclude, and a spiral CT scan is necessary in some cases (see Chapter 14). However, the pleural effusion with pulmonary embolus usually occupies less than 25% of the hemithorax and disappears spontaneously within a couple of weeks. Patients with parapneumonic effusions are usually febrile, and the pleural fluid differential white blood cell count reveals predominantly neutrophils and a very low percentage of eosinophils.

The differential is somewhat different for the late pleural effusion occurring after CABG, and the main diagnoses to consider are congestive heart failure, chylothorax, tuberculosis, malignancy, constrictive pericarditis, and pulmonary embolus. As with the early effusion, the diagnosis of congestive heart failure is eliminated if the patient has an exudative pleural effusion and the diagnosis of chylothorax is excluded if the patient's pleural fluid is clear. With a lymphocyte-predominant pleural effusion, one must exclude tuberculosis. Because the adenosine deaminase (ADA) level is less than 40 IU per L in patients with pleural effusions after CABG (12) and is above this level in patients with tuberculous pleuritis, demonstration of an ADA below 40 IU per L virtually excludes the diagnosis of tuberculous pleuritis. Patients with constrictive pericarditis will usually have other signs and symptoms such as bilateral pedal edema and ascites.

Treatment

Most patients with a pleural effusion after CABG will have complete resolution of their effusion with one to three therapeutic thoracenteses (4, 11). When a patient is identified with a large pleural effusion after CABG, a thoracentesis should be performed to exclude the other diagnoses in the differential outlined earlier. Because the therapy of choice is a therapeutic thoracentesis in this situation, it is recommended that the initial thoracentesis be a therapeutic thoracentesis.

If the other diagnostic possibilities are excluded and the fluid recurs, a second and then a third therapeutic thoracentesis are indicated. Many patients are also given nonsteroidal antiinflammatory agents (NSAIDS) or oral prednisone, but there are no controlled studies documenting the efficacy of this approach. In like manner, chemical pleurodesis has been successful in some patients. Before one becomes too aggressive in managing this condition, it is important to realize that most patients will do well with no more than a couple of thoracenteses. In our prospective study, we followed 32 patients with pleural effusions occupying more than 25% of the hemithorax for 6 months. By the 6-month time point, only five of the 37 patients (14%) reported dyspnea, and only two had received a thoracentesis between 3 and 6 months postoperatively (4).

On occasion, the effusion persists despite several therapeutic thoracenteses. We have subjected eight such patients to thoracoscopy in recent years. At thoracoscopy, several patients had thin sheets of fibrous tissue that coated the lung and prevented it from expanding (9). It is likely that this sheet of fibrous tissue "trapped" the lung and prevented it from reexpanding. After the fibrous tissue coating the visceral pleura was removed, the lung expanded and the effusion did not recur (9). However because most had a mechanical or a chemical pleurodesis at the same time, one cannot be certain that the decortication was responsible for the effusion not recurring.

In view of the above-mentioned series, thoracoscopy is recommended for an effusion after CABG that continues to recur for several months despite several therapeutic thoracentesis. At thoracoscopy, any fibrous tissue coating the visceral pleura should be removed and the parietal pleura should be abraded to create a pleurodesis.

POSTCARDIAC INJURY (DRESSLER'S) SYNDROME

The postcardiac injury syndrome is characterized by the onset of fever, pleuropericarditis, and parenchymal infiltrates in the weeks following injury to the pericardium or myocardium (13, 14). This syndrome has been described following myocardial infarction, cardiac surgery, blunt chest trauma, percutaneous left ventricular puncture, pacemaker implantation, and angioplasty.

Incidence

The incidence of the postcardiac injury syndrome was thought by Dressler to be 3% to 4% after an acute myocardial infarction (13). Subsequent studies have demonstrated that the incidence is probably less than 1% (15), but the incidence is much higher in patients with large transmural infarctions in which the pericardium is involved (16). In one series, 15% of patients with an acute myocardial infarction and pericarditis developed the postmyocardial infarction syndrome during the follow-up period (16). The incidence of the syndrome is much higher following surgical procedures involving the pericardium (14, 17) than after an acute myocardial infarction. Engle et al. (14) reported that 30% of 257 children undergoing cardiac operations developed the syndrome. Miller et al. (18) reported an incidence of 17.8% in 944 patients undergoing cardiac surgery at Johns Hopkins Hospital during a 1-year period.

Etiologic Factors

The cause of the syndrome is unknown, but it appears to have an immunologic basis. Damage to the pericardium may initiate the immunologic events in susceptible individuals. In patients undergoing surgical procedures involving the pericardium, a close relationship exists between the development of the syndrome and the presence of antimyocardial antibodies. Engle et al. (14) prospectively followed 257 patients undergoing cardiac operations and found that 67 (26%) had high titers of antimyocardial antibodies, and all of these patients developed the syndrome. None of the 102 patients without a rise in antibody titers developed the syndrome, and only four of 93 patients with intermediate titers developed the syndrome. In a second study conducted by De Scheerder et al. (19), antibodies to actin and myosin were measured preoperatively and postoperatively in 62 patients undergoing CABG. Eight patients (13%) developed the postcardiac injury syndrome, and all eight had more than a 60% increase in their antibodies to both actin and myosin postoperatively. Thirty-eight patients did not develop the syndrome, and none of these patients had more than a 50% rise in either of the antibodies. The remaining patients developed an incomplete syndrome and had intermediate increases in their antibody titers. No such clearcut relationship has been demonstrated between antimyocardial antibodies and the syndrome in patients with myocardial infarction. Liem et al.

(15) were unable to find any association between the development of the syndrome and the presence of antimyocardial muscle antibodies in 136 patients with an acute myocardial infarction. In postoperative patients, it is unclear whether the antimyocardial antibodies precipitate or result from the syndrome.

Other factors also appear to be associated with the development of the postcardiac injury syndrome. Epidemiologic studies indicate that there is a seasonal variation in the postcardiac injury syndrome, with the highest incidence corresponding to the time of the highest prevalence of viral infection in the community (20). It has been hypothesized that a concurrent viral infection may trigger the immune response (19). In patients undergoing cardiac surgery, the incidence is approximately the same after all types of surgery (18). Younger patients and patients who are asymptomatic preoperatively are more likely to develop the syndrome (18). There is also a higher incidence of the syndrome if the patient has a history of pericarditis or if the patient had taken corticosteroids previously (18).

Clinical Manifestations

The postcardiac injury syndrome is characterized by fever, chest pain, pericarditis, pleuritis, and pneumonitis occurring after cardiac trauma or an acute myocardial infarction. The symptoms following myocardial infarction usually develop in the second or third week; an occasional patient develops symptoms within the first week (21), and a larger percentage develops symptoms only after the third week. The syndrome is seen at an average of 3 weeks following cardiac operations but can occur any time between 3 days and 1 year (22). The two cardinal symptoms of the syndrome are fever and chest pain (13, 22). The chest pain often precedes the onset of fever and varies from crushing and agonizing, mimicking myocardial ischemia, to a dull ache, to pleuritic chest pain (13). Almost all patients have a pericardial friction rub, and many also have a pericardial effusion. As many as 75% of patients with these syndromes have pulmonary infiltrates, either linear or in patches, mostly located in the base of the lungs (23). Laboratory evaluation reveals a peripheral leukocytosis (10,000 to

20,000 per mm^3) and an elevated erythrocyte sedimentation rate in most patients (13, 22).

Pleural involvement is common in the postcardiac injury syndrome. Dressler reported that 68% of 35 patients with the postmyocardial infarction syndrome had pleural effusions (13). Stelzner et al. (23) reported that 29 of 35 patients (83%) had a pleural effusion. The effusion was unilateral in 18 and bilateral in 11 the patients (23). In general, the pleural effusion is small, and pericarditis is the dominant feature. The pleural fluid is an exudate with a normal pH and a normal glucose level (23). The pleural fluid is frankly bloody in about 30% of patients, and the differential WBC may reveal predominantly polymorphonuclear leukocytes or mononuclear cells, depending on the acuteness of the process (23).

Diagnosis

The diagnosis of the syndrome should be considered in any patient who develops a pleural effusion following myocardial infarction or a cardiac operation, particularly when signs of pericarditis are present. The diagnosis of the syndrome is established by the clinical picture and by ruling out congestive heart failure, pulmonary embolism, and pneumonia. Congestive heart failure as a cause of the pleural effusion is excluded by the demonstration of an exudative pleural fluid. A spiral CT or a perfusion lung scan should be obtained to exclude the diagnosis of pulmonary embolization. It is important not to diagnose pulmonary embolism mistakenly rather than the postmyocardial infarction syndrome because anticoagulation is contraindicated in the postmyocardial infarction syndrome (13). Patients with the syndrome are at risk for developing hemopericardium. One report suggested that the diagnosis of the syndrome could be established by demonstrating a high titer of antimyocardial antibodies and a low complement level in the pleural fluid (24).

Treatment

This syndrome usually responds to treatment with antiinflammatory agents such as aspirin or indomethacin. In the more severe forms of the syndrome, corticosteroids may be necessary (25). It is important to establish the diagnosis of the postcardiac injury syndrome in patients who have undergone CABGs because the pericarditis may cause graft occlusion. Urschel et al. (22) reported that graft occlusion occurred in 12 of 14 patients (86%) who developed the syndrome after CABGs and who were treated symptomatically. When 31 subsequent patients were treated with prednisone, 30 mg per day for a week and tapering doses for 5 weeks thereafter, in addition to aspirin 600 mg q.i.d., only 5 (16%) of the grafts became occluded (22).

PERICARDIAL DISEASE

A substantial percentage of patients with pericardial disease develop a pleural effusion, which is usually left sided. Weiss and Spodick (26) reviewed the charts of 133 consecutively discharged patients with pericardial effusion. Thirty-five of the patients (26%) had a roentgenographically demonstrable pleural effusion and no other lung disease. Twenty-one of the patients had inflammatory pericardial disease without congestive heart failure, and 15 of these patients had only a left-sided pleural effusion, three had more fluid on the left than on the right, and in three, the effusions were the same size on both sides. Of the five patients with inflammatory pericarditis and congestive heart failure, the effusions were equal bilaterally in two, greater on the right side in two, and left sided in one. Two of the three patients with constrictive pericarditis had a unilateral left-sided effusion. Tomaselli et al. (27) reviewed 30 cases of constrictive pericarditis and found that a pleural effusion was present in 18 (60%). In 12 of the 18 patients, the effusion was bilateral and approximately symmetric. Three effusions were left sided, and three were right sided. We described one patient with constrictive pericarditis who had a large unilateral right-sided pleural effusion, which we attributed to the transdiaphragmatic transfer of his ascitic fluid (28).

The mechanism responsible for the pleural effusion associated with pericardial disease is not clear. The obvious explanation is that the pulmonary and systemic capillary pressures are elevated secondary to the pericardial disease, resulting in a transudative pleural effusion. It is still not clear why the effusions are more commonly left sided in patients with inflammatory pericardial disease or why at least some patients with constrictive pericarditis have exudative pleural effusions (27). The pericardial inflammation itself is probably related to the development of the pleural effusion (26).

The characteristics of the pleural fluid seen in conjunction with pericardial disease are not well described. Tomaselli et al. (27) reported that the fluid was exudative in three patients and transudative in one patient with constrictive pericarditis. We described one patient with a large right-sided pleural effusion with constrictive pericarditis who had a pleural fluid protein of 4.0 g per dL (28). In another recent report of two patients with constrictive pericarditis secondary to bromocriptine therapy, the pleural fluid in one had a protein level of 4.0 g per dL (29). I would suspect that the pleural fluid with inflammatory pericardial disease is also exudative.

Obviously, the treatment of choice for the pleural effusion secondary to pericardial disease is to treat the pericardial disease.

REFERENCES

1. American Heart Association. *1999 Heart and stroke statistical update.* Dallas, TX: American Heart Association, 1998.
2. Peng M-J, Vargas FS, Cukier A, et al. Postoperative pleural changes after coronary revascularization. *Chest* 1992;101:327–330.
3. Vargas FS, Cukier A, Hueb W, et al. Relationship between pleural effusion and pericardial involvement after myocardial revascularization. *Chest* 1994;105:1748–1752.
4. Rodriguez RM, Moyers JP, Rogers JT, et al. Prevalence and clinical course of pleural effusion at 30 days post coronary artery bypass surgery. *Chest* 1999;116:282S.
5. Rodriguez RM, Moyers JP, Rogers JT, et al. Incidence of pleural effusions 30 days post coronary artery bypass surgery. *Chest* 1998;114:387S.
6. Hurlbut D, Myers ML, Lefcoe M, et al. Pleuroplumonary morbidity: internal thoracic artery versus saphenous vein graft. *Ann Thorac Surg* 1990;50:959–964.
7. Daganou M, Dimopoulou I, Michalopoulos N, et al. Respiratory complications after coronary artery bypass surgery with unilateral or bilateral internal mammary artery grafting. *Chest* 1998;113:1285–1289.
8. Sadikot RT, Rogers JT, Cheng D-S, et al. Pleural fluid characteristics of patients with symptomatic pleural effusion post coronary artery bypass surgery. *Arch Intern Med* 2000;160:2665–2668.

9. Lee YC, Vaz MAC, Ely KA, et al. Symptomatic persistent post-coronary artery bypass graft pleural effusions requiring operative treatment–clinical and histologic features. *Chest* 2001 (*in press*).
10. Kim YK, Mohsenifar Z, Koerner SK. Lymphocytic pleural effusion in postpericardiotomy syndrome. *Am Heart J* 1988;115:1077–1079.
11. Light RW, Rogers JT, Cheng D-S, et al. Large pleural effusions occurring after coronary artery bypass grafting. *Ann Intern Med* 1999;130:891–896.
12. Lee YC, Rogers JT, Rodriguez RM, et al. Adenosine deaminase (ADA) levels in non-tuberculous lymphocytic pleural effusions. *Chest* 2000;118:1315.
13. Dressler W. The post-myocardial infarction syndrome. *Arch Intern Med* 1959;103:28–42.
14. Engle MA, Zabriskie JB, Senterfit LB, et al. Postpericardiotomy syndrome: a new look at an old condition. *Mod Concepts Cardiovasc Dis* 1975;44:59–64.
15. Liem KL, ten Veen JH, Lie KI, et al. Incidence and significance of heart-muscle antibodies in patients with acute myocardial infarction and unstable angina. *Acta Med Scand* 1979;206:473–475.
16. Toole JC, Silverman ME. Pericarditis of acute myocardial infarction. *Chest* 1975;67:647–653.
17. McCabe JC, Ebert PA, Engle MA, et al. Circulating heart-reactive antibodies in the post-pericardiotomy syndrome. *J Surg Res* 1973;14:158–164.
18. Miller RH, Horneffer PJ, Gardner TJ, et al. The epidemiology of the postpericardiotomy syndrome: a common complication of cardiac surgery. *Am Heart J* 1988;116:1323–1329.
19. De Scheerder I, De Buyzere M, Robbrecht J, et al. Postoperative immunologic response against contractile proteins after coronary bypass surgery. *Br Heart J* 1986;56:440–444.
20. Khan AH. The postcardiac injury syndromes. *Clin Cardiol* 1992;15:67–72.
21. Kossowsky WA, Epstein PJ, Levine RS. Post-myocardial infarction syndrome: an early complication of acute myocardial infarction. *Chest* 1973;63:35–40.
22. Urschel HC Jr, Razzuk MA, Gardner M. Coronary artery bypass occlusion secondary to post-cardiotomy syndrome. *Ann Thorac Surg* 1976;22:528–531.
23. Stelzner TJ, King TE Jr, Antony VB, et al. The pleuropulmonary manifestations of the postcardiac injury syndrome. *Chest* 1983;84:383–387.
24. Kim S, Sahn SA. Postcardiac injury syndrome. An immunologic pleural fluid analysis. *Chest* 1996;109:570–572.
25. Gregoratos G. Pericardial involvement in acute myocardial infarction. *Cardiol Clin* 1990;8:601–618.
26. Weiss JM, Spodick DH. Association of left pleural effusion with pericardial disease. *N Engl J Med* 1983;308:696–697.
27. Tomaselli G, Gamsu G, Stulbarg MS. Constrictive pericarditis presenting as pleural effusion of unknown origin. *Arch Intern Med* 1989;149:201–203.
28. Sadikot RT, Fredi JL, Light RW. A 43-year-old man with a large recurrent right-sided pleural effusion. *Chest* 2000;117:1191–1194.
29. Champagne S, Coste E, Peyriere H, et al. Chronic constrictive pericarditis induced by long-term bromocriptine therapy: report of two cases. *Ann Pharmacother* 1999;33:1050–1054.

17

Pleural Disease in Obstetrics and Gynecology

In this chapter, the pleural effusions seen in the practice of obstetrics and gynecology are discussed. The ovarian hyperstimulation syndrome occurring before pregnancy, fetal pleural effusions, postpartum pleural effusion, Meigs' syndrome, and finally, the pleural effusions secondary to endometriosis are addressed.

OVARIAN HYPERSTIMULATION SYNDROME

The ovarian hyperstimulation syndrome (OHSS) is a serious complication of ovulation induction with human chorionic gonadotropin (hCG) and occasionally clomiphene. This syndrome is characterized by ovarian enlargement, ascites, pleural effusion, hypovolemia, hemoconcentration, and oliguria (1). A rare complication is the occurrence of thromboembolism related to hemoconcentration (1). The severe form with ascites or pleural effusion, or both, occurs in approximately 3% of patients undergoing ovulation induction for *in vitro* fertilization, but radiologically evident pleural effusions develop in only about 1% (2).

Pathogenesis

OHSS has two primary components: (a) enlargement of the ovaries accompanied by the formation of follicular, luteal, and hemorrhagic ovarian cysts and edema of the stroma, and (b) an acute shift of fluid out of the intravascular space (2). The syndrome is more frequent in cycles resulting in pregnancy (3). The exact pathogenesis of this syndrome is not clear. At one time, it was thought that the ovarian hyperstimulation syndrome resulted from high local concentrations of estrogen in the ovaries causing altered capillary permeability and ascites, which, in turn, led to the pleural effusion. This does not appear to be the sole explanation, however, because the syndrome can still be produced in rabbits when the ovaries are exteriorized (4). This indicates that there must be systemic effects involved in the fluid shifts into the peritoneal and pleural cavities. It is now believed that the syndrome is precipitated by an ovarian product, vasoactive peptide, or cytokine that has been released into the peritoneal cavity by the ovary, or that has gained access to the systemic circulation directly from the corpus luteum or serosal vessels. Two likely candidates are interleukin 6 (IL-6) and vascular endothelial growth factor (VEGF). IL-6 has been shown to be markedly elevated in the follicular fluid and ascites, as well as in the serum and pleural fluid from patients with severe OHSS (5). VEGF is thought to be the major capillary permeability factor in OHSS ascites, because the addition of specific antibodies against VEGF is able to neutralize 70% of capillary permeability activity (6). However, the pleural fluid levels of VEGF are comparable in patients with OHSS (7) and in patients with congestive heart failure (8).

There are probably two factors responsible for the accumulation of pleural fluid with OHSS. In patients with bilateral effusions, the probable mechanism is a generalized capillary leak syndrome. In patients with large right-sided pleural effusions, it is probable that the fluid moves directly from the peritoneal space to the pleural space. Evidence supporting this mechanism is the fact that the effusions are frequently large and right sided, many patients have ascites, and the observation in one patient that the pleural fluid IL-6 level was more than 100 times higher than the simultaneously obtained serum level (9). Obviously, the pleural fluid in this case was not due to a generalized capillary leak syndrome.

Clinical Manifestations

Patients with OHSS initially develop abdominal discomfort and distention, followed by nausea, vomiting, and diarrhea. As the syndrome worsens, the patients develop evidence of ascites and then hydrothorax or breathing difficulties. In the most severe stages, the patients develop increased blood viscosity owing to hemoconcentration, coagulation abnormalities, and diminishing renal function (2). Respiratory symptoms develop 7 to 14 days after the hCG injection (3).

The pleural effusions with OHSS are usually right sided. In the series of 33 patients with pleural effusions reported by Abramov et al. (10), 17 effusions (52%) were right sided, nine (27%) were bilateral, and seven (21%) were unilateral left sided. At times, a pleural effusion may be the sole manifestation of OHSS (11). The pleural effusion can be a significant problem, as evidenced by one patient (12) who had 8,500 mL pleural fluid aspirated from her pleural space over 14 days. The pleural fluid in patients with OHSS is an exudate. In the series of Abramov et al. (13), the mean pleural fluid protein was 4.1 g per dL, whereas the mean plasm protein was 4.4 g per dL.

The incidence of the syndrome can be reduced if the serum estrogen levels and the number of ovarian follicles are monitored. If the serum estrogen levels are very high or if there are more than 15 ovarian follicles with a high proportion of small and intermediate size follicles, hCG should be withheld (1).

Diagnosis and Treatment

The treatment of the ovarian hyperstimulation syndrome is primarily supportive. Hemoconcen-

tration should be treated with intravenous fluids, because hypovolemia can lead to renal failure and even death. If the patient has a large pleural effusion and is dyspneic, a therapeutic thoracentesis should be performed.

FETAL PLEURAL EFFUSION

The ability to diagnose fetal abnormalities prenatally has been extended by diagnostic ultrasound. One abnormality now diagnosed on occasion is fetal pleural effusion. The prevalence of fetal pleural effusion is approximately one in 10,000 deliveries (14). The prevalence is approximately twice as high in boys as in girls (15).

If the fetal pleural effusion is untreated, there is a high mortality rate. In one series of untreated patients, the mortality rate was 37% for 54 untreated fetuses (14). The high perinatal mortality rate in cases of fetal pleural effusion is related to three factors: development of nonimmune hydrops, prematurity, and pulmonary hypoplasia (14). The intrathoracic compression of the developing lung produces pulmonary hypoplasia. This pulmonary hypoplasia can sometimes result in perinatal death.

Pathogenesis and Clinical Manifestations

The pathogenesis of the fetal pleural effusion is not known and is possibly multifactorial. There is some evidence that the fetal pleural effusions are actually chylothoraces. Benacerraf and Frigoletto (16, 17) analyzed the pleural fluid from two fetuses and reported abundant lymphocytes in both, but one had almost all T lymphocytes, whereas the other had a mixture of T and B lymphocytes. The presence of the lymphocytes was suggestive of a chylous effusion. In addition, most neonatal pleural effusions, which in many cases are continuations of fetal pleural effusions, are chylothoraces (18). Analysis of the pleural fluid for chylomicrons is not useful in the diagnosis of fetal chylothorax because the fetuses are not eating any lipids.

In a recent review of isolated fetal pleural effusion, 82 cases were found in the medical literature (14). The fetal pleural effusions were bilateral in 28 of 82 cases (58%), right sided in 14 (17%), and left sided in 20 (24%) (14).

Polyhydramnios was noted in 35 of 82 (42%). The reason for the polyhydramnios is not clear, but it has been suggested that the increased intrathoracic pressure may interfere with normal fetal swallowing.

Treatment

The optimal management for fetuses with pleural effusions is controversial (14). If the pleural effusions are not treated, some resolve spontaneously whereas others deteriorate to generalized hydrops. Some infants die from pulmonary hypoplasia after delivery, whereas others survive. As mentioned earlier, in a recent review, the mortality rates of those treated surgically and those treated conservatively were comparable (14). In a second review, however, the percentage of fetuses with a good outcome was significantly higher if they were subjected to invasive treatment (19).

The following management scheme, as recommended by Hagay et al. (14), is suggested for the management of fetal pleural effusion. When a pleural effusion is discovered in a fetus, a repeat ultrasound is obtained in 2 to 3 weeks. If the effusion has decreased in size, then the fetus is followed with scans every 2 to 3 weeks. If the effusion is stable or if the effusion has increased in size, then a diagnostic amniocentesis should be performed for chromosomal analysis and culture of amniotic fluid to screen for bacterial or viral infection. At the same time, a diagnostic thoracentesis should be performed and the pleural fluid sent for culture, cell analysis, and biochemical study. The lung size and the fetal lung distendability are assessed through ultrasound before and after the thoracentesis. Fetuses who have less than normal lung expansion are then subjected to surgical intervention.

The possible surgical interventions for fetal pleural effusion are pleuroamniotic shunt or repeated therapeutic thoracentesis. Rodeck et al. (20) reported their results with the implantation of pleuroamniotic shunts in eight human fetuses with pleural effusion. These shunts were established with double-pigtail nylon catheters with external and internal diameters of 0.21 and 0.15 mm, respectively. The shunts were introduced transamniotically under ultrasound visu-

alization through the fetal midthoracic wall into the effusion. All eight fetuses in this series had large pleural effusions with hydramnios. Twelve pleuroamniotic shunts were placed in these fetuses. One shunt was noted to be free in the amniotic cavity 1 week after insertion and a second shunt was inserted. The remaining 11 shunts functioned until delivery (median 2.5 weeks; range 1 to 14 weeks). In six fetuses, the pleural effusions almost completely resolved and the hydramnios disappeared. Three of the six fetuses had hydrops that resolved after the insertion of the shunt. All six infants survived, and five had no respiratory difficulty at birth. Fetal hydrothoraces did not resolve in two patients, both of whom had hydrops and died shortly after delivery. In a second study, Blott et al. (21) inserted shunts into 11 fetuses between 24 and 35 weeks' gestation and reported that the effusions were successfully drained in all cases and that eight of the 11 fetuses survived.

An alternative approach to the management of the fetal pleural effusion is to perform serial thoracenteses. Benacerraf et al. (16, 17) performed three to five thoracenteses on two fetuses between 20 and 24 weeks' gestation with massive pleural effusions. The effusion did not recur after the last thoracentesis and normal babies resulted from both pregnancies.

Prognosis

The prognosis of fetuses who have pleural effusion and who receive pleuroamniotic shunting appears to be good. Thompson et al. (22) studied 17 infants who had undergone pleuroamniotic shunting for a fetal pleural effusion at a median age of 12 months. They reported that respiratory symptoms and respiratory function were no different in these 17 infants than in a control group (22).

POSTPARTUM PLEURAL EFFUSION

Pleural effusions may develop in the immediate postpartum period or a week or more after delivery. The pathogenesis of the pleural effusions at these two different times periods is different.

Immediate Postpartum

The prevalence of small pleural effusions in the immediate postpartum period is uncertain (23, 24). Hughson et al. (23) retrospectively studied 112 patients who had delivered vaginally and had posteroanterior and lateral chest radiographs within 24 hours of delivery. They reported that 46% of the patients had small pleural effusions, which were bilateral in 75%. The same workers then conducted a prospective study of 30 similar patients who were requested to have a lateral decubitus radiograph if fluid was suggested on the standard radiographs. In this group of 30 women, 20 (67%) had a pleural effusion, and in 11, the effusion was bilateral. Ten of the women had a decubitus radiograph, and free fluid was demonstrated in seven. The results by Hughson et al. (23), however, could not be duplicated by Udeshi et al. (24), who prospectively studied 50 women within 1 to 45 hours of delivery by ultrasound. These workers reported that only one patient (2%) had a pleural effusion and that this patient had severe preeclampsia with clinically apparent pulmonary edema (24). In a subsequent study, Wallis et al. (25) prospectively studied 34 patients with preeclampsia with ultrasound and reported that six (26.5%) of the patients had a pleural effusion. There was no difference in the severity of the preeclampsia between those women with and without pleural effusion (25). Because ultrasound is more sensitive than the chest radiograph, it is likely that the true incidence is closer to that reported by the latter two groups. The mechanism responsible for the pleural effusion is unknown. No therapeutic intervention is necessary in the absence of symptoms or signs of illness (23).

Delayed Postpartum

There have been two reports (26, 27) with a total of four patients that have documented the occurrence of a systemic illness, with pleural effusions and pulmonary infiltrates occurring in the first few weeks after delivery. All four of the patients had biologically false-positive tests for syphilis early in the course of their pregnancy. Three of the four patients had severe preeclampsia and had a cesarean section. All four patients had either lupus anticoagulant or anticardiolipin antibodies, or both, in conjunction with a negative antinuclear antibody test (26, 27). Two of the four patients had serious cardiac manifestations, and two of the four patients had intravascular thrombosis within 4 weeks of delivery. Patients who experience pleuropulmonary complications in the first few weeks after delivery should be evaluated for antiphospholipid antibodies. Patients with positive assays may benefit from immunosuppressive therapy and prophylactic anticoagulation to prevent thromboembolic disease (26, 27).

MEIGS' SYNDROME

Meigs originally described a syndrome characterized by the presence of ascites and pleural effusions in patients with benign solid ovarian tumors (28). When the ovarian tumor was removed, the ascites and the pleural effusion both resolved. Subsequent to this original report, it has become apparent that a similar syndrome can occur with benign cystic ovarian tumors, with benign tumors of the uterus (fibromyomata), with low-grade ovarian malignant tumors without evidence of metastases (29), and with endometrioma (30). Meigs still prefers to reserve his name for only those cases in which the primary neoplasm is a benign solid ovarian tumor (29). Nevertheless, I classify any patient with a pelvic neoplasm associated with ascites and pleural effusion, in whom surgical extirpation of the tumor results in permanent disappearance of the ascites and pleural effusion, as having Meigs' syndrome.

Etiologic Factors

The pathogenesis of the ascitic fluid in patients with Meigs' syndrome appears to be a generalized secretion of fluid from the primary tumor. Such tumors secrete a large amount of fluid even when they have been resected and placed in dry containers (29). Only large tumors appear to be associated with free peritoneal fluid at the time of surgical procedures. Samanth and Black (31) found that only tumors with diameters greater than 11 cm were associated with free peritoneal fluid. Approximately 15% of patients with ovarian fibromas have free ascitic fluid (32), but not all patients with ascites have pleural effusions. The genesis of the pleural fluid in Meigs' syndrome is similar to that with ascites and cirrhosis (see Chapter 6); that is, fluid passes through pores in the diaphragm (33). Evidence for this pathogenesis includes the similar characteristics of the ascitic and pleural fluids, the rapid reaccumulation of the fluid following thoracentesis, and the absence of pleural effusions in some patients with ovarian tumors and ascites (32). Other investigators have concluded that the pleural fluid arises from the transdiaphragmatic transfer of ascitic fluid by the lymphatic vessels (32, 34, 35).

The tumor most commonly responsible for Meigs' syndrome is the ovarian fibroma, followed by ovarian cysts, thecomas, granulosal cell tumors, and leiomyomas of the uterus (29).

Clinical Manifestations

Patients with Meigs' syndrome usually have a chronic illness characterized by weight loss, pleural effusion, ascites, and a pelvic mass (32). It is important to remember that not all such patients have disseminated pelvic malignant disease. Patients with Meigs' syndrome may even have markedly elevated serum CA 125 levels (36). The pleural effusion is right sided in about 70% of patients, is left sided in 10%, and is bilateral in 20% (35). The only symptom referable to the pleural effusion is shortness of breath. The ascites may not be evident on physical examination.

The pleural fluid is usually an exudate. Although several authors have stated that the pleural fluid with Meigs' syndrome is a transudate (32, 37), this opinion appears to be based on the gross appearance of the fluid rather than on its protein levels. Most pleural fluids secondary to Meigs' syndrome have a protein level above 3.0 g per dL (32, 37–40). The pleural fluid usually has a low WBC (fewer than 1,000 per mm^3) and occasionally is bloody (32, 40). At times, the level of CA 125 in the pleural fluid is elevated and should not be taken as an indication of malignancy (41).

Diagnosis and Management

The diagnosis of Meigs' syndrome should be considered in all women who have pelvic masses, ascites, and pleural effusions. If in such patients the cytologic examination of the ascitic and pleural fluid is negative, an exploratory laparotomy or at least a diagnostic laparoscopy should be performed with surgical removal of the primary neoplasm. The diagnosis is confirmed when the ascites and the pleural fluid resolve postoperatively and do not recur. Postoperatively, the pleural fluid disappears from the chest rapidly and is usually completely gone within 2 weeks (39).

ENDOMETRIOSIS

At times, severe endometriosis is complicated by massive ascites (42). In a substantial proportion of patients a pleural effusion is also present. Muneyyirci-Delale et al. (42) presented four cases and reviewed the literature with 23 additional cases and found that eight of the 27 patients (30%) also had a pleural effusion. The pleural effusion was described as a bloody exudate and in one instance had an elevated pleural fluid level of CA 125 (42). The pleural effusion is thought to be due to ascitic fluid gaining entrance to the pleural cavity through the diaphragm, as in Meigs' syndrome.

Most patients initially present with abdominal distention, pain, anorexia, and nausea. Because significant weight loss occurs in many of the patients, the usually presumptive diagnosis is malignancy. However, a large proportion also have clinical manifestations of endometriosis, such as progressive dysmenorrhea and cul-de-sac and uterosacral ligament nodularity. Some patients have exacerbation of their symptoms coincident with menses.

The treatment of the massive ascites, pleural effusion, and endometriosis is difficult. Hormonal therapy [progestational agents, danazol, or luprolide acetate (Lupron)] fails in at least 50% of cases. The most common treatment is total abdominal hysterectomy and bilateral salpingo-oophorectomy, but this is difficult owing to the pelvic endometriosis (42).

REFERENCES

1. Rizk B, Aboulghar M. Modern management of ovarian hyperstimulation syndrome. *Hum Reprod* 1991;6: 1082–1087.
2. Levin MF, Kaplan BR, Hutton LC. Thoracic manifestations of ovarian hyperstimulation syndrome. *Canad Assoc Radiol J* 1995;46:23–26.
3. Gregory WT, Patton PE. Isolated pleural effusion in severe ovarian hyperstimulation: a case report. *Am J Obstet Gynecol* 1999;180:1468–1471.
4. Polishuk WZ, Schenker JG. Ovarian overstimulation syndrome. *Fertil Steril* 1969;20:241–249.
5. Loret de Mola JR. Pathophysiology of unilateral pleural effusions in the ovarian hyperstimulation syndrome. *Hum Reprod* 1999;14:272–273.
6. Elchalal U, Schenker JG. The pathophysiology of ovarian hyperstimulation syndrome—views and ideas. *Hum Reprod* 1997;12:1129–1137.
7. Chen CD, Wu MY, Chen HF, et al. Prognostic importance of serial cytokine changes in ascites and pleural effusion in women with severe ovarian hyperstimulation syndrome. *Fertil Steril* 1999;72:286–292.
8. Cheng C-S, Rodriguez RM, Perkett EA, et al. Vascular endothelial growth factor in pleural fluid. *Chest* 1999;115:760–765.
9. Loret de Mola JR, Farredondo-Soberon F, Randle CP, et al. Markedly elevated cytokines in pleural effusion during the ovarian hyperstimulation syndrome: transudate or ascites? *Fertil Steril* 1997;67:780–782.
10. Abramov Y, Elchalal U, Schenker JG. Pulmonary manifestations of severe ovarian hyperstimulation syndrome: a multicenter study. *Fertil Steril* 1999;71:645–651.
11. Rabinerson D, Shalev J, Royburt M, et al. Severe unilateral hydrothorax as the only manifestation of the ovarian hyperstimulation syndrome. *Gynecol Obstet Invest* 2000;49:140–142.
12. Yuen BH, McComb P, Sy L, et al. Plasma prolactin, human chorionic gonadotropin, estradiol, testosterone, and progesterone in the ovarian hyperstimulation syndrome. *Am J Obstet Gynecol* 1979;133:316–320.
13. Abramov Y, Elchalal U, Schenker JG. Febrile morbidity in severe and critical ovarian hyperstimulation syndrome: a multicentre study. *Hum Reprod* 1998;13:3128–3131.
14. Hagay Z, Reece A, Roberts A, et al. Isolated fetal pleural effusion: a prenatal management dilemma. *Obstet Gynecol* 1993;81:147–152.
15. Eddleman KA, Levine AB, Chitkara U, et al. Reliability of pleural fluid lymphocyte counts in the antenatal diagnosis of congenital chylothorax. *Obstet Gynecol* 1991;78:530–532.
16. Benacerraf BR, Frigoletto FD Jr. Mid-trimester fetal thoracentesis. *J Clin Ultrasound* 1985;13:202–204.
17. Benacerraf BR, Frigoletto FD Jr, Wilson M. Successful midtrimester thoracentesis with analysis of the lymphocyte population in the pleural effusion. *Am J Obstet Gynecol* 1986;155:398–399.
18. Chernick V, Reed MH. Pneumothorax and chylothorax in the neonatal period. *J Pediatr* 1970;76:624–632.
19. Weber AM, Philipson EH. Fetal pleural effusion: a review and meta-analysis for prognostic indicators. *Obstet Gynecol* 1992;79:281–286.
20. Rodeck CH, Fisk NM, Fraser DI, et al. Long-term in utero drainage of fetal hydrothorax. *N Engl J Med* 1988;319:1135–1138.
21. Blott M, Nicolaides KH, Greenough A. Pleuroamniotic shunting for decompression of fetal pleural effusions. *Obstet Gynecol* 1988;102:288–290.
22. Thompson PJ, Greenough A, Nicolaides KH. Respiratory function in infancy following pleuro-amniotic shunting. *Fetal Diagn Ther* 1993;8:79–83.
23. Hughson WG, Friedman PJ, Feigin DS, et al. Postpartum pleural effusion: a common radiologic finding. *Ann Intern Med* 1982;97:856–858.
24. Udeshi UL, McHugo JM, Crawford JS. Postpartum pleural effusion. *Br J Obstet Gynaecol* 1988;95:894–897.
25. Wallis MG, McHugo JM, Carruthers DA, et al. The prevalence of pleural effusions in pre-eclampsia: an ultrasound study. *Br J Obstet Gynaecol* 1989;96: 431–433.
26. Kochenour NK, Branch DW, Rote NS, et al. A new postpartum syndrome associated with antiphospholipid antibodies. *Obstet Gynecol* 1987;69:460–468.
27. Ayres MA, Sulak PJ. Pregnancy complicated by antiphospholipid antibodies. *South Med J* 1991;84: 266–269.
28. Meigs JV, Cass JW. Fibroma of the ovary with ascites and hydrothorax. *Am J Obstet Gynecol* 1937;33:249–267.
29. Meigs JV. Pelvic tumors other than fibromas of the ovary with ascites and hydrothorax. *Obstet Gynecol* 1954;3:471–486.
30. Yu J, Grimes DA. Ascites and pleural effusions associated with endometriosis. *Obstet Gynecol* 1991;78: 533–534.
31. Samanth KK, Black WC III. Benign ovarian stromal tumors associated with free peritoneal fluid. *Am J Obstet Gynecol* 1970;107:538–545.
32. Meigs JV. Fibroma of the ovary with ascites and hydrothorax. Meigs' syndrome. *Am J Obstet Gynecol* 1954;67:962–987.
33. Kirschner PA. Porous diaphragm syndromes. *Chest Surg Clin N Am* 1998;8:449–472.
34. Lemming R. Meigs' syndrome and pathogenesis of pleurisy and polyserositis. *Acta Med Scand* 1960;168:197–204.
35. Majzlin G, Stevens FL. Meigs' syndrome: case report and review of literature. *J Int Coll Surg* 1964;42:625–630.
36. Lin JY, Angel C, Sickel JZ. Meigs syndrome with elevated serum CA 125. *Obstet Gynecol* 1992;80:563–566.
37. O'Flanagan SJ, Tighe BF, Egan TJ, et al. Meigs' syndrome and pseudo-Meigs' syndrome. *J R Soc Med* 1987;80:252–253.
38. Hurlow RA, Greening WP, Krantz E. Ascites and hydrothorax in association with stroma ovarii. *Br J Surg* 1976;63:110–112.
39. Jimerson SD. Pseudo-Meigs' syndrome: an unusual case with analysis of the effusions. *Obstet Gynecol* 1973;42:535–537.
40. Neustadt JE, Levy RC. Hemorrhagic pleural effusion in Meigs' syndrome. *JAMA* 1968;204:179–180.
41. Timmerman D, Moerman P, Vergote I. Meigs' syndrome with elevated serum CA 125 levels: two case reports and review of the literature. *Gynecol Oncol* 1995;59: 405–408.
42. Muneyyirci-Delale O, Neil G, Serur E, et al. Endometriosis with massive ascites. *Gynecol Oncol* 1998;69:42–46.

18

Pleural Disease Due to Collagen Vascular Diseases

RHEUMATOID PLEURITIS

Rheumatoid disease is occasionally complicated by an exudative pleural effusion that characteristically has a low pleural fluid glucose level.

Incidence

Patients with rheumatoid arthritis (RA) have an increased incidence of pleural effusion. In a review of 516 patients with RA, Walker and Wright found 17 cases of pleural effusions (3.3%) without other obvious causes (1). Pleural effusions were more common in men (7.9%) than in women (1.6%). These authors also found a high incidence of chest pain in their patients with RA; 28% of the men and 18% of the women gave a history of pleuritic chest pain (1). In a separate study, Horler and Thompson (2) studied 180 patients with rheumatoid disease and found that nine (5%) had an otherwise unexplained pleural effusion. In this latter study, eight of 52 men (15%) but only one of 128 women (1%) had rheumatoid pleural effusions.

Pathologic Features

Examination of the pleural surfaces in patients with rheumatoid pleuritis at the time of thoracoscopy reveals a visceral pleura with varying degrees of nonspecific inflammation. In contrast, in most cases the parietal pleural surface has a "gritty" or frozen appearance. The parietal surface looks slightly inflamed and thickened, with numerous small vesicles or granules about 0.5 mm in diameter (3).

Histopathologically, the most constant finding is a lack of a normal mesothelial cell covering (3). Instead there is a pseudostratified layer of epithelioid cells that focally forms multinucleated giant cells of a type different from those of Langerhans or foreign body giant cells (3). The histologic features in nodular areas are those of a rheumatoid nodule with palisading cells, fibrinoid necrosis, and both lymphocytes and plasma cells (4, 5). This picture is virtually diagnostic of rheumatoid pleuritis. This specific histologic picture may not even be seen with tissue obtained from open thoracotomy (6). At times, the thickened pleura contains cholesterol clefts (5).

Clinical Manifestations

Rheumatoid pleural effusions classically occur in the older male patient with RA and subcutaneous nodules. Almost all patients with rheumatoid pleural effusions are older than 35 years of age, approximately 80% are men, and approximately 80% have subcutaneous nodules (1, 2, 6, 7). Typically, the pleural effusion appears when the arthritis has been present for several years. When two series totaling 29 patients are combined (1, 7), the pleural effusion preceded the development of arthritis in two patients by 6 weeks and 6 months, occurred simultaneously (within 4 weeks) with arthritis in 6 patients, and occurred after the development of arthritis in the remaining 21 patients. In this last group of patients, the mean interval between the development of arthritis and the pleural effusion was about 10 years.

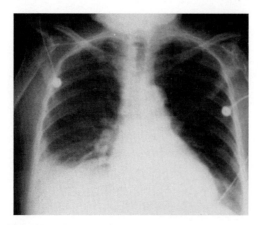

FIG. 18.1. Posteroanterior radiograph from a patient with long-standing rheumatoid arthritis. Note the right pleural effusion and the destructive changes in the shoulders. (Courtesy of Dr. Harry Sassoon.)

The reported frequency of chest symptoms in patients with rheumatoid pleural effusions has varied markedly from one series to another. In one series of 24 patients, 50% of the patients had no symptoms referable to the chest (8). In a second series of 17 patients, 15 complained of pleuritic chest pain (1), whereas in a third series, four of 12 complained of pleuritic chest pain, and of these, three were febrile (7). Other patients complained of dyspnea secondary to the presence of fluid. In one reported patient, the pleural effusion was large enough to cause respiratory failure (9).

The chest radiograph in most patients reveals a small-to-moderate-sized pleural effusion occupying less than 50% of the hemithorax (Fig. 18.1). The pleural effusion is most commonly unilateral, and no predilection exists for either side (6). In approximately 25% of patients, the effusion is bilateral (1). The effusion may eventually alternate from one side to the other or may come and go on the same side. As many as one third of these patients may have associated intrapulmonary manifestations of RA (1).

Diagnosis

The diagnosis of a rheumatoid pleural effusion is not difficult if the patient is a middle-aged man with RA and subcutaneous nodules.

Pleural Fluid Examination

Examination of the pleural fluid is useful in establishing the diagnosis because the fluid is an exudate characterized by a low glucose level (<40 mg per dL), a low pH (<7.20), a high lactate dehydrogenase (LDH) level (>700 IU per L or >2 times the upper limit of normal for serum), low complement levels, and high rheumatoid factor titers (>1:320), which are at least as high as those in serum (7) (see Chapter 4). Occasionally, the pleural fluid glucose is not reduced when the patient is first seen, but serial pleural fluid glucose determinations reveal progressively lower pleural fluid glucose levels. In the patient with arthritis and pleural effusions, the main differential diagnosis is between rheumatoid pleuritis and lupus pleuritis. Patients with lupus pleuritis have higher pleural fluid glucose levels (>60 mg per dL), higher pleural fluid pH (>7.35), and lower pleural fluid LDH levels (<500 IU per L or <2 times the upper limit of normal for serum) than patients with rheumatoid pleuritis (7). Other immunologic tests are discussed in Chapter 4, but they are not generally recommended.

The pleural fluid differential can reveal predominantly polymorphonuclear or mononuclear leukocytes, depending on the acuteness of the process. The cytologic picture from most patients with rheumatoid pleural effusion is very suggestive of the diagnosis (8). The cytological picture with rheumatoid pleuritis is characterized by three distinct features: (a) slender, elongated multinucleated macrophages; (b) round giant multinucleated macrophages; and (c) necrotic background material (8). When Naylor reviewed the cytologic picture of 24 patients seen at the University of Michigan over a 32-year period with rheumatoid pleuritis, the pleural fluid from each patient had a least one of the above-mentioned three characteristics (8). Twenty-three fluids demonstrated granular necrotic material, 17 multinucleated giant macrophages, and 15 elongated macrophages (8). These features were not seen in any of 10,000 other pleural fluids due to diverse causes (8).

The pleural fluid from patients with rheumatoid pleuritis may contain "ragocytes" or RA cells. The term ragocyte was coined by Delbarre et al. (10) who described small, spherical, cytoplasmic inclusions in neutrophilic leukocytes and occasionally in monocytes in unstained wet films of the sediment obtained from the synovial fluid of patients with various types of arthritis. These inclusions were reminiscent of raisin seeds; hence, the adoption of the prefix *rago,* which is derived from the Greek word for grape. The inclusion bodies have been shown to represent phagocytic vacuoles or phagosomes, which are of greater size than normal lysosomes of granular leukocytes (11). The presence of these cells is not useful diagnostically because pleural effusions of other etiologies, particularly those with a low glucose level, contain these cells (8, 12).

Concomitant Infection

When a patient is seen with RA and a pleural effusion characterized by a low glucose level (<20 mg per dL), a low pH (<7.20), and a high LDH level, one must rule out pleural infection, which can produce pleural fluid with the same characteristics (see Chapter 9). Hindle and Yates (13) first reported a pyopneumothorax in a patient with a rheumatoid pleural effusion. At thoracotomy, it was found that a necrobiotic nodule in the visceral pleura had broken down, producing a bronchopleural fistula. Jones and Blodgett (14) subsequently reported that five of 10 patients with rheumatoid pleural effusion followed for a 5-year period developed empyemas. These investigators found that empyemas were more common in patients who had been treated with corticosteroids, and they attributed the pleural infection to the creation of bronchopleural fistula through necrobiotic subpleural rheumatoid nodules.

When a patient with an apparent rheumatoid pleural effusion is seen, it is important to obtain both aerobic and anaerobic cultures of the pleural fluid. In addition, the pleural fluid should be centrifuged, and the sediment should be Gram stained because stains made in this manner are more sensitive than those made on uncentrifuged pleural fluid.

Glucose Levels

The most striking characteristic of the rheumatoid pleural effusion is its low glucose content. In a review of 76 patients with rheumatoid pleuritis, 48 patients (63%) had pleural fluid glucose levels below 20 mg per dL, whereas 63 patients (83%) had pleural fluid glucose levels below 50 mg per dL (6). The explanation for the low pleural fluid glucose in this condition is not known precisely. If the serum level of glucose is increased in patients with rheumatoid pleural effusions, little change is seen in the pleural fluid glucose levels (15–17), but similar results are obtained in patients with low pleural fluid glucose levels from other diseases (18). In contrast, when patients with rheumatoid pleural effusions are given oral urea (17) or intravenous d-xylose (16) loads, the pleural fluid and serum levels of these substances equilibrate over several hours.

Carr and McGuckin have suggested that the rheumatoid inflammatory process alters the normal state of one or more enzymes that constitute the carbohydrate transport mechanism of cellular membranes (17). This interpretation should be viewed with some caution. The relationship between the serum and pleural fluid glucose levels is dictated not only by the ease with which glucose passes from the serum into the pleural fluid but also by the rate at which the pleural surfaces and fluid use the glucose. Because the pleural fluid glucose level falls within 30 minutes from 2,000 to 236 mg per dL after the intrapleural injection of glucose in patients with rheumatoid pleuritis (15), there must be either rapid glucose uptake by the pleura or no great barrier to its diffusion.

The pleural surfaces with rheumatoid pleuritis appear to be active metabolically, as manifested by the high pleural fluid LDH and the low pleural fluid glucose levels, although the metabolic activity of rheumatoid pleural fluid is virtually nil even when glucose is added (16). The thickened pleura in rheumatoid pleuritis probably limits the movement of glucose into the pleural space, and because glucose consumption by the pleural surfaces is high, an equilibrium is formed in which the pleural fluid glucose level is much lower than the serum glucose level.

Cholesterol Levels

Another interesting characteristic of rheumatoid pleural effusions is their tendency to contain cholesterol crystals or high levels of cholesterol. Ferguson (5) first reported on two patients with rheumatoid pleural effusions in whom the pleural fluid contained numerous cholesterol crystals. Subsequently, Naylor (8) reported that five of 24 rheumatoid pleural fluids (21%) contained cholesterol crystals. Some rheumatoid pleural effusions contain high levels of cholesterol without cholesterol crystals (6).

Lillington et al. (6) measured the lipid levels in seven rheumatoid pleural effusions and found levels above 1,000 mg per dL in four of the seven fluids. One of the two patients who I have seen with cholesterol crystals in the pleural fluid had rheumatoid pleuritis. The cholesterol crystals impart a sheen to the fluid when viewed with the naked eye under proper lighting. High cholesterol levels make the pleural fluid turbid. The significance of the presence of high levels of cholesterol or cholesterol crystals in the pleural fluid is unknown. Cholesterol pleural effusions are discussed more extensively in Chapter 23.

Biopsy

Closed pleural biopsies have a limited role in the diagnosis of rheumatoid pleuritis. Although a pleural biopsy specimen may reveal a rheumatoid nodule diagnostic of rheumatoid pleuritis in an occasional patient, the pleural biopsy usually only reveals chronic inflammation or fibrosis. Pleural biopsy is not recommended in the typical case of rheumatoid pleuritis. In atypical cases, however, such as in patients without arthritis or in those with a normal pleural fluid glucose level, thoracoscopy or pleural biopsy should be performed to rule out malignant disease and tuberculosis.

Prognosis and Treatment

The natural history of rheumatoid pleuritis is variable. In the series of Walker and Wright (1), 13 of 17 patients (76%) had spontaneous resolution of their pleural effusions within 3 months, although one of the 13 patients had a subsequent recurrence. One patient had a spontaneous resolution after 18 months of observation, whereas another had a persistent effusion for more than 2 years. One patient developed progressive severe pleural thickening and eventually had to undergo a decortication. The last patient developed an empyema.

Little information is available in the literature on the efficacy of therapy in rheumatoid pleural disease. Some patients have appeared to respond to systemic corticosteroids (1), whereas in others no beneficial effects were observed (19–21). The degree of activity in the pleural space and in the joints is not necessarily parallel. In one report, the administration of methotrexate was associated with improvement in the arthritis but also with the development of a pleural effusion (22). The main goal of therapy should be to prevent the progressive pleural fibrosis that may necessitate a decortication in a small percentage of patients (1, 4, 20, 23, 24). There are no controlled studies evaluating the efficacy of corticosteroids or nonsteroidal antiinflammatory drugs in the treatment of rheumatoid pleural effusion. It is recommended that patients be treated with nonsteroidal antiinflammatory drugs such as aspirin or ibuprofen for 8 to 12 weeks initially. If the pleural effusion persists and if the joint symptoms are not well controlled, then appropriate therapy should be directed toward the rheumatologic problem. If the only symptomatic problem is the pleural disease, then the patient should have a therapeutic thoracentesis and possibly an intrapleural injection of corticosteroids. There have been two reports concerning the intrapleural injection of corticosteroids; the first (21) had two patients, and the intrapleural corticosteroids were ineffective; the second (25) had one patient who seemed to respond to one injection of 120 mg of depomethylprednisolone.

Decortication should be considered in patients with thickened pleura who are symptomatic with dyspnea. Computed tomographic examination is useful in delineating the extent of the pleural thickening. In patients with pleural effusions, the significance of the pleural thickening can be gauged by measuring the pleural pressure serially during a therapeutic thoracentesis (see Chapter 25). If the pleural pressure drops rapidly as pleural fluid is removed, the lung is trapped by the pleural disease (26), and decortication should be considered. The decortication procedure is difficult to perform in patients with rheumatoid pleuritis because it is not easy to develop a plane between the lung and the fibrous peel. Therefore, air leaks persist longer than usual after decortication (24). Nevertheless, decortication can substantially improve the quality of life of some patients with dense pleural fibrosis secondary to rheumatoid disease.

As mentioned earlier, patients with rheumatoid pleural effusions have a high incidence of complicated parapneumonic effusions. The management of such patients is the same as for any patient with complicated parapneumonic effusion (see Chapter 9). The incidence of persistent bronchopleural fistula is higher in the patient with rheumatoid disease, and more exploratory thoracotomies are required (24).

SYSTEMIC LUPUS ERYTHEMATOSUS

Both systemic and drug-induced lupus erythematosus may affect the pleura.

Incidence

The pleura is involved more frequently in systemic lupus erythematosus (SLE) than in any other collagen vascular disease. In a review of 138 patients with SLE, Harvey et al. (27) found that 16% had pleural effusions and that 56% complained of pleuritic chest pain some time during the course of their illness. Winslow et al. (28) reviewed the chest radiographs of 57 cases of SLE and found pleural effusions without other apparent cause in 21 (37%). Alarcon-Segovia and Alarcon (29) reviewed 48 patients with SLE and found that 21 (44%) had pleural effusions some time during their course. These figures may overestimate the incidence of pleural effusions with SLE because almost all of these patients had severe disease. A comparable incidence of pleural effusions has also been reported with drug-induced SLE (30).

Pathologic Features

Surprisingly, little has been written concerning the pathologic features of the pleura with SLE. In an autopsy series of 54 patients with SLE, acute fibrinous pleuritis was seen in about 40% and evidence of previous pleural inflammation in the form of pleural fibrosis and thickening was seen in about 33% (31). Pleural biopsy usually reveals chronic inflammation, although on rare occasions, hematoxylin bodies can be demonstrated in pleural biopsy specimens (32).

Clinical Manifestations

Most patients with pleural effusions secondary to SLE are women (7, 28), and any age group can be affected. Pleuritic chest pain is the most common symptom of the pleural disease. All nine patients in the series by Halla et al. (7) had pleuritic chest pain, as did 12 of the 14 patients in a more recent series (33). Thirteen of the 23 patients (57%) in these two series were febrile. The majority of patients with lupus pleuritis have arthritis or arthralgias before the pleuritis. The pleuritis frequently dominates the clinical picture (33) and may precede any other symptoms (28).

The pleural effusions secondary to SLE are usually small, but, at times, they may occupy nearly the entire hemithorax. The pleural effusions are bilateral in about 50% of patients, left sided only in 17%, right sided only in 17%, and alternate from one side to another in 17% (28). The effusion may be the only abnormality on the chest radiograph, but frequently the cardiac silhouette is enlarged (34). Nonspecific alveolar infiltrates, usually basilar, or atelectasis may also be seen (33, 34).

It is important to recognize that a lupus-like syndrome may develop after taking many different drugs (Table 18.1). The first five drugs in this table have been definitely incriminated in producing the lupus-like syndrome (35). They cause SLE in many individuals and elicit antinuclear antibodies (ANA) in a still higher percentage of patients. The remainder of the drugs occasionally induce a lupus-like syndrome and are not associated with an increase in the ANA (35). The incidence of pleuritic chest pain and pleural effusion is comparable in patients with drug-induced SLE and naturally occurring SLE. The main clinical difference between drug-induced SLE and idiopathic SLE is the lower incidence of renal involvement with the drug-induced SLE.

TABLE 18.1. *Drugs associated with lupus-like syndromes*

Definitely Associated	Possibly Associated
Hydralazine	Carbamazepine
Procainamide	D-Penicillamine
Isoniazid	Ethosuximide
Phenytoin	Ethylphenacemide
Chlorpromazine	Guanoxan
	Griseofulvin
	Mephenytoin
	Methyldopa
	Methylthiouracil
	Methysergide
	Oral contraceptives
	PAS
	Penicillin
	Phenylbutazone
	Primidone
	Propylthiouracil
	Reserpine
	Streptomycin
	Sulfonamides
	Tetracycline
	Troxidone

PAS, para-aminosalicylic acid.

The symptoms associated with drug-induced SLE characteristically abate within days of discontinuing the offending drug (30).

Of course, patients with SLE may have pleural effusions for other reasons than SLE. Patients with the nephrotic syndrome may have hypoproteinemia and pleural effusions on this basis. In addition, patients with SLE may have uremia, pericardial effusions, pneumonia, pulmonary emboli, congestive heart failure, or other disorders that can produce pleural effusions.

Diagnosis

The possibility of lupus pleuritis should be considered in any patient with an exudative pleural effusion of unknown etiology.

Pleural Fluid Examination

The pleural fluid is usually a yellow or serosanguineous exudate. The differential white blood cell count on the pleural fluid may reveal a preponderance of polymorphonuclear leukocytes or mononuclear cells (33).

Halla et al. (7) reported that measurement of the pleural fluid glucose, LDH, and pH levels were useful in distinguishing rheumatoid pleural effusions from lupus effusions. They reported that patients with lupus pleuritis had a pleural fluid glucose level above 80 mg per dL, an LDH level below 500 IU per L and a pH above 7.20, whereas patients with rheumatoid pleuritis had a glucose level below 25 mg per dL, an LDH above 700 IU per L, and a pH below 7.20. These biochemical tests do not always distinguish between lupus and rheumatoid pleuritis because an occasional patient with lupus pleuritis will have a low pleural fluid glucose, a high pleural fluid LDH, or a low pleural fluid pH (33). In one report of a pleural effusion due to procainamide, the pleural fluid was an exudate with a WBC of 53,200 per mm^3, an LDH of 4296 IU per L, a pH of 7.195, and a glucose of 79 mg per dL (36).

Although in the past it was believe that the most useful test for establishing the diagnosis of lupus pleuritis was the measurement of the ANA level in the pleural fluid, this does not appear to be the case. In one study of 82 patients, including eight with known SLE, the pleural fluid ANA levels were less useful than had been reported previously. The pleural fluid ANA titers were increased to 1:320 or above in six patients with lupus pleuritis (37) and were below 1:160 in two patients with SLE and effusions due to other factors. In the six patients with lupus pleuritis, the ANA titers in the pleural fluid and in the serum tended to be within one dilution of each other. However, the pleural fluid ANA titers were above 1:40 in eight of the 74 patients (10.8%) who did not appear to have lupus and in three of the patients the titers were greater than 160. The staining pattern in the patients with lupus pleuritis tended to be homogeneous, whereas it tended to be speckled in the patients without lupus, but again there was some overlap. The patients with lupus also tended to have higher titers for specific ANA to ssDNA, dsDNA, smooth muscle, and ribonucleoprotein (37).

A more recent study evaluated the ANA titers of 126 pleural fluids including seven due to SLE (38). In this study, the ANA tests were performed using a commercially available kit that used an indirect immunofluorescent antibody method with a human epithelial (HEP-2) cell line. Although all the pleural fluids from patients with SLE had titers greater than 1:320, the pleural fluid ANA titer and pattern essentially mimicked the titer and pattern in the serum (38). In addition, the pleural fluid ANA titers were greater than 1:160 in 13 other patients, including 11 patients with malignant effusions, one patient with tuberculous pleuritis, and one patient with an empyema due to amebiasis. In each instance, the pleural fluid ANA titer was within 1 dilution of the serum ANA titer (38).

The demonstration of LE cells in pleural fluid is very suggestive of lupus pleuritis (39). In a recent study, the LE cell test was positive in 8 of 11 patients who were thought to have lupus pleuritis. Moreover, the LE cell test on the pleural fluid was negative in 13 patients with serum and effusion ANA titers greater than 1:160 who were not thought to have SLE. However, because the LE cell tests on the pleural fluid always correlated with the LE test results on the serum, the LE cell test on the pleural fluid provided no additional information (39). There have been false-positive reports with the LE cell test on the pleural fluid (40).

On the basis of the above-mentioned studies, it appears that tests for ANA or LE cells on the pleural fluid add very little to the information obtained on these tests on the serum. Accordingly, they are not recommended.

Biopsy

Pleural biopsy is useful in establishing the diagnosis of lupus pleuritis if immunofluorescence is combined with light-microscopic examination. Chandrasekhar et al. (41) performed immunofluorescent studies on pleural biopsy specimens from 36 patients with exudative pleural effusions. These researchers found that their 3 patients with drug-induced SLE had a specific immunofluorescent pattern characterized by diffuse and speckled staining of the nuclei of the cells in the pleural biopsy with either anti-immunoglobulin G (IgG), anti-IgM, or anti-C3.

Other workers have reported that pleural specimens obtained at autopsy from patients with SLE have the same specific nuclear immunofluores-

cence (42). Many pleural biopsy specimens have positive immunofluorescence outside the nuclei (43); only positive nuclear immunofluorescence is thought to be diagnostic of SLE. It is my impression, however, that these stains are rarely used in establishing the diagnosis of lupus pleuritis.

Treatment

In contrast to rheumatoid pleuritis, the pleuritis with SLE definitely responds to corticosteroid administration. Hunder et al. (44) treated six patients with lupus pleuritis with corticosteroids and reported that the pleural effusions in five of the six patients rapidly cleared once therapy was begun, and the sixth effusion gradually subsided over 6 months. In the series of Winslow et al. (28), 11 patients were treated with corticosteroids and the effusions cleared rapidly in 10 of these patients. In contrast, only 10 of 16 effusions cleared spontaneously without corticosteroids. In view of the responsiveness of the pleuritis to corticosteroids and the much lower incidence of side effects with alternate-day corticosteroid therapy, corticosteroid therapy should be initiated with 80 mg prednisone every other day, with rapid dose tapering once the symptoms are controlled. Of course, if the patient has drug-induced SLE, adequate therapy consists of withdrawing the drug.

At times the pleural effusion is large and does not respond to corticosteroid therapy. In such a situation, the alternatives are similar to those for malignant pleural effusion and include chemical pleurodesis with a tetracycline derivative (45) or the implantation of a pleuroperitoneal shunt.

MIXED CONNECTIVE TISSUE DISEASE

The term mixed connective tissue disease (MCTD) was coined to distinguish the patients with combined clinical features of SLE, scleroderma, and polymyositis-dermatomyositis. A prerequisite for the diagnosis of MCTD is the presence of high titers of autoantibodies against small nuclear ribonucleoprotein (snRNP) (46). Other characteristic laboratory abnormalities in MCTD include high titer (>1:1000) of speckled antibody and high levels of antibody to RNA-sensitive extractable nuclear antigen (ENA) (46). The Sm antibodies and high titers of antinative DNA that are characteristic of SLE are uncommon in MCTD (46).

Most patients are women, and the average age at diagnosis is 37. Common clinical features of MCTD include Raynaud's phenomenon, polyarthritis, sclerodactyly, and inflammatory myositis (46). The pleural effusions are usually small and resolve spontaneously (46). In rare instances, the pleural effusion may be the presenting manifestation of MCTD. The pleural fluid is an exudate with normal glucose and complement levels.

OTHER COLLAGEN VASCULAR DISEASES

Pleural effusions occasionally occur in the course of several other collagen vascular diseases.

Angioimmunoblastic Lymphadenopathy

This disease is characterized by the acute onset of constitutional symptoms, generalized lymphadenopathy, hepatosplenomegaly, anemia, and polyclonal hypergammaglobulinemia (19). Between its original description in 1973 (47) and 1979, more than 200 cases were reported (48). It affects primarily elderly persons of either sex, with the median age of the reported cases exceeding 60 years. Pathologically, this disorder is characterized by extensive infiltration of lymph nodes with atypical lymphocytes, proliferation of arborizing small vessels, and the deposition of amorphous acidophilic material (19). It is thought to be a nonneoplastic hyperimmune proliferation of the B lymphocytes, possibly related to a lack of suppressor T lymphocytes (48, 49). Patients with this disease have a 5% to 20% likelihood of developing an aggressive lymphoma.

Approximately 12% of patients with immunoblastic lymphadenopathy have pleural effusions (49). The pleural fluid is said to be an exudate with a preponderance of mononuclear cells but no other particularly characteristic finding. In one series of 10 patients, 50% had pleural effusions, but the same patients also had ascites

and pedal edema (48). In this series, the characteristics of the pleural fluid were not described, and the pleural effusions might have been transudates. Other findings on the chest radiograph include interstitial infiltrates and mediastinal or hilar adenopathy, each in 15% to 20% of patients (48). The diagnosis is made by biopsy examination of an enlarged lymph node. In general, the prognosis is poor, with more than a 65% mortality rate in 2 years (49). Both corticosteroids and cytotoxic therapy have been tried, with equivocal results (19, 49). In addition danazol, cyclosporine, and interferon alfa have all been reported to have some efficacy, but the prognosis is poor despite therapy.

Sjögren's Syndrome

This syndrome is a chronic inflammatory disease characterized by dryness of the mouth, eyes, and other mucous membranes (19). It is frequently associated with other collagen vascular diseases, most notably RA, but sometimes SLE, dermatomyositis, or scleroderma. Pathologically, lymphocytic infiltration of the lacrimal and salivary glands occurs. It appears that Sjögren's syndrome can have an associated pleural effusion.

In a review of the pulmonary manifestations of Sjögren's syndrome, 31 of 349 patients (9%) had pulmonary involvement, and of these, five (1%) had pleural effusions (50). Of these five patients, three had RA or SLE, but two had no other connective tissue disease (50). In another series, however, none of 62 patients with Sjögren's syndrome had a pleural effusion (51). The pleural fluid has been described in two patients and was a lymphocyte-predominant exudate with normal pH and glucose level and a low adenosine deaminase level (52, 53).

Familial Mediterranean Fever

This disease, also known as familial paroxysmal polyserositis, is a rare cause of paroxysmal attacks of fever and pleuritic chest pain, sometimes with pleural effusion (54, 55). The hallmark of the disease is the recurrent, acute, self-limited febrile episodes of peritonitis, pleuritis, synovitis, or an erysipelas-like syndrome. Familial Mediterranean fever is an autosomal recessive disease that occurs almost exclusively in Armenians and Sephardic Jews who have their origin in the Mediterranean countries.

The initial attack usually occurs before age 20 and is typically dominated by peritoneal symptoms and signs. The initial attack is characterized by pleuritic chest pain and fever in fewer than 10% of patients, but approximately 40% have an attack of febrile pleurisy during the course of their disease (54). Chest radiographs during the acute pleuritic attacks reveal elevation of the ipsilateral diaphragm and frequently small pleural effusions (55). The pleural fluid contains predominantly polymorphonuclear leukocytes (56). The radiographic abnormalities and the symptoms are usually completely gone within 48 hours. Approximately 25% of the patients also have amyloidosis (52). The attacks are recurrent, with irregular intervals of days to months between. Because the administration of colchicine, 0.5 mg orally twice daily, decreases the frequency of the attacks (57, 58), it is worthwhile to establish this diagnosis in patients with recurrent episodes of polyserositis.

Churg-Strauss Syndrome

This syndrome is a disorder characterized by hypereosinophilia and systemic vasculitis occurring in individuals with asthma and allergic rhinitis (59). The American College of Rheumatology has proposed six criteria for the Churg-Strauss syndrome, with four being necessary for the diagnosis with a 85% sensitivity and 99.7% specificity; the six criteria are asthma, eosinophilia greater than 10%, paranasal sinusitis, pulmonary infiltrate, histologic proof of vasculitis, and mononeuritis multiplex (60). Typically, this disease begins with allergic rhinitis, with the subsequent development of asthma and peripheral blood eosinophilia. The systemic vasculitis with the Churg-Strauss syndrome resembles that of periarteritis nodosa, but severe renal disease is uncommon. The classic histologic picture consists of a necrotizing vasculitis, eosinophilic tissue infiltration, and extravascular granulomas,

but all three components are found in a minority of cases. In recent years, it has been suggested that there is an association between the administration of leukotriene receptor antagonists and the development of the Churg-Strauss syndrome (61).

Pleural involvement occurs on occasion with the Churg-Strauss syndrome. In Lanham et al.'s review of the literature in 1984 (59), 18 of 61 patients (30%) in whom chest radiograph results were reported had a pleural effusion. However, in a recent review of 96 patients, pleural effusions were said to be rare (60). The pleural fluid findings with the Churg-Strauss syndrome may be unique. Erzurum et al. (62) reported on one patient with bilateral effusions and pleural fluid with an LDH of 2,856 IU per L, a pH of 7.08, a glucose less than 10 mg per dL, and 10,400 WBC with 95% eosinophils. The only other disease with comparable pleural findings is paragonimiasis.

Patients with Churg-Strauss syndrome respond well to treatment with steroids, although some patients benefit from the addition of immunosuppressive agents. The vasculitic illness is usually of limited duration, but relapses can occur, and they should be detected and treated early (59).

Wegener's Granulomatosis

This disease, characterized by necrotizing granulomatous vasculitis of the small vessels, typically involves the upper and lower respiratory tracts and produces glomerulonephritis (19). Radiologically, the most common patterns in the lung are solitary or multiple nodular densities, either poorly defined or sharply circumscribed (63). An associated small pleural effusion is frequently seen (63, 64).

In one series of 11 patients, six (55%) had small pleural effusions (64), whereas in another series of 18 patients, four (22%) had pleural effusions (63). The pleural fluid in patients with Wegener's granulomatosis has not been well characterized, but it is probably an exudate. Because effective treatment for this disease is now available (19), it is important to consider this diagnosis in patients with parenchymal infiltrates and a pleural effusion. Measurement of serum antineutrophil cytoplasmic antibodies (ANCA) is useful in the diagnosis of Wegener's granulomatosis. There are two major patterns of ANCA immunofluorescence—c-ANCA shows granular staining in the cytoplasm that is accentuated in the cleft between the neutrophil nuclear lobes; p-ANCA shows perinuclear accentuation around the periphery of the neutrophil nucleus. Most patients with Wegener's granulomatosis are c-ANCA positive (65).

Eosinophilia-Myalgia Syndrome

In the late 1980s, an epidemic of the eosinophilia-myalgia syndrome was linked to the dietary ingestion of contaminated l-tryptophan. The clinical manifestations of the eosinophilia-myalgia syndrome include myalgias, arthralgias, skin rashes, muscle pain, edema, fatigue, neuropathy, and marked peripheral eosinophilia (66). A similar syndrome appears sporadically without exposure to contaminated l-tryptophan (67). Over half of the patients with the eosinophilia-myalgia syndrome have respiratory complaints, with dyspnea occurring most frequently.

Pleural effusions can occur with the eosinophilia-myalgia syndrome. In one large series of 1,531 patients, 718 patients had chest radiographs and pleural effusions were present in 12% (68). The pleural effusions are usually bilateral and are sterile eosinophilic exudates (67, 69). Although some patients have improved with the discontinuation of l-tryptophan or corticosteroid therapy, the response is often incomplete and the disease may be chronic and progressive.

Miscellaneous Diseases

Occasionally, patients with other collagen vascular diseases such as scleroderma (70), temporal arteritis (71), ankylosing spondylitis, polyarteritis nodosa, Behçet's syndrome (72), or dermatomyositis have a pleural effusion, but it appears that the pleural effusions in such patients result from complications of the disease, such as heart failure, pneumonia, or pulmonary embolism, rather than from the primary disease.

REFERENCES

1. Walker WC, Wright V. Rheumatoid pleuritis. *Ann Rheum Dis* 1967;26:467–474.
2. Horler AR, Thompson M. The pleural and pulmonary complications of rheumatoid arthritis. *Ann Intern Med* 1959;51:1179–1203.
3. Faurschou P, Francis D, Faarup P. Thoracoscopic, histological, and clinical findings in nine case of rheumatoid pleural effusion. *Thorax* 1985;40:371–375.
4. Feagler JR, Sorensen GD, Rosenfeld MG, et al. Rheumatoid pleural effusion. *Arch Pathol* 1971;92:257–266.
5. Ferguson GC. Cholesterol pleural effusion in rheumatoid lung disease. *Thorax* 1966;21:577–582.
6. Lillington GA, Carr DT, Mayne JG. Rheumatoid pleurisy with effusion. *Arch Intern Med* 1971;128:764–768.
7. Halla JT, Schronhenloher RE, Volanakis JE. Immune complexes and other laboratory features of pleural effusions. *Ann Intern Med* 1980;92:748–752.
8. Naylor B. The pathognomonic cytologic picture of rheumatoid pleuritis. *Acta Cytol* 1990;34:465–473.
9. Pritikin JD, Jensen WA, Yenokida GG, et al. Respiratory failure due to a massive rheumatoid pleural effusion. *J Rheumatol* 1990;17:673–675.
10. Delbarre F, Kahan A, Amor B, et al. La ragocyte synovial: Son intérèt pour le diagnosic des maladies rheumatismales. *Presse Méd* 1964;72:2129–2132.
11. Sahn SA. Immunologic diseases of the pleura. *Clin Chest Med* 1985;6:103–112.
12. Faurschou P. Decreased glucose in RA-cell-positive pleural effusion: correlation of pleural glucose, lactic dehydrogenase and protein concentration to the presence of RA-cells. *Eur J Respir Dis* 1984;65:272–277.
13. Hindle W, Yates DAH. Pyopneumothorax complicating rheumatoid lung disease. *Ann Rheum Dis* 1965;24:57–60.
14. Jones FL, Blodgett RC. Empyema in rheumatoid pleuropulmonary disease. *Ann Intern Med* 1971;74:665–671.
15. Ball GV, Whitfield CL. Studies on rheumatoid disease pleural fluid. *Arthritis Rheumat* 1966;9:846.
16. Dodson WH, Hollingsworth JW. Pleural effusion in rheumatoid arthritis. *N Engl J Med* 1966;275:1337–1342.
17. Carr DT, McGuckin WF. Pleural fluid glucose. *Am Rev Respir Dis* 1968;97:302–305.
18. Russakoff AH, LeMaistre CA, Dewlett HJ. An evaluation of the pleural fluid glucose determination. *Am Rev Respir Dis* 1962;85:220–223.
19. Hunninghake GW, Fauci AS. Pulmonary involvement in the collagen vascular diseases. *Am Rev Respir Dis* 1979;119:471–503.
20. Mays EE. Rheumatoid pleuritis: observations in eight cases and suggestions for making the diagnosis in patients without the "typical findings." *Dis Chest* 1968;53:202–214.
21. Russell ML, Gladman DD, Mintz S. Rheumatoid pleural effusion: lack of response to intrapleural corticosteroid. *J Rheumatol* 1986;13:412–415.
22. Abu-Shakra M, Nicol P, Urowitz MB. Accelerated nodulosis, pleural effusion, and pericardial tamponade during methotrexate therapy. *J Rheumatol* 1994;21: 934–937.
23. Brunk JR, Drash EC, Swineford O. Rheumatoid pleuritis successfully treated with decortication. Report of a case

and review of the literature. *Am J Med Sci* 1966;251: 545–551.

24. Yarbrough JW, Sealy WC, Miller JA. Thoracic surgical problems associated with rheumatoid arthritis. *J Thorac Cardiovasc Surg* 1975;68:347–354.

25. Chapman PT, O'Donnell JL, Moller PW. Rheumatoid pleural effusion: response to intrapleural corticosteroid. *Rheumatology* 1992;19:478–480.

26. Light RW, Jenkinson SG, Minh V, et al. Observations on pleural pressures as fluid is withdrawn during thoracentesis. *Am Rev Respir Dis* 1980;121:799–804.

27. Harvey AM, Shulman LE, Tumulty PA, et al. Systemic lupus erythematosus: review of the literature and clinical analysis of 138 cases. *Medicine* 1954;33:291–437.

28. Winslow WA, Ploss LN, Loitman B. Pleuritis in systemic lupus erythematosus: its importance as an early manifestation in diagnosis. *Ann Intern Med* 1958;49:70–88.

29. Alarcon-Segovia D, Alarcon DG. Pleuro-pulmonary manifestations of systemic lupus erythematosus. *Dis Chest* 1961;39:7–17.

30. Blomgren SE, Condemi JJ, Vaughan JH. Procainamide-induced lupus erythematosus. *Am J Med* 1972;52:338–348.

31. Purnell DC, Baggenstoss AH, Olsen AM. Pulmonary lesions in disseminated lupus erythematosus. *Ann Intern Med* 1955;42:619–628.

32. Gueft B, Laufer A. Further cytochemical studies in systemic lupus erythematosus. *Arch Pathol* 1954;57:201–226.

33. Good JT Jr, King TE, Antony VB, et al. Lupus pleuritis: clinical features and pleural fluid characteristics with special reference to pleural fluid antinuclear antibodies. *Chest* 1983;84:714–718.

34. Gould DM, Dayes ML. Roentgenologic findings in systemic lupus erythematosus. *J Chronic Dis* 1955;2:136–145.

35. Harpey J-P. Lupus-like syndromes induced by drugs. *Ann Allergy* 1974;33:256–261.

36. Smith PR, Nacht RI. Drug-induced lupus pleuritis mimicking pleural space infection. *Chest* 1992;101: 268–269.

37. Khare V, Baethge B, Lang S, et al. Antinuclear antibodies in pleural fluid. *Chest* 1994;106:866–871.

38. Wang DY, Yang PC, Yu WL, et al. Serial antinuclear antibodies titre in pleural and pericardial fluid. *Eur Respir J* 2000;15:1106–1110.

39. Wang DY, Yang PC, Yu WL, et al. Comparison of different diagnostic methods for lupus pleuritis and pericarditis: a prospective three-year study. *J Formos Med Assoc* 2000;99:375–380.

40. Chao TY, Huang SH, Chu CC. Lupus erythematosus cells in pleural effusions: diagnostic of systemic lupus erythematosus? *Acta Cytol* 1997;41:1231–1233.

41. Chandrasekhar AJ, Robinson J, Barr L. Antibody deposition in the pleura: a finding in drug-induced lupus. *J Allergy Clin Immunol* 1978;61:399–402.

42. Pertschuk LP, Moccia LF, Rosen Y, et al. Acute pulmonary complications in systemic lupus erythematosus. Immunofluorescence and light microscopic study. *Am J Clin Pathol* 1977;68:553–557.

43. Andrews BS, Arora NS, Shadforth MF, et al. The role of immune complexes in the pathogenesis of pleural effusions. *Am Rev Respir Dis* 1981;124:115–120.

44. Hunder GG, McDuffie FC, Hepper NGG. Pleural fluid complement in systemic lupus erythematosus and rheumatoid arthritis. *Ann Intern Med* 1972;76:357–362.

45. McKnight KM, Adair NE, Agudelo CA. Successful use of tetracycline pleurodesis to treat massive pleural effusion secondary to systemic lupus erythematosus. *Arthritis Rheum* 1991;34:1483–1484.

46. Prakash UB. Respiratory complications in mixed connective tissue disease. *Clin Chest Med* 1998;19:733–746.

47. Lukes RJ, Tindle BH. Immunoblastic lymphadenopathy: a hyperimmune entity resembling Hodgkin's disease. *N Engl J Med* 1975;292:1–8.

48. Cullen MH, Stansfeld AG, Oliver RT, et al. Angio-immunoblastic lymphadenopathy: report of ten cases and review of the literature. *Q J Med* 1979;181:151–177.

49. Shaw RA, Schonfeld SA, Whitcomb ME. A perplexing case of hilar adenopathy. *Chest* 1981;80:736–740.

50. Strimlan CV, Rosenow EC, Divertie MG, et al. Pulmonary manifestations of Sjögren's syndrome. *Chest* 1976;70:354–361.

51. Bloch KJ, Buchanan WW, Wohl MJ, et al. Sjögren's syndrome. *Medicine* 1965;44:187–231.

52. Alvarez-Sala R, Sanchez-Toril F, Garcia-Martinez J, et al. Primary Sjögren syndrome and pleural effusion. *Chest* 1989;96:1440–1441.

53. Ogihara T, Nakatani A, Ito H, et al. Sjögren's syndrome with pleural effusion. *Intern Med* 1995;34:811–814.

54. Sohar E, Gafni J, Pras M, et al. Familial Mediterranean fever. *Am J Med* 1967;43:227–253.

55. Ehrenfeld EN, Eliakim M, Rachmilewitz M. Recurrent polyserositis (familial Mediterranean fever; periodic disease). *Am J Med* 1961;31:107–123.

56. Merker H-J, Hersko C, Shibolet S. Serosal exudates in familial Mediterranean fever. *Am J Clin Pathol* 1967;48:23–29.

57. Zemer D, Revach M, Pras M, et al. A controlled trial of colchicine in preventing attacks of familial Mediterranean fever. *N Engl J Med* 1974;291:932–934.

58. Dinarello CA, Wolff SM, Goldfinger SE, et al. Colchicine therapy for familial Mediterranean fever. A double-blind trial. *N Engl J Med* 1974;291:934–937.

59. Lanham JG, Elkon KB, Pusey CD, et al. Systemic vasculitis with asthma and eosinophilia: a clinical approach to the Churg-Strauss syndrome. *Medicine* 1984;63: 65–81.

60. Guillevin L, Cohen P, Gayraud M, et al. Churg-Strauss syndrome. Clinical study and long-term follow-up of 96 patients. *Medicine (Baltimore)* 1999;78:26–37.

61. Wechsler ME, Garpestad E, Flier SR, et al. Pulmonary infiltrates, eosinophilia, and cardiomyopathy following corticosteroid withdrawal in patients with asthma receiving zafirlukast. *JAMA* 1998;279:455–457.

62. Erzurum SE, Underwood GA, Hamilos DL, et al. Pleural effusion in Churg-Strauss syndrome. *Chest* 1989;95:1357–1359.

63. Fauci AS, Wolff SM. Wegener's granulomatosis: studies in eighteen patients and a review of the literature. *Medicine* 1973;52:535–561.

64. Gonzales L, Van Ordstrand HS. Wegener's granulomatosis: review of 11 cases. *Radiology* 1973;108:295–300.

65. Homer RJ. Antineutrophil cytoplasmic antibodies as markers for systemic autoimmune disease. *Clin Chest Med* 1998;19:627–639.

66. Martin RW, Duffy J, Engel AG, et al. The clinical spectrum of the eosinophilia-myalgia syndrome associated with l-tryptophan ingestion. *Ann Intern Med* 1990;113:124–134.

67. Killen JW, Swift GL, White RJ. Eosinophilic fasciitis with pulmonary and pleural involvement. *Postgrad Med J* 2000;76:36–37.

68. Swygert LA, Maes EF, Sewell LE, et al. Eosinophilia-myalgia syndrome. Results of national surveillance. *JAMA* 1990;264:1698–1703.

69. Strumpf IJ, Drucker RD, Ander KH, et al. Acute eosinophilic pulmonary disease associated with the ingestion of l-tryptophan-containing products. *Chest* 1991;99:8–13.

70. Thompson AE, Pope JE. A study of the frequency of pericardial and pleural effusions in scleroderma. *Br J Rheumatol* 1998;37:1320–1323.

71. Garcia-Alfranca F, Solans R, Simeon C, et al. Pleural effusion as a form of presentation of temporal arteritis. *Br J Rheumatol* 1998;37:802–803.

72. Tunaci A, Berkmen YM, Gokmen E. Thoracic involvement in Behçet's disease: pathologic, clinical, and imaging features. *AJR Am J Roentgenol* 1995;164:51–56.

19

Pleural Effusion Due to Drug Reactions

Adverse reactions to drugs produce only a small percentage of all pleural effusions. Because the pleural disease in most cases rapidly resolves when the drug is discontinued, however, it is important to consider the possibility of drug-induced pleural disease in all patients with pleural effusions. The lupus-like syndromes associated with various drugs are described in Chapter 18. In this chapter, the pleural diseases resulting from the administration of nitrofurantoin, dantrolene, methysergide, bromocriptine, amiodarone, interleukin-2, procarbazine, methotrexate, and clozapine are discussed. These are the only drugs convincingly incriminated in the production of pleural disease other than drugs that produce the lupus-like syndrome. Additional drugs will probably be implicated in the future.

NITROFURANTOIN

Nitrofurantoin (Furadantin) is widely used in the treatment of urinary tract infections. Israel and Diamond first reported that the administration of nitrofurantoin could be associated with the development of an acute febrile illness with pulmonary infiltrates and pleural effusion (1). A subsequent review of the literature and the records of the company that produces nitrofurantoin in 1969 revealed that approximately 200 cases of this syndrome had been reported (2). There have now been over 2,000 cases reported (3). It is thought that nitrofurantoin injures the lung through the production of oxygen radicals (4).

Pulmonary reactions to nitrofurantoin may develop in two distinct patterns characterized by the length of treatment before the development of the syndrome (4). The acute presentation occurs within 1 month of initiating therapy with the drug. The symptoms with the acute presentation include dyspnea, nonproductive cough, and fever. The chest radiograph is usually abnormal. In one series of 335 patients (5), 186 (56%) had infiltrates, 65 (19%) had infiltrates and effusion, 14 (3%) had only an effusion, and 70 (21%) had a normal chest radiograph.

Most patients with acute pleuropulmonary reactions to nitrofurantoin have both peripheral eosinophilia (>350 per mm^3) and lymphopenia ($<1,000$ per mm^3) (6). The only reported pleural fluid analysis showed 17% eosinophils in the patient's pleural fluid (6).

The chronic syndrome occurs when the patient has been taking nitrofurantoin for 2 months to 5 years and is much less frequent than the acute syndrome. The presentation is insidious, with the gradual onset of dyspnea on exertion and a nonproductive cough (4). Patients with the chronic syndrome always have abnormal chest radiographs; diffuse bibasilar infiltrates are the most common abnormality (5). Pleural effusions, which are less common with the chronic form, occur in fewer than 10% of patients. No patients with the chronic syndrome have had a pleural effusion without an infiltrate (4).

The diagnosis of nitrofurantoin pleuropulmonary reaction should be suspected in all patients with a pleural effusion who are taking nitrofurantoin. If the drug is discontinued, the patient with the acute syndrome usually improves clinically within 1 to 4 days, and the chest radiograph becomes normal within a week (5). Symptoms and signs with the chronic syndrome resolve much more slowly (5).

DANTROLENE

Dantrolene sodium (Dantrium) is a long-acting skeletal muscle relaxant used in treating patients with spastic neurologic disorders. The chemical structure of dantrolene is similar to that of nitrofurantoin (7, 8). The chronic administration of dantrolene can lead to an eosinophilic pleural effusion (7, 8). At my previous institution, the Veterans Affairs Medical Center in Long Beach, we saw more than 10 instances of pleural effusions due to dantrolene during a 10-year period. This institution had a large population of patients with spinal cord injury for whom dantrolene was frequently prescribed. In one report, four patients developed an eosinophilic pleural effusion 2 months to 3 years after the initial administration of dantrolene (7). In one case, the eosinophilic effusion developed 12 years after dantrolene therapy was initiated (8). The pleural effusions in all patients were unilateral, and no associated pulmonary infiltrates were seen. In the reported series of four patients, one had a pericardial friction rub and another had a pericardial rub with a pericardial effusion (7). Two of the patients were febrile, and two had pleuritic chest pain.

All reported patients have had at least 5% eosinophils in their peripheral blood (7). The pleural fluid is an exudate with normal glucose and amylase levels. The differential white blood cell count on the pleural fluid has revealed at least 35% eosinophils in all cases. When dantrolene is discontinued, the patients improve symptomatically within days, but it takes several months for the pleural effusions to resolve completely. The mechanism by which dantrolene produces the eosinophilic pleural effusion is unknown.

METHYSERGIDE

Methysergide (Sansert) is a serotonin antagonist used to treat migraine headaches. The association of methysergide administration with the development of retroperitoneal fibrosis and fibrosing

mediastinitis is well established (9). One report described 13 cases of "pleurisy" secondary to methysergide treatment (10). It is not clear what these authors meant by the term pleurisy, but apparently all the patients had pleural effusions or pleural thickening (10). The pleurisy developed 1 month to 3 years after methysergide therapy was initiated, and in five patients, it was bilateral. Only one of the 13 patients had concomitant retroperitoneal fibrosis. Although no description of the pleural fluid was included in this report, in another report of a patient with bilateral pleural effusions, the fluid was bloody on one side and clear on the other (11). When methysergide was discontinued, the patients' symptoms and signs improved. At follow-up 6 months or more after discontinuation of the drug, pleural fibrosis was not detectable or was slight in seven patients, moderate in three patients, and severe in two patients. The two patients with severe fibrosis were those who had continued to take methysergide for the longest period (18 and 36 months) after the onset of this pleurisy (10). Therefore, the occurrence of a pleural effusion or pleural thickening in a patient taking methysergide is a strong indication for the prompt discontinuation of the drug.

ERGOT ALKALOIDS

Ergot alkaloid drugs such as bromocriptine, ergotamine, dihydroergotamine, nicergoline, pergolide, and dopergine are sometimes used in the long-term treatment of Parkinson's disease. The long-term administration of any of these drugs can lead to pleuropulmonary changes (12–17). Rinne reviewed the chest radiographs of 123 patients taking bromocriptine for Parkinson's disease and found that seven patients (6%) had pleural effusions, pleural thickening, and pulmonary infiltrates (12).

As of 1988, there had been a total of 23 patients reported who developed pleuropulmonary disease while taking bromocriptine (13). All the patients have been men, and the majority have had a history of long-term cigarette smoking. The prevalence of symptomatic pleuropulmonary disease among individuals taking bromocriptine is 2% to 5% (13). Patients had taken the drug for

6 months to 4 years before symptoms developed. The chest radiograph reveals unilateral or bilateral pleural thickening or effusion with or without pulmonary infiltrates. An occasional patient has only pulmonary infiltrates. Analysis of the pleural fluid reveals an exudate with predominantly lymphocytes and frequently eosinophils (13, 18). The erythrocyte sedimentation rate (ESR) is sometimes markedly elevated in these patients (17). There is some suggestion that patients taking bromocriptine-type drugs are more likely to develop pleural disease if they have a history of exposure to asbestos (17, 19).

The natural history of pleuropulmonary disease during treatment with ergot alkaloids is unclear. The disease progresses only in some of the patients who continue taking the drug (13). On discontinuation, the majority of patients improve, but complete resolution of the process is rare. It is recommended that annual chest radiographs be obtained in patients who are taking ergot alkaloids on a long-term basis. If the radiograph reveals pleural or parenchymal infiltrates, strong consideration should be given to stopping the ergot alkaloids and using an alternative drug for the treatment of the Parkinson's disease.

AMIODARONE

Amiodarone is an antiarrhythmic drug that may produce severe and potentially lethal pulmonary toxicity. The current incidence of pulmonary toxicity in patients receiving amiodarone is 5% to 10% (20), and 5% to 10% of those with pulmonary toxicity die of pulmonary fibrosis. The pulmonary toxicity is characterized by the insidious onset of nonproductive cough, dyspnea, weight loss, and, occasionally, fever. The chest radiograph reveals parenchymal infiltrates, which are predominantly interstitial (20). The toxicity rarely begins before 2 months of therapy, and it rarely occurs in patients receiving less than 400 mg per day.

Pleural effusions occur as a manifestation of amiodarone toxicity, but they are uncommon (21–23). Gonzalez-Rothi et al. (21) reviewed 11 cases of pleural disease attributed to amiodarone and found that all 11 had concomitant parenchymal involvement. Subsequently, a case has been reported in which there was no parenchymal involvement (22). The pleural fluid is an exudate (21–23) and may have predominantly lymphocytes (23), macrophages (22), or polymorphonuclear leukocytes (21). Pleural fluid eosinophilia has not been reported with amiodarone toxicity. The pleural abnormalities resolve when the amiodarone is discontinued.

INTERLEUKIN-2

Recombinant interleukin-2 (IL-2) is sometimes used in the treatment of malignancy, most commonly melanoma or renal cell carcinoma. The administration of IL-2 is accompanied by multiple acute but generally reversible toxic effects, including fever, chills, lethargy, diarrhea, anemia, thrombocytopenia, eosinophilia, confusion, and diffuse erythroderma, among others (24).

One of the primary side effects of IL-2 administration is the development of pulmonary infiltrates and pleural effusion (24, 25). Vogelzang et al. (24) reviewed the chest radiographs of 54 patients who were receiving high-dose IL-2 with or without lymphokine-activated killer cell therapy for advanced cancer and reported that 28 (52%) had a pleural effusion (24). Other abnormalities on the chest radiograph included pulmonary edema in 41% and focal infiltrates in 22%. The abnormalities were more frequent in patients receiving bolus rather than constant intravenous therapy (24). These pulmonary reactions were clinically significant in that 19 patients (35%) either developed dyspnea at rest or required intubation. The pleural effusions tend to resolve, but they persisted in 17% of patients 4 weeks following therapy. In a second study, 26 of 54 patients (48%) developed a pleural effusion after IL-2 therapy (25). In this series, 80% of the patients had either alveolar edema or interstitial edema. Two of the patients without parenchymal infiltrates had a pleural effusion (25).

The pathogenesis of the pleural effusion with IL-2 therapy is probably related to the generalized capillary leak syndrome that sometimes occurs after IL-2 therapy. It is likely that the pleural fluid originates from the leaky capillaries in the lung. Therefore, the pleural fluid would be expected to be an exudate, but to my knowledge, there is no published description of the pleu- ral fluid characteristics. It is unclear as to why the pleural effusion persists so much longer than does the pulmonary edema.

PROCARBAZINE

Procarbazine hydrochloride (Matulane), a me- thylhydralazine derivative, is effective in the treatment of Hodgkin's disease and other lym- phomas. Two detailed case reports have de- scribed pleuropulmonary reactions consisting of chills, cough, dyspnea, and bilateral pulmonary infiltrates with pleural effusions occurring after treatment with procarbazine (26, 27). In both instances, rechallenge with procarbazine again produced the infiltrates and pleural effusions. Both patients had peripheral eosinophilia. When the drug was discontinued, the patients' symp- toms and radiologic changes resolved within sev- eral days (26, 27). This syndrome appears to be identical to that associated with nitrofurantoin.

METHOTREXATE

One report exists of pleural effusion occurring after methotrexate therapy for trophoblastic tu- mors (28). Walden et al. treated 317 patients with methotrexate, 50 mg intramuscularly, followed by folinic acid for trophoblastic disease and re- ported that 14 of the patients developed pleuritic chest pain after the second to the fifth injection (28). Four of the patients also developed pleu- ral effusions, but no peripheral eosinophilia was noted. In a second report, pleural disease was re- ported in 18 of 210 patients (9%) being treated for osteogenic sarcoma with high-dose methotrexate (29). Most of the patients had severe chest pain. The mechanism of the pleuritis in those patients is unknown.

CLOZAPINE

Clozapine is an antipsychotic drug that is used in the treatment of severely ill schizophrenic pa- tients. There have been at least three reports of pleural effusions that have been attributed to clo- zapine (30–32). The pleural effusions develop within 7 to 14 days of starting the drug and

resolve when the drug is discontinued. Some but not all patients have had a concomitant skin rash or peripheral eosinophilia. Although there are no reports of the characteristics of the pleural fluid, concomitant pericardial fluid in one patient had a protein level of 5.5 g per dL and a lactate dehy- drogenase (LDH) level of 2,018 IU per L (32).

OTHER DRUGS

Several other drugs have been incriminated in causing pleural effusions.

Dapsone. The sulfone syndrome consists of a constellation of symptoms secondary to a hy- persensitivity reaction to dapsone. The clinical manifestations include fever, malaise, acute hepatitis, exfoliative dermatitis, and hemolytic anemia (33). The syndrome typically develops 2 to 6 weeks after the institution of dapsone therapy. There is one report in which a pa- tient had a large unilateral right-sided exuda- tive pleural effusion (33).

Metronidazole. Kristenson and Fryden (34) re- ported an interesting patient who developed fever and pleural effusions on two different occasions within a day of starting a course of oral metronidazole. On the initial occasion pulmonary infiltrates were also present.

Mitomycin. Small pleural effusions are frequently present in patients who have interstitial infil- trates secondary to mitomycin (35).

Isotretinoin. There is one report (36) of a 49-year- old woman who developed an eosinophilic pleural effusion 7 months after starting isotre- tinoin for systemic sclerosis. When the isotre- tinoin was discontinued, the chest radiograph became normal within 3 months. There is an- other case report of a similar case (37), and the manufacturer of isotretinoin has on file three other cases of pleural effusion occurring in pa- tients who took isotretinoin for acne.

Propylthiouracil. Middleton et al. (38) have re- ported one patient who developed left pleuritic chest pain and an eosinophilic pleural effusion 3 weeks after starting propylthiouracil (PTU). A thoracentesis 5 weeks after starting therapy revealed 16% eosinophils. The patient contin- ued taking the PTU for 2 more weeks, and the effusion enlarged and the eosinophils increased to 45%. The effusion then resolved after PTU was discontinued (38).

Simvastatin. Simvastatin is a member of the statin family of drugs used to treat hypercholesterolemia. There is one case report of a patient who developed a moderate-sized right-sided pleural effusion and interstitial infiltrates after taking simvastatin for 6 months. Thoracoscopy revealed no pleural abnormalities. He had concomitant marked elevations of his liver function tests. The patient improved after the simvastatin was stopped and prednisone was administered (39).

Warfarin. There is one case report of a patient who developed a dry cough, low-grade fever, right-sided exudative pleural effusion with 57% eosinophils, and blood eosinophilia 9 months after starting warfarin. When the warfarin was discontinued, the peripheral eosinophilia decreased somewhat, and when it was reinstituted, the peripheral eosinophilia again increased and a pleural effusion developed on the left. When the warfarin was discontinued a second time, the peripheral eosinophilia and the pleural effusions gradually resolved (40).

Gliclazide. There is one case report of a diabetic who developed a moderate-sized pleural effusion 2 weeks after beginning therapy with gliclazide, a new oral hypoglycemic agent. The patient had a peripheral eosinophil count of 20%, and the pleural fluid was an exudate with 80% eosinophils. When gliclazide was discontinued, the effusion resolved (41).

REFERENCES

1. Israel HL, Diamond P. Recurrent pulmonary infiltration and pleural effusion due to nitrofurantoin sensitivity. *N Engl J Med* 1962;266:1024–1026.
2. Hailey FJ, Glascock HW Jr, Hewitt WF. Pleuropneumonic reactions to nitrofurantoin. *N Engl J Med* 1969;281:1087–1090.
3. Rosenow EC III. Drug-induced bronchopulmonary pleural disease. *J Allergy Clin Immunol* 1987;80:780–787.
4. Cooper JA, White DA, Matthay RA. Drug-induced pulmonary disease. *Am Rev Respir Dis* 1986;133:488–505.
5. Holmberg L, Boman G. Pulmonary reactions to nitrofurantoin: 447 cases reported to the Swedish adverse drug reaction committee, 1966–1976. *Eur J Respir Dis* 1981;62:180–189.
6. Geller M, Flaherty DK, Dickie HA, et al. Lymphopenia in acute nitrofurantoin pleuropulmonary reactions. *J Allergy Clin Immunol* 1977;59:445–448.
7. Petusevsky ML, Faling J, Rocklin RE, et al. Pleuropericardial reaction to treatment with dantrolene. *JAMA* 1979;242:2772–2774.
8. Mahoney JM, Bachtel MD. Pleural effusion associated with chronic dantrolene administration. *Ann Pharmacother* 1994;28:587–589.
9. Graham JR. Cardiac and pulmonary fibrosis during methysergide therapy for headache. *Am J Med Sci* 1967;254:1–12.
10. Kok-Jensen A, Lindeneg O. Pleurisy and fibrosis of the pleura during methysergide treatment of hemicrania. *Scand J Respir Dis* 1970;51:218–222.
11. Hindle W, Posner E, Sweetnam MT, et al. Pleural effusion and fibrosis during treatment with methysergide. *Br Med J* 1970;1:605–606.
12. Rinne UK. Pleuropulmonary changes during long-term bromocriptine treatment for Parkinson's disease. *Lancet* 1981;1:44.
13. McElvaney NG, Wilcox PG, Churg A, et al. Pleuropulmonary disease during bromocriptine treatment of Parkinson's disease. *Arch Intern Med* 1988;148:2231–2236.
14. Bhatt MH, Keenan SP, Fleetham JA, et al. Pleuropulmonary disease associated with dopamine agonist therapy. *Ann Neurol* 1991;30:613–616.
15. Frans E, Dom R, Demedts M. Pleuropulmonary changes during treatment of Parkinson's disease with a long-acting ergot derivative, cabergoline. *Eur Respir J* 1992;5:263–265.
16. Ling LH, Ahlskog JE, Munger TM, et al. Constrictive pericarditis and pleuropulmonary disease linked to ergot dopamine agonist therapy (cabergoline) for Parkinson's disease. *Mayo Clin Proc* 1999;74:371–375.
17. De Vuyst P, Pfitzenmeyer P, Camus P. Asbestos, ergot drugs and the pleura. *Eur Respir J* 1997;10:2695–2698.
18. Kinnunen E, Viljanen A. Pleuropulmonary involvement during bromocriptine treatment. *Chest* 1988;94:1034–1036.
19. Knoop C, Mairesse M, Lenclud C, et al. Pleural effusion during bromocriptine exposure in two patients with pre-existing asbestos pleural plaques: a relationship? *Eur Respir J* 1997;10:2898–2901.
20. Martin WJ II, Rosenow EC III. Amiodarone pulmonary toxicity. *Chest* 1988;93:1067–1074.
21. Gonzalez-Rothi RJ, Hannan SE, Hood I, et al. Amiodarone pulmonary toxicity presenting as bilateral exudative pleural effusions. *Chest* 1987;92:179–182.
22. Stein B, Zaatari GS, Pine JR. Amiodarone pulmonary toxicity. Clinical, cytologic and ultrastructural findings. *Acta Cytol* 1987;31:357–361.
23. Akoun GM, Cadranel JL, Blanchette G, et al. Pleural T-lymphocyte subsets in amiodarone-associated pleuropneumonitis. *Chest* 1989;95:596–597.
24. Vogelzang PJ, Bloom SM, Mier JW, et al. Chest roentgenographic abnormalities in IL-2 recipients. Incidence and correlation with clinical parameters. *Chest* 1992;101:746–752.
25. Saxon RR, Klein JR, Bar MH, et al. Pathogenesis of pulmonary edema during interleukin-2 therapy: correlation of chest radiographic and clinical findings in 54 patients. *AJR Am J Roentgenol* 1991;156:281–285.

26. Jones SE, Moore M, Blank N, et al. Hypersensitivity to procarbazine (Matulane) manifested by fever and pleuropulmonary reaction. *Cancer* 1972;29:498–500.

27. Ecker MD, Jay B, Keohane MF. Procarbazine lung. *AJR Am J Roentgenol* 1978;131:527–528.

28. Walden PAM, Mitchell-Heggs PF, Coppin C, et al. Pleurisy and methotrexate treatment. *Br Med J* 1977;2:867.

29. Urban C, Nirenberg A, Caparros B, et al. Chemical pleuritis as the cause of acute chest pain following high-dose methotrexate treatment. *Cancer* 1983;51:34–37.

30. Thompson J, Chengappa KN, Good CB, et al. Hepatitis, hyperglycemia, pleural effusion, eosinophilia, hematuria and proteinuria occurring early in clozapine treatment. *Int Clin Psychopharmacol* 1998;13:95–98.

31. Stanislav SW, Gonzalez-Blanco M. Papular rash and bilateral pleural effusion associated with clozapine. *Ann Pharmacother* 1999;33:1008–1009.

32. Catalano G, Catalano MC, Frankel Wetter RL. Clozapine induced polyserositis. *Clin Neuropharmacol* 1997;20:352–356.

33. Corp CC, Ghishan FK. The sulfone syndrome complicated by pancreatitis and pleural effusion in an adolescent receiving dapsone for treatment of acne vulgaris. *J Pediatr Gastroenterol Nutr* 1998;26:103–105.

34. Kristenson M, Fryden A. Pneumonitis caused by metronidazole. *JAMA* 1988;260:184.

35. Gunstream SR, Seidenfield JJ, Sobonya RE, et al. Mitomycin-associated lung disease. *Cancer Treat Rep* 1983;67:301–304.

36. Bunker CB, Sheron N, Maurice PD, et al. Isotretinoin and eosinophilic pleural effusion [Letter]. *Lancet* 1989;1: 435–436.

37. Milleron BJ, Valcke J, Akoun GM, et al. Isotretinoin-related eosinophilic pleural effusion. *Chest* 1996; 110:1128.

38. Middleton KL, Santella R, Couser JI Jr. Eosinophilic pleuritis due to propylthiouracil. *Chest* 1993;103:955–956.

39. De Groot RE, Willems LN, Dijkman JH. Interstitial lung disease with pleural effusion caused by simvastin. *J Intern Med* 1996;239:361–363.

40. Kuwahara T, Hamada M, Inoue Y, et al. Warfarin-induced eosinophilic pleurisy. *Intern Med* 1995;34:794–796.

41. Tzanakis N, Bouros D, Siafakas N. Eosinophilic pleural effusion due to gliclazide. *Respir Med* 2000;94:94.

Pleural Effusion Due to Miscellaneous Diseases

ASBESTOS EXPOSURE

The exposure to asbestos definitely appears to be associated with the occurrence of benign exudative pleural effusions.

Incidence

Epler et al. reviewed the medical histories of 1,135 asbestos workers whom they had followed for several years and found that 35 of the workers (3%) had pleural effusions for which there was no other ready explanation (1). In contrast, no unexplained effusions were seen in the control group of 717 subjects. These authors found a direct relationship between the level of asbestos exposure and the development of a pleural effusion. In patients with heavy, moderate, and mild asbestos exposure, the incidence of pleural effusion was 9.2, 3.9, and 0.7 effusions per 1,000 person-years, respectively (1). Pleural effusions occur sooner after asbestos exposure than do pleural plaques or pleural calcification. In the foregoing series, many patients developed pleural effusions within 5 years of the initial exposure, and almost all did so within 20 years of the initial exposure. This finding is in direct contrast to the occurrence of pleural plaques and pleural calcifications, which usually do not occur until at least 20 years after the initial exposure. Other investigators, however, have reported a much longer period between the initial exposure and the development of the effusion. Hillerdal and Ozesmi (2) reviewed 60 patients with asbestos pleural effusions and found that the mean latency after the

initial exposure was 30 years and that only four of their patients had developed a pleural effusion within 10 years of the initial exposure.

Pathogenesis and Pathologic Features

The pathogenesis of the pleural effusion that occurs after asbestos exposure is not known but is probably similar to that of pleural plaques, which are described in Chapter 24. In the series of Epler et al., 20% of the affected individuals had pleural plaques (1), whereas in the Hillerdal and Ozesmi series (2), 39 of 60 patients (65%) had bilateral pleural plaques. It is likely that the presence of submicroscopic asbestos particles in the pleural space provides a constant stimulation to the pleural mesothelial cells (3). When mesothelial cells are cultured in the presence of asbestos particles, they synthesize and release a protein fraction with chemotactic activity for neutrophils, which appears to be interleukin-8 (IL-8) (4). When crocidolite is instilled into the pleural spaces of rabbits, chemotactic activity rapidly appears in the pleural fluid and this chemotactic activity is significantly inhibited by a neutralizing antibody to human IL-8 (4). In addition, when rat mesothelial cells are incubated in the presence of crocidolite or chrysotile asbestos fibers, they secrete the fibroblast chemoattractant fibronectin (5).

The gross pathologic findings in patients with pleural effusions secondary to asbestos are not well-defined. Mattson performed a thoracoscopy on nine patients with asbestos pleural effusion and found that the lung surface was completely normal in all patients but the parietal pleura was inflamed (6). In contrast, Gaensler and Kaplan reported that both the visceral pleura and the parietal pleura of their patients were thickened, and an irregular pleural symphysis was seen in all patients (7). Perhaps the difference between these series is that pleural disease had been present longer in the second group. Microscopic examination of the pleura reveals chronic fibrosing pleuritis with varying degrees of inflammation and vascularity, depending on the acuteness of the process (7, 8).

Clinical Manifestations

Patients with pleural effusions secondary to asbestos have surprisingly few symptoms (1, 2). In Hillerdal's series of 60 patients, 47% had no symptoms, 34% had chest pain, 6% had dyspnea, and the remainder had various other symptoms (2). Mattson reported that his patients often complained of feeling heavy in their chest (6). Most of Gaensler's patients complained of pleuritic chest pain or progressive dyspnea, but these patients were referred for symptoms rather than having their disorder diagnosed on the basis of serial chest radiographs (7).

The chest radiograph usually reveals a small-to moderate-sized pleural effusion, which is bilateral in about 10% of patients (1). Many patients have pleural plaques, whereas fewer than 5% have pleural calcifications, and approximately 50% have some evidence of parenchymal asbestosis (1, 7).

The pleural fluid that is associated with asbestos pleural effusion is an exudate that is serous or serosanguineous (6). The pleural fluid white blood cell count (WBC) can be as high as 28,000 per mm^3, and the pleural fluid differential WBC can reveal either predominantly polymorphonuclear leukocytes or mononuclear cells (2). Pleural fluid eosinophilia appears to be a characteristic of asbestos pleural effusions. In one series, more than 50% eosinophils were found in five of 11 asbestos pleural effusions, and an additional two effusions had more than 15% eosinophils (6). In a second series (2), 26% of 66 asbestos effusions had pleural fluid eosinophilia. Most asbestos pleural effusions contain mesothelial cells (2).

Diagnosis

The diagnosis of asbestos pleural effusion is one of exclusion. Patients with a strong history of exposure to asbestos and a pleural effusion should be closely evaluated for mesothelioma or metastatic bronchogenic carcinoma because these diseases occur much more commonly in individuals exposed to asbestos. If these diseases as well as tuberculosis and pulmonary embolism are ruled out, the patient probably has an asbestos pleural effusion and should be watched. The occupational history of any patient with an undiagnosed exudative pleural effusion should be evaluated for exposure to asbestos. If such exposure is found and the patient is asymptomatic with a small pleural effusion, the effusion is probably due to asbestos exposure.

Prognosis

The natural history of the patient with an asbestos pleural effusion is one of chronicity with frequent recurrences and sometimes the development of fibrosis of the parietal pleura (1, 6–8). The pleural effusion on the average lasts several months, but eventually, it clears and leaves no residual pleural disease in the majority of patients (2). In the series of 35 patients followed by Epler et al. for a mean period of 9.7 years, 29% of the patients developed recurrent benign effusions, more commonly on the contralateral side (1). In about 20% of patients, massive pleural fibrosis follows the asbestos pleural effusion, whereas in an additional 20%, the ipsilateral costophrenic angle remains blunted after the effusion has resolved. At times, malignant mesotheliomas follow asbestos pleural effusions. Three of the 61 patients (5%) in the series of Epler et al. developed a mesothelioma during the follow-up period. These mesotheliomas occurred 6, 9, and 16 years after the initial pleural effusion (1).

POSTLUNG TRANSPLANTATION

Pleural effusions are common after lung transplantation. Normally, 80% of the fluid that enters the interstitial spaces of the lungs is cleared from the lung via the lymphatics, whereas 20%

is cleared through the pleural space (see Chapter 2). In the patient with a lung transplant, however, the lymphatics are transected, and, accordingly, almost all the fluid that enters the lung exits through the pleural space. The continuity of the lymphatics is restored within 2 to 4 weeks after lung transplantation (9).

Pleural effusions usually are not evident in the immediate posttransplant period because the patients have chest tubes. The amount of fluid that drains through the chest tube may be very large, particularly if the patient has the reperfusion syndrome. In one patient with a severe reperfusion syndrome, the chest tube drained more than 600 mL per hour (10). Most patients do not have large amounts of chest tube drainage. Judson et al. performed serial analyses on the chest tube drainage from seven patients who had undergone lung transplantation (11). They reported that the mean output from the chest tube fell from 400 mL per day on day 1 to 200 mL per day on day 4 and that these mean outputs were similar to those seen in patients undergoing coronary artery bypass or other cardiothoracic surgeries (11). The pleural fluid on day 1 is a bloody neutrophil–predominant exudate, which by day 7 is still bloody with a mean protein of 2.0 g per dL and a mean lactate dehydrogenase (LDH) level of 677 IU per L (upper limit of normal 300 IU per L). Over this same time period, the mean WBC decreased from 10,600 cells per mm^3 to 637 cells per mm^3 and the percentage of neutrophils decreased from 90 to 49 (11).

It appears that patients who develop complications after their lung transplants are likely to have a pleural effusion. In one series in children, radiologic findings were correlated with histopathologic diagnoses in 62 instances (12): Pleural effusions occurred with 14 of 19 (74%) episodes of acute rejection, seven of eight (88%) instances of chronic rejection, six of 11 (55%) episodes of infection, three of four (75%) instances with lymphoproliferative diseases, and 15 of 20 (75%) episodes in which the histopathology was nonspecific. The high prevalence of effusion with the different entities after transplantation is probably due to the fact that a larger percentage of interstitial fluid exits through the pleural space in the patient with lung transplantation.

After lung transplantation, patients are at risk of developing empyema. In one series of 392 patients from the University of Pittsburgh, empyema developed in 14 patients (3.6%) at a mean time of 46 days after transplantation (13). Four of the 14 patients (29%) died from complicating pneumonia or sepsis, or both (13). The pleural effusion that accompanies acute lung rejection is a lymphocyte-predominant exudative pleural effusion (14).

The omental flap used to prevent dehiscence of the bronchial anastomosis may result in a pseudoeffusion on the chest radiograph. The omentum with its blood supply is introduced into the chest cavity through a small incision in the diaphragm. It is particularly likely to mimic an effusion on a supine radiograph (15).

POSTBONE MARROW TRANSPLANTATION

Pleural effusions can occur on rare occasions as a complication after bone marrow transplantation. Seber et al. (16) reviewed the medical records of 1,905 patients who received bone marrow transplants between 1974 and 1993 at the University of Minnesota. They found seven patients who had unexplained multiple effusions involving two or more of the pleural, pericardial, or peritoneal cavities. The pleura was involved in all patients. All of these cases of polyserositis occurred in recipients of allogeneic transplants. The pleural fluid was characterized by a WBC below 1,000 cells per mm^3 and a protein level below 3.0 g per dL. Because all patients had concomitant severe graft-versus-host disease, the effusions were also attributed to graft-versus-host disease (16).

YELLOW NAIL SYNDROME

The yellow nail syndrome consists of the triad of deformed yellow nails, lymphedema, and pleural effusions. Until 1986, only 97 patients had been reported with this syndrome (17). About twice as many women as men are affected (18). Eighty-nine percent of the reported cases have had yellow nails, and the yellow nails were the presenting manifestation in 37%. Lymphedema of various degrees was encountered in 80% of the reported cases and was the initial manifestation in 34%. Pleural effusions were found in 36% of all cases (17). The three separate entities may become manifest at widely varying times. For example, one patient developed lymphedema in childhood, chronic nail changes at age 78, and a pleural effusion in her ninth decade (19). An occasional patient with the yellow nail syndrome also has a pericardial effusion (20, 21) or chylous ascites (21).

The basic abnormality in this syndrome appears to be hypoplasia of the lymphatic vessels. Lymphangiograms of the lower extremity demonstrate hypoplasia of at least some lymphatic vessels in most patients with the syndrome (19). Emerson has postulated that pleural effusions may develop when a lower respiratory tract infection or pleural inflammation damages previously adequate but impaired lymphatic vessels (22). Subsequently, the lymphatic drainage of the pleural space is insufficient to maintain a fluid-free pleural space. In one report, biopsy of the parietal pleura revealed abnormally dilated lymphatics, neogenesis of lymphatic channels, and edematous tissues in some areas, suggesting some deficit in lymphatic drainage (23). The albumin turnover in the pleural fluid is not greatly decreased in patients with this syndrome, however (24).

With this syndrome, the nails are yellow, thickened, and smooth and may show transverse ridging (25). They are excessively curved from side to side, and the actual color is pale yellow to greenish. Onycholysis (separation of nail from bed) is frequently present, and nail growth is slow (25).

The pleural effusions are bilateral in about 50% of patients and vary in size from small to massive (25). Once pleural effusions have occurred with this syndrome, they persist and recur rapidly after a thoracentesis (19). The pleural fluid is usually a clear yellow exudate with a normal glucose level and predominantly lymphocytes in the pleural fluid differential WBC (19, 22, 25). The pleural fluid LDH tends to be low relative to the pleural fluid protein level. The pleural biopsy reveals fibrosis, nonspecific inflammation, or lymphocytic cellular infiltrates, none of which are diagnostic of the disease (18).

The diagnosis is made when a patient has a chronic pleural effusion in conjunction with yellow nails or lymphedema. No specific treatment exists for the syndrome, but if the effusion is large and produces dyspnea, pleurodesis with a tetracycline derivative or thoracoscopy with pleural abrasion should be considered (23, 25, 26). One patient with pleural effusion secondary to the yellow nail syndrome has been treated successfully with a pleuroperitoneal shunt (27).

SARCOIDOSIS

Sarcoidosis is occasionally complicated by a pleural effusion (28–31). The incidence of pleural effusion with sarcoidosis is probably about 1% to 2% (28, 30), although it has been reported to be as high as 7% (28). Patients with sarcoid pleural effusion usually have extensive parenchymal sarcoidosis and frequently also have extrathoracic sarcoidosis (28). The symptoms of pleural involvement with sarcoidosis are variable; many patients have no symptoms (28), although an equal number have pleuritic chest pain or dyspnea.

The pleural effusions with sarcoidosis are bilateral in approximately one third of cases. The pleural effusions are usually small but may be large. The pleural fluid is generally an exudate with predominantly small lymphocytes on the differential WBC (28, 30, 31). In one case, 90% of the cells in the pleural fluid were eosinophils at the time of the initial thoracentesis. In one report, all seven patients were described as having transudative pleural effusions with no pleural fluid protein concentration above 2.5 g per dL (29). This report is so much at variance with other reports (28, 30, 31) concerning the protein levels in the pleural fluid, however, that it can probably be ignored. Needle biopsy of the pleura or open pleural biopsy reveals noncaseating granulomas in the pleura.

The diagnosis of a sarcoid pleural effusion should be suspected in any patient with bilateral parenchymal infiltrates and a pleural effusion. A pleural biopsy demonstrating noncaseating granulomas is further support for the diagnosis, but most patients with pleural effusions and noncaseating granulomas on their pleural biopsy have tuberculosis rather than sarcoidosis. Fungal disease involving the pleura (see Chapter 11) must also be considered when noncaseating granulomas are seen on pleural biopsy examination. If a patient has typical, symmetric bilateral hilar adenopathy, parenchymal infiltrates, a negative purified protein derivative (PPD) test, and noncaseating granulomas in tissue besides the pleura, however, he or she probably has sarcoidosis. An elevated serum angiotensin-converting enzyme level gives strong support to the diagnosis. The administration of corticosteroids to patients with pleural sarcoidosis leads to a rapid amelioration of symptoms (if any) and a resolution of the pleural effusion (31).

Necrotizing sarcoid granulomatosis is a disease in which the primary pathologic abnormality is a sarcoid-like granuloma, which is also characterized by vasculitis and necrosis (32). By 1989, about 80 cases had been described. Clinically, patients may be asymptomatic or may present with cough, fever, sweats, malaise, dyspnea, hemoptysis, or pleuritic pain. Extrapulmonary findings are usually absent. Roentgenographically, the majority of patients manifest multiple well-defined nodules or ill-defined opacities. There seems to be a greater pleural component with necrotizing sarcoid granulomatosis than with typical sarcoid. In one recent report, seven patients presented with pleuritic chest pain (32). Pleural involvement was seen on computed tomography (CT) scanning in six patients, and two patients had pleural effusion. The pleural fluid findings with necrotizing sarcoid granulomatosis have not been described. The prognosis of patients with necrotizing sarcoid granulomatosis is favorable, and most patients improve rapidly after corticosteroid therapy is initiated (32).

UREMIA

In 1836, Richard Bright noted, when reviewing patients who died of nephritis, that "of all the membranes, the pleura has decidedly been most often diseased" (33). Seventy-one of his 100 cases demonstrated pleural involvement at autopsy; 41 had serous effusion, 16 showed evidence of recent inflammation, and 40 had old adhesions. In more recent series, fibrinous pleuritis has been found in approximately 20% of patients who died of uremia (34). During life, this fibrinous pleuritis can be manifested as pleuritic chest pain with pleural rubs (35), pleural effusions (35–37), or progressive pleural fibrosis producing severe restrictive ventilatory dysfunction (37–39). The pathogenesis of the pleural disease associated with uremia is not known, but it is probably similar to that for the pericarditis that is seen with uremia. The pleural effusion and the restrictive pleuritis have been likened to the hemorrhagic pericarditis and constrictive pericarditis seen with uremia.

The incidence of pleural effusions with uremia is approximately 3% (36). No close relationship exists between the degree of uremia and the occurrence of a pleural effusion (36). More than 50% of these patients are symptomatic, with fever (50%), chest pain (30%), cough (35%), and dyspnea (20%) being the most common symptoms (36). The pleural effusions are bilateral in about 20% of patients and may be large. In a series of 14 patients with uremic pleural effusions, more than 50% of the hemithorax was occupied by pleural fluid in six patients (43%) (36). Another patient had opacification of the entire hemithorax, with mediastinal shift contralaterally.

There is a high incidence of pleural effusions in patients who are receiving chronic hemodialysis. Coskun et al. (40) reviewed the thoracic CT findings of 117 uremic patients on long-term hemodialysis and reported that a pleural effusion was present in 51%. The effusions were bilateral in 63%. Jarratt and Sahn reviewed the medical records of hospitalized patients who had received hemodialysis for at least 3 months and reported that 21% had pleural effusion (41). They had a total of 100 patients with pleural effusions while receiving dialysis, and the effusions had the following etiologies: heart failure, 46; uremia, 16; parapneumonic, 15; atelectasis, 11; and miscellaneous, 12 (41).

The pleural fluid in uremic pleuritis is an exudate that is frequently serosanguineous or frankly hemorrhagic (35–37). The glucose level is normal, and the differential WBC reveals predominantly lymphocytes in the majority of patients (36). In one series of seven patients, the mean WBC was 1,231 cells per mm^3, the mean neutrophil percentage was 22, the mean protein was 3.9, and the mean LDH was slightly more than 50% the upper limit of normal for serum (41). Pleural biopsy specimens invariably reveal chronic fibrinous pleuritis.

The diagnosis of uremic pleuritis is one of exclusion in the patient with chronic renal failure (42). Specifically, fluid overload (in such a case the fluid is a transudate), chronic pleural infection, malignant disease, and pulmonary embolism need to be excluded. There is one report (43) that suggests that measurement of the pleural fluid levels of neopterin might be useful in diagnosing uremic pleural effusions. In this report, eight of nine patients (89%) with a uremic pleural effusion had a pleural fluid neopterin level above 200 nmol per L, whereas none of 85 other patients with pleural effusions of varying etiologies had levels this high (43).

Dialysis is the treatment of choice for patients with uremic pleuritis. With dialysis, the effusion gradually disappears within 4 to 6 weeks in about 75% of patients. In the remaining 25%, the effusion persists, progresses, or recurs.

In an occasional patient, the pleural thickening is progressive and leads to severe restrictive ventilatory dysfunction and marked shortness of breath (37–39). At least three such patients have undergone a decortication procedure, and the operation was not complicated by severe bleeding in any of these patients (37–39). All three patients reported marked symptomatic improvement, and one patient's vital capacity increased from 850 mL preoperatively to 1,600 mL 9 months postoperatively. Based on these reports and the progressive nature of uremic pleuritis, decortication should be considered in uremic patients with pleural thickening and severe respiratory symptoms.

TRAPPED LUNG

A fibrous peel may form over the visceral pleura in response to pleural inflammation. This peel can prevent the underlying lung from expanding (44,45). Therefore, the lung is said to be trapped. When the lung is trapped, the pleural pressure becomes more negative as the chest wall is pulled in. The negative pleural pressure increases pleu-

ral fluid formation and decreases pleural fluid absorption (see Fig. 2.1) resulting in a chronic pleural effusion.

The incidence of pleural effusion secondary to trapped lung is not known, but it is probably much higher than is generally recognized. The event producing the initial pleural inflammation is usually pneumonia or a hemothorax, but spontaneous pneumothorax, thoracic operations including coronary artery bypass surgery (46), uremia, and collagen vascular disease can cause the initial pleural inflammation. The pleural effusion in some patients with malignancy is due to a trapped lung (47). The presence of a transudative pleural effusion for many months on occasion can lead to the formation of a visceral pleural peel and a trapped lung.

Patients with pleural effusions secondary to trapped lung have either shortness of breath due to restrictive ventilatory dysfunction or an asymptomatic pleural effusion. Symptoms of acute pleural inflammation such as pleuritic chest pain or fever are distinctly uncommon, but the patient often gives a history of such events in the past. One characteristic of the pleural effusion secondary to trapped lung is that the amount of fluid is remarkably constant from one study to another (44). Following thoracentesis, the fluid reaccumulates rapidly to its previous level.

Although one would expect that the pleural fluid with trapped lung would be exudative because the pleural surfaces are involved, the pleural fluid is usually a borderline exudate. The ratio of pleural fluid to serum protein is about 0:5, and the ratio of the pleural fluid LDH level to the serum LDH level is about 0:6. The pleural fluid glucose level is normal, and the pleural fluid WBC is usually less than 1,000 per mm^3, with the differential WBC revealing predominantly mononuclear cells.

The diagnosis of pleural effusion secondary to trapped lung should be suspected in any patient with a stable chronic pleural effusion, particularly in a patient with a history of pneumonia, pneumothorax, hemothorax, or thoracic operation. The injection of 200 to 400 mL air at the time of a diagnostic thoracentesis frequently permits demonstration of the thickened visceral pleura. Measurements of the pleural pressure as fluid is withdrawn during therapeutic thoracentesis (see Chapter 25) are useful in supporting this diagnosis. The initial pleural pressure is low, and the rate of decline of pleural pressure as fluid is removed is high in patients with trapped lung. If the initial pleural pressure is below $-10\,cm\,H_2O$, or if the pleural pressure falls more than 20 cm H_2O per 1,000 mL fluid removed, the diagnosis is suggested if the patient does not have bronchial obstruction (45).

The definitive diagnosis of trapped lung requires a thoracotomy and decortication, with the demonstration that the underlying lung will expand to fill the pleural space. This operation also cures the patient, but such a surgical procedure is probably not indicated in the asymptomatic or minimally symptomatic patient with trapped lung. Such patients can be observed if the clinical picture, pleural fluid findings, and pleural pressure measurements are compatible with the diagnosis (45).

THERAPEUTIC RADIATION EXPOSURE

Pleural effusions can occur as a complication of radiotherapy to the chest. Bachman and Macken followed 200 patients treated with between 4,000 and 6,000 rads to the hemithorax for breast carcinoma (48). These researchers reported that 11 patients (5.5%) developed pleural effusions with no other obvious explanation. The pleural effusions, therefore, were attributed to the radiation (48). All patients developed their pleural effusions within 6 months of completing radiation therapy, and every patient had concomitant radiation pneumonitis (48). The pleural fluid with radiation pleuritis has not been well characterized, but one report described the fluid as an exudate with many vacuolated mesothelial cells (49). Most pleural effusions were small, but at least one occupied nearly 50% of the hemithorax. In four of the 11 patients, the fluid gradually disappeared spontaneously in 4 to 23 months. In the remaining patients, the pleural effusions persisted, gradually decreasing in size over the follow-up period of 10 to 40 months.

Pleural effusions can also occur as a late complication of radiotherapy to the chest. Morrone et al. (50) reported one case of bilateral pleu-ral effusion that developed in a patient 19 years after receiving mediastinal radiotherapy for Hodgkin's disease. The effusions were exudates with predominantly lymphocytes. Thoracoscopy revealed that there were enlarged lymphatic vessels in the visceral pleura. In a second report, a patient developed bilateral pleural effusions 8 years after receiving radiotherapy for Hodgkin's disease. In this instance, thoracoscopy demonstrated diffuse thickening of the pleura (51).

DROWNING

Individuals who drown have a substantial amount of pleural fluid at autopsy. Morild reviewed the autopsies of 133 individuals who had drowned between 1987 and 1991 (52). He found that pleural effusions were present in 71 of the patients (53%). The mean amount of fluid was 433 mL, with a maximum of more than 3,000 mL. Effusions were more common if the patient had been in the water for more than 8 hours and were more common with saltwater drowning (52). Although there are no reports of pleural effusion occurring in patients who survive near-drowning, it is likely that some have pleural effusion because one of the patients who died in Morild's series had 900 mL of pleural fluid and had been in the water only 6 to 7 minutes (52).

AMYLOIDOSIS

On rare occasions, amyloidosis can produce an exudative pleural effusion (53–55). Most pleural effusions seen in patients with amyloidosis are transudates and are secondary to the cardiomyopathy associated with that disease. The pleural biopsy may be positive for amyloid even though the pleural fluid is transudative (55). Knapp et al. (53) reported two patients with amyloidosis secondary to multiple myeloma who had pleural biopsies that demonstrated amyloid. The pleural effusion was exudative in one of the two patients. Graham and Ahmad (54) reported on one patient with an exudative pleural effusion and a positive pleural biopsy for amyloid who had primary amyloidosis. The mechanism for the exudative pleural effusion with pleural amyloidosis is unknown, but it is possibly related to obstruction of the lymphatics in the parietal pleura by the amyloid infiltration.

MILK OF CALCIUM PLEURAL EFFUSION

Milk of calcium is a colloidal suspension of precipitated calcium salts. It has been seen in various cystic spaces, such as the gallbladder, renal calyceal diverticula, adrenal cysts, and breast cysts (56). Milk of calcium can also collect in the pleural space. The radiographic picture is characteristic, showing a half-moon or hemispherical calcium-fluid level (56).

Im et al. reported five patients with pleural milk of calcium who showed a loculated pleural collection with double contour on radiography and homogeneous calcification on CT scan (56). Four of the five patients gave a history of pleurisy more than 10 years previously. Aspirated materials from the pleural space consisted of thick yellow fluid containing gritty particles. The concentration of calcium in the aspirated material was greater than 500 mg per dL (56). The five patients were essentially asymptomatic from the milk of calcium fluid collections and received no therapy for the pleural effusion (56).

ELECTRICAL BURNS

Individuals who have suffered major electrical burns may develop a pleural effusion secondary to the burn. If the contact point for the electrical burn is over the chest, the underlying pleura is damaged. Accordingly, a pleural effusion develops within the first week of the accident, and an accompanying pneumonitis may be seen (57). The pleural fluid is an exudate that gradually resolves over a period of several months.

EXTRAMEDULLARY HEMATOPOIESIS

Extramedullary hematopoiesis occurs as a compensatory phenomenon in various diseases in which there is inadequate production or excessive destruction of blood cells. Although the liver and the spleen are the most common sites of extramedullary hematopoiesis, foci can occur in many other organs, including the paravertebral areas of the thorax and the pleura.

An occasional patient with extramedullary hematopoiesis will develop a symptomatic pleural effusion (58–60). The diagnosis of extramedullary hematopoiesis is suggested in the patient with severe anemia by the presence of immature blood cells and megakaryocytes in the pleural fluid. Many patients also have multiple paravertebral masses (58). Patients with pleural effusions secondary to extramedullary hematopoiesis have been managed successfully by both chemical pleurodesis (58) and radiotherapy to the masses of hematopoietic tissue (60).

RUPTURE OF A MEDIASTINAL CYST

On rare occasions, pleural effusions result from rupture of a benign germ cell tumor or a bronchogenic cyst into the pleural space (61–63). In one series of 17 cystic mediastinal teratomas, four of the patients had preoperative rupture with pleural effusion (62). Chemical analysis of the pleural fluid is confusing at times in these cases. Hiraiwa et al. (61) reported one patient who developed a right pleural effusion after rupture of a benign mediastinal teratoma in which the pleural fluid carcinoembryonic antigen (CEA) level was elevated to 160 g per L. I have seen another case in which the pleural fluid amylase level was elevated owing to high amylase levels in the germ cell tumor. Khalil et al. (63) reported two cases of bronchogenic cysts with associated pleural effusion. No description of the fluid was provided (63).

ACUTE RESPIRATORY DISTRESS SYNDROME

There appears to be a high prevalence of small pleural effusions in patients with the acute respiratory distress syndrome (ARDS). The usual origin of the pleural fluid in patients with the ARDS is probably the interstitial spaces of the lung. Tagliabue et al. reviewed the CT findings in 74 patients with ARDS (64). They reported that pleural effusions were present in 37 (50%). On the chest radiograph, the effusion was apparent in 25 of the 37 (41%). The effusions were bilateral in 21, unilateral and right-sided in six, and unilateral and left-sided in ten. The effusions were small in 22 and moderate in 15. In a second study,

Talmor et al. (65) prospectively studied 199 patients with ARDS in a surgical intensive care unit who required positive end-expiratory pressure (PEEP). These investigators found that 19 patients (10%) who had unsatisfactory oxygenation status had effusions visible on the supine chest radiograph. When chest tubes were inserted into these patients, their oxygenation status and their lung compliance improved (65). Fartoukh et al. (66) demonstrated that a diagnostic thoracentesis is indicated for patients in the intensive care unit who have a pleural effusion because the results of the diagnostic thoracentesis frequently changed the management of the patient. Patients with ARDS with significant pleural fluid should undergo a thoracentesis in order to delineate the characteristics of the pleural fluid. If the patient is having trouble with oxygenation or with being weaned from the ventilator, a therapeutic thoracentesis should be performed.

WHIPPLE'S DISEASE

Whipple's disease is characterized by weight loss, diarrhea, arthralgias, and abdominal pain. Whipple's disease is due to chronic infection with the bacterium *Tropheryma whippelii* (67). At times, patients with Whipple's disease have pleural effusions, but the pleural effusions are usually not an important manifestation of the disease. In one case, polymerase chain reaction (PCR) on the cells from a pleural effusion demonstrated *T. whippelii*–specific rRNA (68).

SYPHILIS

On rare occasions, syphilis can cause a pleural effusion. There was one case report (69) of a patient with an exudative pleural effusion with predominantly lymphocytes in the fluid and granuloma on the pleural biopsy who turned out to have syphilis (69).

IATROGENIC PLEURAL EFFUSIONS

At times, physicians are responsible for the development of pleural effusions in their patients. The iatrogenic effusions secondary to various pharmaceutical agents, radiation therapy, endoscopic esophageal sclerotherapy, the ovarian hyperstimulation syndrome, and fluid overload are discussed elsewhere in this book, as are those that occur following coronary artery bypass surgery and abdominal surgery. In this section, I discuss the iatrogenic pleural effusions that result from misplacement of percutaneously inserted catheters or enteral feeding tubes, those associated with translumbar aortography, and those resulting from rupture of silicone bag mammary prosthesis.

Superior Vena Cava Perforation by a Central Catheter

An uncommon but potentially fatal iatrogenic cause of pleural effusion is the misplacement of a percutaneously inserted catheter into the mediastinum or the pleural space. As of 1995, there had been 35 reports describing 69 patients with central venous catheter–induced hydrothorax (70). The incidence of this complication has been estimated to be as high as 0.5% (70). The two major risk factors for the development of this complication are (1) catheter insertion from the left and (2) large-bore catheters (71).

The average time interval from catheter placement to the onset of symptoms is 2.0 days, with a range of 1 to 60 days (71). The more common clinical symptoms and signs are dyspnea (82%), chest pain (46%), respiratory failure (18%), hypotension (13%), and cardiac arrest (5%). The chest radiograph may reveal unilateral or bilateral pleural effusions with or without a widened mediastinum. A unilateral pleural effusion may be ipsilateral or contralateral to the catheter's insertion site (71).

The pleural fluid may be pure blood resulting from laceration or puncture of one of the vessels (72). More frequently, the pleural fluid reflects the characteristics of the infusate. If the patient is receiving an intravenous fat emulsion, the pleural fluid may appear milky and is easily confused with a chylothorax (73). If the patient is receiving 5% dextrose-containing solutions, the pleural fluid glucose level is invariably higher than the simultaneous serum glucose level (71). The pleural fluid protein and LDH levels are usually very low (70).

The diagnosis should be suspected in any patient with a central line who has a large pleural effusion. If aspiration of the central catheter yields blood, a perforation may still be present (74). Analysis of the pleural fluid usually confirms the diagnosis. The treatment is to remove the catheter immediately. If the patient is in respiratory distress, a therapeutic thoracentesis should be performed. If fresh blood is present, a chest tube should be inserted immediately, and if bleeding persists, an exploratory thoracotomy may be necessary (72).

Perforation of Pleura with a Nasogastric Tube

The development of soft, flexible, small-bore polyurethane feeding tubes has made nasogastric and nasoenteric feeding more practical and comfortable for patients. The increasing awareness by physicians of the importance of malnutrition and metabolic support has led to an increase in the use of such tubes. Their use has been associated with significant pleural complications, however. In an 11-month period in one institution, there were four instances in which nasogastric tubes were placed in the tracheobronchial tree for an incidence of about 0.3% of all intensive care unit patients who received nasogastric tubes (75). These tubes are often inserted into patients who have taken an overdose. Because such patients are obtunded, sometimes the tubes enter the pleural space. There have been several instances in which charcoal has been instilled into the pleural space (76).

Pneumothorax is the most common complication (77), but the infusion of the enteral formula into the pleural space or the development of an empyema also occurs relatively frequently (77). The stylets used for ease of insertion provide stiffness and strength to the tubing and allow easier advancement of the device. With the stylet in place, the tubing becomes stiff and is able to perforate structures relatively easily. There are frequently no clinical clues that the tube has entered the bronchial tree instead of the esophagus. The risk of this complication is much greater if the patient has an endotracheal tube in place or if he or she is obtunded (77). To prevent this complication, these tubes should only be inserted by experienced individuals, and the tube should be removed immediately if the patient starts coughing. If any resistance is felt, no further attempts should be made to advance the tube. Before feeding is initiated, the position of the tip of the tube should be confirmed radiographically (78). The standard tests for the placement of nasogastric tubes such as the insufflation of air with auscultation over the left upper quadrant or the aspiration of fluid are often misleading with the small nasogastric tubes (78).

If the tube enters the pleural space and the enteral solutions or charcoal is infused, tube thoracostomy should be performed after the nasogastric tube has been removed. In such a situation, the possibility of an empyema should be evaluated because the incidence of empyema is high when these small tubes enter the pleural space (77).

Translumbar Aortography

Pleural effusion may also complicate translumbar aortographic examination (79). Small pleural effusions requiring decubitus radiographs for their demonstration frequently occur after translumbar aortographic studies (79) and are thought to be secondary to the passage of the needle through the most inferior part of the pleural space. An exudative pleural effusion may result from irritation of the pleural space by the extravasated contrast medium. The pleural effusion following translumbar aortographic examination is sometimes frankly bloody and probably results from blood leaking from the aorta into the pleural space. In such situations, a therapeutic thoracentesis is usually sufficient treatment because the leak stops spontaneously (79).

After Mammaplasty

There have been at least four case reports of a pleural effusion developing after rupture of a silicone bag mammary prosthesis (80–82). One patient developed left-sided pleuritic chest pain 24 hours after she had sustained a blow of moderate severity on the left anterior chest wall. Five years previously, she had undergone bilateral augmentation mammoplasties with insertion of silicone bag prostheses. On physical examination, the breasts appeared equal in size. The chest radiograph revealed a large left pleural effusion. Thoracentesis revealed slightly turbid fluid with a protein level of 4.6 g per dL and an LDH level of 372 IU per L. A subsequent pleural biopsy revealed a dense mixed cellular infiltrate with several granulomas with large multinucleated giant cells suggestive of a foreign body reaction. Two liters of pleural fluid were aspirated, and an oily layer was observed on the top of the fluid, which was consistent with the presence of silicone gel in the aspirate. After the aspiration, the pleural effusion did not recur. Two other patients (81, 82) developed pleural effusions approximately 1 year after their implants had ruptured. In one patient, there was viscid, yellowish pasty material that could only be obtained with a 14-gauge needle (81). The other fluid was yellow, and scanning electron microscopy was necessary to demonstrate material with the electron energy pattern of silicone (82). These three reports demonstrate that silicone can reach the pleural space, but once there, it does not elicit much of an inflammatory reaction.

REFERENCES

1. Epler GR, McLoud TC, Gaensler EA. Prevalence and incidence of benign asbestos pleural effusion in a working population. *JAMA* 1982;247:617–622.
2. Hillerdal G, Ozesmi M. Benign asbestos pleural effusion: 73 exudates in 60 patients. *Eur J Respir Dis* 1987;71:113–121.
3. Sargent EN, Jacobson G, Gordonson JS. Pleural plaques: a signpost of asbestos dust inhalation. *Semin Roentgenol* 1977;12:287–297.
4. Boylan AM, Ruegg C, Kim KJ, et al. Evidence of a role for mesothelial cell–derived interleukin 8 in the pathogenesis of asbestos-induced pleurisy in rabbits. *J Clin Invest* 1992;89:1257–1267.
5. Kuwahara M, Kuwahara M, Verma K, et al. Asbestos exposure stimulates pleural mesothelial cells to secrete the fibroblast chemattractant, fibronectin. *Am J Respir Cell Mol Biol* 1994;10:167–176.
6. Mattson S-B. Monosymptomatic exudative pleurisy in persons exposed to asbestos dust. *Scand J Respir Dis* 1975;56:263–272.
7. Gaensler EA, Kaplan AI. Asbestos pleural effusion. *Ann Intern Med* 1971;74:178–191.
8. Hillerdal G. Non-malignant asbestos pleural disease. *Thorax* 1981;36:669–675.
9. Ruggiero R, Fietsam R Jr, Thomas GA, et al. Detection of canine allograft lung rejection by pulmonary lymphoscintigraphy. *J Thorac Cardiovasc Surg* 1994;108:253–258.
10. Raju S, Heath BJ, Warren ET, et al. Single- and double-

11. Judson MA, Handy JR, Sahn SA. Pleural effusions following lung transplantation. Time course, characteristics, and clinical implications. *Chest* 1996;109:1190–1194.
12. Medina LS, Siegel MJ, Bejarano PA, et al. Pediatric lung transplantation: radiographic-histopathologic correlation. *Radiology* 1993;187:807–810.
13. Nunley DR, Grgurich WF, Keenan RJ, et al. Empyema complicating successful lung transplantation. *Chest* 1999;115:1312–1315.
14. Judson MA, Handy JR, Sahn SA. Pleural effusion from acute lung rejection. *Chest* 1997;111:1128–1130.
15. O'Donovan PB. Imaging of complications of lung transplantation. *Radiographics* 1993;13:787–796.
16. Seber A, Khan SP, Kersey JH. Unexplained effusions: association with allogeneic bone marrow transplantation and acute or chronic graft-versus-host disease. *Bone Marrow Transplant* 1996;17:207–211.
17. Nordkild P, Kromann-Andersen H, Struve-Christensen E. Yellow nail syndrome—the triad of yellow nails, lymphedema, and pleural effusions. *Acta Med Scand* 1986;219:221–227.
18. Cordasco EM Jr, Beder S, Coltro A, et al. Clinical features of the yellow nail syndrome. *Cleve Clin J Med* 1990;57:472–476.
19. Beer DJ, Pereira W Jr, Snider GL. Pleural effusion associated with primary lymphedema: a perspective on the yellow nail syndrome. *Am Rev Respir Dis* 1978;117:595–599.
20. Morandi U, Golinelli M, Brandi L, et al. "Yellow nail syndrome" associated with chronic recurrent pericardial and pleural effusions. *Eur J Cardiothorac Surg* 1995;9:42–44.
21. Malek NP, Ocran K, Tietge UJ, et al. A case of the yellow nail syndrome associated with massive chylous ascites, pleural and pericardial effusions. *Gastroenterology* 1996;34:763–766.
22. Emerson PA. Yellow nails, lymphoedema, and pleural effusions. *Thorax* 1966;21:247–253.
23. Lewis M, Kallenbach J, Zaltzman M, et al. Pleurectomy in the management of massive pleural effusion associated with primary lymphoedema: demonstration of abnormal pleural lymphatics. *Thorax* 1983;38:637–639.
24. Mambretti-Zumwalt J, Seidman JM, Higano N. Yellow nail syndrome: complete triad with pleural protein turnover studies. *South Med J* 1980;73:995–997.
25. Hiller E, Rosenow EC III, Olsen AM. Pulmonary manifestations of the yellow nail syndrome. *Chest* 1972;61:452–458.
26. Jiva TM, Poe RH, Kallay MC. Pleural effusion in yellow nail syndrome: chemical pleurodesis and its outcome. *Respiration* 1994;61:300–302.
27. Brofman JD, Hall JB, Scott W, et al. Yellow nails, lymphedema and pleural effusion. Treatment of chronic pleural effusion with pleuroperitoneal shunting. *Chest* 1990;97:743–745.
28. Chusid EL, Siltzbach LE. Sarcoidosis of the pleura. *Ann Intern Med* 1974;81:190–194.
29. Wilen SB, Rabinowitz JG, Ulreich S, et al. Pleural involvement in sarcoidosis. *Am J Med* 1974;57:200–209.
30. Beekman JF, Zimmet SM, Chun BK, et al. Spectrum of pleural involvement in sarcoidosis. *Arch Intern Med* 1976;136:323–330.

31. Nicholls AJ, Friend JAR, Legge JS. Sarcoid pleural effusion: three cases and review of the literature. *Thorax* 1980;35:277–281.

32. Chittock DR, Joseph MG, Paterson NA, et al. Necrotizing sarcoid granulomatosis with pleural involvement. Clinical and radiographic features. *Chest* 1994;106:672–676.

33. Bright R. Tabular view of the morbid appearance in 100 cases connected with albuminous urine, with observations. *Guys Hosp Rep* 1836;1:380–400.

34. Hopps HC, Wissler RW. Uremic pneumonitis. *Am J Pathol* 1955;31:261–273.

35. Nidus BD, Matalon R, Cantacuzino D, et al. Uremic pleuritis: a clinicopathological entity. *N Engl J Med* 1969;281:255–256.

36. Berger HW, Rammohan G, Neff MS, et al. Uremic pleural effusion: a study in 14 patients on chronic dialysis. *Ann Intern Med* 1975;82:362–364.

37. Galen MA, Steinberg SM, Lowrie EG, et al. Hemorrhagic pleural effusion in patients undergoing chronic hemodialysis. *Ann Intern Med* 1975;82:359–361.

38. Gilbert L, Ribot S, Frankel H, et al. Fibrinous uremic pleuritis: a surgical entity. *Chest* 1975;67:53–56.

39. Rodelas R, Rakowski TA, Argy WP, et al. Fibrosing uremic pleuritis during hemodialysis. *JAMA* 1980;243:2424–2425.

40. Coskun M, Boyvat F, Bozkurt B, et al. Thoracic CT findings in long-term hemodialysis patients. *Acta Radiol* 1998;40:181–186.

41. Jarratt MJ, Sahn SA. Pleural effusions in hospitalized patients receiving long-term hemodialysis. *Chest* 1995;108:470–474.

42. Maher JF. Uremic pleuritis. *Am J Kidney Dis* 1987;10:19–22.

43. Chiang CS, Chiang CD, Lin JW, et al. Neopterin, soluble interleukin-2 receptor and adenosine deaminase levels in pleural effusions. *Respiration* 1994;61:150–154.

44. Moore PJ, Thomas PA. The trapped lung with chronic pleural space, a cause of recurring pleural effusion. *Mil Med* 1967;132:998–1002.

45. Light RW, Jenkinson SG, Minh V, et al. Observations on pleural pressures as fluid is withdrawn during thoracentesis. *Am Rev Respir Dis* 1980;121:799–804.

46. Lee YC, Vaz MAC, Ely KA, et al. Symptomatic persistent postcoronary artery bypass graft pleural effusions requiring operative treatment—clinical and histologic features. *Chest* 2001 (*in press*).

47. Pien GW, Gant M, Washam C, et al. Use of an implantable pleural catheter for "trapped lung" syndrome in patients with malignant pleural effusion. *Chest* 2001 (*in press*).

48. Bachman AL, Macken K. Pleural effusions following supervoltage radiation for breast carcinoma. *Radiology* 1959;72:699–709.

49. Fentanes de Torres E, Guevara E. Pleuritis by radiation: report of two cases. *Acta Cytol* 1981;25:427–429.

50. Morrone N, Silva Volpa VLG, Dourado AM, et al. Bilateral pleural effusion due to mediastinal fibrosis induced by radiotherapy. *Chest* 1993;104:1276–1278.

51. Rodriguez-Garcia JL, Fraile G, Moreno MA, et al. Recurrent massive pleural effusion as a late complication of radiotherapy in Hodgkin's disease. *Chest* 1991;100:1165–1166.

52. Morild I. Pleural effusion in drowning. *Am J Forensic Med Pathol* 1995;16:253–256.

53. Knapp MJ, Roggli VL, Kim J, et al. Pleural amyloidosis. *Arch Pathol Lab Med* 1988;112:57–60.

54. Graham DR, Ahmad D. Amyloidosis with pleural involvement. *Eur Respir J* 1988;1:571–572.

55. Kavuru MS, Adamo JP, Ahmad M, et al. Amyloidosis and pleural disease. *Chest* 1990;98:20–23.

56. Im JG, Chung JW, Han MC. Milk of calcium pleural collections: CT findings. *J Comput Assist Tomogr* 1993;17:613–616.

57. Baxter CR. Present concepts in the management of major electrical injury. *Surg Clin North Am* 1970;50:1401–1418.

58. Peng MJ, Kuo HT, Chang MC. A case of intrathoracic extramedullary hematopoiesis with massive pleural effusion: successful pleurodesis with intrapleural minocycline. *J Formos Med Assoc* 1994;93:445–447.

59. Bartlett RP, Greipp PR, Tefferi A, et al. Extramedullary hematopoiesis manifesting as a symptomatic pleural effusion. *Mayo Clin Proc* 1995;70:1161–1164.

60. Garcia-Riego A, Cuinas C, Vilanova JJ, et al. Extramedullary hematopoietic effusions. *Acta Cytol* 1998;42:1116–1120.

61. Hiraiwa T, Hayashi T, Kaneda M, et al. Rupture of a benign mediastinal teratoma into the right pleural cavity. *Ann Thorac Surg* 1991;51:110–112.

62. Choi SJ, Lee JS, Song KS, et al. Mediastinal teratoma: CT differentiation of ruptured and unruptured tumors. *AJR Am J Roentgenol* 1998;171:591–594.

63. Khalil A, Carette MF, Milleron B, et al. Bronchogenic cyst presenting as mediastinal mass with pleural effusion. *Eur Respir J* 1995;8:2185–2187.

64. Tagliabue M, Casella TC, Zincone GE, et al. CT and chest radiography in the evaluation of adult respiratory distress syndrome. *Acta Radiol* 1994;35:230–234.

65. Talmor M, Hydo L, Gershenwald JG, et al. Beneficial effects of chest tube drainage of pleural effusion in acute respiratory failure refractory to positive end-expiratory pressure ventilation. *Surgery* 1998;123:137–143.

66. Fartoukh M, Azoulay E, Galliot R, et al. Clinically documented pleural effusions in medical ICU patients. How useful is routine thoracentesis? *Intensive Care Med* 2001 (*in press*).

67. Riemer H, Hainz R, Stain C, et al. Severe pulmonary hypertension reversed by antibiotics in a patient with Whipple's disease. *Thorax* 1997;52:1014–1015.

68. Muller C, Stain C, Burghuber O. *Tropheryma whippelii* in peripheral blood mononuclear cells and cells of pleural effusion. *Lancet* 1993;341:701.

69. Impens N, Warson F, Roels P, et al. A rare cause of pleurisy. *Eur J Respir Dis* 1986;68:388–389.

70. Duntley P, Siever J, Forwess ML, et al. Vascular erosion by central venous catheters. Clinical features and outcome. *Chest* 1992;101:1633–1638.

71. Thurnheer R, Speich R. Impending asphyxia in a 27-year-old woman 14 days after a gynecologic operation. *Chest* 1995;107:1169–1171.

72. Holt S, Kirkman N, Myerscough E. Haemothorax after subclavian vein cannulation. *Thorax* 1977;32:101–103.

73. Wolthuis A, Landewe RB, Theunissen PH, et al. Chylothorax or leakage of total parenteral nutrition? *Eur Respir J* 1998;12:1233–1235.

74. Kollef MH. Fallibility of persistent blood return for confirmation of intravascular catheter placement in patients with hemorrhagic thoracic effusions. *Chest* 1994;106:1906–1908.

75. Bankier AA, Wiesmayr MN, Henk C, et al. Radiographic detection of intrabronchial malpositions of nasogastric

tubes and subsequent complications in intensive care unit patients. *Intensive Care Med* 1997;23:406–410.

76. Sabga E, Dick A, Lertzman M, et al. Direct administration of charcoal into the lung and pleural cavity. *Ann Emerg Med* 1997;30:695–697.

77. Roubenoff R, Ravich WJ. Pneumothorax due to nasogastric feeding tubes. Report of four cases, review of the literature, and recommendations for prevention. *Arch Intern Med* 1989;149:184–188.

78. Miller KS, Tomlinson JR, Sahn SA. Pleuropulmonary complications of enteral tube feedings. *Chest* 1985;88:231–233.

79. Bilbrey GL, Hedberg CL. Hemorrhagic pleural effusion secondary to aortography: a case report. *J Thorac Cardiovasc Surg* 1967;54:85–89.

80. Stevens UM, Burdon JG, Niall JF. Pleural effusion after rupture of silicone bag mammary prosthesis. *Thorax* 1987;42:825–826.

81. Taupmann RE, Adler S. Silicone pleural effusion due to iatrogenic breast implant rupture. *South Med J* 1993;86:570–571.

82. Hirmand H, Hoffman LA, Smith JP. Silicone migration to the pleural space associated with silicone-gel augmentation mammaplasty. *Ann Plast Surg* 1994;32:645–647.

21

Pneumothorax

A pneumothorax is air in the pleural space, that is, air between the lung and the chest wall. Pneumothoraces can be divided into *spontaneous pneumothoraces*, which occur without antecedent trauma or other obvious cause, and *traumatic pneumothoraces*, which occur from direct or indirect trauma to the chest. A subcategory of traumatic pneumothorax is *iatrogenic pneumothorax*, which occurs as an intended or inadvertent consequence of a diagnostic or therapeutic maneuver. Spontaneous pneumothoraces are further divided into *primary* and *secondary spontaneous pneumothoraces*. Primary spontaneous pneumothoraces occur in otherwise healthy individuals, whereas secondary spontaneous pneumothoraces occur as a complication of underlying lung disease, most commonly chronic obstructive pulmonary disease (COPD).

PRIMARY SPONTANEOUS PNEUMOTHORAX

Incidence

Probably, the most complete figures on the incidence of primary spontaneous pneumothorax come from a study of the residents of Olmsted County, Minnesota, where complete medical records are kept on all residents. Between 1959 and 1978, 77 cases of primary pneumothorax occurred among the county's population, which averaged 60,000 over this period. The age-adjusted incidence of primary spontaneous pneumothorax was 7.4 per 100,000 per year for men and 1.2 per 100,000 per year for women (1). If these figures are extrapolated to the entire population of 250 million in the United States, one can antici-

pate about 10,000 new cases of primary spontaneous pneumothorax per annum.

Etiologic Factors

Primary spontaneous pneumothorax results from rupture of subpleural emphysematous blebs that are usually located in the apices of the lung (2, 3). In one older study, Gobbel et al. operated on 31 patients with primary spontaneous pneumothorax and found subpleural blebs or bullae in each patient (2). In a more recent study, Lesur et al. (3) obtained computed tomography (CT) scans on 20 young (mean age 27) patients with spontaneous pneumothorax and could demonstrate apical subpleural emphysematous lesions in 16 of the 20 (80%). In another recent study, Bense et al. obtained CT scans on 27 nonsmoking patients with primary spontaneous pneumothorax and reported that 22 (81%) had emphysema-like changes mostly in the upper lobes (4). It appears that the apical blebs present on direct visualization and the emphysema-like changes seen on CT scan represent the same abnormality.

The pathogenesis of these subpleural blebs is probably related to airway inflammation. One factor strongly associated with the development of a primary spontaneous pneumothorax is cigarette smoking, which certainly can produce airway inflammation. When the smoking habits of 505 patients from four separate studies are analyzed (5–8), 461 of the patients (91%) were smokers. Furthermore, the occurrence of a spontaneous pneumothorax appears to be related to the level of cigarette smoking. Compared with nonsmokers, the relative risk of a pneumothorax in men is seven times higher in light smokers

(1 to 12 cigarettes per day), 21 times higher in moderate smokers (13 to 22 cigarettes per day), and 102 times higher in heavy smokers (>22 cigarettes per day). For women, the relative risk is 4, 14, and 68 times higher in light, moderate, and heavy smokers than in nonsmokers, respectively (8). Disease of the small airways related to the smoking probably contributes to the development of the subpleural blebs.

Two studies concluded that spontaneous pneumothoraces were more likely to develop following days when there are broad swings in the atmospheric pressure (9, 10). It was postulated that the air in the apical blebs was not in free communication with the airways. Therefore, when the atmospheric pressure falls, the distending pressure of the bleb may increase and could result in its rupture (9). It should be noted that two other studies found no relationship between change in the atmospheric pressure and the occurrence of a spontaneous pneumothorax (11, 12). In one study, however, there was a significant relationship between thunderstorms and the occurrence of pneumothoraces (11).

Patients with primary spontaneous pneumothorax are usually taller and thinner than control patients. In a study of military recruits with pneumothorax, Withers et al. found that those with pneumothoraces were 2 inches taller and 25 pounds lighter than the average military recruit (13). Because the gradient in pleural pressure is greater from the lung base to the lung apex in taller individuals (see Chapter 2), the alveoli at the lung apex are subjected to a greater mean distending pressure in taller individuals. Over a long period, this phenomenon could lead to the formation of subpleural blebs in taller individuals who are genetically predisposed to bleb formation.

There seems to be some familial tendency for the development of primary spontaneous pneumothorax. In one study of primary spontaneous pneumothorax in the Israeli Defense Forces, 11.5% of 286 patients had a positive family history for primary spontaneous pneumothorax (14). A more in-depth analysis of 15 families suggested that the mode of inheritance for the tendency for pneumothorax was either autosomal dominant with incomplete penetrance or X-linked recessive (15). In another report of

patients with familial pneumothorax, individuals with human leukocyte antigen (HLA) haplotype A_2,B_{40} were found to be much more likely to have a pneumothorax (16). Other studies of familial pneumothorax have been unable to document any association with the HLA haplotypes (17).

There is a very high prevalence of bronchial abnormalities in nonsmoking patients with spontaneous pneumothorax. Bense et al. (18) performed fiberoptic bronchoscopy on 26 people who had never smoked but who had a history of spontaneous pneumothorax. They reported that 25 of 26 (96%) of the patients had bronchial abnormalities bilaterally. In comparison, only one of 41 control patients had such abnormalities (18). The bronchial abnormalities included disproportionate bronchial anatomy (smaller than normal dimensions and deviating anatomic arrangements of the airways at various locations), an accessory bronchus, or a missing bronchus. The most common abnormality was the disproportionate bronchial anatomy (18).

Pathophysiologic Features

The pressure in the pleural space is negative with reference to the atmospheric pressure during the entire respiratory cycle. The negative pressure is due to the inherent tendency of the lungs to collapse and of the chest wall to expand. The resting volume of the lung, the functional residual capacity (FRC), is the volume at which the outward pull of the chest wall is equal to, but opposite in direction to, the inward pull of the lung. In Fig. 21.1, the FRC is at 36% of the vital capacity.

The alveolar pressure is always greater than the pleural pressure owing to the elastic recoil of the lung. Therefore, if a communication develops between an alveolus and the pleural space, air will flow from the alveolus into the pleural space until a pressure gradient no longer exists or until the communication is sealed. Because the thoracic cavity is below its resting volume and the lung is above its resting volume, with a pneumothorax, the thoracic cavity enlarges and the lung becomes smaller.

The influence of a pneumothorax on the volumes of the hemithorax and lung is illustrated

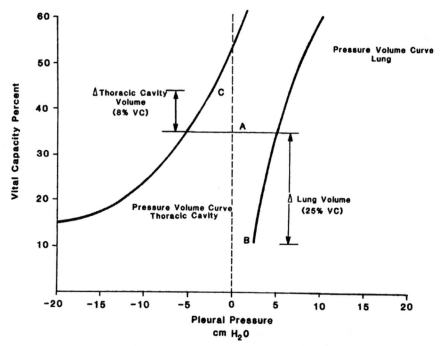

FIG. 21.1. Influence of a pneumothorax on the volumes of the lung and hemithorax. See text for details.

in Fig. 21.1. In the example, enough air entered the pleural space to increase the pleural pressure from -5 to -2.5 cm H_2O at end expiration. The end-expiratory volume of the lung (point B) decreased from 36% to 11% of the vital capacity, whereas the end-expiratory volume of the hemithorax (point C) increased from 36% to 44% of the vital capacity. The total volume of the pneumothorax is equal to 33% of the vital capacity, of which 25% represents a decrease in lung volume and 8% represents an increase in the volume of the hemithorax.

The main physiologic consequences of a pneumothorax are a decrease in the vital capacity and a decrease in PaO_2. In the otherwise healthy individual, the decrease in the vital capacity is well tolerated. If the patient's lung function is compromised before the pneumothorax, however, the decrease in the vital capacity may lead to respiratory insufficiency with alveolar hypoventilation and respiratory acidosis.

Most patients with a pneumothorax have a reduced PaO_2 and an increased alveolar-arterial oxygen difference [P(A − a)O$_2$]. In one series of 12 patients, the PaO_2 was below 80 mm Hg in nine (75%) and was below 55 mm Hg in two patients (19). In the same series, ten of the 12 patients (83%) had an increased P(A − a)O$_2$. As one would expect, the patients with secondary spontaneous pneumothorax and patients with larger pneumothoraces tended to have a greater decrease in the PaO_2 (19). Similar findings are present in animals with pneumothoraces. When a pneumothorax was induced in awake, standing dogs by the intrapleural injection of 50 mL per kg N_2, the mean PaO_2 fell from 86 to 51 mm Hg (20).

The reduction in PaO_2 appears to be due to both anatomic shunts and areas of low ventilation-perfusion ratios in the partially atelectatic lung. When Norris et al. gave 100% oxygen to their 12 patients, the average anatomic shunt was over 10% (19). The larger pneumothoraces were associated with greater shunts. Pneumothoraces occupying less than 25% of the hemithorax are not associated with increased shunts.

In the study on dogs conducted by Moran et al. (20), the relative perfusion of the lungs was not altered when pneumothorax was induced, but the ventilation to the ipsilateral lung was reduced, resulting in low ventilation-perfusion ratios on the side with the pneumothorax. Anthonisen reported that lungs with pneumothorax demonstrated uniform airway closure at low lung volumes, and he suggested that airway closure is the chief cause of ventilation maldistribution in spontaneous pneumothorax (21).

The PaO_2 usually improves with treatment. In the animal study of Moran et al. in which the mean PaO_2 dropped from 86 to 51 mm Hg with the introduction of a pneumothorax, the PaO_2 returned to baseline immediately after reexpansion (20). In humans treated for pneumothorax, the normalization of the PaO_2 takes longer. Three patients with an initial anatomic shunt above 20% had a reduction of at least 10% in their shunt 30 to 90 minutes after the removal of intrapleural air, but it still remained above 5% in all patients (19). Three additional patients with anatomic shunts of 10% to 20% had no change in their shunts when the air was removed (19). The delay in improvement in humans as compared with animals may be related to the duration of the pneumothorax.

When resected specimens from the lungs of patients with spontaneous pneumothorax are examined, there is frequently an eosinophilic pleuritis (22). In addition, some patients have mild pulmonary vascular and perivascular eosinophilia (22). Many patients also have pulmonary artery intimal fibrosis and pulmonary vein intimal fibrosis (23). The eosinophilic pleuritis is probably directly related to the air in the pleural space, and the presence of abnormalities in the pulmonary vessels should not serve as an indication to investigate the patient for pulmonary vascular disease.

The pathophysiologic features of tension pneumothorax are discussed later in this chapter.

Clinical Manifestations

The peak age for the occurrence of a primary spontaneous pneumothorax is in the early 20s, and primary spontaneous pneumothorax rarely occurs after age 40. The main symptoms associated with the development of primary spontaneous pneumothorax are chest pain and dyspnea.

In the series of 39 patients reported by Vail et al. (24), every patient had chest pain or dyspnea, and both symptoms were present in 25 of the 39 patients (64%). Seremetis (7) reported chest pain in 140 of 155 patients (90%). The chest pain usually has an acute onset and is localized to the side of the pneumothorax. On rare occasions, the patient has neither chest pain nor dyspnea. In the series of Seremetis (7), five patients (3%) complained only of generalized malaise. On rare occasions, the pneumothorax is discovered on a routine chest radiograph (25). Horner's syndrome has been reported as a rare complication of spontaneous pneumothorax and is thought to be due to traction on the sympathetic ganglion produced by shift of the mediastinum (26).

Primary spontaneous pneumothorax usually develops while the patient is at rest. In the series of 219 patients of Bense et al. (27), 87% of the patients were at rest at the onset of symptoms and no patients were exerting themselves heavily when symptoms began. Other series have reported comparable findings (5, 7).

Many patients with spontaneous pneumothorax do not seek medical attention immediately after the development of the symptoms. Eighteen percent of the patients in one series had symptoms for more than a week before seeking medical attention (7), whereas 46% in a second series waited more than 2 days before seeing a physician (5). Patients with symptoms for more than 3 days should not have negative pressure applied to their chest tubes in view of the higher incidence of reexpansion pulmonary edema with prolonged pneumothorax (see Chapter 25).

Physical Changes

Physical examination of patients with primary spontaneous pneumothorax reveals vital signs that are usually normal with the exception of a moderate tachycardia. If the pulse rate exceeds 140 or if hypotension, cyanosis, or electromechanical dissociation is present, a tension pneumothorax should be suspected (see the section later in this chapter on tension pneumothorax). Examination of the chest reveals that the side with the pneumothorax is larger than the contralateral side and moves less during the respiratory cycle. Tactile fremitus is absent, the percussion note is hyperresonant, and the breath sounds are absent or reduced on the affected side. The trachea may be shifted toward the contralateral side. With right-sided pneumothoraces, the lower edge of the liver may be shifted inferiorly.

Electrocardiographic Changes

Patients with spontaneous pneumothorax may show electrocardiographic changes due to the pneumothorax. In a study of 7 patients with spontaneous left pneumothorax, Walston et al. (28) found that a rightward shift of the frontal QRS axis, a diminution of precordial R voltage, a decrease in QRS amplitude, and precordial T-wave inversion could all occur. In a second study of patients with right-sided pneumothorax, prominent R wave voltage in lead V_2 with loss of S-wave voltage, mimicking posterior myocardial infarction, and reversible reduced QRS voltage have been reported (29). In addition, marked PR segment elevation in the inferior leads with reciprocal PR-segment depression in aVR has been reported (30). These changes should not be mistaken for an acute non–Q wave myocardial infarction.

Diagnosis

In a young, thin, tall man, the diagnosis is usually suggested by the clinical history and physical examination. The diagnosis is established by demonstrating a pleural line on the chest radiograph (Fig. 3.12). Because expiratory chest radiographs have little or no advantage over inspiratory chest radiographs in making the diagnosis of pneumothorax (31), they are not recommended. The diagnosis of pneumothorax can also be established with ultrasound (32).

Approximately 10% to 20% of patients have an associated pleural effusion, which is usually small and is manifested radiographically as an air–fluid level (7, 24). The pleural fluid with pneumothorax is characterized by eosinophilia, and the median percentage of eosinophils exceeds 20% after 1 day and 60% after 7 days (33). There is a significant correlation between the interleukin-5 (IL-5) levels in the pleural fluid and pleural fluid eosinophilia (33).

Quantitation

One should estimate the amount of lung collapse when treating a patient with a pneumothorax. The volume of the lung and the hemithorax are roughly proportional to the cube of their diameters. Thus, one can estimate the degree of collapse by measuring an average diameter of the lung and the hemithorax, cubing these diameters, and finding the ratios. For example, in Fig. 3.10, the average diameter of the hemithorax is about 10 cm, and the distance between the lung and chest wall is 4 cm. Therefore, the ratio of the diameters cubed $6^3 : 10^3$ equals 22% and about an 80% pneumothorax is present, although it appears substantially less severe at first glance.

Collins et al. (34) have described an alternate method for estimating the percentage of collapse. With their method, the distance between the apex of the partially collapsed lung and the apex of the thoracic cavity (distance A), and the midpoints of the upper (distance B) and lower (distance C) halves of the collapsed lung and the lateral chest wall were measured in centimeters. They found that the percentage pneumothorax size could be calculated by the formula

$$\% \text{ pneumothorax} = 4.2 + [4.7 \times (A + B + C)]$$

When the volume calculated from a helical CT was compared with the volume measured with this formula, the correlation coefficient in 20 patients was 0.98 (34). Even though the correlation coefficient was very high, improvements can be made in the above-mentioned formula because it does not take into account the patient's size. Obviously, a very large person will have a smaller pneumothorax in relation to the overall size of the lung than a small person with identical distances between the lung and the chest wall.

Recurrence Rates

A patient who has had a primary spontaneous pneumothorax is at risk of having a recurrence. Sadikot et al. (35) followed 153 patients with primary spontaneous pneumothorax for a mean of 54 months and found that the recurrence rate was 54.2%. In this study, the recurrence rates were less in men (46%) than in women (71%) and were less in individuals who stopped smoking (40%) than in those who continued smoking (70%). There was not a significant relationship between the size of the original pneumothorax or the treatment of the original pneumothorax and the recurrence rates. Twenty-four of their patients (16%) had a pneumothorax on the contralateral side; in only one patient did the pneumothoraces occur simultaneously (35). Gobbel et al. (2) followed a group of 119 patients with spontaneous pneumothorax for a mean of 6 years. These investigators found that, of the 110 patients who did not have a thoracotomy at the time of their initial pneumothorax, 57 (52%) had an ipsilateral recurrence. Once a patient had second and third pneumothoraces without thoracotomy, the incidence of subsequent recurrence was 62% and 83%, respectively.

Older studies suggested that there is substantial risk of recurrence over many years. In the series of Gobbel et al. (2), the average interval between the first and the second pneumothorax was 2.3 years, although the average interval for recurrence in the series of Seremetis was 17 months (7). However, more recent studies have suggested that most recurrences occur within the first year (36–38).

Attempts have been made to predict which patients with a primary spontaneous pneumothorax are more likely to have recurrence. If one could predict which patients are more likely to have a recurrence, then those patients could be treated more aggressively at the time of their first pneumothorax. Mitlehner et al. (38) assessed the usefulness of the chest CT in predicting recurrence, with the hypothesis being that those individuals with the most numerous and the largest bullae would be those who would be most likely to develop a recurrence. They obtained CT scans on 35 patients with primary spontaneous pneumothorax, of whom six (17%) had a recurrence during the mean follow-up period of 9.6 months. They were unable to find a relationship between the size of blebs or the number of blebs and recurrences (38). Abolnik et al. (14) did report that taller, thinner individuals were more likely to have a recurrence.

Treatment

Therapy for the patient with primary spontaneous pneumothorax has two goals: (a) to rid the pleural space of its air and (b) to decrease the likelihood of a recurrence.

Several different treatments can be used for the management of a patient with a primary spontaneous pneumothorax. These include observation; supplemental oxygen; simple aspiration; tube thoracostomy with or without the instillation of a sclerosing agent; medical thoracoscopy with the insufflation of talc; video-assisted thoracoscopy with stapling of blebs, instillation of a sclerosing agent, or pleural abrasion; and open thoracotomy. In selecting the appropriate treatment for any given patient, it should be remembered that a primary spontaneous pneumothorax is mainly a nuisance and is rarely life-threatening to the patient.

Observation

If the communication between the alveoli and the pleural space is eliminated, the air in the pleural space will be reabsorbed for the reasons discussed in Chapter 2. The rate of spontaneous absorption is slow, however. Kircher and Swartzel (39) estimated that 1.25% of the volume of the hemithorax was absorbed each 24 hours. Therefore, a pneumothorax occupying 15% of the hemithorax would take 12 days to be completely reabsorbed.

It is recommended that only patients with pneumothoraces occupying less than 15% of the hemithorax be considered for this type of treatment. If the patient is hospitalized, supplemental oxygen should be administered to increase the rate of pleural air absorption.

Supplemental Oxygen

The administration of supplemental oxygen accelerates the rate of pleural air absorption in experimental and clinical situations. Chernick and Avery (40) administered humidified 100% oxygen to rabbits with experimentally induced pneumothoraces and found that the oxygen increased the rate of air absorption by a factor of 6. Northfield (41) reported that the rate of absorption was increased fourfold when patients were treated with high-flow supplemental oxygen via face mask. It is recommended that hospitalized patients with any type of pneumothorax who are not subjected to aspiration or tube thoracostomy be treated with supplemental oxygen at high concentrations.

Aspiration

The initial treatment for most patients with primary spontaneous pneumothoraces greater than 15% of the volume of the hemithorax should probably be simple aspiration (42, 43). With this procedure, a 16-gauge needle with an internal polyethylene catheter is inserted into the second anterior intercostal space at the midclavicular line after local anesthesia. An alternate site is selected if the pneumothorax is loculated or if adhesions are present. After the needle is inserted, it is extracted from the cannula. Alternatively, one can use one of the commercially available thoracentesis trays such as the Arrow-Clark Thoracentesis Kit manufactured by Arrow International or the Argyle Turkel Safety Thoracentesis Set distributed by Sherwood. These kits have an outer cannula with an inner needle. If they are used, it is important to make a large enough skin incision so that the catheter does not become crumpled during its insertion.

A three-way stopcock and a 60-mL syringe are then attached to the catheter. Air is manually withdrawn until no more can be aspirated. If no resistance has been felt after a total of 4 L has been aspirated, it is assumed that no expansion has occurred, and a tube thoracostomy is performed. After no more air can be aspirated, the stopcock is closed and the catheter is secured to the chest wall. After 4 hours of observation, a chest radiograph should be obtained. If adequate expansion persists, the catheter be can removed and the patient discharged. Patients should return in 24 to 72 hours for a follow-up chest radiograph.

When two large series are combined (42, 43), 73 of 103 (71%) patients with spontaneous pneumothorax were successfully managed with this technique. The advantages to this technique are that it is simple and it is less traumatic than the insertion of a larger chest tube. Additionally, the patient need not be hospitalized and, therefore, this treatment is much less costly. The rate of recurrence appears comparable when patients are managed with simple aspiration and tube thoracostomy.

Tube Thoracostomy

If simple aspiration is unsuccessful, then tube thoracostomy should be performed if thoracoscopy is not readily available. With tube thoracostomy, the chest tube should be positioned in the uppermost part of the pleural space, where residual air accumulates. This procedure permits the air in the pleural space to be evacuated rapidly. The management of chest tubes in general is discussed in Chapter 26. Tube thoracostomy effectively evacuates the pleural air if the tube is properly inserted. In one series of 81 patients, only three patients (4%) had persistent air leaks after several days of chest tube drainage (7). The average duration of hospitalization in this series was only 4 days, with a range of 3 to 6 days. Although one might think that the placement of chest tubes would irritate the pleura and produce at least a partial pleurodesis, diminishing the likelihood of a recurrent pneumothorax, the incidence of recurrent pneumothorax is similar whether the initial episode is treated by bed rest alone or by tube thoracostomy (7).

When patients with spontaneous pneumothorax are managed with tube thoracostomy, several questions need to be addressed, such as what size of tube, whether the patient can be managed as an outpatient, whether to apply suction, when to remove the tube, and when to resort to more aggressive therapy. Although one older study (44) concluded that the success rates were poor when patients with spontaneous pneumothorax were treated with small chest tubes (13 F), subsequent studies have reported that most pneumothoraces are effectively managed with small chest tubes. In another study, Minami et al. treated

71 episodes of spontaneous pneumothorax using a small caliber catheter (No. 5.5 or 7.0 F) connected to a Heimlich valve (45). They reported that the treatment was successful in 60 patients (84.5%) and ineffective in the remaining 11 patients. Only six of these latter 11 patients were successfully managed when a large chest tube was placed (45). When patients with pneumothorax are treated with tube thoracostomy, small tubes (9 to 14 F) should be tried initially because their insertion is much less traumatic than that of a larger tube. They are best inserted using a guidewire technique, as described in Chapter 25. If the lung does not reexpand with the small tube, then a larger tube can be inserted; however, it appears that most patients can be successfully managed with the small tube.

Patients with primary spontaneous pneumothorax can be managed with tube thoracostomy on an outpatient basis (46, 47). Ponn et al. (46) inserted 12 F or 16 F short catheters in 96 patients with spontaneous pneumothorax. To prevent kinking, the tube was placed intracorporeally for most of its length, with only 1 or 2 cm plus the flared end left outside the body. A Heimlich valve is connected and secured with tape. An occlusive dressing covers the entry site, and a gauze sponge is secured over the open end of the valve with a rubber band. Patients return every 2 to 5 days for physical examination and a chest radiograph. Using this procedure, 92 of 96 patients (96%) were treated successfully. Campisi and Voitk successfully treated 14 of 14 patients using a similar procedure (47). The cost reduction associated with outpatient management is obvious; most patients with primary spontaneous pneumothorax who are subjected to tube thoracostomy should be treated as outpatients.

It is recommended that no suction be applied to chest tubes inserted for spontaneous pneumothorax. The chest tubes can either be connected to a Heimlich valve or an underwater seal. Two studies (44, 48) have concluded that the rate at which the lung reexpands is similar whether or not suction is applied. Because the risk of reexpansion pulmonary edema is greater when suction is applied to the chest tube (49), and because the suction appears to offer no benefit, suction is not recommended. If the lung does not

expand after 24 hours of waterseal drainage or Heimlich valve drainage, suction should be applied to the chest tube. A Heimlich valve comes with some of the commercially available kits (see Chapter 25). It is important to hook up the Heimlich valve in the right direction or a tension pneumothorax can result (50).

The chest tube should remain in place for 24 hours after the lung reexpands and the air leak ceases. If the chest tubes are removed too soon after the lung reexpands and the air leak ceases, there is a high likelihood of an early recurrence. Sharma et al. (48) reported a recollapse rate of 25% in 20 patients in whom the chest tubes were removed within 6 hours of lung expansion, but they also reported a recollapse rate of 0% in 20 patients in whom the chest tubes were removed 48 hours after lung expansion.

The duration of the chest tube drainage can be reduced by using a device such as the Pleupump (51) to quantify the amount of air exiting the pleural space. When no air has exited the pleural space for 24 hours, the tube is clamped and is removed if the lung remains expanded. Engdahl and Boe reported that the mean duration of chest tube drainage decreased from 8.1 to 4.8 days when this procedure was used (51).

Not all primary spontaneous pneumothoraces are treated successfully with a small chest tube. If the patient is initially treated with a small caliber chest tube and the lung does not expand within 48 hours, a larger chest tube should be placed. If the lung has not expanded or a bronchopleural fistula persists after 3 or 4 days, consideration should be given to more invasive therapy such as thoracoscopy or thoracotomy. The insertion of additional chest tubes is not recommended (52).

Tube Thoracostomy with Instillation of a Sclerosing Agent

Approximately 50% of patients with an initial primary spontaneous pneumothorax have a recurrence whether they are treated with observation or tube thoracostomy. Efforts have been made to diminish the recurrence rates by injecting various agents into the pleural space in an attempt to create an intense inflammatory reaction that would obliterate the pleural space.

Many different materials including quinacrine (53), talc in a slurry (54), olive oil (55), and tetracycline (37, 56) have been instilled through the chest tube at the time of the initial pneumothorax in an effort to create a pleurodesis and prevent a recurrence.

The two agents that appear to be the best sclerosing agents are talc in a slurry and the tetracycline derivatives. Most commonly, when talc is used as an agent to effect a pleurodesis, it is insufflated at the time of thoracoscopy or thoracotomy (see the discussion below). There have been two reports (54, 57), however, with a total of 32 patients in which 5 to 10 g of talc suspended in 250 mL saline was administered intrapleurally. The recurrence rate in these 32 patients was less than 10%.

The primary drawback to talc is that there have been four reports with a total of 17 patients developing the acute respiratory distress syndrome (ARDS) following the instillation of talc slurry intrapleurally (58). Several of the patients died. Although most of the cases occurred in patients who were being treated for malignant pleural effusions rather than pneumothorax, the fact that ARDS and death do occur after talc slurry intrapleurally should make one hesitant to use it for a benign condition in young healthy individuals.

An alternative agent for pleurodesis in patients with pneumothorax is a tetracycline derivative. In the Veterans Administration (VA) cooperative study on pneumothorax, 229 patients who were being treated with tube thoracostomy for spontaneous pneumothorax were randomized to receive 1,500 mg of tetracycline or nothing through their chest tube. During the 5-year study period, the 25% recurrence rate in the tetracycline group was significantly less than the 41% recurrence rate in the control group (37). In a second study, Alfageme et al. (59) reported that the recurrence rate was 9% in 66 patients treated with tetracycline intrapleurally, whereas the recurrence rate was 36% for the 79 patients treated with observation or chest tubes only (59).

In summary, the evidence presented earlier suggests strongly that the intrapleural injection of tetracycline or talc in a slurry in patients with spontaneous pneumothorax significantly reduces the subsequent recurrence rates. Which patients with spontaneous pneumothorax should receive the intrapleural injection of an agent in an attempt to produce a pleurodesis and decrease recurrence rates? It is recommended that all patients with primary or secondary spontaneous pneumothorax who are treated with tube thoracostomy receive an agent unless they will be subjected to thoracoscopy or thoracotomy.

What agent should be used? At the present time, the recommended agent for an attempted pleurodesis through a chest tube is a tetracycline derivative. If it were not for the reported cases of the ARDS after the administration of talc in a slurry to patients with malignant pleural effusions, talc in a slurry would be the recommended agent. Parenteral tetracycline is no longer available owing to increasingly stringent manufacturing requirements for parenteral antibiotics. Tetracycline derivatives appear comparable in effectiveness to tetracycline. In the rabbit model, minocycline (60) or doxycycline (61) are as effective as tetracycline in producing a pleurodesis at approximately one fourth the dose of tetracycline. Intrapleural doxycycline is also an effective treatment for malignant pleural effusion (see Chapter 7). Accordingly, 500 mg of doxycycline intrapleurally is recommended for patients with spontaneous pneumothorax who are treated with chest tubes. An alternative agent is minocycline (300 mg intrapleurally). Bleomycin should not be used because it is ineffective in producing a pleurodesis in rabbits (62) and is expensive.

The intrapleural injection of tetracycline derivatives is an intensely painful experience for many patients. In the VA cooperative study (37), over 50% of the patients reported severe pain at the time of the tetracycline injection, and 70% of the individuals stated that the pain was greater at the time of the tetracycline injection than at either the onset of the pneumothorax or at the time the chest tube was placed. The intrapleural administration of 100 mg of lidocaine (Xylocaine) was not effective in ameliorating the intense chest pain. However, some have recommended that when a tetracycline derivative is administered intrapleurally for pneumothorax, the injection be preceded by 4 mg per kg of Xylocaine up to a maximal dose of 250 mg (63). The patient should also be premedicated with an agent such as a short-acting benzodiazepine (e.g., midazolam).

It is recommended that the tetracycline derivative be injected as soon as the lung has reexpanded. The patient should be positioned so that the tetracycline comes into contact with the apical pleura. In experimental animals, the presence of a small pneumothorax at the time of the injection does not decrease the efficacy of the pleurodesis (64). A persistent air leak is not a contraindication to tetracycline injection. There is, however, no evidence that the intrapleural injection of tetracycline leads to an earlier closure of the bronchopleural fistula (37, 65).

Autologous Blood Patch for Persistent Air Leak

In the past few years, there have been several articles that have reported that an autologous blood patch is an effective treatment for a persistent air leak in patients with spontaneous pneumothorax. With this technique, 50 mL of blood is drawn from a vein and then promptly injected, without anticoagulation, through the chest tube into the pleural space (66). When three studies (66–68) are combined, air leaks ceased in 52 of 67 patients (78%) at 48 hours. Although no controlled studies have been performed, it appears that this treatment might have merit because the air leaks in only 65% of the 39 patients in the VA cooperative study ceased within 5 days (as opposed to 2 days). It is possible that the blood-patch technique might also decrease the incidence of recurrence. In the study of Cagirici, there were no recurrences in any of the 32 patients treated with the blood-patch technique during a follow-up of 12 to 48 months (67). When the blood-patch technique has been used in patients undergoing needle aspiration of the lung, it was ineffective in preventing pneumothorax in two studies (69, 70), but it was effective in preventing larger pneumothoraces in the most recent study (71).

Intrapleural Fibrin Glue for Persistent Air Leak

There has been one recent article (72) that suggested that the intrapleural administration of a large amount of diluted fibrin glue might be effective in patients with persistent air leaks. Kinoshita et al. diluted both the compounds used with the regular fibrin glue to 60 mL and then injected the 120 mL total into 40 high-risk patients with persistent bronchopleural fistula. They reported that the bronchopleural fistula closed after one injection in 35 patients, after two injections in four patients, and after three injections in one patient. The air leaks ceased within 12 hours of injection. During the follow-up period of 2.5 to 6.5 years, the pneumothorax recurred in five patients (12.5%), but an additional single treatment with fibrin glue resulted in resolution of the pneumothorax with no further recurrences (72). If these results can be duplicated by others, the intrapleural administration of fibrin glue represents a significant advance in the treatment of high-risk patients with pneumothorax.

Medical Thoracoscopy

Medical thoracoscopy is performed with the patient under local anesthesia, usually combined with conscious sedation. In contrast, video-assisted thoracoscopic surgery (VATS) is performed almost exclusively under general anesthesia with double-lumen endotracheal intubation, which allows single-lung ventilation and the collapse of the lung on the operated side (73). There are strong advocates for using medical thoracoscopy for the treatment of primary spontaneous pneumothorax (73, 74). Tschopp et al. (74) treated 89 patients for persistent or recurrent spontaneous pneumothorax from 1986 to 1994 with talc insufflation at the time of medical thoracoscopy. They reported that the initial medical thoracoscopy was successful in 80 patients (90%), and that the subsequent recurrence rate was six of 80 patients (7.5%). One advantage that medical thoracoscopy has over VATS is that it is much less expensive. Nevertheless, in general, medical thoracoscopy with talc insufflation is not recommended because of the possible development of ARDS after the use of talc intrapleurally.

Video-Assisted Thoracoscopic Surgery

Over the past few years thoracoscopy has become much more popular in this country due primarily to better instrumentation. With the advent of VATS, there has been renewed interest in the use of thoracoscopy for the management of patients with pneumothorax. The visibility of the entire thoracic cavity obtained with VATS compares favorably with that obtained by direct view through a limited axillary, inframammary, or lateral thoracotomy (75). At the present time, the same procedures can be performed through the thoracoscope, as can be done with a full thoracotomy, namely, wedge resection of bullae or blebs, ablation of blebs with laser or electrocoagulation, insufflation of talc, parietal pleurectomy, or pleural scarification. The advantages of VATS over full thoracotomy are obvious: rapid full expansion of the lung, decreased postoperative pain, shorter postoperative hospital stay, and the avoidance of a painful thoracotomy wound. General anesthesia is recommended for VATS (75).

VATS is effective in the treatment of spontaneous pneumothorax and the prevention of recurrent pneumothorax. With VATS, there are two primary objectives: (a) to treat the bullous disease responsible for the pneumothorax and (b) to create a pleurodesis. At the present time, the most common means by which the bullae are treated is with an endoscopic stapling device. The primary disadvantage of the endo stapler is its expense. The Endo:GIA model costs about $500, and additional cartridges (of which an average of two per procedure are used) each costs $500 (76). Previously, the bullae were treated with electrocoagulation, which was associated with a higher recurrence rate (77). An alternative method of dealing with the apical bullae is to ligate the bullae with a Roeder loop (78). However, Inderbitzi et al., who have reported one of the largest series using VATS for the treatment of pneumothorax, have reported a relatively high recurrence rate after use of the loop and recommend that it be abandoned in favor of wedge resection with the endo stapler (78).

Since the last edition of this book, there have been several series, each with over 100 patients, in which patients with spontaneous pneumothorax were treated with VATS. In general, VATS with stapling of bullae is very effective at managing spontaneous pneumothorax, with an overall recurrence rate of about 5% (79–83). Yim and Liu (79) treated 483 patients with VATS using mechanical pleurodesis plus some other procedures such as endo stapling or endoloop for management of the bullae. They reported that their median postoperative hospital stay was only 3 days and the recurrence rate was 1.74%, with a mean follow-up of 20 months (79). Cardillo et al. (80) used VATS to treat 432 patients with primary spontaneous pneumothorax between 1992 and 1998. They used subtotal pleurectomy to induce a pleurodesis in some patients and talc insufflation in others. The conversion rate to open procedures was 2.3%, most often due to extensive pleural adhesions. The mean time to chest tube removal was 5.4 days, and the mean hospital stay was 6.1 days. The recurrence rate was 4.4%, with a mean follow-up of 38 months (80). Waller (81) performed VATS with stapled bullectomy and parietal pleurectomy on 173 patients with spontaneous pneumothorax. In this series, 6.6% of the patients required reoperation for treatment failures, but with increasing experience, there was a significant decrease in treatment failures (81). Inderbitzi et al. used VATS to treat 79 patients between June 1990 and June 1993 for spontaneous pneumothorax. If the patients had a secondary spontaneous pneumothorax or if no bullous lesion was found, they also received an apical parietal pleurectomy. The recurrence rate in the 72 patients with follow-up was 8.3%. Because most of the recurrences occurred in patients who had not received the parietal pleurectomy, it appears that the pleurectomy does decrease the rate of recurrence (78).

Once the lesion in the lung is treated, some attempt should probably be made to create a pleurodesis. The primary alternatives are mechanical abrasion of the pleura, partial parietal pleurectomy, and talc insufflation. Of these three, mechanical abrasion of the pleura is the simplest, and because there is no evidence that talc insufflation or partial pleurectomy is better, it is the method of choice.

Which patients with spontaneous pneumothorax should be subjected to VATS? In some centers, all patients with spontaneous pneumothorax are subjected to thoracoscopy (84). This approach seems overly aggressive because approximately 50% of patients with an initial pneumothorax never have a recurrence even with no treatment. In my opinion, the indications for thoracoscopy in patients with primary spontaneous pneumothorax are as follows: (a) a failed aspiration of a pneumothorax, (b) an unexpanded lung after 3 days of tube thoracostomy, (c) a persistent bronchopleural fistula after 3 days, (d) a recurrent pneumothorax after chemical pleurodesis, or (e) an occupation or an avocation such as airplane piloting or deep sea diving in which the occurrence of the pneumothorax is dangerous to the patient. Of course the availability of VATS or medical thoracoscopy will influence the decision as to which procedure to select. In general, VATS is preferred to medical thoracoscopy because medical thoracoscopy involves the insufflation of talc with its attendant risks.

Open Thoracotomy

The indications for open thoracotomy are the same as those for thoracoscopy. If VATS is available, thoracotomy is recommended only after thoracoscopy has failed. The reason for this recommendation is that the hospitalization is shorter and the postoperative pain is less severe after thoracoscopy (76, 85). It should be mentioned, however, that some surgeons still prefer axillary mini-thoracotomy to VATS for the treatment of spontaneous pneumothorax (86, 87). The reason for this preference is that time is saved because double-lumen intubation is not required, the operating time is short, there is a good cosmetic result, and it is less expensive (87).

At thoracotomy, the apical pleural blebs are oversewn and the pleura is scarified. This procedure is effective in controlling the pneumothorax and diminishing the rate of recurrence. In one large series in which 362 patients underwent parietal pleurectomy, only two documented ipsilateral recurrences were reported, with an average follow-up of 4.5 years in 310 patients (88). The low rates of morbidity and mortality of the procedure are attested to in the same article (88). Only one operative death was reported in the 362 operative procedures, and the average postoperative period of hospitalization was only 6 days. Various methods proposed for scarification of the pleura range from visceral and parietal pleurectomy to mere abrasion of the pleura with dry sponges. All of these procedures appear to be

effective (5), but because pleural abrasion with dry gauze is less traumatic than pleurectomy and does not affect a potential later thoracotomy, it is the procedure of choice.

In summary, most patients with primary spontaneous pneumothorax should be managed initially as an outpatient with simple aspiration. If the simple aspiration is ineffective or if the patient has a recurrent pneumothorax, then either VATS or tube thoracostomy with a small chest tube is recommended. The intrapleural injection of a tetracycline derivative at this time decreases the likelihood of a recurrence, but it is painful for the patient. If the lung does not reexpand or if an air leak persists for 3 days, thoracoscopy with endo stapling of bullae and pleural scarification is indicated. Thoracoscopy is also indicated if the patient has a recurrent pneumothorax after receiving a tetracycline intrapleurally. Thoracotomy with oversewing of the apical blebs and pleural scarification is indicated if thoracoscopy is not available or if it is unsuccessful.

SECONDARY SPONTANEOUS PNEUMOTHORAX

Secondary spontaneous pneumothoraces are more serious than primary spontaneous pneumothoraces because they decrease the pulmonary function of a patient with already compromised pulmonary function. The secondary spontaneous pneumothoraces that occur in patients with the acquired immunodeficiency syndrome (AIDS), cystic fibrosis, or tuberculosis are discussed in separate sections.

Incidence

The incidence of secondary spontaneous pneumothorax is similar to that of primary spontaneous pneumothorax. In the study from Olmsted County, Minnesota, the incidence was 6.3 and 2.0 per 100,000 per year for men and women, respectively (1). If these figures are extrapolated to the entire population of the United States, about 10,000 new cases of secondary spontaneous pneumothorax will be seen each year.

Etiologic Factors

Most secondary spontaneous pneumothoraces are due to COPD or *Pneumocystis carinii* infection in patients with AIDS (89, 90), although almost every lung disease has been reported to be associated with secondary spontaneous pneumothorax. Between 1983 and 1991, 120 patients with a spontaneous pneumothorax were seen at Parkland Memorial Hospital in Dallas, Texas, and 32 (27%) occurred in patients with AIDS (90). In a recent series of 505 patients from Israel with secondary spontaneous pneumothorax, the etiologies were as follows: COPD, 348; tumor, 93; sarcoidosis, 26; tuberculosis, 9; other pulmonary infections, 16; and miscellaneous, 13 (91).

One unique condition associated with secondary spontaneous pneumothorax is pulmonary lymphangioleiomyomatosis (LAM), which is discussed in more detail in Chapter 23. This rare condition is characterized by peribronchial, perivascular, and perilymphatic proliferation of abnormal smooth muscle cells. LAM almost exclusively affects women of childbearing age and presents with slowly progressive breathlessness, chylothorax, recurrent spontaneous pneumothorax, or hemoptysis (92). There is a high incidence of spontaneous pneumothorax with LAM. When two recent series (92, 93) with a total of 104 patients are combined, 71 of the patients (68%) had experienced at least one episode of spontaneous pneumothorax.

There appears to be a tendency for patients with more severe COPD to develop spontaneous pneumothorax. In the VA cooperative study, which included 171 patients with secondary spontaneous pneumothorax, 51 of the patients (30%) had an FEV_1 of less than 1,000 mL and 56 of the patients (33%) had an FEV_1/FVC of less than 0.40 (37).

Clinical Manifestations

In general, the clinical symptoms associated with secondary spontaneous pneumothorax are more severe than those associated with primary spontaneous pneumothorax. Most patients with secondary spontaneous pneumothorax have dyspnea (94, 95), which frequently seems out of proportion to the size of the pneumothorax (96). In one series of 57 patients with COPD, all complained of shortness of breath, whereas 42 of 57 (74%) had chest pain on the side of the pneumothorax (94). In addition, five patients were cyanotic and four patients were hypotensive.

The occurrence of a pneumothorax in a patient with underlying lung disease is a serious setback. Because the pulmonary reserve of these patients is already diminished, the partial or total loss of the function of a lung can be life-threatening. In one series of 18 patients in whom arterial blood gases were obtained at the time of admission, the mean PaO_2 was 48 mm Hg and the mean $PaCO_2$ was 58 mm Hg (94). In the VA cooperative study, the PaO_2 was below 55 mm Hg in 20 of 118 (17%) and was below 45 mm Hg in 5 of 118 (4%). The $PaCO_2$ exceeded 50 mm Hg in 19 of 118 (16%) and exceeded 60 mm Hg in 5 of 118 (4%) (37).

A substantial mortality rate is associated with secondary spontaneous pneumothorax. When three series totaling 120 patients are combined, the mortality rate was 16% (94, 96, 97). Causes of death included sudden death before chest tubes could be inserted in three patients, respiratory failure within the first 24 hours of treatment in three patients, late respiratory failure in three patients, and massive gastrointestinal bleeding in three patients. In the VA cooperative study, none of the 185 patients with secondary spontaneous pneumothorax died from a recurrent ipsilateral pneumothorax. However, the overall mortality rate in the 5-year follow-up period was 43% (37). The high mortality rate probably reflects the severity of the underlying disease. The leading causes of death were COPD, lung cancer, pneumonia, and heart disease (37).

The physical examination of patients with secondary spontaneous pneumothorax is less helpful than in primary spontaneous pneumothorax. These patients already have hyperexpanded lungs, decreased tactile fremitus, hyperresonant percussion notes, and distant breath sounds over both lung fields. Accordingly, when a pneumothorax develops, side-to-side differences in the physical examination may not be apparent. The possibility of a pneumothorax should be considered in any patient with COPD who has increasing shortness of breath, particularly if chest pain is also present.

Diagnosis

As with primary spontaneous pneumothorax, the diagnosis of secondary spontaneous pneumothorax is established by the chest radiograph. In patients with COPD, the radiographic appearance of the pneumothorax is altered by the loss of elastic recoil of the lung and the presence of air trapping. Normal areas of the lung collapse more completely than diseased areas with large bullae or severe emphysema in the absence of adhesions. In addition, the deflation of the diseased lung is limited by its decreased elastic recoil.

The diagnosis of pneumothorax is established by the demonstration of a visceral pleural line. It is sometimes difficult to see this line because the lung is hyperlucent and little difference exists in radiodensity between the pneumothorax and the emphysematous lung. Frequently, the presence of the pneumothorax is overlooked on the initial chest radiograph. One must distinguish a spontaneous pneumothorax from a large, thin-walled, air-containing bulla. The pleural line with a pneumothorax is usually oriented in convex fashion toward the lateral chest wall, whereas the apparent pleural line with a large bulla is usually concave toward the lateral chest wall. If there is any doubt as to whether the patient has a pneumothorax or a giant bulla, CT should be obtained because the two conditions are easily differentiated with this procedure (98). It is important to make the distinction between a large bulla and a pneumothorax, because only the pneumothorax should be treated with tube thoracostomy.

In patients with cystic lung disease, the presence of cysts and pleural adhesions sometimes makes it difficult to determine whether a pneumothorax is present on the routine chest radiographs. If patients with cystic lung disease present with increased shortness of breath, the possibility of a pneumothorax should be considered, particularly if the hemithoraces are asymmetric in size. In such cases, the CT scan will delineate whether a pneumothorax is present and will also assist in selecting the appropriate site for chest tube placement (99).

Occasionally, secondary spontaneous pneumothoraces result from primary carcinoma of the lung with bronchial obstruction. One must recognize the radiologic signs of bronchial obstruction in these patients because the insertion of chest tubes is contraindicated. When a patient has a totally collapsed lung, one should search for air bronchograms in the lung. Air bronchograms are absent when there is an endobronchial obstructing lesion, but otherwise they are present (100). If no air bronchograms are present, a bronchoscopic examination should be performed before a chest tube is inserted.

Recurrence Rates

The recurrence rates for secondary spontaneous pneumothorax appear to be somewhat higher than those for primary spontaneous pneumothorax (36, 37, 101). Videm et al. (101) followed a total of 303 patients for a median period of 5.5 years and reported that 24 of the 54 patients (44%) with COPD had a recurrence. In patients without COPD, 96 of 249 (39%) had a recurrence (101). In the VA cooperative study, 92 patients with secondary spontaneous pneumothorax were treated with chest tubes without pleural sclerosis and the recurrence rate was 47% with a median follow-up of 3 years.

Treatment

The goals of treatment of the patient with secondary spontaneous pneumothorax, as with primary spontaneous pneumothorax, are to rid the pleural space of air and to decrease the likelihood of a recurrence. Achievement of these goals is more important in the patient with secondary spontaneous pneumothorax, however. A primary spontaneous pneumothorax or its recurrence is mostly just a nuisance. In contrast, the occurrence of a pneumothorax in a patient with lung disease may be life-threatening, even though the mortality rate from recurrent pneumothorax is low (37).

The treatment options for the patient with a secondary spontaneous pneumothorax are the same as those for a patient with a primary spontaneous pneumothorax, as discussed earlier in this chapter. The recommendations for the treatment of the patient with a secondary spontaneous pneumothorax differ from those of the patient with a primary spontaneous pneumothorax in the following ways.

Nearly every patient with a secondary spontaneous pneumothorax should initially be hospitalized and managed by tube thoracostomy (52). Aspiration of the pneumothorax is not recommended because it is less likely to be successful (102, 103) and does nothing to diminish the likelihood of a recurrence. Even if the pneumothorax is small, its evacuation can lead to a rapid improvement in symptoms. Arterial blood gases usually improve within 24 hours of instituting tube thoracostomy (97). If the patient has respiratory failure necessitating mechanical ventilation, a chest tube should definitely be placed because the pneumothorax is likely to enlarge during mechanical ventilation.

Tube thoracostomy is less efficacious in secondary pneumothorax than in primary pneumothorax, however. In primary spontaneous pneumothorax, the lung usually expands, and the air leak ceases within 3 days. In secondary spontaneous pneumothorax due to COPD, the mean time for the lung to expand is 5 days. In about 20% of patients with secondary spontaneous pneumothorax, the lung remains unexpanded or the air leak persists after 7 days (90, 97, 98, 100, 101).

Once the lung has expanded, it is recommended that attempts be made to prevent the recurrence of a pneumothorax (52). This can be done with thoracoscopy, mini-thoracotomy, or the instillation of a sclerosant through the chest tube. If thoracoscopy is available, it is the procedure of choice because thoracoscopy with the stapling of blebs and pleural abrasion reduces the likelihood of recurrence to under 5%. A good alternative to thoracoscopy is the mini-thoracotomy, which is at least as effective as thoracoscopy. If these procedures are not available, or if the patient refuses or is too sick to undergo surgery, then doxycycline can be injected through the chest tube, as described earlier. However, the intrapleural injection of a tetracycline derivative will only decrease the recurrence rate from about 50% to 30% (37).

When one contemplates an attempt to prevent a recurrent pneumothorax, the effect that the agent will have on a future lung transplant should be considered if the patient has a disease such as LAM, cystic fibrosis, interstitial pulmonary fibrosis, or COPD that might be managed with lung transplantation. In the past, patients were excluded from lung transplantation if attempts at pleurodesis had been made on the side of the proposed transplant owing to the increased difficulty of the procedure and the risk of excessive bleeding. However, a recent consensus conference statement on lung transplantation concluded that pleurodesis was not a contraindication to lung transplantation in patients with cystic fibrosis (104). In one study, the outcome of 18 patients with a previous intrapleural procedure was compared with 18 paired controls without previous intrapleural procedures and there was no difference in the two groups (105).

If the lung does not expand within 72 hours or if there is a persistent air leak for more than 3 days, strong consideration should be given to performing thoracoscopy (106, 107). At thoracoscopy, the blebs are excised with a stapling instrument and some other procedure is done to create a pleurodesis. In one study 22 patients with secondary spontaneous pneumothorax due to COPD with a mean age of 70 and a mean preoperative FEV_1 of 48% of predicted were subjected to VATS for either persistent air leak (18 patients) or recurrent pneumothorax (four patients) (106). The mean duration of the procedure was only 57 minutes, and only one patient required mechanical ventilation during the immediate postoperative period. The mean duration of postoperative hospitalization was 9 days. The fact that the mean hospitalization was 18 days before surgery suggests that the hospitalization would have been shortened if the procedure had been performed sooner. VATS failed in four of the 22 patients (18%), in that there was a large air leak postoperatively that necessitated thoracotomy. There were two deaths in this series; one patient developed a contralateral tension pneumothorax and a subsequent fatal myocardial infarction, and the other developed bronchopneumonia after revisional thoracotomy and died in respiratory failure. None of the surviving patients had a recurrent pneumothorax (106).

The series of Waller et al. detailed earlier (106) documents that elderly patients with severe

COPD and pneumothorax can be managed successfully with VATS with acceptable rates of morbidity and mortality. Since VATS has such good results, it is recommended that it be attempted if the lung remains unexpanded or if there is a persistent air leak after 3 days. If facilities are available for VATS, it is advisable to attempt it relatively early rather than attempting to reexpand the lung with several chest tubes. Indeed, some authors have recommended that all patients with secondary spontaneous pneumothorax undergo VATS (52, 107). If the patient is a good operative candidate and if thoracoscopy is readily available, I would agree with this recommendation.

PNEUMOTHORAX SECONDARY TO ACQUIRED IMMUNODEFICIENCY SYNDROME

Patients with AIDS and *P. carinii* infection have a relatively high incidence of spontaneous pneumothorax. Most patients with AIDS who have a spontaneous pneumothorax have a history of *P. carinii* infection, are on prophylactic pentamidine, and have a recurrence of their *P. carinii* infection (108–110). Pulmonary tuberculosis and pulmonary cryptococcosis are also associated with spontaneous pneumothorax in patients with AIDS. In one series, 13 of 35 patients (37%) with spontaneous pneumothorax and AIDS had tuberculosis (111). Most patients have a $CD4^+$ count less than 100 per μL (110). The reported prevalence of pneumothorax in patients who have a history of *P. carinii* infection and who receive prophylactic pentamidine has varied widely. In one series of 408 patients who were receiving prophylactic pentamidine therapy in San Francisco, there were 17 cases (4%) of spontaneous pneumothorax but only about one fourth of the 408 patients had had *P. carinii* pneumonia previously (112). Renzi et al. (113) reported that five of 48 patients (10%) with a history of *P. carinii* infection who were receiving prophylactic pentamidine therapy developed a spontaneous pneumothorax. In another small series of hemophiliacs who were infected with human immunodeficiency virus (HIV) and who were receiving prophylactic pentamidine, four of 13 patients (31%) developed a spontaneous pneumo-

thorax (114). At some medical centers where large numbers of patients with AIDS are treated, pneumothoraces in AIDS patients account for a sizable percentage of all spontaneous pneumothoraces. For example, at Parkland Memorial Hospital in Dallas, Texas, 32 of 120 cases (27%) of spontaneous pneumothorax between 1983 and 1991 occurred in patients with AIDS (90).

The explanation for the high incidence of spontaneous pneumothorax in these patients appears to be the presence of multiple subpleural lung cavities, which are associated with subpleural necrosis (115–118). These bullous changes and pulmonary cysts develop due to repeated episodes of inflammation and cytotoxic effects of HIV on pulmonary macrophages (116). Most patients have radiologic evidence of fibrocystic parenchymal disease (Fig. 21.2) (115). If these patients are subjected to surgery, there is diffuse involvement of the lung parenchyma with greater involvement in the upper lobe than in the lower lobe. Areas of necrosis are usually present in consolidated areas of the lung, and these areas are exceedingly friable and prone to laceration with the slightest manipulation. Emphysematous blebs are located on the surface of the lungs, and the apex of the lungs contains multiple cysts based on consolidated parenchyma (119). Microscopically, the tissue specimens invariably reveal extensive necrosis with a complete loss of the inherent architecture (119). When patients are studied prospectively,

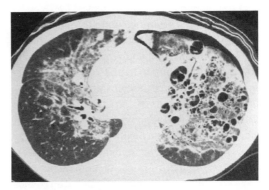

FIG. 21.2. CT scan of patient with AIDS and *P. carinii* infection. Note the numerous cysts in the left lung and the large subpleural cyst anteriorly in the left lung, which is probably responsible for the pneumothorax seen anteriorly. (Courtesy of Dr. David P. Naidich.)

those with a lower diffusion capacity are more likely to develop a spontaneous pneumothorax (113). The reason for the relationship between the aerosolized pentamidine and the occurrence of the pneumothorax is not clear, but it probably is related to the fact that the aerosolized pentamidine does not reach the periphery of the upper lobes. Accordingly, a low-grade infection persists and destroys the lung, leading to the development of the cysts and the bronchopleural fistulas.

The occurrence of a spontaneous pneumothorax in a patient with AIDS and *P. carinii* infection is ominous prognostically. In one series, the in-hospital mortality rate was 50% in 32 patients with *P. carinii* infection and spontaneous pneumothorax (120). In a second series, 17 of 22 patients (77%) with spontaneous pneumothorax died, with a mean survival of 147 days after the diagnosis of the pneumothorax (119). In another series, the in-hospital mortality rate was 10 of 35 (29%) for patients with spontaneous pneumothorax (121). However, the in-hospital mortality rate was only 6% in the patients reported by Wait (122) who were managed with VATS.

Once a patient with AIDS and *P. carinii* infection has a spontaneous pneumothorax, he or she is very likely to have a recurrent pneumothorax or a contralateral pneumothorax. In one series of 20 patients, contralateral pneumothoraces occurred in 13 (65%) and ipsilateral recurrences occurred in 13 (65%) (108). In another series of 22 patients, eight (36%) had synchronous or sequential bilateral pneumothoraces (119).

Owing to the necrotic lung surrounding the ruptured cavity, the spontaneous pneumothorax associated with AIDS and *P. carinii* infection is notoriously difficulty to treat. Conservative therapy consisting of tube thoracostomy is rarely successful. In one report of 20 patients, the median length of hospitalization was 42 days and a chest tube was required for a median of 20 days but was successful in only four patients. In this series, the pneumothorax resolved in 11 patients with sclerotherapy, whereas five patients required thoracotomy (108). In a second series, 35 patients were treated with chest tubes and tetracycline and doxycycline pleurodesis, and this treatment was effective in only nine (26%) (121).

In view of the poor results with tube thoracostomy alone, alternate procedures are necessary. It is recommended that alternate therapies be initiated if the patient still has an air leak after 3 days, because the leak will probably not close spontaneously. The simplest alternative is to attach a Heimlich valve to the chest tube and send the patient home while not worrying about the closure of the bronchopleural fistula (110, 123, 124). This treatment gets the patient home fastest and is associated with the least morbidity. It is not always successful, however, in that in some patients the Heimlich valve cannot handle the air flow through the large bronchopleural fistula and the lung does not remain expanded. Trachiotis and associates (110) discharged eight patients with 10 pneumothoraces and reported that there was no incidence of morbidity or mortality related to the Heimlich valve. Two patients died in a hospice, and the others were successfully managed as outpatients.

If the patient cannot be managed with a Heimlich valve, or if definitive treatment of the pneumothorax is desired, the treatment of choice is probably VATS. The optimal procedure to perform with VATS remains to be defined. Wait performed VATS with the insufflation of 5 to 10 g of asbestos-free talc without treating the air leaks directly and reported success in 30 of 32 patients (94%) (122). The mean hospital stay after VATS was 3.9 days, and no patient was discharged with a Heimlich valve (122).

An alternative aggressive approach is thoracotomy with stapling of blebs and pleural abrasion (125–127). Crawford et al. (126) reported successful management for 13 of 14 patients using thoracotomy with direct closure of the bronchopleural fistula and parietal pleurectomy. Horowitz and Oliva (127) reported the successful management of seven of seven patients with this procedure. Because the incidence of contralateral pneumothorax is so high in these patients, one group has recommended the use of a median sternotomy incision with bilateral pleurodesis for those patients who require surgery (125).

Pleural sclerosis has a limited role in the management of the secondary pneumothorax in patients with AIDS because it is usually ineffective

(108, 121). The reason for its ineffectiveness is unknown, but it is probably related to the size of the bronchopleural fistula or the inability of the immunocompromised host to mount a brisk inflammatory response. If pleurodesis is attempted through a chest tube, doxycycline is recommended. There has been one report in which six of seven spontaneous pneumothoraces in patients with AIDS were managed successfully with intrapleural doxycycline (128).

PNEUMOTHORAX SECONDARY TO CYSTIC FIBROSIS

Secondary spontaneous pneumothorax is also frequent with cystic fibrosis, a disease with a high prevalence of severe COPD. Spector and Stern (129) reviewed 1,268 patients with cystic fibrosis who were followed between 1959 and 1987 in the University Hospitals of Cleveland. They reported that 99 of the patients (8%) had at least one episode of spontaneous pneumothorax. The median age of the patients at the time of their initial pneumothorax was 17 years (129). Approximately 16% to 20% of patients with cystic fibrosis who are older than 18 years of age will experience a pneumothorax at some time in their lives.

The treatment of the secondary spontaneous pneumothorax associated with cystic fibrosis is similar to the treatment of that associated with COPD. Because the recurrence rate approaches 50% (130), consideration should be given to preventing a recurrence. Almost all patients should initially be treated with tube thoracostomy. If the air leak ceases and the lung remains expanded, consideration should be given to the prevention of a recurrence with either thoracoscopy or the intrapleural injection of a sclerosant. Because many patients with cystic fibrosis are candidates for lung transplantation, one has to consider the effect of the preventive measures on the subsequent lung transplantation. As discussed earlier, it appears that efforts to create a pleurodesis do not preclude a lung transplantation and do not add appreciably to the complications (104, 105). Accordingly, the procedure of choice for prevention is tube thoracostomy with the stapling of blebs and pleural abrasion. Thoracoscopy should also

be performed if the air leak persists or the lung remains unexpanded for 3 days after tube thoracostomy is performed. Indeed, one can make a good case for thoracoscopy for all cases of pneumothorax secondary to cystic fibrosis as soon as the patient is stabilized with tube thoracostomy.

PNEUMOTHORAX SECONDARY TO TUBERCULOSIS

The prevalence of secondary spontaneous pneumothorax in patients hospitalized with pulmonary tuberculosis is between 1% and 3% (131). In a recent series from Spain, tuberculosis was the second leading cause of secondary spontaneous pneumothorax after COPD (132). All patients with pneumothorax secondary to tuberculosis should be treated with tube thoracostomy. In one series of 28 patients, 11 were treated by observation or repeated pleural aspiration, and seven of the 11 (64%) died. In contrast, of the 17 patients treated with chest tubes, only one (6%) died. Once chest tubes are placed in such patients, a long period of chest tube drainage can be anticipated. The duration of tube thoracostomy ranged from 5 days to 6 months, with a mean duration of 50 days in the above-mentioned series (131). The literature on the use of VATS to treat pneumothoraces secondary to tuberculosis is quite limited, but Andres and associates did report success with VATS in three patients (133).

CATAMENIAL PNEUMOTHORAX

A catamenial pneumothorax occurs in conjunction with menstruation and is usually recurrent (134). It is unusual, with only 80 cases reported up to 1996 (135). The initial pneumothorax usually does not occur until the woman is in her 20s. Patients with catamenial pneumothorax classically develop chest pain and sometimes dyspnea within 24 to 48 hours of the onset of the menstrual flow (134). Catamenial pneumothorax may be more likely if the patient's menstrual period is preceded by mental or physical stress. These pneumothoraces are usually right sided, but left-sided and even bilateral pneumothoraces have been reported (135).

Pathogenesis

The pathogenesis of catamenial pneumothorax is not definitely known. When Maurer et al. (136) initially described the syndrome, they hypothesized that air gained access to the peritoneal cavity during menstruation and then entered the pleural cavity through a diaphragmatic defect, because their initial patient had a diaphragmatic defect. However, in a subsequent review by Lillington et al. (134) of 18 patients who had undergone thoracotomy, only three patients had diaphragmatic defects, whereas six had pleural or diaphragmatic endometriosis. These reviewers concluded that the most plausible explanation was leakage of air from the lung owing to subpleural endometrial implants. Joseph and Sahn (135) more recently reviewed the literature on catamenial pneumothorax and found 61 patients who had undergone thoracotomy or thoracoscopy. Eight of the patients (13%) had pleural endometriosis, 16 (26%) had diaphragmatic defects, 14 (23%) had cysts or blebs, and 15 (25%) had no abnormal findings (135). It is likely that either of the mechanisms can be responsible for the syndrome. There is one case report in which a woman simultaneously had a catamenial pneumothorax and air under her diaphragm on three different occasions (137).

Diagnosis and Treatment

The diagnosis of catamenial pneumothorax is not difficult if the possibility is considered. Any woman over the age of 20 years who develops a pneumothorax during the first 48 hours of her menstrual flow should be considered to have a probable catamenial pneumothorax. The medical treatment of catamenial pneumothorax is aimed at treating the endometriosis by suppressing the ectopic endometrium (134, 135, 138). This can be accomplished by suppressing ovulation using oral contraceptives or by suppressing the production of gonadotropins by using danazol or gonadotropin-releasing hormone (GnRH). With medical therapy, the recurrence rate within the first year is about 50% (135). The surgical treatment for catamenial pneumothorax is thoracoscopy with closure of the diaphragmatic defects,

stapling of any blebs in the lung, and pleural abrasion. If facilities for thoracoscopy are not available, then the same procedures can be performed with a thoracotomy (134, 139). There has been one case reported in which recurrent pneumothoraces developed after thoracoscopy with pleural abrasion and thoracotomy with partial pleurectomy and plication of the diaphragm; however, after bilateral tubal ligation, there were no recurrences (140).

NEONATAL PNEUMOTHORAX

Spontaneous pneumothorax occurs more commonly in the newborn period than at any other age. In radiologic surveys, a pneumothorax is present shortly after birth in 1% to 2% of all infants (141), and a symptomatic pneumothorax is present in approximately 0.5% (141). Spontaneous neonatal pneumothorax is twice as common in boys as in girls, and the infants are usually full term or post term (141). In most instances, the baby has a history of fetal distress requiring resuscitation or a difficult delivery with evidence of aspiration of meconium, blood, or mucus (141).

The incidence of pneumothorax in infants with the respiratory distress syndrome (RDS) is high (141, 142). The more severe the RDS, the more likely the infant is to develop a pneumothorax. In one series of 295 infants with RDS, 19% developed a pneumothorax (142). Pneumothorax developed in only 3.5% of those not requiring respiratory assistance, but it occurred in 11% of those requiring continuous positive airway pressure and in 29% of those requiring intermittent positive-pressure ventilation with positive end-expiratory pressures (142).

Pathogenesis

The pathogenesis of neonatal pneumothorax in infants without RDS is related to the mechanical problems of first expanding the lung. Karlberg (143) has demonstrated transpulmonary pressures averaging 40 cm H_2O during the first few breaths of life, with occasional transpulmonary pressures as high as 100 cm H_2O. At birth, the alveoli usually open in rapid sequence, but if bronchial obstruction occurs from the aspiration of blood, meconium, or mucus, high transpulmonary pressures may lead to rupture of the lung (141). A transpulmonary pressure of 60 cm H_2O ruptures adult lungs (141), whereas a transpulmonary pressure of only 45 cm H_2O ruptures neonatal rabbit lungs (144). There has been one family reported in which the maternal grandfather, a maternal aunt, and an older sister, along with the patient had spontaneous neonatal pneumothorax (145).

In infants with RDS, the pneumothoraces also occur due to high transpulmonary pressures. With the infant breathing spontaneously, abnormally negative transpulmonary pressures can be generated because of the reduced lung volumes and the noncompliant lung. Intermittent positive-pressure ventilation is even more likely to produce high transpulmonary pressures and pneumothorax.

Clinical Manifestations

Depending on the size of the pneumothorax, the signs vary from none to severe acute respiratory distress. In the infant with a small pneumothorax, no clinical signs or mild apneic spells with some irritability or restlessness may be present. Large pneumothoraces incur varying degrees of respiratory distress, and, in severe cases, marked tachypnea (up to 120 per minute), grunting, retractions, and cyanosis are present (141). The detection of pneumothorax by physical examination is often difficult because abnormal physical signs are often not found. The most reliable sign is a shift of the apical heart impulse away from the side of the pneumothorax. Because breath sounds are widely transmitted in the small neonatal thorax, appreciation of diminished breath sounds on the affected side is difficult (141).

In infants who develop pneumothorax as a complication of RDS, the onset of the pneumothorax is frequently heralded by a change in the vital signs (142). In the series of Ogata et al. (142) of 49 infants with pneumothorax complicating RDS, cardiac arrest marked the development of the pneumothorax in 12 (24%). Most of the other babies had a decrease in the pulse of 10 to 90 beats per minute, a decrease in the blood pressure of 8 to 22 mm Hg, or a decrease in the respiratory rate of 8 to 20 breaths per minute (142). Although the PaO_2 decreased with the development of pneumothorax, no consistent changes were seen in the pH or $PaCO_2$. The infant with RDS who develops hypotension as a result of a pneumothorax is at high risk of having an intraventricular hemorrhage. In one series, 32 of 36 infants (89%) with pneumothorax associated with hypotension had a grade 3 or 4 intraventricular hemorrhage. In contrast, only three of 31 (10%) infants with pneumothorax and normal blood pressure developed an intraventricular bleed (146). It is hypothesized that the hypotension results in a cerebral infarction, with the intraventricular hemorrhage occurring after the systemic blood pressure has been raised to normal values (146). The infants who developed hypotension had a higher mortality rate and more residual brain damage than did those who maintained their blood pressure (146).

Diagnosis

The diagnosis of pneumothorax should be entertained in any neonate with respiratory distress or in any infant with RDS who deteriorates clinically. A radiograph of the chest is essential to differentiate pneumothorax from pneumomediastinum, hyaline membrane disease, aspiration pneumonia, congenital cyst of the lung, lobar emphysema, and diaphragmatic hernia. A clinically significant pneumothorax should be evident on a high-quality anteroposterior or posteroanterior chest radiograph (141). Transillumination of the chest with a high-intensity transilluminating light is also a rapid, accurate, and easy way to make the diagnosis of pneumothorax in the neonate (147).

Treatment

The neonate without RDS who is asymptomatic or is mildly symptomatic can be treated by close observation, and the pneumothorax resolves in the majority of patients over a few days. Close observation is necessary because of the possibility that the pneumothorax will enlarge or that a tension pneumothorax (see the section later in this chapter) will develop (141). Supplemental oxygen can increase the speed at which the pneumothorax is absorbed, but it should be administered

with care, particularly in the preterm infant because of the dangers of retrolental fibroplasia
(141). A chest tube should be inserted in the
neonate who is more than mildly symptomatic.
With tube thoracostomy, the air leak almost always stops within 24 hours (141). When the leak
has stopped for 24 hours, the chest tube can be
safely removed.

Tube thoracostomy should almost always be
performed in infants with RDS and pneumothorax because the pneumothorax compromises the
patient's already poor ventilatory status and often
increases in size. Usually, the air leak is small,
and intermittent positive-pressure ventilation can
maintain adequate gas exchange. In certain patients, however, air leaks are so large that most
of the ventilation delivered by the respirator exits the lung through the bronchopleural fistula. In
such patients, high-frequency ventilation may be
the only method by which adequate gas exchange
can be maintained (148). (See the discussion of
bronchopleural fistulas at the end of this chapter.)

IATROGENIC PNEUMOTHORAX

The incidence of iatrogenic pneumothorax is
high and is likely to increase as the use of invasive procedures becomes more widespread. In
Olmsted County, Minnesota, between 1950 and
1974, 102 instances of iatrogenic pneumothorax
were reported, as compared with 77 cases of primary and 64 cases of secondary spontaneous
pneumothorax (1). In the VA cooperative study
on spontaneous pneumothoraces, data were collected on the incidence of iatrogenic pneumothoraces at the same time (149). These investigators
reported that during the 4-year study period, there
were 538 instances of iatrogenic pneumothorax
and 520 instances of spontaneous pneumothorax.
This study probably underestimates the relative
incidence of iatrogenic pneumothorax because
some of the medical centers did not appear to be
diligent in searching for iatrogenic pneumothoraces. The major causes of iatrogenic pneumothorax in this latter study are shown in Table 21.1.

There is a substantial rate of morbidity and
even some deaths associated with iatrogenic
pneumothorax. Despars et al. (150) reviewed the
cases of iatrogenic pneumothoraces at the VA

TABLE 21.1. *Leading causes of iatrogenic pneumothorax in the veterans administration cooperative study*

Procedure	Number	Percent
Transthoracic needle aspiration	128	24
Subclavian needle stick	119	22
Thoracentesis	101	20
Pleural biopsy	45	8
Positive pressure ventilation	38	7
Supraclavicular needle stick	24	5
Nerve block	16	3
Miscellaneous	5	1

Medical Center in Long Beach, California, and
reported that between October 1983 and December 1988, there were 105 cases of iatrogenic pneumothorax in comparison to 90 cases of spontaneous pneumothorax. The most common cause
of iatrogenic pneumothorax was transthoracic
needle aspiration (35), followed by thoracentesis
(30), subclavian venipuncture (23), and positive-
pressure ventilation (7). There was substantial
morbidity from the iatrogenic pneumothoraces
in this series. The majority of patients (65 of
98) were treated with large chest tubes that were
in place 4.7 ± 3.9 days. Nine of the patients required a second chest tube. Two patients died
from the iatrogenic pneumothorax (150).

At present, the leading cause of iatrogenic
pneumothorax is transthoracic needle aspiration
of lung masses. The incidence of iatrogenic pneumothorax with this procedure in three series, each
with over 300 patients, ranged from 20% to 40%
(151–153). The percentage of patients undergoing needle aspiration of the lung who are
treated with chest tubes ranges from 2% to 8%
(151–153). The two primary factors related to the
development of the pneumothorax are the depth
of the lesion and the severity of the underlying
lung disease (151, 153). In one study, the incidence of pneumothorax was 15% if no aerated
lung was traversed and approximately 50% if
aerated lung was penetrated (153). In this same
study, the incidence of pneumothorax was 49%
if emphysema was present on the CT scan and
35% if emphysema was absent. Patients with emphysema were three times more likely to receive
chest tubes than were patients without emphysema (153). As of yet, no method to decrease the
incidence of the pneumothorax has been found.

Positioning the patient with the biopsied lung inferior is not effective (152, 154), even though it is in animals. Similarly, the use of a blood patch technique was ineffective in decreasing the incidence of pneumothorax in two studies (69, 70), but it did decrease the incidence of large pneumothoraces in a third study (71). A preliminary study suggested that the use of fibrin glue as a sealant might decrease the incidence of pneumothorax after lung aspiration. In a prospective randomized study in patients with COPD, 26 patients received 1 mL of fibrin glue as the needle was withdrawn, while 32 control patients received nothing. The incidence of pneumothorax was 19.2% in the group that received the fibrin glue compared with 40.6% in the control group. In the group that received the fibrin glue, one patient (3.8%) received a chest tube, whereas six patients (18%) in the control group received a chest tube (155). If these results can be confirmed, the routine use of fibrin glue at the time of needle aspiration of the lung may be warranted.

The second leading cause of iatrogenic pneumothorax is probably the insertion of a central line (149). The reported incidence of iatrogenic pneumothorax following subclavian vein catheterization has varied from 0 to 12% (156–160), with the average being about 2%. The importance of monitoring the incidence of complications in individual institutions is demonstrated by the report of Lockwood (156). In this report, the incidence of pneumothorax fell dramatically from 12% once training programs were initiated (156). Because more than 1 million subclavian catheters are inserted annually in the United States, this procedure is responsible for a substantial number of pneumothoraces. Pneumothoraces appear to be more common with internal jugular cannulations as opposed to subclavian cannulations and with Swan-Ganz catheters as opposed to central venous catheters. It is important to note that the pneumothorax following subclavian vein catheterization may not be apparent on the immediate postprocedure radiograph (161).

Thoracentesis is probably the third leading cause of iatrogenic pneumothorax. At present, the incidence of pneumothorax after thoracentesis is about 5%, with about 20% to 50% of those with a pneumothorax requiring a chest tube (162–164). The incidence of pneumothorax is higher if the patients have COPD. Most of the patients who have a pneumothorax after thoracentesis aspirated air at the time of the thoracentesis or have undergone more than one attempt at thoracentesis (164). If tactile fremitus is present over the upper lung field after thoracentesis, if the patient is not symptomatic, and if the physician does not suspect a pneumothorax, a chest radiograph after thoracentesis is not indicated (162, 164).

Although mechanical ventilation was the leading cause of iatrogenic pneumothorax in the 1970s (165), it is probably now only the third or fourth leading cause of iatrogenic pneumothorax. The relative decrease in the incidence of iatrogenic pneumothorax caused by mechanical ventilation probably is due to a combination of two factors. First, procedures such as transthoracic needle aspiration and subclavian vein catheterization were used much less commonly 20 years ago. Second, newer ventilatory modes have made it possible to ventilate patients with lower peak inspiratory pressures and lower mean airway pressures (150). In a series of 553 patients requiring ventilatory support from nearly 25 years ago, the incidence of iatrogenic pneumothorax was 4% (166). In this series, the frequency of pneumothorax was increased if the patient had aspiration pneumonia (37%), COPD (8%), intubation of the right main stem bronchus (13%), or treatment with positive end-expiratory pressure (15%) (166).

The incidence of pneumothorax is relatively high in patients with ARDS. Weg et al. (167) reported that the incidence of pneumothorax was 9.2% in a series of 644 patients with ARDS. Although the occurrence of pneumothoraces in this situation in the past had been attributed to high inspiratory pressures or mean airway pressures, these pressures were very similar in patients with and without pneumothorax in Weg's series. In this series, the mortality rate was not significantly different in those with and without pneumothorax. The presence of mediastinal emphysema may precede the development of the pneumothorax. In one series of 20 patients who developed a pneumothorax while on mechanical ventilation, previous chest radiographs had shown the presence of mediastinal emphysema in 10 (50%) (168).

Other procedures associated with iatrogenic pneumothorax and their approximate incidence are pleural biopsy, 10% (169); transbronchial lung biopsy, 1–2% (170, 171); laparoscopy, 0.2% (172); and liver biopsy, 0.35% (173). The reported incidences are probably minimum percentages because the authors of articles are usually more experienced in the various procedures they describe than is the average physician. Iatrogenic pneumothorax may occur following tracheostomy, when air passes into the mediastinum and pleural space by the cervical fascial planes. Iatrogenic pneumothorax also frequently complicates cardiopulmonary resuscitation. In an autopsy series, 12 patients had tension pneumothoraces that were undiagnosed during life, and nine of these patients had undergone cardiopulmonary resuscitation (174). Resuscitation-related rib fractures were found in only three of the nine patients.

Physicians treating heart-lung transplant recipients should be aware of the fact that these patients do not have an intact mediastinum. Because they are likely to undergo procedures that are associated with iatrogenic pneumothorax such as transthoracic needle aspiration, bronchoscopy, thoracentesis, and central line insertion, they may develop life-threatening bilateral pneumothoraces. Paranjpe et al. (175) reported that 15 of 72 heart-lung transplant recipients developed iatrogenic pneumothoraces, and the pneumothoraces were bilateral in six of the patients. Lee and associates reported the development of a contralateral tension pneumothorax following the unilateral chest tube drainage of bilateral pneumothoraces (176).

Clinical Manifestations

The clinical manifestations of iatrogenic pneumothorax depend both on the patient's condition and on the initiating procedure. If the pneumothorax occurs as a complication of mechanical ventilation, the patient is likely to demonstrate a sudden clinical deterioration. A sensitive indicator of the development of a pneumothorax in such patients is an increasing peak and plateau pressure on the respirator if the patient is on volume-controlled ventilation, or a decreasing tidal volume if the patient is on pressure support. The development of a pneumothorax during cardiopulmonary resuscitation is heralded by more difficulty in ventilating the patient. In contrast, many patients who develop pneumothorax after thoracentesis, pleural biopsy, transbronchial biopsy, or percutaneous lung aspiration have no symptoms referable to the pneumothorax.

Diagnosis

The diagnosis of iatrogenic pneumothorax should be suspected in any patient treated by mechanical ventilation. The presence of mediastinal emphysema should serve as an indicator to look closely for a pneumothorax (169). Recognition of the pneumothorax in the patient on mechanical ventilation is more difficult because the chest radiographs are obtained with the patient supine or semisupine. When the patient is in this position, the most superior part of the chest (where the air accumulates) is the anterior costophrenic sulcus. In one series of 112 pneumothoraces seen on supine radiographs, the most common location of air was anteromedially (38%), followed by subpulmonic 26%, apicolateral 22%, and posteromedial 11% (177). Air in the anterior costophrenic sulcus is manifested as hyperlucency over the upper abdominal quadrants (177). Pneumothoraces are frequently not recognized on the supine radiographs. Kollef (178) prospectively reviewed all 464 medical intensive care unit admissions at Fitzsimons Army Medical Center over a 1-year period and reported that nine of 28 pneumothoraces (32%) were not originally recognized. Three of these nine patients subsequently went on to develop a tension pneumothorax.

The occurrence of an iatrogenic pneumothorax should also be suspected in patients who become more short of breath after a medical or surgical procedure associated with the development of an iatrogenic pneumothorax. The signs and symptoms of the pneumothorax are similar to those of primary and secondary pneumothorax, and the diagnosis is confirmed by chest radiographs.

Treatment

The treatment of iatrogenic pneumothorax differs from that of spontaneous pneumothorax in that recurrence is not likely, and, therefore, one need not try to create a pleurodesis, as is done frequently with spontaneous pneumothorax. When a pneumothorax occurs during positive-pressure ventilation, tube thoracostomy should be performed immediately in most cases to prevent the development of a tension pneumothorax. With mechanical ventilation, positive pressure in the alveoli leads to increased entry of air into the pleural space and the likelihood that a tension pneumothorax will develop. The chest tube should be left in place for at least 48 hours after the air leak stops if the patient continues to receive mechanical ventilation. At times, an ipsilateral recurrent pneumothorax develops in a patient on mechanical ventilation while the chest tube is still in place. This development is usually due to placement of the chest tube in a fissure (179). Malpositioning of the chest tube is suggested if the chest tube is perpendicular to the lateral chest wall; the chest tube should be relatively parallel to the chest wall (179). Bronchopleural fistulas and mechanical ventilation are discussed later in this chapter.

When an iatrogenic pneumothorax develops after a procedure, symptoms vary from none to severe respiratory distress. In general, if the patient has no symptoms or just mild symptoms and the pneumothorax occupies less than 40% of the hemithorax, the patient can be managed with observation. The administration of supplemental oxygen will increase the rate at which air is absorbed from the pleural space (see Chapter 2) (41). If the patient is more than mildly symptomatic, if the pneumothorax occupies more than 40% of the hemithorax, or if the pneumothorax continues to enlarge, however, one should consider removing the intrapleural air.

In general, most iatrogenic pneumothoraces should first be treated with aspiration. If the initial aspiration is unsuccessful, then a Heimlich valve should be attached to the catheter. Only when the lung does not expand and remain expanded with the Heimlich valve is a larger chest tube inserted. Delius et al. (180) treated 79 needle-induced iatrogenic pneumothoraces by aspiration through an 8 F radiopaque Teflon catheter. The initial aspiration was successful in 59 (75%), and an additional nine patients (15%) were successfully managed with a Heimlich valve attached to this small catheter (180). Patients can be managed as outpatients with small intrapleural catheters and Heimlich valves (181). In general, the patient is more likely to require a chest tube if he or she has COPD (182).

TRAUMATIC (NONIATROGENIC) PNEUMOTHORAX

Traumatic pneumothorax can result from either penetrating or nonpenetrating chest trauma.

Mechanism

The mechanism of the pneumothorax is easily understood with penetrating chest trauma because the wound allows air to enter the pleural space directly through the chest wall. In addition, the visceral pleura is frequently penetrated, allowing air to enter the pleural space from the alveoli. With nonpenetrating trauma, the ribs may become fractured or dislocated, and the visceral pleura may thereby be lacerated, leading to a pneumothorax. In the majority of patients with pneumothorax secondary to nonpenetrating trauma, however, no associated rib fractures occur (183). The mechanism of the pneumothorax in such patients is thought to be as follows (183). With sudden chest compression, the alveolar pressure increases and may cause alveolar rupture. Air then enters the interstitial spaces and dissects either toward the visceral pleura or toward the mediastinum to produce mediastinal emphysema. A pneumothorax results when either the visceral or the mediastinal pleura ruptures.

Incidence and Diagnosis

The diagnosis of traumatic pneumothorax should be considered in any patient who suffers significant trauma. In most instances, the initial chest radiograph on trauma patients is obtained in the supine position and small pneumothoraces may not be apparent. These supine chest radiographs are insensitive in diagnosing both pneumothorax and hemothorax. In one series of 103 patients with blunt chest trauma, thoracic CT scans revealed pneumothorax in 44 patients compared with 17 patients on the supine chest radiograph (184). In the same series, the CT revealed hemothorax in 44 patients compared with 23 patients on the supine chest radiograph (184). In view of this series, a case can be made for obtaining a thoracic CT in all severely injured patients with blunt chest trauma.

Pneumothoraces seen only on the CT are labeled as occult pneumothoraces. Overall, about 5% of multiple trauma patients have a pneumothorax and about 40% of the pneumothoraces are occult. For example, in one series of 2,048 multiple trauma patients, there were 90 patients (4.4%) who had a pneumothorax (185). Thirty-five of these pneumothoraces (38.8%) were not identified on the admission chest radiograph but were subsequently identified on CT scans of the chest or abdomen (185). In a second series of 457 patients with multisystem injuries undergoing abdominal CT scans, the incidence of pneumothorax was 5.7% and none of the pneumothoraces was evident on the chest radiograph (186).

Treatment

Most traumatic pneumothoraces should be treated with tube thoracostomy. If the lung does not expand or an air leak persists, VATS should be performed within the first few days to evaluate the reason for the air leak (187). Tube thoracostomy may not be necessary for patients with small pneumothoraces or those with occult pneumothoraces. Knottenbelt and van der Spuy observed 333 patients with small (<1.5 cm from lung to chest wall) pneumothoraces due to chest trauma and reported that only 33 required subsequent drainage for an enlarging pneumothorax (188). Ordog et al. (189) observed 47 patients with small pneumothoraces (<20%) secondary to stab wounds of the chest and reported that only 32% required a chest tube or showed progression of the pneumothorax within 24 hours. They recommend that such patients be admitted to the hospital and have repeat radiographs at 6 hours, 24 hours, and again at 48 hours. The patients are then discharged if the pneumothorax is unchanged or shows evidence of resolving (189). If a hemopneumothorax is present, one chest tube should be placed in the superior part of the hemithorax to evacuate the air

and another should be placed in the inferior part of the hemithorax to remove the blood (see Chapter 22). With traumatic pneumothorax, the lung expands and the air leak usually ceases within 72 hours.

Most patients with occult pneumothoraces need not be treated with tube thoracostomy (186, 190, 191). Wolfman et al. (191) classified occult pneumothoraces as minuscule (<1 cm in greatest anteroposterior thickness and seen on no more than four contiguous CT images), anterior (>1 cm but not extending beyond the midcoronal line), and anterolateral (extending posteriorly beyond the midcoronal line). Of the 28 occult pneumothoraces in their series, six were minuscule, 14 were anterior, and eight were anterolateral. The patients with the minuscule and the anterior occult pneumothoraces were less likely to receive tube thoracostomy (191). Some patients who have an occult pneumothorax and receive mechanical ventilation have been managed without tube thoracostomy (192). Nevertheless, it is recommended that all patients with occult pneumothorax who receive mechanical ventilation be treated with tube thoracostomy owing to the possibility of the development of a tension pneumothorax, which could be fatal. All other patients with occult pneumothoraces can probably be observed with tube thoracostomy being performed only if the pneumothorax is enlarging.

Whenever a patient with a traumatic pneumothorax is seen, two uncommon diagnostic possibilities, both indications for immediate thoracic operation, should be considered. One is fracture of the trachea or a major bronchus; the second is traumatic rupture of the esophagus. Bronchial rupture should be suspected in patients with persistent air leak following a traumatic pneumothorax, particularly if there is subcutaneous emphysema, pneumomediastinum, deep cervical emphysema, hemoptysis, or rib or clavicular fractures (193, 194). The possibility of bronchial rupture should be assessed in such patients with fiberoptic bronchoscopy. Thoracic CT scan does not definitively establish the diagnosis in most patients (194). The treatment of choice is surgical repair.

Traumatic rupture of the esophagus usually produces a hydropneumothorax. Therefore, if a patient with a traumatic pneumothorax also has a pleural effusion, the possibility of esophageal rupture should be entertained. A reliable screening test for esophageal rupture is measurement of the pleural fluid amylase level (195). If the patient's pleural fluid amylase level is elevated, contrast radiographic studies of the esophagus should be performed.

If a patient has suffered a traumatic pneumothorax, how long should they wait before they travel by air? The Aerospace Medicine Association has suggested that patients should be able to fly 2 to 3 weeks after radiologic resolution of the pneumothorax (196). The following study appears to have validated these recommendations. Cheatham and Safcsak (197) studied 12 consecutive patients with recent traumatic pneumothorax who desired to travel by commercial airline. Ten patients waited at least 14 days and all were asymptomatic in flight. One of two patients who flew earlier than 14 days developed respiratory distress in-flight with symptoms suggesting a recurrent pneumothorax.

TRAUMATIC PNEUMOTHORAX SECONDARY TO DRUG ABUSE

Intravenous drug abuse has become endemic in many urban areas. It appears that there is a high incidence of traumatic pneumothorax in intravenous drug users. Douglass and Levison (198) reviewed 525 diagnoses of pneumothorax between January 1, 1982 and December 31, 1984 at the Detroit Receiving Hospital. They reported that 113 (21.5%) occurred because of drug abuse. The user or a companion had attempted to inject the drug into the subclavian or internal jugular vein. It has been recommended that intravenous drug users with traumatic pneumothorax be managed with tube thoracostomy (198). In the series of Douglass and Levison, the average number of days for chest tube management was 4.4. It is probable, however, that many such cases could be managed with simple aspiration.

PNEUMOTHORAX *EX VACUO*

Pneumothorax *ex vacuo* is said to occur when patients develop a pneumothorax secondary to acute bronchial obstruction. The theory is that the acute collapse of the lung results in negative intrapleural pressure, which leads to the accumulation of gas that originated in the ambient tissues and blood in the pleural space (199).

It is not obvious to me that this entity actually exists. In order for air to come out of the tissues and into the pleural space, the pleural pressure would have more negative than -60 cm H_2O (see Chapter 2). To my knowledge, the pleural pressure has never been measured in such a purported instance of pneumothorax *ex vacuo*, and most patients who have been thought to have this condition have other possible explanations for their pneumothorax.

TENSION PNEUMOTHORAX

A tension pneumothorax is said to be present when the intrapleural pressure exceeds atmospheric pressure throughout expiration and often during inspiration as well. The mechanism by which a tension pneumothorax develops is probably related to some type of one-way valve process in which the valve is open during inspiration and closed during expiration. During inspiration, owing to the action of the respiratory muscles, the pleural pressure becomes negative, and air moves from the alveoli into the pleural space. Then, during expiration, with the respiratory muscles relaxed, the pleural pressure becomes positive. A one-way valve mechanism must be implicated; otherwise, on expiration, when the pleural pressure is positive with respect to the alveolar pressure, gas would flow from the pleural space into the alveoli, and no positive pressure would develop in the pleural space. Of course, if the patient is on mechanical ventilation and positive end-expiratory pressure, a one-way valve need not be postulated because the alveolar pressure is positive throughout the respiratory cycle.

Pathophysiologic Features

The development of a tension pneumothorax is usually heralded by a sudden deterioration in the cardiopulmonary status of the patient. The precise explanation for sudden deterioration is not known, but it is probably related to the combination of a decreased cardiac output due to impaired venous return and marked hypoxemia (200). Older studies in unventilated animals suggested that the primary pathophysiologic abnormality was a precipitous fall in the PaO_2 to below 30 mm Hg (201, 202). However, more recent studies in ventilated animals have suggested that the primary problem is decreased cardiac output. Carvalho et al. (203) induced right-sided tension pneumothoraces with mean pleural pressures of +10 and then +25 cm H_2O in 10 mechanically ventilated adult sheep. The mean cardiac output in these animals fell from 3.5 L per minute to approximately 1.2 L per minute, and the mean blood pressure fell from 80 mm Hg to less than 50 mm Hg as the pleural pressure increased from −5 to +25 cm H_2O (203). The decrease in the PaO_2 was much less life-threatening; the PaO_2 was 150 mm Hg at baseline and fell to 59 mm Hg when the pleural pressure was 25 cm H_2O (203). The inspiratory airway pressure nearly doubled from 19 to 35 cm H_2O (203). However, studies by Barton et al. (204) in ventilated swine suggested that the fall in the SaO_2 was at least as important as the fall in cardiac output. They measured the cardiac output and the SaO_2 as 100 mL aliquots of air were introduced into the pleural space. They found that when the mean intrapleural pressure had increased to 11 mm Hg with the introduction of 700 mL of air, the mean cardiac output had fallen from 2.8 to 1.9 L per minute, the mean arterial pressure had fallen only from 90 to 73 mm Hg, but the SaO_2 had fallen from 97% to 55% (204).

In humans, for obvious reasons, there have not been systematic studies of the blood gases or the hemodynamics associated with tension pneumothorax. Beards and Lipman (205) did report on the hemodynamics of three patients receiving mechanical ventilation who developed tension pneumothorax. In their three patients, the cardiac indices, which were 7.3, 4.8, and 3.6 baseline, fell to 3.0, 3.1, and 1.4 L per minute m^2 with the development of a tension pneumothorax, whereas the baseline mean arterial pressures, which were 97, 96, and 68, respectively, fell to 33, 68, and 57, respectively. The oxygenation status did not deteriorate nearly as dramatically (205). The patients in this study did not have consistent changes

in their heart rates (205). In another report a 67-year-old man with COPD developed a tension pneumothorax while on mechanical ventilation. This patient's cardiac output fell from 7.11 to 3.80 L per minute and the stroke volume fell from 56 to 27 mL, whereas the pulse increased from 127 to 142 (206). In the same patient, the PaO_2 fell from 76 mm Hg to 47 mm Hg with the development of the tension pneumothorax.

In summary, the disastrous effect of a tension pneumothorax in patients appears to be the result of the combination of a marked decrease in the cardiac output and in the PaO_2. In patients, the decrease in the cardiac output is most life-threatening, but the marked decrease in the PaO_2 should not be ignored.

Clinical Manifestations

Although tension pneumothorax occasionally evolves from a spontaneous pneumothorax, it is much more frequent in patients who develop pneumothorax while receiving mechanical ventilation or during cardiopulmonary resuscitation. The clinical status of patients with tension pneumothorax is striking. The patient appears distressed with rapid labored respirations, cyanosis, and usually profuse diaphoresis, hypotension, and marked tachycardia. Arterial blood gases reveal marked hypoxemia and sometimes respiratory acidosis. The physical findings are those of any large pneumothorax, but in addition, the involved hemithorax is larger than the contralateral hemithorax with the interspaces widened. The trachea is usually shifted toward the contralateral side.

Diagnosis and Treatment

The diagnosis of tension pneumothorax should be suspected in patients receiving mechanical ventilation, in those with a pneumothorax, or in patients whose condition suddenly deteriorates after a procedure known to cause a pneumothorax. If difficulty is encountered in the ventilation of a patient during cardiopulmonary resuscitation or a patient has electromechanical dissociation, a tension pneumothorax should also be suspected. In a series of 3,500 autopsies, unsuspected tension pneumothorax was found in 12 patients; ten of these had been supported by mechanical ventilators, and nine had undergone cardiopulmonary resuscitation (174). There is one report of three cases of tension pneumothorax that occurred during hyperbaric oxygen therapy for acute carbon monoxide poisoning (206). The presence of a chest tube in a patient with a pneumothorax does not preclude the possibility of a tension pneumothorax because the chest tube might be malpositioned (207). There is a report of two cases of tension pneumothorax that occurred when the Heimlich valve used for treating pneumothorax was attached backwards (208).

It is important to assess carefully the chest radiograph for pneumothorax in patients who are receiving mechanical ventilation. Patients with unrecognized pneumothoraces who are receiving mechanical ventilation are those most likely to develop a tension pneumothorax. Kollef (178) reviewed 464 medical intensive care unit admissions at Fitzsimons Army Medical Center over a 1-year period and reported that 28 patients acquired a pneumothorax during their stay in the intensive care unit. The pneumothorax was not originally recognized in nine of the patients, and three of these patients (33%) subsequently developed a tension pneumothorax. In a second series, Tocino et al. (177) reported that a pneumothorax was originally missed in 34 of 112 patients in an intensive care unit and 16 of these 34 patients developed tension pneumothorax. The diagnosis of pneumothorax on the supine chest radiograph is discussed earlier in this chapter in the section on iatrogenic pneumothorax.

Tension pneumothorax is a medical emergency. Although the diagnosis of tension pneumothorax can be established radiographically by demonstrating severe contralateral mediastinal shift and ipsilateral diaphragmatic depression, valuable time should not be wasted on radiologic studies because the clinical situation and the physical findings are usually sufficient to establish the diagnosis. When the diagnosis is suspected, the patient should immediately be given a high concentration of supplemental oxygen to combat the hypoxia. Then, the elevated pressure in the pleural space must be eliminated. Optimally, this is done with a silicon catheter such as that advocated for thoracentesis (see Chapter 25). Ideally, the catheter should be attached to a three-way stopcock and a 50-mL syringe partially filled with sterile saline solution. After the catheter is inserted into the pleural space, it is connected through the three-way stopcock to the syringe. Then the stopcock is opened to the syringe, and the plunger is withdrawn. A rush of air bubbling outward through the fluid in the syringe establishes the diagnosis of tension pneumothorax.

If a tension pneumothorax is confirmed, the catheter should be left in place and in communication with the atmosphere until air ceases to exit through the syringe. Additional air can be withdrawn from the pleural space with the syringe and the three-way stopcock. If a tension pneumothorax is present, preparations should be made for the immediate insertion of a large chest tube. If no bubbles escape from the syringe, the patient does not have a tension pneumothorax, and the catheter should be withdrawn from the pleural space.

BRONCHOPLEURAL FISTULAS

Bronchopleural fistula constitutes a serious and sometimes fatal disorder that usually occurs after pulmonary surgery or as a complication of an underlying pulmonary disease. Bronchopleural fistulas occurring concomitantly with spontaneous pneumothorax have been discussed earlier in this chapter. In this section, the problem of bronchopleural fistulas in patients on mechanical ventilation and in patients after pulmonary surgery is discussed.

Bronchopleural Fistulas and Mechanical Ventilation

The management of a patient on mechanical ventilation with a large bronchopleural fistula is frequently difficult. In general, hypoxia rather than hypercapnia is the main threat to the patient because the air that leaves the bronchopleural fistula has a carbon dioxide level comparable to that in mixed expired air (209). In other words, the air that exits through the chest tube is effective in removing carbon dioxide from the patient. Indeed, Prezant et al. (210) reported on a patient whose total ventilatory requirements could be maintained through a chronic bronchopleural fistula. At times, however, when a high percentage of the minute ventilation exits through the bronchopleural fistula, the patient's oxygenation may suffer (211).

The first question that must be addressed when dealing with a patient with a bronchopleural fistula who is receiving mechanical ventilation is the management of the chest tubes. How much suction? How many chest tubes? It appears that the level of flow through the fistula is decreased when the side with the fistula is placed in the dependent position (212). The number and size of the chest tubes should be sufficient to effect a complete expansion of the underlying lung. The amount of suction should probably be established on an individual basis. Powner et al. (213) have shown that the level of suction at which the flow through the bronchopleural fistula is minimized varies from patient to patient. In some patients, the flow is minimized at no suction, whereas in others, it is minimized at an intermediate level (10 to 15 cm H_2O), and in still others, it is minimized with high suction (25 cm H_2O).

One approach to decreasing the flow through a bronchopleural fistula is to place the patient on a high-frequency jet ventilator. Although high-frequency ventilation appears to decrease the flow through the fistula and improve gas exchange in the experimental model (214), it is not recommended because it has not been demonstrated to be effective in patients. Two separate studies in adults (215, 216) demonstrated no benefits of high-frequency ventilation compared with conventional mechanical ventilation with respect to the flow through the bronchopleural fistula or gas exchange. In infants, Gonzalez et al. (217) applied conventional ventilation at a rate of 60 per minute and high-frequency jet ventilation with a rate of 420 per minute to six infants with continuously bubbling chest tubes. They recommended that jet ventilation be used in such instances because the mean flow through the bronchopleural fistula dropped from 227 to 104 mL per minute as the infants were switched to the jet ventilator. The PaO_2 dropped from 49 to 44 mm Hg when the patients were switched to the jet ventilator, however. Therefore, it is difficult to agree with their recommendation.

Multiple agents and devices, including silver nitrate, Gelfoam, cyanoacrylate-based agents, and fibrin agents, have been passed through a bronchoscope in attempts to occlude the bronchopleural fistula (218). The cyanoacrylate agents have been recently improved with an additive that slows drying time to permit greater time for modeling of the agent into the fistula site (218) and show the most promise. There are, however, no sizable series on the use of any of these agents in the treatment of bronchopleural fistula in patients on mechanical ventilation.

Different agents such as tetracycline derivatives, talc, and fibrin glue have also been injected into the pleural space in an attempt to effect closure of the bronchopleural fistula. The most promising agent is dilute fibrin glue. Kinoshita et al. injected fibrin glue into the pleural spaces of five patients with persistent bronchopleural fistula receiving mechanical ventilation. They reported that the bronchopleural fistula closed within 12 hours in four of the five patients (72).

Postoperative Bronchopleural Fistulas

After pulmonary resections of lesser magnitude than a pneumonectomy, there is frequently an air leak from the residual raw parenchymal surface. If the lung has expanded and the pleural space is obliterated, the leak usually stops in 2 or 3 days. The persistence of a leak beyond 7 days is considered abnormal and generally used to define a "prolonged" air leak (219). One can try various maneuvers empirically, such as increasing or decreasing the suction, conversion to waterseal drainage only, or the placement of additional tubes, to speed closure of the fistula. A recent article suggested that flutter valves were more effective than waterseal systems for the management of postoperative air leaks (220). Prolonged air leaks are a very frequent problem after lung volume reduction surgery. In one study, prolonged air leaks occurred in 35 of 197 patients (15.2%) undergoing lung volume reduction surgery, but only three leaks persisted after 14 days (221).

A bronchopleural fistula is observed in approximately 1% to 4% of patients after a pneumonectomy or a lobectomy and less often after a segmentectomy or lesser procedure (219).

In patients with lung cancer, significant risk factors for the development of a bronchopleural fistula include residual carcinomatous tissue at the bronchial stump, preoperative irradiation, and diabetes mellitus (222). A bronchopleural fistula is more common after resections for inflammatory disease of the lung, especially in patients with active tuberculosis and positive sputum culture (219).

After pulmonary surgery, a bronchopleural fistula may develop immediately or weeks to months later. The early appearance of a fistula (e.g., 1 to 6 days) frequently is due to a technically poor closure of the bronchial stump. After a pneumonectomy, the early fistula is massive and persistent. The patient frequently develops massive subcutaneous emphysema and may exhibit varying degrees of respiratory insufficiency (219).

When the bronchial leak occurs later in the postoperative course (e.g., 7 to 10 days), it may be caused by failure of healing because of inadequate viable tissue coverage of the stump, or as the result of infection of the fluid within the space and rupture of the empyema through the suture line of the bronchial stump. At this stage, the patient coughs up variable quantities of serosanguineous, frothy fluid from the respiratory tract. The patient should be placed with the affected side down to decrease the danger of flooding the remaining lung.

When a bronchopleural fistula occurs more than 2 weeks after pneumonectomy, it is usually due to rupture of a frank empyema through the bronchial stump, although, at times, it may be due to failure of healing of the bronchial stump (219). The patient appears chronically ill with a cough and fever. Thoracentesis reveals that the pleural fluid is infected.

The management of a postoperative bronchopleural fistula depends on the time of its development and its underlying cause. If the bronchopleural fistula occurs early in the postoperative period, it can sometimes be managed with reoperation and repair of the bronchial stump. If primary repair of the bronchial stump is attempted, it is imperative that the new bronchial suture line be covered. This can be done with a transposed muscle flap (223), the pericardial fat pad, or an omental pedicle flap (219). With direct closure, the bronchial stump should be shortened as much as possible (224).

If primary repair of the bronchopleural fistula is not attempted or is unsuccessful, the patient should be treated with a chest tube. Several studies have reported on the implantation of different materials in the bronchus through a bronchoscope in an attempt to close the air leak. When the patient has undergone less than a pneumonectomy, a Fogarty balloon catheter is passed down the working channel of the bronchoscope, and systematic occlusion of all lung segments on the side of the air leak is undertaken. The segment or segments leading to the fistula can be noted by observing decreases or disappearance of the air leak (225). Materials placed in the appropriate bronchus to close the fistula have included Gelfoam (225), doxycycline and blood (226), fibrin glue (227, 228) and vascular occlusion coils (229). Fibrin glue appears to be the most promising material. Hollaus et al. (228) applied fibrin glue to 45 patients with bronchopleural fistula after pneumonectomy (40 patients) or lobectomy (five patients). They reported that nine of 29 patients who were treated only endoscopically were cured. Small fistulas (<3 mm) were particularly likely to respond. The ultimate place of this approach in the management of patients with a postoperative bronchopleural fistula remains to be determined.

Bronchopleural fistulas that occur late after surgery are almost always associated with empyema. Such fistulas are discussed in Chapter 9 in the section on postpneumonectomy empyema.

REFERENCES

1. Melton LJ, Hepper NGG, Offord KP. Incidence of spontaneous pneumothorax in Olmsted County, Minnesota: 1950 to 1974. *Am Rev Respir Dis* 1979;120: 1379–1382.
2. Gobbel WG Jr, Rhea WG Jr, Nelson IA, et al. Spontaneous pneumothorax. *J Thorac Cardiovasc Surg* 1963;46:331–345.
3. Lesur O, Delorme N, Fromaget JM, et al. Computed tomography in the etiologic assessment of idiopathic spontaneous pneumothorax. *Chest* 1990;98:341–347.
4. Bense L, Lewander R, Eklund G, et al. Nonsmoking, non-alpha 1-antitrypsin deficiency–induced emphysema in nonsmokers with healed spontaneous pneumothorax, identified by computed tomography of the lungs. *Chest* 1993;103:433–438.
5. O'Hara VS. Spontaneous pneumothorax. *Mil Med* 1978;143:32–35.

6. Jansveld CAF, Dijkman JH. Primary spontaneous pneumothorax and smoking. *Br Med J* 1975;4: 559–560.

7. Seremetis MG. The management of spontaneous pneumothorax. *Chest* 1970;57:65–68.

8. Bense L, Eklund G, Wiman LG. Smoking and the increased risk of contracting spontaneous pneumothorax. *Chest* 1987;92:1009–1012.

9. Scott GC, Berger R, McKean HE. The role of atmospheric pressure variation in the development of spontaneous pneumothoraces. *Am Rev Respir Dis* 1989;139:659–662.

10. Bense L. Spontaneous pneumothorax related to falls in atmospheric pressure. *Eur J Respir Dis* 1985;65:544–546.

11. Smit HJ, Deville WL, Schramel FM, et al. Atmospheric pressure changes and outdoor temperature changes in relation to spontaneous pneumothorax. *Chest* 1999;116:676–681.

12. Suarez-Varela MM, Martinez-Selva MI, Llopis-Gonzalez A, et al. Spontaneous pneumothorax related with climatic characteristics in the Valencia area. *Eur J Epidemiol* 2000;16:193–198.

13. Withers JN, Fishback ME, Kiehl PV, et al. Spontaneous pneumothorax. *Am J Surg* 1964;108:772–776.

14. Abolnik IZ, Lossos IS, Gillis D, et al. Primary spontaneous pneumothorax in men. *Am J Med Sci* 1993;305:297–303.

15. Abolnik IZ, Lossos IS, Zlotogora J, et al. On the inheritance of primary spontaneous pneumothorax. *Am J Med Genet* 1991;40:155–158.

16. Sharpe IK, Ahmad M, Braun W. Familial spontaneous pneumothorax and HLA antigens. *Chest* 1980;78:264–268.

17. Lenler-Petersen P, Grunnet N, Jespersen TW, et al. Familial spontaneous pneumothorax. *Eur Respir J* 1990;3:342–345.

18. Bense L, Eklung G, Wiman LG. Bilateral bronchial anomaly. A pathogenetic factor in spontaneous pneumothorax. *Am Rev Respir Dis* 1992;146:513–516.

19. Norris RM, Jones JG, Bishop JM. Respiratory gas exchange in patients with spontaneous pneumothorax. *Thorax* 1968;23:427–433.

20. Moran JF, Jones RH, Wolfe WG. Regional pulmonary function during experimental unilateral pneumothorax in the awake state. *J Thorac Cardiovasc Surg* 1977;74:396–402.

21. Anthonisen NR. Regional function in spontaneous pneumothorax. *Am Rev Respir Dis* 1977;115:873–876.

22. Luna E, Tomashefski JF Jr, Brown D, et al. Reactive eosinophilic pulmonary vascular infiltration in patients with spontaneous pneumothorax. *Am J Surg Pathol* 1994;18:195–199.

23. Cyr PV, Vincic L, Kay JM. Pulmonary vasculopathy in idiopathic spontaneous pneumothorax in young subjects. *Arch Pathol Lab Med* 2000;124:717–720.

24. Vail WJ, Alway AE, England NJ. Spontaneous pneumothorax. *Dis Chest* 1960;38:512–515.

25. Maeda A, Ishioka S, Yoshihara M, et al. Primary spontaneous pneumothorax detected during a medical checkup. *Chest* 1999;116:847–848.

26. Aston SJ, Rosove M. Horner's syndrome occurring with spontaneous pneumothorax. *N Engl J Med* 1972;287:1098.

27. Bense L, Wiman LG, Hedenstierna G. Onset of symptoms in spontaneous pneumothorax: correlations to physical activity. *Eur J Respir Dis* 1987;71:181–186.

28. Walston A, Brewer DL, Kitchens CS, et al. The electrocardiographic manifestations of spontaneous left pneumothorax. *Ann Intern Med* 1974;80:375–379.

29. Alikhan M, Biddison JH. Electrocardiographic changes with right-sided pneumothorax. *South Med J* 1998;91: 677–680.

30. Strizik B, Forman R. New ECG changes associated with a tension pneumothorax. *Chest* 1999;115:1742–1744.

31. Seow A, Kazerooni EA, Pernicano PG, et al. Comparison of upright inspiratory and expiratory chest radiographs for detecting pneumothoraces. *AJR Am J Roentgenol* 1996;166:313–316.

32. Dulchavsky SA, Hamilton DR, Diebel LN, et al. Thoracic ultrasound diagnosis of pneumothorax. *J Trauma* 1999;47:970–971.

33. Smit HJ, van den Heuvel MM, Barbierato SB, et al. Analysis of pleural fluid in idiopathic spontaneous pneumothorax; correlation of eosinophil percentage with the duration of air in the pleural space. *Respir Med* 1999;93:262–267.

34. Collins CD, Lopez A, Mathie A, et al. Quantification of pneumothorax size on chest radiographs using interpleural distances: regression analysis based on volume measurements from helical CT. *AJR Am J Roentgenol* 1995;165:1127–1130.

35. Sadikot RT, Greene T, Meadows K, et al. Recurrence of primary spontaneous pneumothorax. *Thorax* 1997;52:805–809.

36. Lippert HL, Lund O, Blegvad S, et al. Independent risk factors for cumulative recurrence rate after first spontaneous pneumothorax. *Eur Respir J* 1991;4:324–331.

37. Light RW, O'Hara VS, Moritz TE, et al. Intrapleural tetracycline for the prevention of recurrent spontaneous pneumothorax. *JAMA* 1990;264:2224–2230.

38. Mitlehner W, Friedrich M, Dissmann W. Value of computer tomography in the detection of bullae and blebs in patients with primary spontaneous pneumothorax. *Respiration* 1992;59:221–227.

39. Kircher LT Jr, Swartzel RL. Spontaneous pneumothorax and its treatment. *JAMA* 1954;155:24–29.

40. Chernick V, Avery ME. Spontaneous alveolar rupture at birth. *Pediatrics* 1963;32:816–824.

41. Northfield TC. Oxygen therapy for spontaneous pneumothorax. *Br Med J* 1971;4:86–88.

42. Harvey J, Prescott RJ. Simple aspiration versus intercostal tube drainage for spontaneous pneumothorax in patients with normal lungs. British Thoracic Society Research Committee. *Br Med J* 1994; 309:1338– 1339.

43. Andrivet P, Djedaini K, Teboul J-L, et al. Spontaneous pneumothorax. Comparison of thoracic drainage vs immediate or delayed needle aspiration. *Chest* 1995;108:335–340.

44. So SY, Yu DYC. Catheter drainage of spontaneous pneumothorax: suction or no suction, early or late removal. *Thorax* 1982;37:46–48.

45. Minami H, Saka H, Senda K, et al. Small caliber catheter drainage for spontaneous pneumothorax. *Am J Med Sci* 1992;404:345–347.

46. Ponn RB, Silverman HJ, Federico JA. Outpatient chest tube management. *Ann Thorac Surg* 1997;64:1437–1440.

47. Campisi P, Voitk AJ. Outpatient treatment of spontaneous pneumothorax in a community hospital using a Heimlich flutter valve: a case series. *J Emerg Med* 1997;15:115–119.

48. Sharma TN, Agnihotri SP, Jain NK, et al. Intercostal tube thoracostomy in pneumothorax: factors influencing re-expansion of lung. *Indian J Chest Dis Allied Sci* 1988;30:32–35.

49. Shaw TJ, Caterine JM. Recurrent re-expansion pulmonary edema. *Chest* 1984;86:784–786.

50. Lizotte PE, Whitlock WL, Prudhomme JC, et al. Tension pneumothorax complicating small-caliber chest tube insertion. *Chest* 1990;97:759–760.

51. Engdahl O, Boe J. Quantification of aspirated air volume reduces treatment time in pneumothorax. *Eur Resp J* 1990;3:649–652.

52. Baumann MH, Strange C, Heffner JE, et al. Management of spontaneous pneumothorax: an ACCP Delphi Consensus Statement. *Chest* 2001 (*in press*).

53. Larrieu AJ, Tyers GFO, Williams EH, et al. Intrapleural instillation of quinacrine for treatment of recurrent spontaneous pneumothorax. *Ann Thorac Surg* 1979;28:146–150.

54. Almind M, Lange P, Viskum K. Spontaneous pneumothorax: comparison of simple drainage, talc pleurodesis, and tetracycline pleurodesis. *Thorax* 1989;44:627–630.

55. Ofoegbu RO. Pleurodesis for spontaneous pneumothorax: experience with intrapleural olive oil in high risk patients. *Am J Surg* 1980;140:679–681.

56. Goldszer RC, Bennett J, VanCampen J, et al. Intrapleural tetracycline for spontaneous pneumothorax. *JAMA* 1979;241:724–725.

57. Spector ML, Stern RC. Pneumothorax in cystic fibrosis: a 26-year experience. *Ann Thorac Surg* 1989;47:204–207.

58. Light RW. Diseases of the pleura: the use of talc for pleurodesis. *Curr Opinion* 2000;6:255–258.

59. Alfageme I, Moreno L, Huetas C, et al. Spontaneous pneumothorax. Long-term results with tetracycline pleurodesis. *Chest* 1994;106:347–350.

60. Light RW, Wang N-S, Sassoon CSH, et al. Comparison of the effectiveness of tetracycline and minocycline as pleural sclerosing agents in rabbits. *Chest* 1994;106:577–582.

61. Wu W, Teixeira LR, Light RW. Doxycycline pleurodesis in rabbits. Comparison of results with and without chest tube. *Chest* 1998;114:563–568.

62. Vargas FS, Wang N-S, Lee HM, et al. Effectiveness of bleomycin in comparison to tetracycline as pleural sclerosing agent in rabbits. *Chest* 1993;104:1582–1584.

63. Sherman S, Ravikrishnan KP, Patel AS, et al. Optimum anesthesia with intrapleural lidocaine during chemical pleurodesis with tetracycline. *Chest* 1988;93:533–536.

64. Xie C, Teixeira LR, McGovern JP, et al. Effect of pneumothorax on pleurodesis induced with talc in rabbits. *Chest* 1998;114:1143–1146.

65. Wang YT, Ng KY, Poh SC. Intrapleural tetracycline for spontaneous pneumothorax with persistent air leak. *Singapore Med J* 1988;29:72–73.

66. Robinson CL. Autologous blood for pleurodesis in recurrent and chronic spontaneous pneumothorax. *Can J Surg* 1987;30:428–429.

67. Cagirici U, Sahin B, Cakan A, et al. Autologous blood patch pleurodesis in spontaneous pneumothorax with persistent air leak. *Scand Cardiovasc J* 1998;32:75–78.

68. Ando M, Yamamoto M, Kitagawa C, et al. Autologous blood-patch pleurodesis for secondary spontaneous pneumothorax with persistent air leak. *Respir Med* 1999;93:432–434.

69. Bourgouin PM, Shepard JA, McLoud TC, et al. Transthoracic needle aspiration biopsy: evaluation of the blood patch technique. *Radiology* 1988;166:93–95.

70. Herman SJ, Weisbrod GL. Usefulness of the blood patch technique after transthoracic needle aspiration biopsy. *Radiology* 1990;176:395–397.

71. Lang EK, Ghavami R, Schreiner VC, et al. Autologous blood clot seal to prevent pneumothorax at CT-guided lung biopsy. *Radiology* 2000;216:93–96.

72. Kinoshita T, Miyoshi S, Katoh M, et al. Intrapleural administration of a large amount of diluted fibrin glue for intractable pneumothorax. *Chest* 2000;117:790–795.

73. Loddenkemper R. Thoracoscopy—state of the art. *Eur Respir J* 1998;11:213–221.

74. Tschopp JM, Brutsche M, Frey JG. Treatment of complicated spontaneous pneumothorax by simple talc pleurodesis under thoracoscopy and local anaesthesia. *Thorax* 1997;52:329–332.

75. Landreneau RJ, Hazelrigg SR, Mack MJ, et al. Video-assisted thoracic surgery for pulmonary and pleural disease. In: Shields TW, ed. *General thoracic surgery,* 4th ed. Malvern, PA: Williams & Wilkins, 1994:508–528.

76. Hazelrigg SR, Landreneau RJ, Mack M, et al. Thoracoscopic stapled resection for spontaneous pneumothorax. *Thorac Cardiovasc Surg* 1993;105:389–393.

77. Takeno Y. Thoracoscopic treatment of spontaneous pneumothorax. *Ann Thorac Surg* 1993;56:688–690.

78. Inderbitzi RGC, Leiser A, Furrer M, et al. Three years' experience in video-assisted thoracic surgery (VATS) for spontaneous pneumothorax. *Thorac Cardiovasc Surg* 1994;107:1410–1415.

79. Yim AP, Liu HP. Video assisted thoracoscopic management of primary spontaneous pneumothorax. *Surg Laparosc Endosc* 1997;7:236–240.

80. Cardillo G, Facciolo F, Giunti R, et al. Videothoracoscopic treatment of primary spontaneous pneumothorax: a 6-year experience. *Ann Thorac Surg* 2000;69:357–361.

81. Waller DA. Video-assisted thoracoscopic surgery for spontaneous pneumothorax—a 7-year learning experience. *Ann R Coll Surg Engl* 1999;81:387–392.

82. Bertrand PC, Regnard JF, Spaggiari L, et al. Immediate and long-term results after surgical treatment of primary spontaneous pneumothorax by VATS. *Ann Thorac Surg* 1996;61:1641–1645.

83. Berrisford RG, Page RD. Video assisted thoracic surgery for spontaneous pneumothorax. *Thorax* 1996;51 [Suppl 2]:S23–S28.

84. Schramel FM, Sutedja TG, Braber JC, et al. Cost-effectiveness of video-assisted thoracoscopic surgery versus conservative treatment for first time or recurrent spontaneous pneumothorax. *Eur Respir J* 1996;9:1821–1825.

85. Radberg G, Dernevik L, Svanvik J, et al. A comparative retrospective study of thoracoscopy versus thoracotomy for the treatment of spontaneous pneumothorax. *Surg Laparosc Endosc* 1995;5:90–93.

86. Kim KH, Kim HK, Han JY, et al. Transaxillary minithoracotomy versus video-assisted thoracic surgery for spontaneous pneumothorax. *Ann Thorac Surg* 1996;61:1510–1512.

87. Dusmet M, Corpataux JM. The axillary minithoracotomy is a cost-effective alternative to VATS for bullectomy in recurrent pneumothorax. *Am J Respir Dis Crit Care Med* 2000;161:A268.

88. Deslauriers J, Beaulieu M, Després J-P, et al. Transaxillary pleurectomy for treatment of spontaneous pneumothorax. *Ann Thorac Surg* 1980;30:569–574.

89. O'Rourke JP, Yee ES. Civilian spontaneous pneumothorax. Treatment options and long-term results. *Chest* 1989;96:1302–1306.

90. Wait MA, Estrera A. Changing clinical spectrum of spontaneous pneumothorax. *Am J Surg* 1992; 164: 528–531.

91. Weissberg D, Refaely Y. Pneumothorax. *Chest* 2000; 117:1279–1285.

92. Urban T, Lazor R, Lacronique J, et al. Pulmonary lymphangioleiomyomatosis. A study of 69 patients. *Medicine (Baltimore)* 1999;78:321–337.

93. Chu SC, Horiba K, Usuki J, et al. Comprehensive evaluation of 35 patients with lymphangioleiomyomatosis. *Chest* 1999;115:1041–1052.

94. Dines DE, Clagett OT, Payne WS. Spontaneous pneumothorax in emphysema. *Mayo Clin Proc* 1970;45: 481–487.

95. Tanaka F, Itoh M, Esaki H, et al. Secondary spontaneous pneumothorax. *Ann Thorac Surg* 1993;55:372–376.

96. Shields TW, Oilschlager GA. Spontaneous pneumothorax in patients 40 years of age and older. *Ann Thorac Surg* 1966;2:377–383.

97. George RB, Herbert SJ, Shames JM, et al. Pneumothorax complicating pulmonary emphysema. *JAMA* 1975;234:389–393.

98. Bourgouin P, Cousineau G, Lemire P, et al. Computed tomography used to exclude pneumothorax in bullous lung disease. *J Can Assoc Radiol* 1985;36: 341–342.

99. Phillips GD, Trotman-Dickenson B, Hodson ME, et al. Role of CT in the management of pneumothorax in patients with complex cystic lung disease. *Chest* 1997;112:275–278.

100. Fraser RS, Muller NL, Colman N, et al. *Diagnosis of diseases of the chest*, 4th ed, vol IV. Philadelphia: WB Saunders, 2000:2781–2794.

101. Videm V, Pillgram-Larsen J, Ellingsen O, et al. Spontaneous pneumothorax in chronic obstructive pulmonary disease: complications, treatment, and recurrences. *Eur J Respir Dis* 1987;71:365–371.

102. Ng AW, Chan KW, Lee SK. Simple aspiration of pneumothorax. *Singapore Med J* 1994;35:50–52.

103. Seaton D, Yoganathan K, Coady T, et al. Spontaneous pneumothorax: marker gas technique for predicting outcome of manual aspiration. *Br Med J* 1991;302:262–265.

104. Yankaskas MR, Mallory GB Jr, and the Consensus Committee. Lung transplantation in cystic fibrosis. *Chest* 1998;113:217–226.

105. Dusmet M, Winton TL, Kesten S, et al. Previous intrapleural procedures do not adversely affect lung transplantation. *J Heart Lung Transplant* 1996;15: 249–254.

106. Waller DA, Forty J, Soni AK, et al. Videothoracoscopic operation for secondary spontaneous pneumothorax. *Ann Thorac Surg* 1994;57:1612–1615.

107. Deslauriers J. The management of spontaneous pneumothorax [Editorial]. *Can J Surg* 1994;37:182.

108. Sepkowitz KA, Telzak EE, Gold JW, et al. Pneumothorax in AIDS. *Ann Intern Med* 1991;114:455–459.

109. Coker RJ, Moss F, Peters B, et al. Pneumothorax in patients with AIDS. *Respir Med* 1993;87:43–47.

110. Trachiotis GD, Vricella LA, Alyono D, et al. Management of AIDS-related pneumothorax. *Ann Thorac Surg* 1996;62:1608–1613.

111. Tumbarello M, Tacconelli E, Pirronti T, et al. Pneumothorax in HIV-infected patients: role of *Pneumocystis carinii* pneumonia and pulmonary tuberculosis. *Eur Respir J* 1997;10:1332–1335.

112. Leoung GS, Feigal DW Jr, Montgomery AB, et al. Aerosolized pentamidine for prophylaxis against *Pneumocystis carinii* pneumonia. *N Engl J Med* 1990;323:769–775.

113. Renzi PM, Corbeil C, Chasse M, et al. Bilateral pneumothoraces hasten mortality in AIDS patients receiving secondary prophylaxis with aerosolized pentamidine. Association with a lower D_{co} prior to receiving aerosolized pentamidine. *Chest* 1992;102:491–496.

114. Cuthbert AC, Wright D, McVerry BA. Pneumothorax in pentamidine-treated haemophiliacs [Letter]. *Lancet* 1991;337:918.

115. Newsome GS, Ward DJ, Pierce PF. Spontaneous pneumothorax in patients with acquired immunodeficiency syndrome treated with prophylactic aerosolized pentamidine. *Arch Intern Med* 1990;150:2167–2168.

116. Shanley DJ, Luyckx BA, Haggerty MF, et al. Spontaneous pneumothorax in AIDS patients with recurrent *Pneumocystis carinii* pneumonia despite aerosolized pentamidine prophylaxis. *Chest* 1991;99:502–504.

117. Scannell KA. Pneumothoraces and *Pneumocystis carinii* pneumonia in two AIDS patients receiving aerosolized pentamidine. *Chest* 1990;97:479–480.

118. Beers MF, Sohn M, Swartz M. Recurrent pneumothorax in AIDS patients with *Pneumocystis* pneumonia. A clinicopathologic report of three cases and review of the literature. *Chest* 1990;98:266–270.

119. Gerein AN, Brumwell ML, Lawson LM, et al. Surgical management of pneumothorax in patients with acquired immunodeficiency syndrome. *Arch Surg* 1991;126:1272–1276.

120. Ingram RJ, Call S, Andrade A, et al. Management and outcome of pneumothoraces in patients infected with human immunodeficiency virus. *Clin Infect Dis* 1996;23:624–627.

121. Wait MA, Dal Nogare AR. Treatment of AIDS-related spontaneous pneumothorax. *Chest* 1994;106:693–696.

122. Wait MA. AIDS-related pneumothorax. *Ann Thorac Surg* 1997;64:290–291.

123. Driver AG, Peden JG, Adams HG, et al. Heimlich valve treatment of *Pneumocystis carinii*–associated pneumothorax. *Chest* 1991;100:281–282.

124. Walker WA, Pate JW, Amundson D, et al. AIDS-related bronchopleural fistula. *Ann Thorac Surg* 1993;55:1048.

125. Byrnes TA, Brevig JK, Yeoh CB. Pneumothorax in patients with acquired immunodeficiency syndrome. *J Thorac Cardiovasc Surg* 1990;98:546–550.

126. Crawford BK, Galloway AC, Boyd AD, et al. Treatment of AIDS-related bronchopleural fistula by pleurectomy. *Ann Thorac Surg* 1992;54:212–213.

127. Horowitz MD, Oliva H. Pneumothorax in AIDS patients: operative management. *Am Surg* 1993;59:200–204.

128. Read CA, Reddy VD, O'Mara TE, et al. Doxycycline pleurodesis for pneumothorax in patients with AIDS. *Chest* 1994;105:823–825.

129. Spector ML, Stern RC. Pneumothorax in cystic fibrosis: a 26-year experience. *Ann Thorac Surg* 1989;47:204–207.

130. Luck SR, Raffensperger JG, Sullivan HJ, et al. Management of pneumothorax in children with chronic pulmonary disease. *J Thorac Cardiovasc Surg* 1977;74:834–839.

131. Wilder RJ, Beacham EG, Ravitch MM. Spontaneous pneumothorax complicating cavitary tuberculosis. *J Thorac Cardiovasc Surg* 1962;43:561–573.

132. Blanco-Perez J, Bordon J, Pineiro-Amigo L, et al. Pneumothorax in active pulmonary tuberculosis: resurgence of an old complication? *Respir Med* 1998;92:1269–1273.

133. Andres B, Lujan J, Robles R, et al. Treatment of primary and secondary spontaneous pneumothorax using videothoracoscopy. *Surg Laparosc Endosc* 1998;8:108–112.

134. Lillington GA, Mitchell SP, Wood GA. Catamenial pneumothorax. *JAMA* 1972;219:1328–1332.

135. Joseph J, Sahn SA. Thoracic endometriosis syndrome: new observations from an analysis of 110 cases. *Am J Med* 1996;100:164–170.

136. Maurer ER, Schaal JA, Mendez FL. Chronic recurrent spontaneous pneumothorax due to endometriosis of the diaphragm. *JAMA* 1958;168:2013–2014.

137. Downey DB, Towers MJ, Poon PY, et al. Pneumoperitoneum with catamenial pneumothorax. *AJR Am J Roentgenol* 1990;155:29–30.

138. Dotson RL, Peterson CM, Doucette RC, et al. Medical therapy for recurring catamenial pneumothorax following pleurodesis. *Obstet Gynecol* 1993;82[4 Pt 2 Suppl]:656–658.

139. Stern H, Toole AL, Merino M. Catamenial pneumothorax. *Chest* 1980;78:480–482.

140. Eckford SD, Westgate J. A cure for pneumothorax during menstruation. *Lancet* 1996;347:734.

141. Chernick V, Reed MH. Pneumothorax and chylothorax in the neonatal period. *J Pediatr* 1970;76:624–632.

142. Ogata ES, Gregory GA, Kitterman JA, et al. Pneumothorax in the respiratory distress syndrome: incidence and effect on vital signs, blood gases, and pH. *Pediatrics* 1976;58:177–183.

143. Karlberg P. Respiratory studies in newborns. II. Pulmonary ventilation and mechanics of breathing in the first minutes of life including the onset of respiration. *Acta Paediatr* 1962;51:121–136.

144. Adler SM, Wyszogrodski I. Pneumothorax as a function of gestational age: clinical and experimental studies. *J Pediatr* 1975;87:771–775.

145. Engdahl MS, Gershan WM. Familial spontaneous pneumothorax in neonates. *Pediatr Pulmonol* 1998;25:398–400.

146. Mehrabani D, Gowen CW Jr, Kopelman AE. Association of pneumothorax and hypotension with intraventricular haemorrhage. *Arch Dis Child* 1991;66:48–51.

147. Kuhns LR, Bednarek FJ, Wyman ML, et al. Diagnosis of pneumothorax or pneumomediastinum in the neonate by transillumination. *Pediatrics* 1975;56:355–360.

148. Carlon GC, Kahn RC, Howland WS, et al. Clinical experience with high frequency jet ventilation. *Crit Care Med* 1981;9:1–6.

149. Sassoon CSH, Light RW, O'Hara VS, et al. Iatrogenic pneumothorax: etiology and morbidity. *Respiration* 1992;59:215–220.

150. Despars JA, Sassoon CSH, Light RW. Significance of iatrogenic pneumothoraces. *Chest* 1994;105:1147–1150.

151. Vitulo P, Dore R, Cerveri I, et al. The role of functional respiratory tests in predicting pneumothorax during lung needle biopsy. *Chest* 1995;109:612–615.

152. Collings CL, Westcott JL, Banson NL, et al. Pneumothorax and dependent versus nondependent patient position after needle biopsy of the lung. *Radiology* 1999;210:59–64.

153. Cox JE, Chiles C, McManus CM, et al. Transthoracic needle aspiration biopsy: variables that affect risk of pneumothorax. *Radiology* 1999;212:165–168.

154. Berger R, Smith D. Efficacy of the lateral decubitus position in preventing pneumothorax after needle biopsy of the lung. *South Med J* 1988;81:1140–1143.

155. Petsas T, Siamblis D, Giannakenas C, et al. Fibrin glue for sealing the needle track in fine-needle percutaneous lung biopsy using a coaxial system: Part II—clinical study. *Cardiovasc Intervent Radiol* 1995;18:378–382.

156. Lockwood AH. Percutaneous subclavian vein catheterization. Too much of a good thing? *Arch Intern Med* 1984;144:1407–1408.

157. Farrell J, Walshe J, Gellens M, et al. Complications associated with insertion of jugular venous catheters for hemodialysis: the value of postprocedural radiograph. *Am J Kidney Dis* 1997;30:690–692.

158. Damascelli B, Patelli G, Frigerio LF, et al. Placement of long-term central venous catheters in outpatients: study of 134 patients over 24,596 catheter days. *AJR Am J Roentgenol* 1997;168:1235–1239.

159. Miller JA, Singireddy S, Maldjian P, et al. A reevaluation of the radiographically detectable complications of percutaneous venous access lines inserted by four subcutaneous approaches. *Am Surg* 1999;65:125–130.

160. Ray S, Stacey R, Imrie M, et al. A review of 560 Hickman catheter insertions. *Anaesthesia* 1996;51:981–985.

161. Tyburski JG, Joseph AL, Thomas GA, et al. Delayed pneumothorax after central venous access: a potential hazard. *Am Surg* 1993;59:587–589.

162. Capizzi SA, Prakash UB. Chest roentgenography after outpatient thoracentesis. *Mayo Clin Proc* 1998;73:948–950.

163. Colt HG, Brewer N, Barbur E. Evaluation of patient-related and procedure-related factors contributing to pneumothorax following thoracentesis. *Chest* 1999;116:134–138.

164. Doyle JJ, Hnatiuk OW, Torrington KG, et al. Necessity of routine chest roentgenography after thoracentesis. *Ann Intern Med* 1996;124:816–820.

165. Steier M, Ching N, Bonfils-Roberts E, et al. Iatrogenic cause of pneumothorax: increasing incidence with advances in medical care. *NY State J Med* 1973;173:1296–1298.

166. De Latorre FJ, Tomasa A, Klamburg J, et al. Incidence of pneumothorax and pneumomediastinum in patients with aspiration pneumonia requiring ventilatory support. *Chest* 1977;72:141–144.

167. Weg JG, Anzueto A, Balk RA, et al. The relation of pneumothorax and other air leaks to mortality in the acute respiratory distress syndrome. *N Engl J Med* 1998;338:341–346.

168. Gammon RB, Shin MS, Buchalter SE. Pulmonary barotrauma in mechanical ventilation. Patterns and risk factors. *Chest* 1992;102:568–572.

169. Poe RH, Israel RH, Utell MJ, et al. Sensitivity, specificity, and predictive values of closed pleural biopsy. *Arch Intern Med* 1984;144:325–328.

170. Frazier WD, Pope TL Jr, Findley LJ. Pneumothorax following transbronchial biopsy. *Chest* 1990;97:539–540.

171. Blasco LH, Hernandez IMS, Garrido VV, et al. Safety of the transbronchial biopsy in outpatients. *Chest* 1991;99:562–565.

172. Richard HM 3rd, Stancato-Pasik A, Salky BA, et al. Pneumothorax and pneumomediastinum after laparoscopic surgery. *Clin Imaging* 1997;21:337–339.

173. Tobkes AI, Nord HJ. Liver biopsy: review of methodology and complications. *Dig Dis* 1995;13267–13274.

174. Ludwig J, Kienzle GD. Pneumothorax in a large autopsy population. *Am J Clin Pathol* 1978;70:24–26.

175. Paranjpe DV, Wittich GR, Hamid LW, et al. Frequency and management of pneumothoraces in heart-lung transplant recipients. *Radiology* 1994;190:255–256.

176. Lee YC (Gary), McGrath GB, Chin WS, et al. Contralateral tension pneumothorax following unilateral chest tube drainage of bilateral pneumothoraces in a heart-lung transplant patient. *Chest* 1999;116:1131–1133.

177. Tocino IM, Miller MH, Fairfax WR. Distribution of pneumothorax in the supine and semirecumbent critically ill adult. *AJR Am J Roentgenol* 1985;144:901–905.

178. Kollef MH. Risk factors for the misdiagnosis of pneumothorax in the intensive care unit. *Crit Care Med* 1991;19:906–910.

179. Heffner JE, McDonald J, Barbieri C. Recurrent pneumothoraces in ventilated patients despite ipsilateral chest tubes. *Chest* 1995;108:1053–1058.

180. Delius RE, Obeid FN, Horst HM, et al. Catheter aspiration for simple pneumothorax. Experience with 114 patients. *Arch Surg* 1989;124:833–836.

181. Gurley MB, Richli WR, Waugh KA. Outpatient management of pneumothorax after fine-needle aspiration: economic advantages for the hospital and patient. *Radiology* 1998;209:717–722.

182. Anderson CLV, Crespo JCA, Lie TH. Risk of pneumothorax not increased by obstructive lung disease in percutaneous needle biopsy. *Chest* 1994;105:1705–1708.

183. Macklin MI, Macklin CC. Malignant interstitial emphysema of the lungs and mediastinum as important occult complication in many respiratory diseases and other conditions: interpretation of clinical literature in light of laboratory experiment. *Medicine* 1944;23:281–356.

184. Trupka A, Waydhas C, Hallfeldt KK, et al. Value of thoracic computed tomography in the first assessment of severely injured patients with blunt chest trauma: results of a prospective study. *J Trauma* 1997;43:405–411.

185. Bridges KG, Welch G, Silver M, et al. CT detection of occult pneumothorax in multiple trauma patients. *J Emerg Med* 1993;11:179–186.

186. Garramone RR Jr, Jacobs LM, Sahdev P. An objective method to measure and manage occult pneumothorax. *Surg Gynecol Obstet* 1991;173:257–261.

187. Carrillo EH, Schmacht DC, Gable DR, et al. Thoracoscopy in the management of posttraumatic persistent pneumothorax. *J Am Coll Surg* 1998;186:636–639.

188. Knottenbelt JD, van der Spuy JW. Traumatic pneumothorax: a scheme for rapid patient turnover. *Br J Accident Surg* 1990;21:77–80.

189. Ordog GJ, Wasserberger J, Balasubramanium S, et al. Asymptomatic stab wounds of the chest. *J Trauma* 1994;36:680–684.

190. Brasel KJ, Stafford RE, Weigelt JA, et al. Treatment of occult pneumothoraces from blunt trauma. *J Trauma* 1999;46:987–990.

191. Wolfman NT, Myers WS, Glauser SJ, et al. Validity of CT classification on management of occult pneumothorax: a prospective study. *AJR Am J Roentgenol* 1998;171:1317–1320.

192. Collins JC, Levine G, Waxman K. Occult traumatic pneumothorax: immediate tube thoracostomy versus expectant management. *Am Surg* 1992;58:743–746.

193. Lin MY, Wu MH, Chan CS, et al. Bronchial rupture caused by blunt chest injury. *Ann Emerg Med* 1995;25:412–415.

194. Kunisch-Hoppe M, Hoppe M, Rauber K, et al. Tracheal rupture caused by blunt chest trauma: radiological and clinical features. *Eur Radiol* 2000;10:480–483.

195. Sherr HP, Light RW, Merson MH, et al. Origin of pleural fluid amylase in esophageal rupture. *Ann Intern Med* 1972;76:985–986.

196. Air Transport Medicine Committee. Aerospace Medical Association. Medical guidelines for air travel. *Aviat Space Environ Med* 1996;67[Suppl]:B1–B8.

197. Cheatham ML, Safcsak K. Air travel following traumatic pneumothorax: when is it safe? *Am Surg* 1999;65:1160–1164.

198. Douglass RE, Levison MA. Pneumothorax in drug abusers: an urban epidemic. *Am Surg* 1986;52:377–380.

199. Woodring JH, Baker MD, Stark P. Pneumothorax ex vacuo. *Chest* 1996;110:1102–1105.

200. Light RW. Tension pneumothorax. *Intensive Care Med* 1994;20:468–469.

201. Rutherford RB, Hurt HH, Brickman RD, et al. The pathophysiology of progressive, tension pneumothorax. *J Trauma* 1968;8:212–227.

202. Gustman P, Yerger L, Wanner A. Immediate cardiovascular effects of tension pneumothorax. *Am Rev Respir Dis* 1983;127:171–174.

203. Carvalho P, Hilderbrandt J, Charan NB. Changes in bronchial and pulmonary arterial blood flow with progressive tension pneumothorax. *J Appl Physiol* 1996;81:1664–1669.

204. Barton ED, Rhee P, Hutton KC, et al. The pathophysiology of tension pneumothorax in ventilated swine. *J Emerg Med* 1997;15:147–153.

205. Beards SC, Lipman J. Decreased cardiac index as an indicator of tension pneumothorax in the ventilated patient. *Anaesthesia* 1994;49:137–141.

206. Murphy DG, Sloan EP, Hart RG, et al. Tension pneumothorax associated with hyperbaric oxygen therapy. *Am J Emerg Med* 1991;9:176–179.

207. McConaghy PM, Kennedy N. Tension pneumothorax due to intrapulmonary placement of intercostal chest drain. *Anaesth Intensive Care* 1995;23:496–498.

208. Mainini SE, Johnson FE. Tension pneumothorax complicating small-caliber chest tube insertion. *Chest* 1990;97:759–760.

209. Bishop MJ, Benson MS, Pierson DJ. Carbon dioxide excretion via bronchopleural fistulas in adult respiratory distress syndrome. *Chest* 1987;91:400–402.

210. Prezant DJ, Aldrich TK, Fell SC, et al. The maintenance of total ventilatory requirements through a chronic bronchopleural cutaneous fistula. *Am Rev Respir Dis* 1987;136:1001–1002.

211. Feeley TW, Keating D, Nishimura T. Independent lung ventilation using high-frequency ventilation in the management of a bronchopleural fistula. *Anesthesiology* 1988;69:420–422.

212. Lau KY. Postural management of bronchopleural fistula. *Chest* 1988;94:1122.

213. Powner DJ, Cline CD, Rodman GH. Effect of chest-tube suction on gas flow through a bronchopleural fistula. *Crit Care Med* 1985;13:99–101.

214. Orlando R III, Gluck EH, Cohen M, et al. Ultra-high-frequency jet ventilation in a bronchopleural fistula model. *Arch Surg* 1988;123:591–593.

215. Albelda SM, Hansen-Flaschen JH, Taylor E, et al. Evaluation of high frequency jet ventilation in patients with bronchopleural fistulas by quantitation of the air leak. *Anesthesiology* 1985;63:551–554.

216. Bishop MJ, Benson MS, Sato P, et al. Comparison of high-frequency jet ventilation with conventional mechanical ventilation for bronchopleural fistula. *Anesth Analg* 1987;66:833–838.

217. Gonzalez F, Harris T, Black P, et al. Decreased gas flow through pneumothoraces in neonates receiving high-frequency jet versus conventional ventilation. *J Pediatr* 1987;110:464–466.

218. Baumann MH, Sahn SA. Medical management and therapy of bronchopleural fistulas in the mechanically ventilated patient. *Chest* 1990;97:721–728.

219. Shields TW, Ponn RB. Complications of pulmonary resection. In: Shields TW, LoCicero J III, Ponn RB, eds. *General thoracic surgery*, 5th ed. Philadelphia: Lippincott Williams & Wilkins, 2000:481–505.

220. Waller DA, Edwards JG, Rajesh PB. A physiological comparison of flutter valve drainage bags and underwater seal systems for postoperative air leaks. *Thorax* 1999;54:442–443.

221. Rice TW, Kirby TTJ. Prolonged air leak. *Chest Surg Clin N Am* 1992;2:803–811.

222. Asamura H, Naruke T, Tsuchiya R, et al. Bronchopleural fistulas associated with lung cancer operations. Univariate and multivariate analysis of risk factors, management, and outcome. *J Thorac Cardiovasc Surg* 1992;104:1456–1464.

223. Arnold PG, Pairolero PC. Intrathoracic muscle flaps. An account of their use in the management of 100 consecutive patients. *Ann Surg* 1990;211:656–662.

224. De Maeseneer N, Van Hee R, Schoofs E, et al. The management of bronchopleural fistulas. *Acta Chir Belg* 1987;87:269–274.

225. Jones DP, David I. Gelfoam occlusion of peripheral bronchopleural fistulas. *Ann Thorac Surg* 1986;42:334–335.

226. Lan R-S, Lee C-H, Tsai Y-H, et al. Fiberoptic bronchial blockade in a small bronchopleural fistula. *Chest* 1987;92:944–946.

227. Torre M, Quaini E, Ravini M, et al. 1987: Endoscopic gluing of bronchopleural fistula. Updated in 1994. *Ann Thorac Surg* 1994;58:901–902.

228. Hollaus PH, Lax F, Janakiev D, et al. Endoscopic treatment of postoperative bronchopleural fistula: experience with 45 cases. *Ann Thorac Surg* 1998;66:923–927.

229. Salmon CJ, Ponn RB, Westcott JL. Endobronchial vascular occlusion coils for control of a large parenchymal bronchopleural fistula. *Chest* 1990;98:233–234.

22

Hemothorax

Hemothorax is the presence of a significant amount of blood in the pleural space. Most hemothoraces result from penetrating or nonpenetrating chest trauma. An occasional hemothorax results from iatrogenic manipulation such as the placement of central venous catheters percutaneously by the subclavian or internal jugular route or from translumbar aortography. On rare occasions, a hemothorax results from a medical condition such as pulmonary embolism or rupture of an aortic aneurysm.

Blood may enter the pleural space from injury to the chest wall, diaphragm, lung, or mediastinum. Blood entering the pleural space coagulates rapidly. Presumably as a result of physical agitation produced by movement of the heart and the lungs, the clot may be defibrinated. Loculation occurs early in the course of hemothorax, as with empyema.

When a diagnostic thoracentesis in a medical patient reveals pleural fluid that appears to be pure blood, a hematocrit should always be obtained on the pleural fluid. Frequently, even though the pleural fluid appears to be blood, the hematocrit on the pleural fluid is less than 5%. A hemothorax should be considered to be present only when the pleural fluid hematocrit is equal to or greater than 50% of the peripheral blood hematocrit.

TRAUMATIC HEMOTHORAX

Traumatic hemothoraces are a frequent occurrence, particularly in centers that treat victims of trauma. In one Houston hospital, more than 300 patients with hemothorax due to penetrating trauma were seen in a 1-year period (1). The relative incidence of hemothorax due to penetrating and blunt thoracic trauma depends on whether the medical center cares primarily for victims of automobile accidents or of stab and gunshot wounds.

There is a high incidence of hemothorax with blunt trauma. In a retrospective analysis of 515 cases of blunt chest trauma, 193 patients (37%) had hemothoraces (2). In patients with rib fractures, hemothorax is more common if the fracture is displaced (3). Pneumothorax occurring concomitantly with hemothorax is common whether the trauma is blunt or penetrating (Fig. 22.1). In a series of 114 patients with hemothorax secondary to blunt trauma, 71 (62%) also had pneumothorax (4). In another series of 373 patients with hemothorax secondary to penetrating trauma, 307 (83%) also had pneumothorax (1).

Diagnosis

The diagnosis of a traumatic hemothorax should be suspected in any patient with penetrating or nonpenetrating trauma to the chest. The diagnosis is usually established by the demonstration of a pleural effusion with a chest radiograph or with ultrasound. As an initial screening test, surgeon-performed ultrasonography appears to be as sensitive as a supine chest radiograph in detecting hemothorax. In one study of 360 patients, 39 of 40 effusions were detected by ultrasound and 37 were detected by chest radiograph. The performance time for ultrasonography was significantly faster than that for chest radiography (1.3 versus 14.2 minutes) (5).

A case can be made for obtaining chest CT scans in all patients with severe chest injuries.

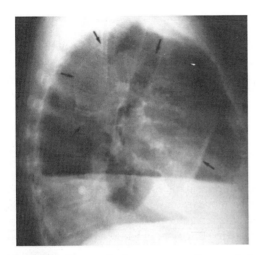

FIG. 22.1. Traumatic hemopneumothorax. Lateral chest radiograph, obtained from a patient shortly after he was stabbed in the chest, that shows a pleural effusion and a pneumothorax. The pleural line *(arrows)* is easily seen outlining the lung. (Courtesy of Dr. Harry Sassoon.)

Trupka et al. (6) obtained supine chest radiographs and chest CT scans in 103 patients with severe chest injuries and reported that the chest radiograph missed hemothoraces in 21 patients, lung contusion in 33 patients, and pneumothorax in 27 patients. A different conclusion could be reached from the study by Ma and Mateer of 240 patients with chest trauma. In this study, 25 of 26 hemothoraces (96%) were detected each by ultrasound and by supine chest radiographs (7).

Treatment

The treatment of choice for patients with traumatic hemothorax is the immediate insertion of a chest tube. In the past, it was believed by some that the insertion of a chest tube would decrease pleural pressure and would thereby augment the pleural bleeding. If the bleeding originates from lacerated pleura, however, apposition of the pleural surfaces will produce a tamponade and will stop the bleeding (8). If the bleeding is from larger vessels, the slight decrease in the pleural pressure with a chest tube is insignificant in comparison to the transvascular pressure (8). The advantages of the immediate institution of tube

thoracostomy are as follows: (a) it allows more complete evacuation of the blood from the pleural space; (b) it stops the bleeding if the bleeding is from pleural lacerations; (c) it allows one to quantitate easily the amount of continued bleeding; (d) it may decrease the incidence of subsequent empyema because blood is a good culture medium (9); (e) the blood drained from the pleural space may be autotransfused (1); and (f) the rapid evacuation of pleural blood decreases the incidence of subsequent fibrothorax (10).

Large-bore chest tubes (size 36 to 40 F) should be inserted in patients with hemothorax because the blood frequently clots. Beall et al. (9) recommend inserting the chest tube high (fourth or fifth intercostal space) in the midaxillary line because the diaphragm may be elevated by the trauma. Immediate thoracotomy is indicated for suspected cardiac tamponade, vascular injury, pleural contamination, debridement of devitalized tissue, sucking chest wounds, or major bronchial air leaks (11). Vascular injury is suggested if the initial chest tube output is more than 1,500 mL.

Continued pleural hemorrhage is another indication for immediate thoracotomy. There is no precise criterion for the amount of pleural bleeding that should serve as an indication for thoracotomy, because each case must be considered individually (8); however, if the bleeding is more than 200 mL per hour and shows no signs of slowing, thoracotomy should be seriously considered. Approximately 20% of patients with hemothorax require thoracotomy (1, 3, 4, 9). Chest tubes should be removed as soon as they stop draining or cease to function because they can serve as conduits for pleural infection. The majority of patients with a traumatic hemothorax can be discharged from the hospital within 48 hours if no other serious injuries are present (9).

One must ensure that the bleeding is not from a misplaced central venous catheter (12). Mattox and Fisher (12) reported seven patients with a traumatic hemothorax in whom continued bleeding originated from a misplaced central venous catheter. This diagnosis is readily established by examining the appearance of the pleural drainage when the character of the infusion fluid is changed. If blood is obtained when fluid is withdrawn from the central catheter, the catheter may still be misplaced in the pleural space (13).

Videothoracoscopy may replace thoracotomy in some patients with traumatic hemothorax who otherwise would have been subjected to thoracotomy. Thoracotomy rather than thoracoscopy should be performed if there is exsanguinating hemorrhage through the chest tubes (14). Villavicencio et al. (15) in a literature review found that videothoracoscopy was effective in controlling the bleeding in 33 of 40 (82%) cases. Thoracoscopy was effective in controlling the bleeding when the bleeding arose from intercostal vessels and lung lacerations.

It is recommended that patients who are treated with tube thoracostomy for hemothorax be given antibiotics empirically. Brunner et al. randomly allowed 90 such patients to receive cefazolin or nothing immediately before and then every 6 hours until tube removal. They reported that there were six empyemas and three pneumonias in the control group, but only one pneumonia and no empyema in the group that received the antibiotic (16).

It appears that prehospital autotransfusion has a role in the management of life-threatening hemothorax. Barriot et al. (17) developed a system by which autotransfusions could be administered in ambulances. The system consists of a 28 to 30 F plastic chest tube and an autotransfusion device. The latter is basically a 750-mL bag with filters. The blood drains by gravity into the collection bag and is then reinfused without anticoagulation into a central line. They reported the use of their system on 18 patients in Paris with life-threatening traumatic hemothorax. During transfer to the hospital, the patients received 4.1 ± 0.6 L of autotransfused blood, without anticoagulation. Thirteen of the 18 patients (72%) survived, and there were no complications. They believed that the 13 patients would have died had it not been for the autotransfusions.

Complications of Hemothorax

The four main pleural complications of traumatic hemothorax are the retention of clotted blood in the pleural space, pleural infection, pleural effusion, and fibrothorax.

Retention of Clotted Blood

Although the majority of traumatic hemothoraces are managed nonoperatively by tube thoracostomy, some of these blood collections remain only partially drained. The residual blood, already potentially contaminated by the insertion of the chest tube, may be the nidus for significant complications such as empyema or fibrothorax. Surgical evacuation of retained hemothoraces decreases this risk (18). In a recent study from California, 20 of 703 patients (3%) treated with tube thoracostomy for hemothorax were found to have retention of clotted blood (18). The chest radiograph may be misleading in patients with hemothorax who are suspected of having retention of clotted blood. Velmahos et al. obtained chest CT scans on 58 consecutive patients with hemothorax who had opacification extending above the costophrenic angle on standard chest radiograph one day after tube thoracostomy for hemothorax. They found that the prediction of fluid from the chest radiograph was correct in less than 50% of cases by both the chest surgeon and the radiologist (18). This study suggests that a CT scan should be obtained before an operative procedure is undertaken to remove the clotted blood.

When a patient is identified as having retention of clotted blood in the pleural space, three questions need to be asked. (a) Does the clot need to be removed? (b) If so, when should it be removed? (c) How should it be removed? If the residual clot occupies at least a third of the involved hemithorax 72 hours or more after the initial tube thoracoscopy, it should probably be removed (19). The clot is most easily disrupted and removed by suction 48 to 72 hours after the initial injury. After seven to nine days, the clot adheres to the lung and pleura, making thoracoscopic removal difficult or impossible and increasing the incidence of complications, such as retained collections, persistent pleural drainage, or air leaks (19). Therefore, the optimal time to remove the clotted blood appears to be between 48 and 96 hours.

The optimal method for removal of the clotted blood appears to be thoracoscopy (15, 19). Villavicencio et al. (15) reviewed eight reports with a total of 99 patients who were subjected to videothoracoscopy for retained hemothoraces. Evacuation of the retained hemothorax was successful in 89 (90%) of the cases. An alternative approach to the patient with a retained hemothorax is to insert a second chest tube. A recent randomized study (20) in which 24 patients received a second chest tube and 15 patients underwent videothoracoscopy demonstrated that hospitalizations were significantly shorter (5.4 versus 8.1 days) and the hospital costs were significantly less in the group that received videothoracoscopy. Of the 24 patients that received a second chest tube, 10 (42%) required thoracoscopy or thoracotomy (20).

Some authors have recommended the intrapleural injection of fibrinolytic agents for the treatment of retained hemothorax (21). Inci et al. (21) treated 24 patients with either 250,000 IU streptokinase or 100,000 IU urokinase and each patient received a mean of five doses. Although complete response was demonstrated in 62.5% of the patients, this treatment is not recommended because it is more expensive than thoracoscopy owing to the expense of the fibrinolytic agents and the longer hospitalizations. In addition, there has been one case in which hypoxemic respiratory failure developed after the intrapleural administration of fibrinolytics (22). Nevertheless, if thoracoscopy is not readily available, consideration can be given to intrapleural fibrinolytics or thoracotomy.

Posttraumatic Empyema

The second complication following hemothorax is empyema, occurring in 3% to 4% of cases (23). This complication can be minimized by using meticulously sterile technique while inserting thoracostomy tubes and by ensuring good apposition of the pleural surfaces so that no space remains for the accumulation of fluid or blood. The risk of empyema increases with the presence of persistent bronchopleural fistula, pulmonary contusions, and residual clotted hemothoraces. As mentioned earlier, the administration of antibiotics to patients with hemothorax who are treated with tube thoracostomy significantly reduces the subsequent development of empyema

and pneumonia (16). Patients who are admitted in shock are more likely to develop empyema, as are those with gross contamination of the pleural space at the time of the original injury. Empyema is also more common with associated abdominal injuries (10) and with prolonged pleural drainage (11). The treatment of empyema complicating hemothorax is similar to that of any bacterial infection of the pleural space (see Chapter 9).

Pleural Effusion

The third complication of hemothorax is the occurrence of a pleural effusion when the chest tubes are removed. In the series reported by Wilson et al. (11), 37 of 290 patients (13%) with no residual hemothorax developed pleural effusions after removal of the chest tubes, and 40 of 118 patients with residual hemothorax (34%) had pleural effusions at the time of discharge from the hospital. Of these 77 patients with a pleural effusion after tube thoracostomy, 20 (26%) had empyema, but the pleural effusions resolved in the other 57, leaving no or minimum residual disease (11). This series indicates that pleural effusions are common after tube thoracostomy for hemothorax. When such effusions occur, a diagnostic thoracentesis should be performed to rule out the possibility of a pleural infection. If no pleural infection is present, the pleural effusion usually clears by itself and leaves no residual disease.

Fibrothorax

The fourth complication of hemothorax is the development of diffuse pleural thickening producing a fibrothorax weeks to months after the hemothorax. This complication occurs in less than 1% of patients, even if residual blood is not removed by exploratory thoracotomy (11). Fibrothorax appears to be more common with hemopneumothorax or when pleural infection is present in addition to the hemothorax. The definitive treatment for fibrothorax is decortication of the lung (see Chapter 24). Decortication should be postponed for several months following the injury in most cases because the pleural thickening frequently diminishes with time.

IATROGENIC HEMOTHORAX

When a hemothorax is discovered, the possibility of iatrogenic origin should be considered. The most common causes of iatrogenic hemothorax are the perforation of a central vein by a percutaneously inserted catheter (12, 24) or leaking from the aorta after translumbar aortographic study (25). Iatrogenic hemothorax can also follow thoracentesis or pleural biopsy. Insertion of a Swan-Ganz catheter is occasionally associated with rupture of the pulmonary artery with a resulting hemothorax, and, in such instances, an immediate thoracotomy is necessary if the patient is going to survive (26). Iatrogenic hemothoraces have also been reported after many other procedures, including percutaneous lung aspiration or biopsy, transbronchial biopsy and sclerotherapy for esophageal varices (27). Patients with iatrogenic hemothorax should be managed with chest tubes for the same reasons as are patients with traumatic hemothorax.

NONTRAUMATIC HEMOTHORAX

Nontraumatic hemothoraces are distinctly uncommon. The most common cause is metastatic malignant pleural disease (28), the second most common cause is a complication of anticoagulant therapy for pulmonary emboli (29), and the third leading cause is probably catamenial hemothorax (30). Other causes of spontaneous hemothorax include a complication of a bleeding disorder such as hemophilia or thrombocytopenia (31), a complication of spontaneous pneumothorax, ruptured thoracic aorta, pancreatic pseudocyst (32), rupture of a patent ductus arteriosus (33), rupture of a coarctation of the aorta (33), rupture of a splenic artery aneurysm through the diaphragm (34), rupture of a pulmonary arteriovenous fistula (35), hereditary hemorrhagic telangiectasia (Osler-Rendu-Weber syndrome) (36), intrathoracic extramedullary hematopoiesis (37), chickenpox (38), osteochondroma of the rib (39), and bronchopulmonary sequestration (40). In some patients, the cause of the hemothorax remains unknown despite exploratory thoracotomy (31, 36).

Diagnosis and Treatment

When bloody appearing pleural fluid is obtained during a diagnostic thoracentesis, the hematocrit of the pleural fluid should be determined. If the hematocrit of the pleural fluid is greater than 50% that of the peripheral blood, the patient has a hemothorax. Regardless of how bloody the pleural fluid looks, a hematocrit should be obtained because pleural fluid with a hematocrit of less than 5% may appear to be blood. A chest tube should be inserted into patients with a spontaneous hemothorax to evacuate the blood and to assess the rate of continued bleeding. Thoracotomy should be performed if brisk bleeding (>100 mL per hour) persists.

Hemothorax Complicating Anticoagulant Therapy

Eleven cases of hemothorax complicating anticoagulant therapy had been reported by 1977 (29). Usually, the hemothorax becomes apparent 4 to 7 days after anticoagulant therapy is initiated, but it may occur only after several months (29). Of the 11 patients reported, five were receiving heparin only, four were receiving heparin and warfarin, and two were receiving only warfarin. The coagulation studies in patients with this complication are usually within an acceptable therapeutic range. Hemothoraces have also been observed following systemic therapy with thrombolytics (41). The spontaneous hemothorax is almost always on the side of the original pulmonary embolus (29). The treatment for spontaneous hemothorax complicating anticoagulant therapy is immediate discontinuation of the anticoagulant therapy and insertion of chest tubes in an attempt to remove all the blood in the pleural space (29).

Catamenial Hemothorax

Catamenial hemothorax is a hemothorax than occurs in conjunction with menstruation and it is unusual. By 1993, there had only been 16 cases reported (30). The majority of patients with catamenial hemothorax have associated pelvic and abdominal endometriosis. The right hemithorax is almost always involved, and diaphragmatic fenestrations with communication of pleural and peritoneal fluid have been documented in some of the patients. Most patients with catamenial hemothorax have endometriosis of the pleura if surgical exploration is undertaken. Catamenial hemothorax can be treated by suppressing ovulation using oral contraceptives or progesterone or suppression of gonadotropins using danazol or gonadotropin-releasing hormone (42). However, hormonal therapy frequently fails. In such instances, chemical pleurodesis can be performed, and if this measure fails, total hysterectomy with bilateral oophorectomy can be done (30).

REFERENCES

1. Graham JM, Mattox KL, Beall AC Jr. Penetrating trauma of the lung. *J Trauma* 1979;19:665–669.
2. Shorr RM, Crittenden M, Indeck M, et al. Blunt thoracic trauma. Analysis of 515 patients. *Ann Surg* 1987;206:200–205.
3. Quick G. A randomized clinical trial of rib belts for simple fractures. *Am J Emerg Med* 1990;8:277–281.
4. Drummond DS, Craig RH. Traumatic hemothorax: complications and management. *Am Surg* 1967;33: 403–408.
5. Sisley AC, Rozycki GS, Ballard RB, et al. Rapid detection of traumatic effusion using surgeon-performed ultrasonography. *J Trauma* 1998;44:291–296.
6. Trupka A, Waydhas C, Hallfeldt KK, et al. Value of thoracic computed tomography in the first assessment of severely injured patients with blunt chest trauma: results of a prospective study. *J Trauma* 1997;43:405–411.
7. Ma OJ, Mateer JR. Trauma ultrasound examination versus chest radiography in the detection of hemothorax. *Ann Emerg Med* 1997;29:312–315.
8. Weil PH, Margolis IB. Systematic approach to traumatic hemothorax. *Am J Surg* 1981;142:692–694.
9. Beall AC Jr, Crawford HW, DeBakey ME. Considerations in the management of acute traumatic hemothorax. *J Thorac Cardiovasc Surg* 1966;52:351–360.
10. Griffith GL, Todd EP, McMillin RD, et al. Acute traumatic hemothorax. *Ann Thorac Surg* 1978;26: 204–207.
11. Wilson JM, Boren CH, Peterson SR, et al. Traumatic hemothorax: is decortication necessary? *J Thorac Cardiovasc Surg* 1979;77:489–495.
12. Mattox KL, Fisher RG. Persistent hemothorax secondary to malposition of a subclavian venous catheter. *J Trauma* 1977;17:387–388.
13. Kollef MH. Fallibility of persistent blood return for confirmation of intravascular catheter placement in patients with hemorrhagic thoracic effusions. *Chest* 1994;106:1906–1908.
14. Smith RS, Fry WR, Tsoi EK, et al. Preliminary report on videothoracoscopy in the evaluation and treatment of thoracic injury. *Am J Surg* 1993;166:690–693.
15. Villavicencio RT, Aucar JA, Wall MJ Jr. Analysis of thoracoscopy in trauma. *Surg Endosc* 1999;13:3–9.
16. Brunner RG, Vinsant GO, Alexander RH, et al. The role of antibiotic therapy in the prevention of empyema in patients with an isolated chest injury (ISS 9-10): a prospective study. *J Trauma* 1990;30:1148–1153.
17. Barriot P, Riou B, Viars P. Prehospital autotransfusion in life-threatening hemothorax. *Chest* 1988;93:522–526.
18. Velmahos GC, Demetriades D, Chan L, et al. Predicting the need for thoracoscopic evacuation of residual traumatic hemothorax: chest radiograph is insufficient. *J Trauma* 1999;46:65–70.
19. Carrillo EH, Richardson JD. Thoracoscopy in the management of hemothorax and retained blood after trauma. *Curr Opin Pulm Med* 1998;4:243–246.
20. Meyer DM, Jessen ME, Wait MA, et al. Early evacuation of traumatic retained hemothoraces using thoracoscopy: a prospective, randomized trial. *Ann Thorac Surg* 1997;64:1396–1400.
21. Inci I, Ozcelik C, Ulku R, et al. Intrapleural fibrinolytic treatment of traumatic clotted hemothorax. *Chest* 1998;114:160–165.
22. Frye MD, Jarratt M, Sahn SA. Acute hypoxemic respiratory failure following intrapleural thrombolytic therapy for hemothorax. *Chest* 1994;105:1595–1596.
23. Battistella FD, Benfield JR. Blunt and penetrating injuries of the chest wall, pleura and lungs. In: Shields TW, LoCicero J III, Ponn RB, eds. *General thoracic surgery.* Philadelphia: Lippincott Williams & Wilkins, 2000: 815–831.
24. Krauss D, Schmidt GA. Cardiac tamponade and contralateral hemothorax after subclavian vein catheterization. *Chest* 1991;99:517–518.
25. Bilbrey GL, Hedberg CL. Hemorrhagic pleural effusion secondary to aortography: a case report. *J Thorac Cardiovasc Surg* 1967;54:85–89.
26. Kearney TJ, Shabot MM. Pulmonary artery rupture associated with the Swan-Ganz catheter. *Chest* 1995;108:1349–1352.
27. Hussain A, Raja AJ. Occurrence of hemothorax (unilateral) after sclerotherapy. *Am J Gastroenterol* 1991;86:1553–1554.
28. Berliner K. Hemorrhagic pleural effusion: an analysis of 120 cases. *Ann Intern Med* 1941;14:2266–2284.
29. Rostand RA, Feldman RL, Block ER. Massive hemothorax complicating heparin anticoagulation for pulmonary embolus. *South Med J* 1977;70:1128–1130.
30. Shepard MK, Mancini MC, Campbell GD, et al. Right-sided hemothorax and recurrent abdominal pain in a 34-year-old woman. *Chest* 1993;103:1239–1240.
31. Slind RO, Rodarte JR. Spontaneous hemothorax in an otherwise healthy young man. *Chest* 1974;66:81.
32. Cochran JW. Pancreatic pseudocyst presenting as massive hemothorax. *Am J Gastroenterol* 1978;69: 84–87.
33. Dippel WF, Doty DB, Ehrenhaft JL. Tension hemothorax due to patent ductus arteriosus. *N Engl J Med* 1973;288:353–354.
34. DeFrance JH, Blewett JH Jr, Ricci JA, et al. Massive hemothorax: two unusual cases. *Chest* 1974;66: 82–84.

35. Spear BS, Sully L, Lewis CT. Pulmonary arterio-venous fistula presenting as spontaneous hemothorax. *Thorax* 1975;30:355–356.

36. Martinez FJ, Villanueva AG, Pickering R, et al. Spontaneous hemothorax. Report of 6 cases and review of the literature. *Medicine* 1992;71:354–368.

37. Smith PR, Manjoney DL, Teitcher JB, et al. Massive hemothorax due to intrathoracic extramedullary hematopoiesis in a patient with thalassemia intermedia. *Chest* 1988;94:603–608.

38. Rodriguez E, Martinez MJ, Javaloyas M, et al. Haemothorax in the course of chickenpox. *Thorax* 1986; 41:491.

39. Harrison NK, Wilkinson J, O'Donohue J, et al. Osteochondroma of the rib: an unusual cause of haemothorax. *Thorax* 1994;49:618–619.

40. Laurin S, Aronson S, Schuller H, et al. Spontaneous hemothorax from bronchopulmonary sequestration. *Pediatr Radiol* 1980;10:54–56.

41. Varnholt V, Ringe H, Nietsch L, et al. Hemothorax under thrombolytic therapy with recombinant tissue: plasminogen activator (rt-PA) in a 16-year-old girl. *Eur J Pediatr* 1999;158[Suppl 3]:S140-S142.

42. Joseph J, Sahn SA. Thoracic endometriosis syndrome: new observations from an analysis of 110 cases. *Am J Med* 1996;100:164–170.

23

Chylothorax and Pseudochylothorax

At times, pleural fluid is milky or at least turbid. When the milkiness or turbidity persists after centrifugation, it is almost always due to a high lipid content of the pleural fluid. High levels of lipid accumulate in the pleural fluid in two situations. First, when the thoracic duct is disrupted, chyle can enter the pleural space to produce a chylous pleural effusion. In this situation, the patient is said to have a chylothorax. Second, in long-standing pleural effusions, large amounts of cholesterol or lecithin–globulin complexes can accumulate in the pleural fluid to produce a chyliform pleural effusion. The patient is then said to have a pseudochylothorax. It is important to differentiate these two conditions because their prognosis and management are completely different.

CHYLOTHORAX

A chylothorax is formed when the thoracic duct is disrupted and chyle enters the pleural space.

Pathophysiologic Features

Dietary fats in the form of long-chain triglycerides are transformed into chylomicra and very-low-density lipoproteins. These are secreted into the intestinal lacteals and lymphatics, and are then conveyed to the cisterna chyli, which overlies the anterior surface of the second lumbar vertebra, posterior to and to the right of the aorta. Usually, one major lymphatic vessel, the thoracic duct, leaves the cisterna chyli and passes through the esophageal hiatus of the diaphragm into the thoracic cavity. The thoracic duct ascends extrapleurally in the posterior mediastinum along the right side of the anterior surface of the vertebral column and lies between the azygos vein and the descending aorta in close proximity to the esophagus and the pericardium. At the level of the fourth to sixth thoracic vertebrae, the duct crosses to the left of the vertebral column and continues cephalad to enter the superior mediastinum between the aortic arch and the subclavian artery and the left side of the esophagus.

Once the thoracic duct passes the thoracic inlet, it arches 3 to 5 cm above the clavicle and passes anterior to the subclavian artery, vertebral artery, and thyrocervical trunk to terminate in the region of the left jugular and subclavian veins. Wide anatomic variations may exist in all portions of the thoracic duct. More than one thoracic duct may leave the cisterna chyli. The duct may continue on the right side of the vertebral column to enter the veins in the right subclavian region. Multiple anastomoses usually exist between various lymphatic channels, and direct lymphaticovenous communications with the azygos vein may be present (1, 2).

The drainage from the thoracic duct is called chyle. Chyle appears grossly as a milky, opalescent fluid that usually separates into three layers upon standing: a creamy uppermost layer containing chylomicrons, a milky intermediate layer, and a dependent layer containing cellular elements, most of which are small lymphocytes (3). If the patient has not eaten, however, chyle may be only slightly turbid because its lipid content will be reduced. Chyle is bacteriostatic and does not become infected even when it stands at room temperature for several weeks (4). Lampson (4) reported that *Escherichia coli* and *Staphylococcus aureus* were unable to grow in

100% chyle. Chyle that is extravasated into the pleural cavity is not irritating and usually does not evoke the formation of a pleural peel or a fibroelastic membrane.

Each day between 1,500 and 2,500 mL of chyle normally empty into the venous system (5). The ingestion of fat can increase the flow of lymph in the thoracic duct by 2 to 10 times the resting level for several hours (6). Ingestion of liquid also increases the chyle flow, whereas the ingestion of protein or carbohydrates has little effect on the lymph flow (6). The protein content of chyle is usually above 3 g per dL, and the electrolyte composition of chyle is similar to that of serum (6).

The primary cell in chyle is the small lymphocyte, and lymphocyte counts range from 400 to 6,800 per mm^3 (3). Prolonged drainage of a chylous pleural effusion can result in profound T-lymphocyte depletion. Breaux and Marks (7) reported that the total peripheral lymphocyte count fell from 1,665 per mm^3 to 264 per mm^3 with 14 days of chest tube drainage in one patient with a chylothorax. Almost all the lymphocytes in the pleural fluid were T lymphocytes.

A chylothorax results when the lymphatic duct becomes disrupted. Ligation of the thoracic duct at any point in its course does not produce a chylothorax in experimental animals (5), presumably as a result of the many collateral vessels and lymphaticovenous anastomoses. Ligation of the superior vena cava produces chylothorax about half the time in experimental animals. In the experimental animal, laceration or transection of the thoracic duct does not always produce a chylothorax. Hodges et al. (8) produced a 2.5 cm longitudinal laceration of the thoracic duct in three dogs at the level of T-9 and transected the thoracic duct at this level in another three dogs. They reported that all animals developed a pleural effusion but that the effusion ceased to form after 2 to 5 days in the animals with lacerations and after 4 to 10 days in the animals with transections (8). Lymphangiograms demonstrated that there was no continuity of the thoracic duct in the animals with the transections and the researchers concluded that the lymph was being conveyed by collaterals (8).

TABLE 23.1. *Causes of 143 chylothoraces from five separate series*

		Number	Percentage
Tumor		76	54
Lymphoma	57		
Other	19		
Trauma		36	25
Surgical	31		
Other	5		
Idiopathic		22	15
Congenital	8		
Other	14		
Miscellaneous		9	6

Etiologic Factors

The causes of 143 chylothoraces from five separate series (5, 6, 9–11) are tabulated in Table 23.1. For convenience, the causes of chylothorax can be grouped into four different categories. The cause of over 50% of chylothoraces is tumor, which is in the lymphoma group about 75% of the time. Chylothorax may be the presenting symptom of lymphoma (6, 10, 12). Therefore, a nontraumatic chylothorax is an indication for a diligent search for a lymphoma. In the series of Roy et al. (10), the diagnosis of lymphoma was not established until 6 to 12 months after the appearance of the chylothorax in four patients.

The second leading cause of chylothorax is trauma. This trauma is usually a cardiovascular, pulmonary, or esophageal surgical procedure. Chylothorax appears particularly frequently following operations in which the left subclavian artery is mobilized (12). The incidence of chylothorax after most thoracic surgeries is less than 1.0%. The incidence of chylothorax was 0.5% in one series of 2,660 cardiovascular operations (13), whereas it was 0.74% in a series of 1,744 pleuropulmonary surgeries (14). The incidence of chylothorax following esophageal resection is relatively high; it was 4.0% in one series of 255 cases (15). Dougenis et al. (15) reported that the incidence of chylothorax following esophageal surgery was significantly higher when the main thoracic duct was not ligated at the time of the resection. Accordingly, they recommend ligation of the main thoracic duct when esophageal resections are performed (15). There is one report of a patient who developed thrombosis of the superior vena cava and bilateral chylothoraces as a complication of the LeVeen shunt (16). Chylothorax has also been reported as a complication of coronary artery bypass surgery when the internal mammary artery is harvested (17), heart transplant (18), high translumbar aortography (19), sclerotherapy for esophageal varices (20), thoracolumbar fusion for correction of kyphosis (21), and cervical node dissection (22).

Of course, penetrating trauma to the chest or neck such as gunshot or knife wounds can also sever the thoracic duct and may lead to chylothorax. Trauma in which the spine is hyperextended or a vertebra is fractured is most likely to cause chylothorax, particularly if the injury occurs after the recent ingestion of a fatty meal (22). A chylothorax secondary to closed trauma is usually on the right side, and the site of rupture is most commonly in the region of the ninth or tenth thoracic vertebra (22). Such trauma includes falls from a height, motor vehicle accidents, compression injuries to the trunk, heavy blows to the back or stomach, and childbirth (23). The injury may be less impressive, and chylothoraces have been attributed to coughing, vomiting, and weight lifting. In one well-documented case report, an episode of vigorous stretching while yawning was followed by swelling in the left supraclavicular fossa and the development of bilateral chylothoraces (24).

The third leading cause of chylothorax is idiopathic, including most cases of congenital chylothorax. One should exclude lymphoma as a cause of the chylothorax before it is labeled as idiopathic. Most cases of idiopathic chylothorax in the adult are probably due to minor trauma, such as coughing or hiccuping, after the ingestion of fatty meals.

Chylothorax is the most common form of pleural effusion encountered in the first few days of life (25). The fetal pleural effusion discussed in Chapter 18 is probably also a chylothorax. Neonatal chylothorax is relatively uncommon; during a 22-year period, 12 cases were diagnosed at the Hospital for Sick Children, which is a large pediatric tertiary care center (26). The babies are usually born at full term after normal labor and delivery. The etiology of congenital chylothorax is unknown (27). Abnormalities of the thoracic duct have not been found in most babies who have undergone exploratory thoracotomy (25). Several cases of generalized pleural oozing have been described during surgery (26). It is possible that birth trauma may result in a tear of a major lymphatic channel in at least some individuals. In some cases, a congenital chylothorax is associated with Turner's syndrome, Noonan's syndrome, or Down syndrome (27). Congenital chylothorax is also more common in infants who are hydropic or who have polyhydramnios (26).

Interestingly, mice who lack the integrin $\alpha_9\beta_1$ appear normal at birth but then develop respiratory failure and die between 6 and 12 days of age (28). The respiratory failure is caused by bilateral chylothoraces. Although the thoracic duct appears normal grossly, microscopic examination reveals edema and lymphocytic infiltration in the chest wall (28). Members of the integrin family of adhesion receptors mediate both cell–cell and cell–matrix interactions and have been shown to play vital roles in embryonic development, wound healing, and other biologic processes. It has been postulated that $\alpha_9\beta_1$ deficiency could be one cause of congenital chylothorax (28).

Miscellaneous etiologies comprise the fourth group of chylothoraces. Thrombosis of the superior vena cava or the subclavian vein is becoming one of the more common causes of chylothorax. Berman et al. (29) reviewed the case histories of 37 infants and children with thrombosis of their superior vena cava in a newborn and pediatric intensive care unit and reported that nine (24%) had a chylothorax. Chylothorax can also complicate left subclavian vein thrombosis (30). Cirrhosis is a relatively common cause of chylothorax. Romero et al. (31) analyzed 24 cases of chylothorax occurring at their institution and reported that five (21%) were secondary to cirrhosis. Interestingly, the mean protein level in these five chylothoraces was only 1.7 g per dL (compared to 4.1 g per dL in the other effusions), the mean lactate dehydrogenase (LDH) level was only 96 IU per L (compared with 351 IU per L in

the other chylothoraces) and ascites was present
in three of the five patients (31). On rare occasions, a chylothorax is associated with heart failure or the nephrotic syndrome and the effusion is
also a transudate in these instances (32). In most
patients with the nephrotic syndrome and a chylothorax, the chylothorax is secondary to chylous
ascites, but on occasion, it can be secondary to
superior vena caval thrombosis (33).

Many other causes of chylothorax have been
reported, but even when all are grouped together,
they account for only a small percentage of chylothoraces. The most interesting of these is pulmonary lymphangioleiomyomatosis, which has
associated interstitial parenchymal infiltrates and
is discussed later in this chapter. Other causes
include Gilbert's syndrome (34) (also discussed
later in this chapter), Kaposi's sarcoma in patients with acquired immunodeficiency syndrome
(AIDS) (35, 36), filariasis, giant lymph node hyperplasia (Castleman's disease) (37), lymphangi-
tis of the thoracic duct, obstruction of the superior
vena cava secondary to Behçet's syndrome
(38, 39), tuberculosis (40), sarcoidosis (41) involving the intrathoracic lymph nodes, aneurysms
of the thoracic aorta that erode the duct, abnormalities of the lymphatic vessels such as intestinal lymphangiectasis (42) or reticular hyperplasia (11, 43), radiation-induced mediastinal
fibrosis (44), and hypothyroidism (45).

Clinical Manifestations

The initial symptoms of chylothorax are usually
related to the presence of the space-occupying
fluid in the thoracic cavity, and, therefore, patients have dyspnea. Pleuritic chest pain and fever
are rare because chyle is not irritating to the pleural surface. With traumatic chylothorax, a latent
period of 2 to 10 days usually occurs between the
trauma and the onset of the pleural effusion (22).
There is one case report in which the latent period
was 11 weeks (46). Lymph collects extrapleurally in the mediastinum after the initial thoracic
duct disruption, forms a chyloma, and produces a
posterior mediastinal mass (2). The mediastinal
pleura eventually ruptures, chyle gains access to
the pleural space, and dyspnea is produced by
the chyle compressing the lung. At times, hy-

potension, cyanosis, and extreme dyspnea occur
when the chyloma ruptures into the pleural space.
The ruptured chyloma is no longer visible radiographically.

With nontraumatic chylothorax, the onset of
symptoms is usually gradual. In congenital chylothorax, the infant develops respiratory distress
in the first few days of life; 50% of patients have
symptoms within the first 24 hours, whereas 75%
have symptoms by the end of the first week (25).
The chyle production in a neonate may exceed
250 mL per day (27).

The main threat to life from chylothorax is
malnutrition and a compromised immunologic
status. Because the thoracic duct carries 2,500 mL
of fluid daily that contains substantial amounts
of protein, fats, electrolytes, and lymphocytes,
the patient can become cachectic rapidly if this
amount of chyle is removed daily through chest
tubes or repeated thoracentesis. In addition, the
patients develop lymphopenia and a compromised immunologic status due to the removal of
large numbers of lymphocytes with the chyle.
Over a 14-day period, one patient had over 35
L of fluid withdrawn, which contained 2.3 kg of
fat and 0.7 kg of protein, and during this period,
the peripheral lymphocyte count dropped from
1,665 per mm^3 to 264 per mm^3 (7). Indeed, until
Lampson initially described successful ligation
of the thoracic duct in 1948 (4), the mortality rate
from chylothorax was 50%. When managing a
patient with chylothorax, one should abandon
conservative treatment before the patient becomes too malnourished and immunocompromised.

Diagnosis

The diagnosis of chylothorax is usually not difficult because chyle usually has a distinctive white,
odorless, milky appearance. When such fluid is
found, the main differentiation is between empyema and a pseudochylothorax. The milkiness
with empyema is caused by the suspended white
blood cells, and if such fluid is centrifuged, the
supernatant is clear. The cloudiness of the chyliform pleural effusion from a pseudochylothorax
is also caused by high lipid levels, either cholesterol or lecithin-globulin complexes. Chylous

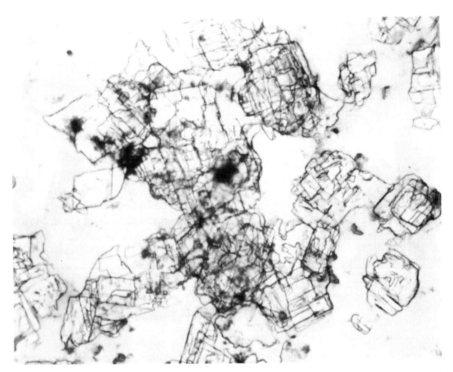

FIG. 23.1. Cholesterol crystals. Typical large polyhedric crystals from a patient with a cholesterol pleural effusion. This patient had a rheumatoid pleural effusion.

and chyliform pleural fluids remain opaque after centrifugation.

If cholesterol crystals are responsible for the turbidity, they may be easily demonstrated by examination of the pleural fluid sediment (Fig. 23.1). If the turbidity is due to high levels of cholesterol, the turbidity will clear when 1 to 2 mL of ethyl ether is added to a test tube of the fluid; if the turbidity is due to chylomicrons or lecithin complexes, the turbidity does not clear (47).

Not all chylous pleural effusions have the typical, milky appearance. With congenital chylothorax, the pleural fluid is initially serous and only turns chylous when milk feedings are started (25). Because congenital chylothorax is the most common cause of pleural effusion in the newborn (25), pleural fluid triglyceride and lipoprotein analyses should be performed in all newborns with pleural effusion. In adults, the pleural fluid does not always look like typical chyle. Staats et al. (9) reported that 20 of 38 cases of chylothorax (53%) were described as other than chylous, whereas

Romero et al. (31) reported that 10 of 24 (42%) patients with chylothorax had nonmilky pleural fluid. In this study of 809 patients with pleural effusions, 24 (3%) of the patients had chylothorax (31). The results of this study suggest that lipid measurements might be indicated in all patients with pleural effusions of unknown etiology in order to rule out the diagnosis of chylothorax.

Triglyceride Measurement

The best way to establish the diagnosis of chylothorax is by measuring the triglyceride and cholesterol levels in the pleural fluid (see Fig. 4.7). If the pleural fluid triglyceride level is above 110 mg per dL and the ratio of the pleural fluid to serum cholesterol is less than 1.0, the diagnosis of chylothorax is established. The cholesterol ratio is used to exclude pseudochylothorax because some patients with chyliform pleural effusions also have triglyceride levels above 110 mg per dL, but their pleural fluid/serum cholesterol ratio will exceed 1:0 (31). Although it has been suggested that in order to establish the diagnosis of chylothorax the pleural fluid triglyceride level should be more than the serum triglyceride level (31), this criterion appears to be unnecessary because there is no relationship between the pleural fluid and the serum triglyceride levels in patients not having a chylothorax (48). The only other situation in which the pleural fluid triglyceride is above 110 mg per dL occurs when intravenous fluid containing high levels of triglycerides leaks from a central vein into the pleural space (49). If there is doubt about the diagnosis of a chylothorax, lipoprotein analysis of the pleural fluid should be performed. The demonstration of chylomicrons in the pleural fluid by lipoprotein analysis establishes the diagnosis of chylothorax (9). One should usually be able to differentiate chylothorax and pseudochylothorax by the clinical course. A chylothorax has an acute onset with normal pleural surfaces, whereas a pseudochylothorax occurs in a patient with a long-standing pleural effusion with thickened pleura (50). If any doubt exists, the pleural fluid should be analyzed for chylomicrons.

Lipophilic Dye Ingestion

Another test for the diagnosis of chylothorax is ingestion of a fatty meal with a lipophilic dye, followed by a thoracentesis 30 to 60 minutes later, to ascertain whether the pleural fluid has changed in color (51). The most commonly used dye is Drug and Cosmetic Green No. 6, a coal-tar dye. One gram of this dye is mixed thoroughly with a quarter pound of butter, and the mixture is spread on a slice of bread. The patient eats the bread, and a thoracentesis performed 30 to 60 minutes later should yield green fluid if a chylothorax is present. I have attempted this test in about six different patients. The greatest problem I had encountered was in maintaining a straight face when I asked the patient to eat the disgusting green mess. Because the diagnosis is usually easily established with triglyceride and lipoprotein analysis, I no longer ask my patients with suspected chylothorax to eat dark green sandwiches.

Treatment

The main danger to patients with chylothorax is that they become malnourished and immunocompromised owing to the removal of large amounts of protein, fat, electrolytes, and lymphocytes from the body with repeated thoracentesis or chest tube drainage. In the past, the mortality rate from chylothorax approached 50%. When managing a patient with chylothorax, one must treat the chylothorax definitively, such as with thoracic duct ligation or pleuroperitoneal shunt implantation, before the patient becomes too cachectic to tolerate the operation. Because the management of chylothorax differs for traumatic, nontraumatic, and congenital chylothoraces, treatment regimens are described separately.

Traumatic Chylothorax

The general aims in treating the patient with traumatic chylothorax are relief of dyspnea by removing the chyle, prevention of dehydration, maintenance of nutrition, and a reduction in the rate of chyle formation. When a postoperative chylothorax is discovered, tube thoracostomy should be performed to remove the chyle and relieve the dyspnea. In this situation, consideration should be given to recycling the chyle to prevent the malnutrition and the immunosuppression. Thomson and Simms (52) reported one case in which the chyle was reinfused directly from the chest tube into the subclavian vein for a total of 18 days. There have been no large series evaluating this procedure, and in the first half of the century, a couple of patients died from "anaphylaxis" soon after chyle infusion was started (52).

When a postoperative chylothorax is managed initially with tube thoracostomy, efforts should be made to decrease the flow of chyle through dietary manipulation. The flow of chyle is minimized if all nourishment by mouth is halted and if the patient's gastrointestinal tract is maintained as empty as possible by constant gastric suction (53). The patient's nutritional status can be maintained with intravenous hyperalimentation (54). In the past, attempts have been made to decrease the lymph flow by providing the fat calories in the diet with medium chain triglycerides (54). These triglycerides have ten or fewer carbon atoms and are absorbed directly into the portal vein and thus gain entrance to the circulatory system without ever entering the thoracic duct (55). Because they are relatively unpalatable and hyperalimentation decreases the flow of chyle much more, hyperalimentation rather than medium-chain triglycerides are recommended when one wishes to reduce the flow of chyle. The flow of chyle is also decreased if the patient stays in bed because any activity of the lower extremities increases the flow of lymph (55). There is one recent report in which the flow of chyle was reduced markedly with inhaled nitrous oxide in a 41-week-old infant with a postoperative chylothorax (56). The reduction in the flow of chyle was thought to be due to alleviation of the central venous hypertension (56).

The defect in the thoracic duct frequently closes spontaneously in traumatic chylothorax. If the thoracic duct is transected in dogs, chyle ceases to enter the pleural space within 10 days as collateral lymphatic channels are formed (8). In a recent series of 22 children with postoperative chylothorax, 19 (86.4%) closed spontaneously (57) when the patients were treated concomitantly with total parenteral nutrition or low-fat enteral diets. The average duration of drainage of these 19 patients was 13.7 days, with a range of 7 to 30 (57). In another series of 47 adults with postoperative chylothorax from the Mayo Clinic (58), the leak closed spontaneously in 7 of 36 patients (19%) who received central hyperalimentation and in six of 11 patients (55%) who were treated with medium-chain triglyceride diets (58).

If large amounts of chyle continue to drain for more than several days postoperatively, a procedure should be performed to treat the chylothorax definitively. The alternatives at this juncture are (a) to insert a pleuroperitoneal shunt, (b) to attempt to create a pleurodesis to obliterate the pleural space through tube thoracostomy, (c) to perform thoracoscopy with pleural abrasion or partial pleurectomy to create a pleurodesis, (d) to perform thoracoscopy with attempted ligation of the thoracic duct, or (e) to perform a thoracotomy with ligation of the thoracic duct.

Pleuroperitoneal Shunt

The optimal method to remove the chyle and alleviate the dyspnea with chylothorax appears to be the insertion of a pleuroperitoneal shunt (59–61) (see the discussion of pleuroperitoneal shunt in Chapter 7). The primary advantage of the pleuroperitoneal shunt is that the lymph is not removed from the body, and, therefore, the patient does not become malnourished or immunocompromised. When the chyle is shunted to the peritoneal cavity, it is absorbed without creating significant ascites (59). A second advantage is that the pleuroperitoneal shunt can be inserted with local anesthesia as opposed to general anesthesia, which is required for thoracic duct ligation. When a pleuroperitoneal shunt is implanted, the defect closes spontaneously in most cases and the shunt can be removed 30 to 90 days after its insertion (62). When the chyle ceases to enter the pleural space, the shunt is removed. The shunt should not be inserted if chylous ascites is present. Little et al. (59) inserted pleuroperitoneal shunts in two patients with chylothoraces postoperatively and reported that the patients had complete resolution of their effusions with subsequent removal of the shunts. In the largest series using the pleuroperitoneal shunt, 16 infants were treated with the shunt and excellent results were obtained in 12 (60). The only patients who did not have favorable outcomes were those whose chylothoraces were from central venous thrombosis (60). Murphy et al. (60) recommend placing the shunt if the drainage persists beyond 5 days. An alternative approach to patients with postoperative chylothorax is to insert the pleuroperitoneal shunt as soon as the diagnosis is made without ever resorting to tube thoracostomy. It is not known how important it is to slow the flow of lymph if a pleuroperitoneal shunt is inserted. At present, I place no dietary restrictions on my patients who have chylothoraces and who are being treated with pleuroperitoneal shunts.

Pleurodesis through a Chest Tube

There are a limited number of reports in which pleurodesis has been attempted by injecting a sclerosing agent through a chest tube. Shimizu et al. (63) reported that six of seven patients (86%) with postoperative chylothorax had a successful pleurodesis after the intrapleural administration of OK-432 one to five times. OK-432 is an immunostimulating agent that is used extensively in Japan for pleurodesis, but the drug is not available in the United States. Adler and Levinsky reported the successful treatment of one patient with a postoperative chylothorax with 10 g talc in a slurry (64). Akaogi et al. (65) reported that two patients with postoperative chylothorax were successfully managed with fibrin glue injected through the chest tube. Others have had a less satisfactory experience with tetracycline (66), nitrogen mustard, or atabrine (67). Tetracycline was ineffective in three patients on whom I attempted pleurodesis. In view of these experiences, pleurodesis by injecting a material through the chest tube is not generally recommended for patients with chylothorax.

Thoracoscopy with Talc Insufflation

There are at least three reports in which more than five patients were treated with talc insufflation at the time of thoracoscopy for chylothorax. Weissberg (68) reported that the intrapleural insufflation of 2 g talc controlled the chylothorax in seven of nine patients. Vargas et al. recently reported the successful treatment of five patients with 2 g insufflated talc at the time of thoracoscopy (69). Graham et al. (70) insufflated talc in eight patients with chylothorax and reported that the treatment was successful in all. Although four of the patients experienced a prolonged course of high output from their chest tubes with relatively slow resolution of the effusions, all had completely resolved by 12 days after the procedure. Therefore, thoracoscopy with the insufflation of talc appears to be an effective treatment for chylothorax. It is not recommended, however, because the intrapleural administration of talc can lead to the development of the acute respiratory distress syndrome (see

Chapter 7). An alternative to thoracoscopy with talc insufflation is thoracoscopy with pleural abrasion or partial parietal pleurectomy.

Ligation of the Thoracic Duct through Thoracotomy

A definitive treatment for postoperative chylothorax is ligation of the thoracic duct. Lampson first demonstrated that a chylothorax could be controlled by ligation of the thoracic duct (4). Ligation of the thoracic duct causes no ill effects, probably on account of the multiple anastomoses among various lymphatic channels and direct lymphaticovenous communications (5, 6). Usually, the side of the chylothorax is ipsilateral to the original surgery, and reoperation can be performed through the original thoracotomy (58). If the chylothorax is unilateral, the thoracotomy should be performed on the side of the fluid (53). If the chylothorax is bilateral, a right thoracotomy should be performed because the duct is more readily approached from that side (53). An alternative approach has been suggested by Mason et al. (71), who recommend that the thoracic duct be ligated just below the diaphragm through an intraabdominal approach.

It has been recommended that a preoperative lymphangiogram be obtained in every case of chylothorax that does not respond to nonoperative management because the site of leak or obstruction can usually be demonstrated by this technique (58). At the time of operation, one should attempt to find the actual point of leakage from the duct and ligate the duct on both sides of the leak (53). In many instances, however, the leak cannot be located, and, therefore, the thoracic duct should be ligated. Several aids for identifying the thoracic duct intraoperatively have been suggested. Probably, the best method is to inject Evans blue dye at a dose of 0.7 to 0.8 mg per kg, the total dose not exceeding 25 mg, into the subcutaneous tissue of the leg. Within 5 minutes, the chyle will be stained blue (53). The patient may also be given butter or cream to eat 3 to 4 hours preoperatively. The objection to this method is that the stomach may not be empty before the induction of anesthesia, although stomach contents may be removed by nasogastric suction (53). If for some reason the thoracic duct cannot be successfully ligated at thoracotomy, a parietal pleurectomy should be performed in order to obliterate the pleural space (6).

If the chylous drainage from the chest tubes persists and the nutritional status of the patient is deteriorating, one must not delay thoracotomy too long. In one series, all three patients with traumatic chylothorax who underwent thoracotomy died in the postoperative period (10). These deaths were attributed to the debilitation of the patients by the time the operation was performed.

Ligation of the Thoracic Duct through Thoracoscopy

With the advent of video-assisted thoracic surgery (VATS), one would expect that ligation of the thoracic duct would be tried with the video-thoracoscope. Thoracoscopy permits the entire pleural space to be visualized, as well as allowing direct suture of a lymphatic leak. Although this technique has not been widely employed for the control of chylothorax, there are anecdotal reports documenting its successful use (72–76). Kent and Pinson (72) successfully ligated the thoracic duct in one patient who developed a chylothorax after a radical neck dissection. Shirai et al. (73) performed thoracoscopy on a patient who developed a chylothorax postoperatively. They were able to identify the site of leakage, and the leakage stopped with the application of fibrin glue. Zoetmulder et al. (74) reported on a 51-year-old patient who developed a chylothorax 4 years after treatment of a soft tissue sarcoma. At thoracoscopy, the thoracic duct leak could be identified and oversewn. The patient also had talc insufflated into her pleural space, and subsequently had no recurrence of her pleural effusion. It is unclear whether the procedure would have been effective if only the talc insufflation had been performed. Peillon et al. (75) used VATS to clip the chylous leak in two patients postoperatively and concluded that VATS therapy was the therapy of choice when medical therapy failed. It remains to be seen whether the endoscopic closure of chylous leaks is more successful or better tolerated than current open techniques (76).

Nontraumatic Chylothorax

In general, the goals of management of nontraumatic chylothorax are the same as for traumatic chylothorax. With nontraumatic chylothorax, however, one must also attempt to establish a cause. If the characteristics of the chyle are transudative, that is, there is a low protein and a low LDH, then the three most likely etiologies are cirrhosis, congestive heart failure, and the nephrotic syndrome (31).

The possibility of lymphoma should be considered in all patients with a nontraumatic chylothorax because it is the most common cause of nontraumatic chylothorax (Table 23.1). Frequently, the patient with lymphoma and chylothorax has no evidence of lymphoma outside the thorax. Computed tomographic (CT) studies of the mediastinum should be performed in all patients with nontraumatic chylothorax to ascertain whether mediastinal lymphadenopathy is present. In women with chylothorax and parenchymal infiltrates, another possibility is pulmonary lymphangioleiomyomatosis (see the section later in this chapter).

Another test that should be obtained on all patients with nontraumatic chylothoraces is a lymphangiogram (77). With the lymphangiogram a total or partial obstruction of lymph flow and the position of the obstacle can be demonstrated. In addition, the lymphangiogram can demonstrate the presence of enlarged lymph nodes or lymphangiectasis that may give a clue as to the etiology of the chylothorax.

The initial management of a patient with a nontraumatic chylothorax should be similar to that of a patient with a traumatic chylothorax. In most cases, a pleuroperitoneal shunt should be inserted. If tube thoracostomy is performed, the gastrointestinal tract should be put at rest and the patient's nutritional status should be maintained by parenteral hyperalimentation. If the chylothorax is due to minor trauma, these measures are usually curative within a week. If CT examination of the mediastinum reveals no lymphadenopathy or other masses and the chylothorax is controlled, no further treatment is indicated. In one series of 35 patients with chylothorax due to tumors, none were successfully managed with chest tubes or repeated pleural aspiration (10). If the chylothorax is not controlled with the pleuroperitoneal shunt, or if the CT study of the mediastinum is positive, the patient should undergo a videothoracoscopy or an exploratory thoracotomy. The mediastinum should then be carefully examined for masses, with lymphoma in mind. In addition, the thoracic duct should be ligated.

If the patient is known to have lymphoma or metastatic carcinoma, then radiation should be given to the mediastinum. Roy et al. (10) reported that radiation therapy to the mediastinum adequately controlled the chylothorax for the remainder of the patient's life in 68% of those with lymphoma and in 50% of those with metastatic carcinoma. If radiotherapy or chemotherapy does not control the chylothorax in patients with known lymphoma or metastatic carcinoma, exploratory thoracotomy is probably not indicated in view of these patients' dismal prognosis (10). If these patients are symptomatic from the chylothorax, however, one should insert a pleuroperitoneal shunt unless the patient also has ascites. An alternative to the pleuroperitoneal shunt is medical thoracoscopy with the instillation of talc. Mares and Mathur (78) reported their experience with this procedure for 24 hemithoraces in 19 patients with lymphoma-related chylothorax in whom chemotherapy or radiation therapy had failed. They reported that none of their patients had a recurrence of their chylothorax during the 90-day follow-up period.

There are special aspects to the treatment of chylothorax associated with some entities. Because patients with chylothorax secondary to the nephrotic syndrome are likely to have chylous ascites, it is important not to place a pleuroperitoneal shunt or ligate the thoracic duct until this possibility is evaluated (79). The chylothorax associated with sarcoidosis is likely to disappear if the patient is treated with corticosteroids (41). Patients with primary intestinal lymphangiectasia frequently have a chylothorax. There is one case report (80) in which the administration of octreotide (50 g tid) led to the resolution of the chylous effusions. The mechanisms by which octreotide, a synthetic somatostatin-like compound, led to the resolution of the chylous effusions is not clear (80).

Congenital Chylothorax

As mentioned earlier in this chapter, chylothorax is the most common type of pleural effusion in infants. Chylothorax in infancy can be fatal. The mortality rate was 30% in one series of 10 patients with congenital chylothorax (81). The three deaths in this series were all ascribed to malnutrition and secondary infection, and the babies who died were the only ones in the series who were subjected to more than 14 thoracenteses. On the other hand, five of the babies (50%) had no recurrence of their chylothorax after one to three thoracenteses, and all seven babies who survived were apparently normal (81). The recommended management of congenital chylothorax, in view of these findings, is as follows. Initially, the baby should be treated conservatively with repeated thoracenteses. In addition, the nutrition for the infant should be provided by total parenteral nutrition (82). If the chylothorax recurs after the third pleural aspiration, a pleuroperitoneal shunt should be inserted (83). Milson et al. (83) implanted pleuroperitoneal shunts in seven infants, one of whom was 7 days old, and reported that the shunt cured the chylothorax in six of the seven patients. Thoracic duct ligation is indicated if the pleuroperitoneal shunting fails. The advantage of the shunt over the thoracic duct ligation is that it is a much simpler procedure.

PULMONARY LYMPHANGIOLEIOMYOMATOSIS

Pulmonary lymphangioleiomyomatosis (LAM) is a rare condition characterized by widespread proliferation of immature smooth muscle throughout the peribronchial, perivascular, and perilymphatic regions of the lung (84, 85). The perilymphatic proliferation of smooth muscle results in lymphatic obstruction, and, accordingly, patients have a high incidence of chylothorax. When two recent series (84, 85) with a total of 104 patients are combined, chylothorax occurred in 28 of the patients (27%). The lymph nodes in the mediastinum and retroperitoneal space may also be infiltrated with immature smooth muscle cells, further impairing lymphatic flow. The thoracic duct may be either obliterated or dilated (86). The proliferation of smooth muscle in the perivascular spaces may obstruct the pulmonary venules and may produce pulmonary hemorrhage, hemoptysis, and pulmonary hemosiderosis. The proliferation of the peribronchial smooth muscles can partially or completely obstruct the airways to cause air trapping, cyst and bullae formation, and a high incidence of pneumothorax (87). Approximately one third of patients have renal angiomyolipoma, which is a benign mesenchymal tumor (84). Usually, the renal angiomyolipoma is discovered before the diagnosis of LAM is made.

It should be noted that there is now an LAM registry in the United States that tracks the outcome of patients with this disease. The contact person is Eugene J. Sullivan, M.D., Cleveland Clinic Foundation, Cleveland, Ohio, (216) 445–2610, e-mail: sullivan@cesmtp.ccf.org (88).

Clinical Manifestations

LAM occurs almost exclusively in women of reproductive age (84). In one series of 69 patients, however, five patients were postmenopausal at disease onset (84) and there is another case report of LAM occurring in a 3-year-old girl (89). The onset of symptoms can occur from age 3 to 70, but most patients are between the ages of 25 and 50 when symptoms begin. Most patients have increasing shortness of breath and or cough, but hemoptysis, pneumothorax, or an incidentally discovered chylothorax can be the presenting manifestation. During the course of their disease, almost all patients have parenchymal infiltrates, about 30% have chylothorax, and about 70% have pneumothorax (84, 85).

Pulmonary LAM is at times part of the syndrome of pulmonary tuberous sclerosis. Tuberous sclerosis is an uncommon, genetically transmitted disease with the classic triad of seizures, adenoma sebaceum, and mental retardation. Only a small percentage of patients with tuberous sclerosis have pulmonary involvement. Clinically, pulmonary tuberous sclerosis is similar to pulmonary LAM. The radiographic and pathologic findings in the lung are identical in both disorders. Lymph nodes are less commonly involved, and chylothorax occurs much less

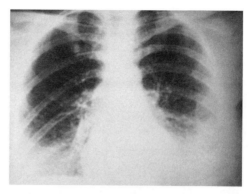

FIG. 23.2. Posteroanterior radiograph from a 37-year-old woman with pulmonary lymphangioleiomyomatosis. Note the reticulonodular pattern and the wide distance between the ribs suggesting hyperinflation. The pleural effusion on the left was a chylothorax. (Courtesy of Dr. Harry Sassoon.)

commonly with pulmonary tuberous sclerosis, however (86, 90). Further support for the relationship between tuberous sclerosis and LAM comes from one report in which estrogen receptors were demonstrated in a woman with tuberous sclerosis and the LAM syndrome (91).

The chest radiograph usually suggests the diagnosis of LAM (Fig. 23.2). A coarse bilateral reticular pattern similar to that of fibrosing alveolitis is seen; however, the lung volumes in LAM are usually increased rather than decreased, as in fibrosing alveolitis and almost every other cause of interstitial lung disease (92). The interstitial lung infiltrates vary in extent, and their distribution may be primarily basal or diffuse. The pleural effusion from the chylothorax may be unilateral or bilateral and is typically large and recurrent. All have been chylous on direct examination. The high-resolution CT scan of patients with LAM is very characteristic (Fig. 23.3) in that there are numerous air-filled cysts surrounded by normal lung parenchyma. The only other disease that has similar findings on the high-resolution CT scan is Langerhans' cell histiocytosis. In the latter disease the lung bases are relatively spared and there are frequently nodules (92). Serial CT scans may be useful in assessing the response to therapy.

Pulmonary function tests in the patient with LAM reveal a normal or reduced vital capacity

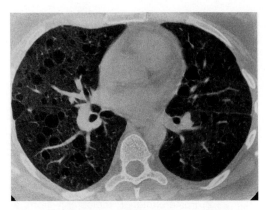

FIG. 23.3. High-resolution CT scan of 48-year-old woman with LAM. Note the numerous thin-walled cysts, rounded and uniform in shape, with normal intervening lung parenchyma.

but an increased total lung capacity. Evidence of moderate to severe obstructive ventilatory dysfunction usually exists, and the diffusing capacity for carbon monoxide is usually reduced (92). Arterial blood gases reveal hypoxia and hypocapnia.

Diagnosis

The diagnosis of pulmonary LAM is frequently delayed. In the series of 32 patients from Stanford and the Mayo Clinic, the diagnosis was delayed an average of 44 months after the initial manifestation of the disease. Only one patient was given a diagnosis of LAM during her initial medical evaluation (93). This diagnosis should be suspected in any woman between the ages of 25 and 50 with a chylothorax, particularly if interstitial infiltrates and increased lung volumes are also present.

Although the diagnosis is strongly suggested by the findings on the high-resolution CT scan, a definitive diagnosis requires tissue confirmation. The tissue can be obtained by transbronchial biopsy, thoracoscopy, or open thoracotomy (84). The diagnosis of LAM is established by the demonstration of the typical histologic pattern of widespread proliferation of immature smooth muscle. This perilymphatic smooth muscle proliferation is generally regarded as a hamartomatous rather than a neoplastic process (86). Characteristically, clefts or spaces between the smooth muscle bundles are lined by endothelium.

Microscopic changes in involved lymph nodes are similar to those in the lung: interlacing bundles of smooth muscle proliferation demarcated by endothelial-lined clefts (86).

It has been shown that the demonstration of the presence of smooth muscle cells that have specific immunoreactivity for the monoclonal antibody HMB45 is specific and highly sensitive for LAM (94). HMB45 is a monoclonal antibody with specific immunoreactivity for malignant melanoma (94). The availability of this test will probably facilitate the use of transbronchial biopsy in making the diagnosis of LAM (95).

Treatment

In the past, it was believed that the prognosis of women with pulmonary LAM was dismal because most patients died within 10 years of the onset of symptoms (90). Recent reports suggest that the prognosis may be somewhat better. In a recent study from France, the Kaplan-Meier plot showed survival probabilities of 91% after 5 years, 79% after 10 years, and 71% after 15 years of disease duration (84). The patients die primarily of progressive respiratory insufficiency (96). Characteristics associated with a poor prognosis include a reduced forced expiratory volume in one second (FEV_1) and forced vital capacity (FVC), an increased total lung capacity (TLC), and a predominantly cystic type of histology as opposed to a predominantly smooth muscle type of histology (97).

Several researchers have suggested that hormonal manipulation may be of value in treating this disease (84). The exclusive occurrence of the disease in women of reproductive age has suggested that the smooth muscle proliferation may be hormonally dependent. The results, however, with hormonal manipulation have not been impressive. Johnson and Tattersfield (98) retrospectively analyzed the rate of decline in pulmonary function of 43 patients with LAM (98). They reported that the mean drop in FEV_1 and diffusing capacity was significantly less in patients receiving progesterone than in those not receiving progesterone, and in postmenopausal as opposed to premenopausal women (98), although there was much overlap between the groups. Urban et al.

reported that hormonal therapy was administered in 57 patients but that only four had a greater than 15% improvement in their FEV_1 (84). The most common treatment regimen is medroxyprogesterone acetate, 400 mg intramuscularly each month.

Therefore, it appears that hormonal manipulations may favorably influence the course of at least some patients. When the diagnosis of LAM is suspected, lung tissue should be obtained for progesterone and estrogen receptor assay, if possible, if for no other reason than to ascertain if there is a relationship between the presence of receptors and the response to therapy. It is recommended that all patients be treated initially with medroxyprogesterone. If the disease progresses, then consideration should be given to performing an oophorectomy or possibly manipulating the estrogen therapy, particularly if estrogen receptors were present.

One possible therapy for LAM is lung transplantation. In 1996, Boehler et al. (99) reported on the results of lung transplantation in 34 patients treated at 16 different lung transplant centers. The actuarial survival calculated by the Kaplan-Meier method was 69% after 1 year and 58% after 2 years. The FEV_1 increased from 24% ± 12% preoperatively to 48% ± 16% 6 months after transplantation (99). LAM recurred in the allograph in one patient. Given the relatively good prognosis of the patients in the study by Urban et al. (84), lung transplantation is not recommended until the patient becomes debilitated from her disease.

GORHAM'S SYNDROME

Gorham's syndrome is a rare disease that can occur at any age but is most often recognized in children or young adults. There is no sex predilection and no inheritance pattern. Other names for Gorham's syndrome include hemangiomatosis, disappearing bone disease, and massive osteolysis. The characteristic lesion of Gorham's syndrome is an intraosseous proliferation of vascular or lymphatic channels that leads to the disappearance of bones. There is a propensity for involvement of the maxilla, shoulder girdle, and pelvis (34).

Patients with Gorham's syndrome have a high incidence of chylothorax. Chylothorax was present in 25 of the 146 cases (17%) of Gorham's syndrome in the literature up until 1994 (34). All the patients with Gorham's syndrome and chylothorax had either rib, scapular, clavicular, or thoracic vertebral bony involvement. Patients with Gorham's syndrome and chylothorax should be treated with a pleuroperitoneal shunt or thoracic duct ligation (34).

CHYLIFORM PLEURAL EFFUSIONS AND PSEUDOCHYLOTHORAX

A chyliform pleural effusion resulting in a pseudochylothorax is a pleural effusion that is turbid or milky from high lipid content not resulting from disruption of the thoracic duct. Some authors have separated pseudochylothoraces into those with cholesterol crystals, designated pseudochylous effusions, and those without cholesterol crystals, designated chyliform pleural effusions (47). Because no practical reason exists for making this distinction, I designate all high-lipid nonchylous effusions as chyliform pleural effusions. Pseudochylothoraces with their associated chyliform pleural fluid are uncommon. Until 1999, only 174 cases had been reported in the international literature (100). Pseudochylothoraces are much less common than chylothoraces. In a series of 53 nontraumatic high-lipid effusions, only six (11%) were chyliform pleural effusions (10).

Pathogenesis

The precise pathogenesis of chyliform pleural effusions is not known (101). Most patients with chyliform pleural effusions have long-standing pleural effusions (mean 5 years), and have thickened and sometimes calcified pleura. Most of the cholesterol in chyliform pleural effusions is associated with high-density lipoproteins in contrast to the cholesterol in acute exudates that is mostly bound to low-density lipoproteins (LDL) (101). It has been hypothesized that the cholesterol that enters the pleural space with acute pleural inflammation becomes trapped in the pleural space and undergoes a change in lipoprotein-binding characteristics (101). The diseased pleura may result in an abnormally slow transfer of cholesterol and other lipids out of the pleural space and may lead to the accumulation of cholesterol in the pleural fluid (50). The origin of the cholesterol and other lipids is not definitely known, but one possibility is from degenerating red and white blood cells in the pleural fluid (50). Most patients with chyliform pleural effusions do not appear to have disturbed cholesterol metabolism because the serum cholesterol levels are usually within normal limits and the patients have no signs of altered cholesterol metabolism such as xanthomas.

Some chyliform pleural effusions contain cholesterol crystals. The factors that dictate whether cholesterol crystals will be present are unknown. Cholesterol crystals have been seen in pleural fluid with cholesterol levels below 150 mg per dL, whereas other pleural fluids with cholesterol levels above 800 mg per dL have had none (50).

Clinical Manifestations

Chyliform pleural effusions are seen in patients with long-standing pleural effusions (50). The mean duration of the effusion is 5 years before it turns chyliform, but some chyliform effusions have developed within a year of onset. The two most common causes of the effusion initially are rheumatoid pleuritis and tuberculosis (50, 102, 103). Patients who have had artificial pneumothoraces for pulmonary tuberculosis and in whom the lung remains atelectatic with a resultant pleural effusion are particularly prone to chyliform pleural effusions (103). In many patients, the etiology of the original pleural effusion remains undetermined. Many pleural effusions secondary to paragonimiasis contain cholesterol crystals (104).

Many patients with chyliform pleural effusions are asymptomatic, or at least are no more symptomatic than when they initially developed the pleural effusion. Because the visceral pleura is usually thickened, the underlying lung contributes minimally to the total ventilation, and the patient may have dyspnea on exertion. Chyliform pleural effusions are usually unilateral.

Diagnosis

The diagnosis of chyliform pleural effusion is not usually difficult. When a patient with a long-standing pleural effusion is found to have turbid or milky pleural fluid, the two other diagnostic possibilities are empyema and chylothorax. In an empyema, centrifugation results in a clear supernatant. The differentiation between chylothorax and pseudochylothorax is not usually difficult; the patient with chylothorax has an acute pleural effusion and normal pleural surfaces, whereas the patient with pseudochylothorax has a chronic pleural effusion and a thickened or calcified pleura.

Analysis of the pleural fluid is useful in the differentiation of chylothorax and pseudochylothorax. If cholesterol crystals are seen on smears of the sediment, the patient has a chyliform pleural effusion. The cholesterol crystals give a distinct, satin-like sheen to the pleural fluid. Microscopically, the cholesterol crystals present a typical rhomboid configuration (Fig. 23.1). If no cholesterol crystals are seen, the patient may still have a chyliform effusion. Pleural fluid cholesterol levels above 200 mg per dL strongly suggest a chyliform effusion (101). The cholesterol levels in the pleural fluid are elevated in high-lipid pleural effusions owing to high numbers of cholesterol crystals or lecithin-globulin complexes (47), but cholesterol levels may also be elevated in chylous pleural effusions (9). Lipoprotein analysis should be performed if any doubt exists as to whether the fluid is chylous or pseudochylous because only chylous pleural fluid contains chylomicrons (9, 50). Some chyliform effusions have high (>250 mg per dL) triglyceride levels (50), so this finding is not diagnostic of chylothorax.

Treatment

When a patient is diagnosed as having a chyliform pleural effusion, the possibility of tuberculosis should always be entertained. If the patient has a history of tuberculosis and has never been treated with antituberculous therapy, isoniazid and rifampin should be given for at least 9 months. Similarly, if the patient has a positive purified protein derivative test, he or she should be treated with these drugs unless he or she has been treated previously or has received the bacille Calmette-Guérin vaccine.

If the patient's exercise capacity is limited by shortness of breath, a therapeutic thoracentesis should be performed. Hillerdal reported that the removal of several hundred milliliters of pleural fluid from patients with pseudochylothorax resulted in a markedly improved exercise tolerance (103). Decortication should be considered if the patient is symptomatic and the underlying lung is believed to be functional (105). The decortication may result in a markedly improved functional status for the patient (105).

REFERENCES

1. Miller JI Jr. Diagnosis and management of chylothorax. *Chest Surg Clin North Am* 1996;6:139–148.
2. Hillerdal G. Chylothorax and pseudochylothorax. *Eur Respir J* 1997;10:1157–1162.
3. Merrigan BA, Winter DC, O'Sullivan GC. Chylothorax. *Br J Surg* 1997;84:15–20.
4. Lampson RS. Traumatic chylothorax: a review of the literature and report of a case treated by mediastinal ligation of the thoracic duct. *J Thorac Surg* 1948;17:778–791.
5. Bower GC. Chylothorax: observations in 20 cases. *Dis Chest* 1964;46:464–468.
6. Williams KR, Burford TH. The management of chylothorax. *Ann Surg* 1964;160:131–140.
7. Breaux JR, Marks C. Chylothorax causing reversible T-cell depletion. *J Trauma* 1988;28:705–707.
8. Hodges CC, Fossum TW, Evering W. Evaluation of thoracic duct healing after experimental laceration and transection. *Vet Surg* 1993;22:431–435.
9. Staats BA, Ellefson RW, Budahn LL, et al. The lipoprotein profile of chylous and non-chylous pleural effusions. *Mayo Clin Proc* 1980;55:700–704.
10. Roy PH, Carr DT, Payne WS. The problem of chylothorax. *Mayo Clin Proc* 1967;42:457–467.
11. Strausser JL, Flye MW. Management of non-traumatic chylothorax. *Ann Thorac Surg* 1981;31:520–526.
12. Miller JI Jr. Anatomy of the thoracic duct and chylothorax. In: Shields TW, Locicero J III, Ponn RB, eds. *General thoracic surgery*, 5th ed. Philadelphia: Lippincott Williams & Wilkins, 2000:747–756.
13. Maloney JV, Spencer FC. The non-operative treatment of traumatic chylothorax. *Surgery* 1956;40:121–128.
14. Terzi A, Furlan G, Magnanelli G, et al. Chylothorax after pleuro-pulmonary surgery: a rare but unavoidable complication. *Thorac Cardiovasc Surg* 1994;42:81–84.
15. Dougenis D, Walker WS, Cameron EW, et al. Management of chylothorax complicating extensive esophageal resection. *Surg Gynecol Obstet* 1992;174:501–506.
16. Warren WH, Altman JS, Gregory SA. Chylothorax secondary to obstruction of the superior vena cava: a complication of the LeVeen shunt. *Thorax* 1990;45:978–979.
17. Zaidenstein R, Cohen N, Dishi V, et al. Chylothorax following median sternotomy. *Clin Cardiol* 1996;19:910–912.
18. Twomey CR. Chylothorax in the adult heart transplant patient: a case report. *Am J Crit Care* 1994;3:316–319.
19. Dupont PA. Chylothorax after high translumbar aortography. *Thorax* 1975;30:110–112.
20. Nygaard SD, Berger HA, Fick RB. Chylothorax as a complication of oesophageal sclerotherapy. *Thorax* 1992;47:134–135.
21. Nagai H, Shimizu K, Shikata J, et al. Chylous leakage after circumferential thoracolumbar fusion for correction of kyphosis resulting from fracture. Report of three cases. *Spine* 1997;22:2766–2769.
22. Thorne PS. Traumatic chylothorax. *Tubercle* 1958;39:29–34.
23. Cammarata SK, Brush RE Jr, Hyzy RC. Chylothorax after childbirth. *Chest* 1991;99:1539–1540.
24. Reilly KM, Tsou E. Bilateral chylothorax: a case report following episodes of stretching. *JAMA* 1975;233:536–537.
25. Chernick V, Reed MH. Pneumothorax and chylothorax in the neonatal period. *J Pediatr* 1970;76:624–632.
26. Van Aerde J, Campbell AN, Smyth JA, et al. Spontaneous chylothorax in newborns. *Am J Dis Child* 1984;138:961–964.
27. van Straaten HL, Gerards LJ, Krediet TG. Chylothorax in the neonatal period. *Eur J Pediatr* 1993;152:2–5.
28. Huang XZ, Wu JF, Ferrando R, et al. Fatal bilateral chylothorax in mice lacking the integrin $\alpha 9\beta_1$. *Mol Cell Biol* 2000;20:5208–5215.
29. Berman W Jr, Fripp RR, Yabek SM, et al. Great vein and right atrial thrombosis in critically ill infants and children with central venous lines. *Chest* 1991;99:963–967.
30. Van Veldhuizen PJ, Taylor S. Chylothorax: a complication of a left subclavian vein thrombosis. *Am J Clin Oncol* 1996;19:99–101.
31. Romero S, Martin C, Hernandez L, et al. Chylothorax in cirrhosis of the liver: analysis of its frequency and clinical characteristics. *Chest* 1998;114:154–159.
32. Villena V, de Pablo A, Martin-Escribano P. Chylothorax and chylous ascites due to heart failure. *Eur Respir J* 1995;8:1235–1236.
33. Hanna J, Truemper E, Burton E. Superior vena cava thrombosis and chylothorax: relationship in pediatric nephrotic syndrome. *Pediatr Nephrol* 1997;11:20–22.
34. Tie MLH, Poland GA, Rosenow EC III. Chylothorax in Gorham's syndrome. A common complication of a rare disease. *Chest* 1994;105:208–213.
35. Pennington DW, Warnock ML, Stulbarg MS. Chylothorax and respiratory failure in Kaposi's sarcoma. *West J Med* 1990;152:421–422.
36. Judson MA, Postic B. Chylothorax in a patient with AIDS and Kaposi's sarcoma. *South Med J* 1990;83:322–324.
37. Blankenship ME, Rowlett J, Timby JW, et al. Giant lymph node hyperplasia (Castleman's disease) presenting with chylous pleural effusion. *Chest* 1997;112:1132–1133.
38. Konishi T, Takeuchi H, Iwata J, et al. Behçet's disease with chylothorax—case report. *Angiology* 1988;39:68–71.

39. Coplu L, Emri S, Selcuk ZT, et al. Life threatening chylous pleural and pericardial effusion in a patient with Behĉet's syndrome. *Thorax* 1992;47:64–65.

40. Vennera MC, Moreno R, Cot J, et al. Chylothorax and tuberculosis. *Thorax* 1983;38:694–695.

41. Parker JM, Torrington KG, Phillips YY. Sarcoidosis complicated by chylothorax. *South Med J* 1994;87:860–862.

42. Dagenais F, Ferraro P, Duranceau A. Spontaneous chylothorax associated with primary lymphedema and a lymphangioma malformation. *Ann Thorac Surg* 1999;67:1480–1482.

43. Bresser P, Kromhout JG, Reekers JA, et al. Chylous pleural effusion associated with primary lymphedema and lymphangioma-like malformations. *Chest* 1993;103:1916–1918.

44. Lee YC, Tribe AE, Musk AW. Chylothorax from radiation-induced mediastinal fibrosis. *Aust N Z J Med* 1998;28:667–668.

45. Kollef MH. Recalcitrant chylothorax and chylous ascites associated with hypothyroidism. *Milit Med* 1993;158:63–65.

46. Milano S, Maroldi R, Vezzoli G, et al. Chylothorax after blunt chest trauma: an unusual case with a long latent period. *Thorac Cardiovasc Surg* 1994;42:187–190.

47. Hughes RL, Mintzer RA, Hidvegi DF, et al. The management of chylothorax. *Chest* 1979;76:212–218.

48. Vaz MAC, Teixeira LR, Vargas FS, et al. Relationship between pleural fluid and serum cholesterol levels. *Chest* 2001 (*in press*).

49. Wolthuis A, Landewe RB, Theunissen PH, et al. Chylothorax or leakage of total parenteral nutrition? *Eur Respir J* 1998;12:1233–1235.

50. Coe JE, Aikawa JK. Cholesterol pleural effusion. *Arch Intern Med* 1961;108:763–774.

51. Klepser RG, Berry JF. The diagnosis and surgical management of chylothorax with the aid of lipophilic dyes. *Dis Chest* 1954;25:409–426.

52. Thomson IA, Simms MH. Postoperative chylothorax: a case for recycling? *Cardiovasc Surg* 1993;1:384–385.

53. Ross JK. A review of the surgery of the thoracic duct. *Thorax* 1961;16:12–21.

54. Valentine VG, Raffin TA. The management of chylothorax. *Chest* 1992;102:586–591.

55. Lichter I, Hill GL, Nye ER. The use of medium-chain triglycerides in the treatment of chylothorax in a child. *Ann Thorac Surg* 1968;4:352–355.

56. Berkenbosch JW, Withington DE. Management of postoperative chylothorax with nitric oxide: a case report. *Crit Care Med* 1999;27:1022–1024.

57. Nguyen DM, Shum-Tim D, Dobell AR, et al. The management of chylothorax/chylopericardium following pediatric cardiac surgery: a 10-year experience. *J Cardiac Surg* 1995;10:302–308.

58. Cerfolio RJ, Allen MS, Deschamps C, et al. Postoperative chylothorax. *J Thorac Cardiovasc Surg* 1996;112:1361–1365.

59. Little AG, Kadowaki MH, Ferguson MK, et al. Pleuroperitoneal shunting: alternative therapy for pleural effusions. *Ann Surg* 1988;208:443–450.

60. Murphy MC, Newman BM, Rodgers BM. Pleuroperitoneal shunts in the management of persistent chylothorax. *Ann Thorac Surg* 1989;48:195–200.

61. Rheuban KS, Kron IL, Carpenter MA, et al. Pleuroperitoneal shunts for refractory chylothorax after operation for congenital heart disease. *Ann Thorac Surg* 1992;53:85–87.

62. Engum SA, Rescorla FJ, West KW, et al. The use of pleuroperitoneal shunts in the management of persistent chylothorax in infants. *J Pediatr Surg* 1999;34:286–290.

63. Shimizu J, Hayashi Y, Oda M, et al. Treatment of postoperative chylothorax by pleurodesis with the streptococcal preparation OK-432. *Thorac Cardiovasc Surg* 1994;42:233–236.

64. Adler RH, Levinsky L. Persistent chylothorax. *J Thorac Cardiovasc Surg* 1978;76:859–863.

65. Akaogi E, Mitsui K, Sohara Y, et al. Treatment of postoperative chylothorax with intrapleural fibrin glue. *Ann Thorac Surg* 1989;48:116–118.

66. Meurer MF, Cohen DJ. Current treatment of chylothorax: a case series and literature review. *Texas Med* 1990;86:82–85.

67. Robinson CLN. The management of chylothorax. *Ann Thorac Surg* 1985;39:90–95.

68. Weissberg D, Ben-Zeev I. Talc pleurodesis. Experience with 360 patients. *J Thorac Cardiovasc Surg* 1993;106:689-695.

69. Vargas FS, Milanez JRC, Filomeno LTB, et al. Intrapleural talc for the prevention of recurrence in benign or undiagnosed pleural effusions. *Chest* 1994;106:1771–1775.

70. Graham DD, McGahren ED, Tribble CG, et al. Use of video-assisted thoracic surgery in the treatment of chylothorax. *Ann Thorac Surg* 1994;57:1507–1511.

71. Mason PF, Ragoowansi RH, Thorpe JA. Postthoracotomy chylothorax—a cure in the abdomen? *Eur J Cardiothorac Surg* 1997;11:567–570.

72. Kent RB 3d, Pinson TW. Thoracoscopic ligation of the thoracic duct. *Surg Endosc* 1993;7:52–53.

73. Shirai T, Amano J, Takabe K. Thoracoscopic diagnosis and treatment of chylothorax after pneumonectomy. *Ann Thorac Surg* 1991;52:306–307.

74. Zoetmulder F, Rutgers E, Baas P. Thoracoscopic ligation of a thoracic duct leakage. *Chest* 1994;106:1233–1234.

75. Peillon C, D'Hont C, Melki J, et al. Usefulness of video thoracoscopy in the management of spontaneous and postoperation chylothorax. *Surg Endosc* 1999;13:1106–1109.

76. Ferguson MK. Thoracoscopy for empyema, bronchopleural fistula, and chylothorax. *Ann Thorac Surg* 1993;56:644–645.

77. Pui MH, Yueh TC. Lymphoscintigraphy in chyluria, chyloperitoneum and chylothorax. *J Nucl Med* 1998;39:1292–1296.

78. Mares DC, Mathur PN. Medical thoracoscopic talc pleurodesis for chylothorax due to lymphoma: a case series. *Chest* 1998;114:731–735.

79. Moss R, Hinds S, Fedullo AJ. Chylothorax: a complication of the nephrotic syndrome. *Am Rev Respir Dis* 1989;140:1436–1437.

80. Ballinger AB, Farthing MJ. Octreotide in the treatment of intestinal lymphangiectasia. *Eur J Gastroenterol Hepatol* 1998;10:699–702.

81. Perry RE, Hodgman J, Cass AB. Pleural effusion in the neonatal period. *J Pediatr* 1963;62:838–843.

82. Fernandez Alvarez JR, Kalache KD, Grauel EL. Management of spontaneous congenital chylothorax: oral

medium-chain triglycerides versus total parenteral nutrition. *Am J Perinatol* 1999;16:415–420.

83. Milson JW, Kron IL, Rheuban KS, et al. Chylothorax: an assessment of current surgical management. *J Thorac Cardiovasc Surg* 1985;89:221–227.

84. Urban T, Lazor R, Lacronique J, et al. Pulmonary lymphangioleiomyomatosis. A study of 69 patients. *Medicine (Baltimore)* 1999;78:321–337.

85. Chu SC, Horiba K, Usuki J, et al. Comprehensive evaluation of 35 patients with lymphangioleiomyomatosis. *Chest* 1999;115:1041–1052.

86. Silverstein EF, Ellis K, Wolff M, et al. Pulmonary lymphangiomyomatosis. *AJR Am J Roentgenol* 1974;120:832–850.

87. Carrington CB, Cugell DW, Gaensler EA, et al. Lymphangioleiomyomatosis. *Am Rev Respir Dis* 1977;116:977–995.

88. Sullivan EJ, Beck GJ, Peavy HH, et al. Lymphangioleiomyomatosis registry. *Chest* 1999;115:301.

89. Nagy B, Nabrady Z, Nemes Z. Pulmonary lymphangiomyomatosis in a preadolescent girl. *N Engl J Med* 1998;338:473–474.

90. Corrin B, Liebow AA, Friedman PJ. Pulmonary lymphangiomyomatosis. *Am J Pathol* 1975;79:348–367.

91. Luna CM, Gene R, Jolly EC, et al. Pulmonary lymphangiomyomatosis associated with tuberous sclerosis. *Chest* 1985;88:473–475.

92. Fraser RS, Muller NL, Colman N, et al. *Diagnosis of diseases of the chest,* 4th ed. Philadelphia: WB Saunders Company, 2000:679–686.

93. Taylor JR, Ryu J, Colby TV, et al. Lymphangioleiomyomatosis: clinical course in 32 patients. *N Engl J Med* 1990;323:1254–1260.

94. Tanaka H, Imada A, Morikawa T, et al. Diagnosis of pulmonary lymphangioleiomyomatosis by HMB45 in

surgically treated spontaneous pneumothorax. *Eur Respir J* 1995;8:1879–1882.

95. Kalassian KG, Doyle R, Kao P, et al. Lymphangioleiomyomatosis: new insights. *Am J Respir Crit Care Med* 1997;155:1183–1186.

96. Miller WT, Cornog JL, Sullivan MA. Lymphangiomyomatosis. *AJR Am J Roentgenol* 1972;111:565–572.

97. Kitaichi M, Nishimura K, Itoh H, et al. Pulmonary lymphangioleiomyomatosis: a report of 46 patients including a clinicopathologic study of prognostic factors. *Am J Respir Crit Care Med* 1995;151:527–533.

98. Johnson SR, Tattersfield AE. Decline in lung function in lymphangioleiomyomatosis: relation to menopause and progesterone treatment. *Am J Respir Crit Care Med* 1999;160:628–633.

99. Boehler A, Speich R, Russi EW, et al. Lung transplantation for lymphangioleiomyomatosis. *N Engl J Med* 1996;335:1275–1280.

100. Garcia-Zamalloa A, Ruiz-Irastorza G, Aguayo FJ, et al. Pseudochylothorax. Report of 2 cases and review of the literature. *Medicine (Baltimore)* 1999;78:200–207.

101. Hamm H, Pfalzer B, Fabel H. Lipoprotein analysis in a chyliform pleural effusion: implications for pathogenesis and diagnosis. *Respiration* 1991;58:294–300.

102. Ferguson GC. Cholesterol pleural effusion in rheumatoid lung disease. *Thorax* 1966;21:577–582.

103. Hillerdal G. Chyliform (cholesterol) pleural effusion. *Chest* 1985;86:426–428.

104. Johnson RJ, Johnson JR. Paragonimiasis in Indochinese refugees: roentgenographic findings with clinical correlations. *Am Rev Respir Dis* 1983;128:534–538.

105. Goldman A, Burford TH. Cholesterol pleural effusion: a report of three cases with a cure by decortication. *Dis Chest* 1950;18:586–594.

24

Other Pleural Diseases

PLEURAL DISEASE DUE TO ASBESTOS EXPOSURE

Exposure to asbestos can cause several different types of pleural disease. First, it can lead to a diffuse malignant mesothelioma, as described in Chapter 8; second, it can lead to a benign pleural effusion, as described in Chapter 20; third, it can bring about the development of pleural plaques or calcification; fourth, it can lead to massive pleural fibrosis; and fifth, it can produce a localized pleural abnormality called "rounded atelectasis," which is easily confused with a parenchymal tumor. Pleural plaques, massive pleural fibrosis, and rounded atelectasis are discussed in this chapter.

PLEURAL PLAQUES

These hyalinized fibrous tissue collections are located predominantly in the parietal pleura at the lateral and posterior intercostal spaces; over the mediastinal pleura, particularly at the pericardium; and over the dome of the diaphragm. These locations generally correspond to areas involved in the clearance of particles from the pleural space by the lymphatics (1). Pleural plaques are one of the earliest and most common manifestations of asbestos exposure and can serve as a marker for clinically relevant asbestos exposure. Although malignant transformation has never been demonstrated in a pleural plaque, the presence of large plaques (>4 cm) has been associated with an increased risk of developing mesothelioma (1). The large plaques serve as an indication of heavy exposure, and it is believed that these plaques do not undergo a malignant transformation.

Prevalence

The prevalence of pleural plaques is somewhat dependent on the population studied. Hillerdal reviewed the chest radiographs of a sizable proportion of the residents of Uppsala, Sweden, and found that the prevalence of pleural plaques in those individuals older than 40 years of age had increased from 0.2% in 1965 to 2.7% in 1985 (2). The prevalence of pleural plaques was 22% in 91 elevator construction workers who probably had been exposed to low levels of asbestos in their work (3). The incidence of pleural plaques at autopsy has varied from 0.5% to 58% (4, 5). When 16 separate studies with a total of 7,085 routine autopsies are combined, the prevalence of pleural plaques was 12.2% (4). The standard chest radiograph can be used to identify between 50% and 80% of the pleural plaques that are actually present (4).

Pleural plaques slowly develop in patients exposed to asbestos. Epler et al. (6) reviewed the chest radiographs of 1,135 patients who had been exposed to asbestos and reported that none of the patients developed pleural plaques during the 10 years after the initial exposure, and the incidence was still only about 10% 20 years after the initial exposure (6). Forty years after the initial exposure, however, over 50% of the patients had radiologically visible pleural plaques. The mean duration between the initial exposure to asbestos and the development of pleural plaques was 33 years in the series of Hillerdal (2). These plaques usually calcify within several years of becoming evident radiologically. Calcification of the pleural plaques rarely occurs within the first 20 years of initial exposure to asbestos, but by 40 years, over one third of these individuals have calcified pleural plaques (6).

Pleural plaques can also develop in individuals who are not occupationally exposed to asbestos. Kilburn et al. (7) reported that the prevalence of pleural abnormalities was 5.4% in the chest radiographs of 280 wives of asbestos workers who were initially exposed to asbestos at least 20 years previously. Churg and DePaoli (8) reported four cases of pleural plaques found at autopsy in individuals who resided in or near the chrysotile mining town of Thetford Mines, Quebec, but who did not work with asbestos. Mineral analysis of the lungs revealed that the individuals with pleural plaques had higher levels of tremolite but comparable levels of chrysotile than did the lungs of nine control subjects without pleural plaques. Constantopoulos et al. (9) reported that the prevalence of pleural calcification was 47% in 688 inhabitants of the Metsovo area in northwest Greece, an area where a solution containing tremolite was used to whitewash the houses.

Pathogenesis

Convincing evidence links pleural plaques to previous asbestos exposure. Kiviluoto (10) reviewed the place of residence of all individuals with bilateral pleural calcification in Finland and demonstrated that almost all such subjects lived near open asbestos pits. Hillerdal reported that 88% of 1,596 adults older than 40 years of age with pleural plaques had an occupational exposure to asbestos (2). Many patients who have pleural plaques at autopsy have a work history in which asbestos exposure would be expected (11, 12). Most pleural plaques contain many submicroscopic asbestos fibers that can be demonstrated by transmission electron microscopic examination, selective area electron diffraction, and microchemical analysis of particles (13, 14).

Ferruginous bodies (asbestos bodies), long considered the histologic hallmark of exposure to asbestos (15), consist of fibers coated by complexes of hemosiderin and glycoproteins and are believed to be formed by macrophages that have phagocytized the particles. Although these bodies have been shown to form from foreign inorganic and organic fibers of many different types, ferruginous bodies in most human lungs have asbestos as a core and are commonly known as *asbestos bodies* (15). Patients with pleural plaques have higher numbers of asbestos bodies in their lungs than do patients without pleural plaques (11, 16, 17). Conversely, the higher the number of asbestos bodies in the lungs, the more likely the presence of pleural plaques (15, 17). It should be noted, however, that the number of asbestos fibers that are uncoated or bare (and visible only on electron microscopy) exceeds the number of asbestos bodies, which are visible by light microscopy, by 5- to 10,000-fold (18).

It appears that the various types of asbestos fibers differ in their ability to induce pleural plaques. Exposure to crocidolite is most frequently associated with the production of pleural plaques. In North America, pleural plaques are more likely to result from tremolite than from chrysotile exposure. Churg et al. (19) correlated the presence of pleural plaques with the fiber type, fiber concentration, and fiber size as determined by analytic electron microscopy in 94 long-term chrysotile miners. They found that patients with pleural plaques had a significantly higher length-width ratio for the tremolite fibers than did those without plaques (19). It is believed by some that a substance other than chrysotile is responsible for pleural plaques in the asbestos mines in Canada (20).

Not all pleural plaques are due to asbestos exposure. Zeolite minerals are aluminum silicates that are widespread in the earth's crust. Erionite is a zeolite that is found in old volcanic sites such as in Turkey, New Zealand, areas of Japan, and in the southwestern United States. In a few villages in Turkey, the mineral has been used in buildings and for road construction, and a large percentage of the population has fiber-related pleural changes (21). One case of diffuse pleural thickening has been attributed to this fiber in Nevada (22). Wollastonite, a silicate that can be fibrous and that is used in ceramics, has been reported to cause pleural plaques (23). Talc, another mineral that is a flaky silicate, has been reported to be associated with plaque formation, but this mineral is often contaminated with amphiboles, so the relationship remains to be proven (24).

The mechanism by which asbestos fibers produce pleural plaques is unknown. Kiviluoto proposed that pleural plaques are formed in response to inflammation of the parietal pleura (10). When an asbestos fiber is inhaled, it passes toward the periphery of the lung. Kiviluoto suggested that the fiber pierces the visceral pleura and then rubs against and irritates the parietal pleura during respiratory movements. The resulting parietal pleural inflammation then gradually evolves into the hyaline plaque, which eventually calcifies. If this theory were correct, however, one would expect to find adhesions between the visceral and parietal pleura in the areas of pleural plaques, as well as long asbestos fibers in the parietal pleura.

Hillerdal has suggested that the short submicroscopic fibers are primarily responsible for the pleural plaques because these fibers can be demonstrated in the plaques (25). He proposes that these short fibers reach the pleural space by penetrating the pulmonary parenchyma and the visceral pleura. These fibers are then removed from the pleural space, as is all particulate matter, by the lymphatic vessels that lie in the parietal pleura. Some fibers are caught in the lymphatic vessels, however, and the presence of the fiber, in conjunction with the appropriate inflammatory cell, causes pleural plaques to form over many years. This hypothesis does not explain several important characteristics of the pleural plaques such as the bilaterality, the symmetric shape, the orientation parallel to the ribs, and sparing of the apices and costophrenic angle (4).

A third hypothesis for the pathogenesis of pleural plaques is that the microfibrils embolize to the parietal pleura by either the parenchymal lymphatic plexus or through the costal vascular supply. Then once present in the parietal pleura, the fiber itself or agents carried by the fiber appear to be responsible for initiating and promoting the inflammatory response. This hypothesis is very compatible with the peculiar characteristics of circumscribed pleural plaques (bilateral, symmetric, and orientated parallel to the ribs) (4).

If asbestos is injected intratracheally, it migrates to the pleura. In one study in rats (26), the asbestos fibers appeared in the pleural space within 3 days after intratracheal injection. Over a 30-day period, there were two peaks in the appearance of the asbestos fibers in the pleural space. The first peak occurred on day 7, at which time the mean length of the fiber was 1.2 μm. The second peak occurred on day 21 when the mean length of the fiber was only 0.3 μm (26).

The intrapleural injection of either crocidolite or chrysotile asbestos fibers leads to the development of a pleural effusion (27, 28). Sahn and Antony (28) injected chrysotile asbestos fibers into normal rabbits, which developed exudative pleural effusions within 4 hours. Over the next 120 hours, there was increasing metabolic activity in the pleural fluid, as evidenced by a falling pH and an increasing Pco_2. The animals developed pleural plaques that were evident by 7 days and completely developed by 1 month. Interestingly, if the rabbits were made neutropenic, they still developed the pleural effusion but subsequently developed marked pleural fibrosis and did not develop pleural plaques. The neutropenic rabbits did not have a macrophage influx as did the normal rabbits. These workers concluded that the pleural macrophage is important in localizing the asbestos fiber and in the ultimate formation of the pleural plaque. When a critical number of macrophages is not present, disorganization and widespread fibrosis occur (28).

Several studies have demonstrated that the exposure of mesothelial cells in cell culture to asbestos particles can induce the cells to produce substances associated with the development of fibrosis. If rat pleural mesothelial cells are exposed to crocidolite or chrysotile asbestos fibers, the asbestos fibers are actively phagocytosed and are incorporated within the phagosomes. Both types of asbestos also stimulate the mesothelial cells to produce fibronectin, a substance with fibroblast chemoattractant activity (29). In contrast, quartz and carbonyl iron particles do not induce similar changes (29). After interaction with cells, asbestos fibers can also trigger a number of signaling cascades involving mitogen-activated protein kinases and nuclear factor kappa-B (30). These signaling cascades can result in the production of various inflammatory mediators such as tumor necrosis factor-α (TNF-α), interleukin-1 (IL-1), IL-6, IL-8, and TGF-β (30). The induction of

TGF-β is particularly noteworthy because it is one of the most fibrogenic agents ever discovered.

Pathologic Features

Macroscopically, pleural plaques appear as discrete, raised, irregularly shaped areas separated by normal or slightly thickened pleura (16). These plaques are always on the parietal pleura and are found most commonly on the posterior wall of the lower half of the pleural space. Pleural plaques on the costal pleura usually have an elliptical shape, running parallel to the ribs superiorly and inferiorly (16). Pleural plaques usually do not occur in the apices of the pleural cavities or in the costophrenic angles (16). The thinner plaques are only slightly raised above the pleural surface and are grayish white in color, whereas the thicker plaques are ivory or cream colored. The diameter of the plaques varies from a few millimeters to 10 cm (16). The pleural plaques are usually multiple, and the costal pleura can look like an archipelago of different-sized plaques (24).

Microscopically, the plaques consist of collagenous connective tissue containing few cells (14, 16). The connective tissue is arranged in a coarse, basket-weave pattern and contains only a few capillaries. Normal mesothelium covers the plaques. The boundary between a plaque and the surrounding normal pleura is always sharply demarcated (16). Elastin stains show the continuity of the lamellae beneath the plaque with the surrounding normal parietal pleural connective tissue. Some calcium deposition is present in a high proportion of plaques (16). Although no asbestos fibers are visible by light microscopy, electron microscopic study demonstrates many submicroscopic fibers in almost all plaques (14).

Radiologic Features

Noncalcified pleural plaques are frequently not visible on the posteroanterior (PA) and lateral chest radiographs (11, 12). The earliest radiologically visible change is a line of increased density adjacent to a rib (Fig. 24.1), usually the seventh or eighth rib (13, 14, 25). As the plaque enlarges,

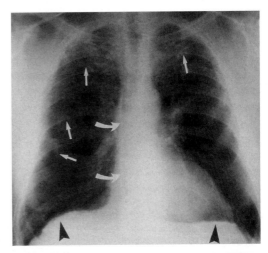

FIG. 24.1. Pleural plaques. Posteroanterior radiograph of a 62-year-old man with prior asbestos exposure and a 40-pack-a-year smoking history shows bilateral calcified pleural plaques *(straight arrows)* and diffuse calcification of the mediastinal *(curved arrows)* and diaphragmatic *(arrowheads)* pleura.

it becomes elliptical and protuberant, with tapering superior and inferior margins typical of an extrapleural lesion. A plaque rarely extends vertically for more than four interspaces. The thickness of the plaque varies from 1 to more than 10 mm but is usually in the range of 1 to 5 mm. Involvement of the apices or the costophrenic angles by pleural plaques is rare. Pleural plaques are usually bilateral and are often symmetric. When the pleural plaques are unilateral, they are left sided about 75% of the time (31). In addition, if the disease is bilateral, there tends to be more disease on the left side (32). The explanation for this left-sided predominance is unknown, but it may be related to the heart obscuring the pleural changes on the left. Gallego recently performed computed tomography (CT) scans on 40 adults with asbestos exposure and reported that the average plaque area on the right of 47.8 cm^2 was not significantly different from the average plaque area on the left of 45.3 cm^2 (33).

On a standard chest radiograph, pleural plaques are most clearly defined when viewed tangentially, that is, in profile along their long axes.

A routine PA chest radiograph distinctly demonstrates a plaque located on the inner surface of the lateral chest wall because the x-ray beam passes through more of the plaque. Noncalcified pleural plaques are best visualized by radiography at 110 to 140 kV, whereas calcification within plaques is best demonstrated at 80 kV.

When the x-ray beam is perpendicular to the plaque, the plaque is presented in a frontal or *en face* orientation. When viewed *en face*, small, noncalcified plaques are difficult to see and are perceived as ill-defined, irregular densities adjacent to the ribs. The en face plaque rarely appears uniformly rounded; rather, it shows a peripheral irregularity of contour that has been likened to the fringe of a map or a lily leaf (13). Because of its faintness in outline, the plaque is often overlooked or is dismissed as an artifact.

Conventional and high-resolution CT scans are more sensitive at detecting pleural plaques than is the standard chest radiograph. In one study of 159 asbestos-exposed workers with a normal chest radiograph, pleural plaques were detected in 59 (37.1%) by CT scan. The conventional CT detected pleural plaques in 58 of the patients, whereas the high-resolution CT detected the pleural plaques in only 48 cases (34). On CT, plaques appear as discrete soft tissue or calcific thickening of the pleural surface (Fig. 24.2). Focal plaques are commonly observed in the posterior and paraspinous regions of the thorax, areas that are poorly seen on chest radiographs.

Differential Radiologic Diagnosis

The greatest problem in the diagnosis of early plaque formation lies in distinguishing plaques from normal companion shadows of the chest wall. At autopsy, some degree of fat accumulation is almost always visible on gross examination along the chest wall in the reflections of the parietal pleura, oriented parallel to the long axes of the ribs on the subpleural osseous surfaces (35). More extensive fat deposits tend to form pads and folds concentrated at the level of the midthoracic wall in the region of the fourth to eighth ribs. Subpleural fat and pleural plaques are frequently indistinguishable on standard chest ra-

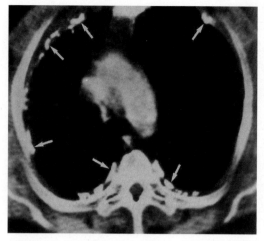

FIG. 24.2. CT scan of patient in Fig. 24.1 after administration of intravenous contrast material shows numerous bilateral calcified pleural plaques *(arrows)*, characteristic of asbestos-related pleural disease.

diographs (35). The chest CT scan is efficient at distinguishing pleural plaques from subpleural fat. If a pleural abnormality is not calcified, a CT scan should probably be obtained to verify that the pleural abnormalities are indeed plaques, particularly if litigation is involved. When two series are combined (35, 36), 87 patients were thought to have pleural plaques on their standard chest radiographs. When they underwent CT examination, however, only 48 of the patients (55%) had pleural plaques, whereas the remainder had fat pads.

On the normal PA chest radiograph, a vertical line of water density may parallel the medial surface of the first three or four ribs along the lateral thoracic wall (13). This line is formed by a combination of muscles, the areolar tissue of the endothoracic fascia, and fat, but it is distinguishable from pleural plaques because plaques rarely extend superior to the third rib and are most prominent at the level of the seventh and eighth ribs. Below the level of the fourth rib, 1 mL is generally considered the maximal acceptable thickness for this normal pleural shadow (14).

The costal slips of origin of the serratus anterior and external abdominal oblique muscles have been confused with pleural plaques because they produce a characteristic rhythmic sequence of shadows between successive intercostal spaces. These anatomic structures are most commonly visible over the eighth rib, but the fifth through the ninth ribs may be involved. These costal slips of muscular origin appear either as one or two distinct triangular shadows or a combination of two opacities superimposed, and they can usually be differentiated from pleural plaques in that the muscle shadow has one sharply defined border and elsewhere fades into the surrounding soft tissues.

The diaphragm is also a common site for pleural plaques. In the PA projection, the plaques usually affect the middle third of each diaphragm and rarely occur within 2.5 cm of the lateral chest wall. Most fibrous plaques are rounded or button-like and may easily be confused with the normal polycyclic outline of the diaphragm because of uneven muscle contraction.

PLEURAL CALCIFICATION

As mentioned earlier in this chapter, pleural plaques often become calcified. Forty years after the initial exposure to asbestos, nearly 40% of individuals have radiologically demonstrable pleural calcification (6). In general, calcified plaques are more striking than uncalcified plaques on the radiograph. When the x-ray beam strikes a plaque tangentially, the calcification is seen as a dense white line, usually discontinuous, paralleling the chest wall, diaphragm, or cardiac border (Figs. 24.1). Because the calcium is deposited near the center of the typical subpleural hyalinized plaque, it is separated from the inner surface of the rib by a line of water density. If the x-ray beam strikes the surface of the calcified plaque en face, it presents an irregular and unevenly dense pattern.

Differential Diagnosis

Asbestos exposure is not the only cause of localized pleural thickening or pleural calcification. Discrete, localized, noncalcified pleural thickening may occur with localized mesothelioma,

metastatic disease, lymphoma, or myeloma (13). Pleural thickening from these diseases is usually unilateral. Localized pleural thickening and callus formation simulating asbestos pleural plaques may occur following rib fractures. The changes in such patients are usually unilateral, and the overlying rib deformity suggests the diagnosis (13). Pleural plaques, which may or may not be calcified, occur in other pneumoconioses including those caused by tremolite talc, mica, Bakelite, calcimine, tin, barite, and silica. Concomitant exposure to asbestos is probably responsible for the pleural plaques seen with such diseases, however (13).

The other main causes of diffuse pleural calcification are long-standing inflammatory diseases, particularly hemothorax, empyema, postpleurodesis, or repeated iatrogenic pneumothorax for tuberculosis therapy. In such instances, the pleural thickening is unilateral, and the calcification is often extensive and sheetlike. The thickening is usually on the visceral pleura, and the calcification occurs in the inner aspect of the pleural thickening (Fig. 24.3).

Significance

Bilateral pleural plaques or calcifications are significant as an index of previous exposure to asbestos. It is controversial whether patients with pleural plaques have an increased risk of lung cancer when the level of smoking is taken into consideration (37). Weiss reviewed the English language literature in 1993 and concluded that the weight of evidence favors the conclusion that persons with asbestos-related pleural plaques do not have an increased risk of lung cancer in the absence of parenchymal asbestosis (38). In 1994, Hillerdal reviewed the incidence of bronchial carcinoma and mesothelioma in 1,596 men with pleural plaques initially detected between 1963 and 1985. He found that 50 bronchial carcinomas occurred, whereas 32.1 were expected, and that 9 mesotheliomas occurred, whereas only 0.8 were expected (39). The risk of cancer and mesotheliomas therefore is probably somewhat increased in patients with pleural plaques, and they should be encouraged to stop smoking.

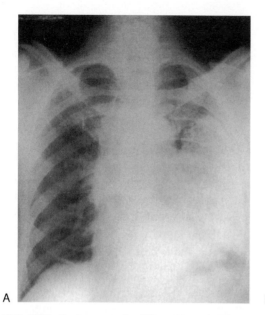 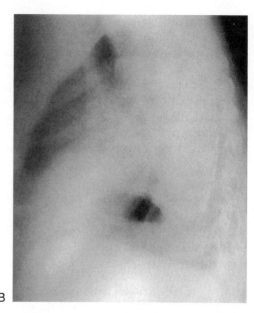

A   B

FIG. 24.3. Posteroanterior **(A)** and lateral **(B)** chest radiographs of a 69-year-old man who sustained a gunshot wound to the left chest 30 years previously show a large irregular dense opacity obscuring much of the left lung on the posteroanterior (PA) view and both lungs on the lateral view. On the lateral view, note the dense calcific opacity conforming to the outline of the pleural space.

It is unclear whether the presence of pleural plaques alone results in a decrease in the pulmonary function tests when there is no parenchymal asbestosis and when smoking is taken into consideration. Schwartz et al. (40) performed spirometry on 1,211 sheet metal workers. They reported that the forced vital capacity (FVC) in the 258 individuals with circumscribed plaque was 3.75 L compared with an FVC of 4.09 in 877 workers without pleural fibrosis. In a subsequent study, this same group was able to demonstrate a significant relationship between the volume of the pleural fibrosis as computed from the three-dimensional reconstruction of the high-resolution CT scan and the total lung capacity (41). The mean total lung capacity, however, of 24 patients with pleural fibrosis was 106% of predicted (41). Fridriksson et al. (42) studied 45 men with asbestos-related pleural plaques of at least 5 mm thickness without parenchymal abnormalities. They found that when the level of smoking was taken into consideration, the mean total lung capacity was 16% below predicted, whereas the vital capacity was 15% below predicted. The lung compliance was decreased by approximately 40%. Patients with calcified pleural plaques had more severe changes in lung physiology than those who had only hyaline plaques. They attributed the functional abnormalities to subclinical parenchymal disease. In a recent study of 51 patients with pleural plaques (32 of which were demonstrable only by CT scan), the presence of the pleural plaque was not associated with any reduction in pulmonary function (43). Certainly, the functional abnormalities produced by pleural plaques alone are not sufficient to produce symptoms. Shih et al. (44) demonstrated that the maximal work capacity was 91.4% of predicted in 20 patients with pleural plaques and no asbestosis of the lung on chest radiograph.

DIFFUSE THICKENING

In addition to the occurrence of parietal pleural plaques, exposure to asbestos may be followed by the development of diffuse pleural fibrosis. Although some authors consider this diffuse pleural fibrosis to be part of the spectrum of parenchymal asbestosis (14), it appears to be a distinct

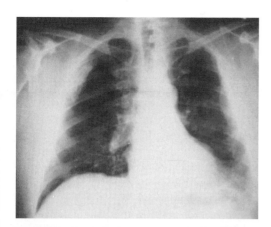

FIG. 24.4. Posteroanterior chest radiograph demonstrating diffuse pleural thickening and blunting of the left costophrenic angle from a patient with a history of asbestos exposure.

entity (2, 45–47). In contrast to pleural plaques, diffuse pleural fibrosis commonly involves the costophrenic angles, is associated with involvement of the visceral pleura with pleural symphysis (Fig. 24.4), and sometimes involves a marked loss of pulmonary function that can lead to hypercapnic respiratory failure (45–47).

The incidence of diffuse pleural fibrosis is much lower than that of pleural plaques. Hillerdal (45), in surveying a group of asbestos workers, found 827 individuals with pleural plaques but only 27 with progressive pleural thickening. Schwartz et al. (40) reviewed the chest radiographs of 1,211 sheet metal workers and reported that 260 had circumscribed plaques, whereas 74 had diffuse thickening. One report suggested that the development of pleural fibrosis was more common with HLA phenotype DQ2 (48).

Although bromocriptine and asbestos exposure can each lead to the development of diffuse pleural fibrosis, it appears that the administration of bromocriptine and a history of asbestos exposure act synergistically to produce diffuse pleural fibrosis (49). Hillerdal et al. (49) reported on a series of 15 patients who had a history of asbestos exposure and who developed diffuse bilateral pleural thickening after taking bromocriptine for Parkinson's disease for 1 to 10 years. The patients complained of malaise, often associated with weight loss, dyspnea, and a disturbing cough. When the bromocriptine was withdrawn, the patients improved clinically. However, in most cases, the diffuse pleural fibrosis and the restrictive lung function defect persisted (49).

The pathogenesis of diffuse pleural thickening is unknown. However, its locale and strong association with interstitial fibrosis suggest that it may be a direct extension of parenchymal fibrosis to the visceral pleura (4). Subpleural interstitial fibrosis has been a constant feature in the limited studies using high-resolution CT (HRCT) in subjects with diffuse pleural disease (50). This does not explain the observation that diffuse pleural fibrosis associated with asbestos exposure frequently follows a benign asbestos pleural effusion (see Chapter 20). Epler et al. (6) reviewed 1,135 asbestos workers and found that of the 44 patients with diffuse thickening greater than 5 mm, almost 50% had had a previous asbestos pleural effusion. Of 35 workers with asbestos effusion, 54% had residual diffuse pleural thickening. Hillerdal documented that the initiating event in 4 of 27 patients with progressive pleural thickening was a benign pleural effusion (45). Diffuse pleural thickening secondary to asbestos exposure almost always involves the costophrenic angle and invariably becomes bilateral, although it may be unilateral at first. This diffuse pleural thickening starts at the bases and progresses at a variable rate. Thickening of the pleural cap may be considerable (45). Although routine radiographs do not demonstrate pleural calcification in the majority of patients, CT scanning often demonstrates pleural calcification (46). Many patients with diffuse pleural fibrosis have no evidence of intrapulmonary fibrosis on a CT scan (46).

Patients with diffuse pleural thickening tend to have symptoms from their pleural disease. In one study, 61 of 64 patients (95%) complained of significant breathlessness on exertion (51). In the same series, 56% of the patients complained of chest pain, which was more frequently precipitated by exertion than by deep inspiration. Six of the patients complained of regular chest pain, which they found to be a constant problem (51).

Patients with diffuse pleural thickening have a significant decrease in the results of their pulmonary function testing (46, 51). In one study of 64 patients with diffuse pleural thickening, the results for various pulmonary functions expressed as a percent of predicted was as follows: FEV_1, 62%; FVC, 77%; TLC, 71%; Dlco, 74%; and Kco 104% (51). In this study, there was no accelerated decline in pulmonary function over a mean follow-up period of 9 years (51). The exercise capacity of some patients with diffuse pleural fibrosis is diminished (44, 52). In one study of 12 patients with diffuse pleural thickening, the mean work capacity was 82.7% of predicted. The intense dyspnea during exercise has been attributed to the rapid shallow breathing pattern that these patients exhibit during exercise. Oxygen desaturation does not occur, and there is no definite evidence that the patients develop respiratory muscle fatigue (52).

The diagnosis of diffuse pleural thickening secondary to asbestos exposure is usually based primarily on the history of exposure. Pleural plaques are present in the majority of patients with diffuse pleural thickening secondary to asbestos exposure (53). In addition, the diffuse thickening secondary to asbestos exposure is usually bilateral and does not involve nodular invasion of the lung (53). One must worry about the possibility of mesothelioma in patients with diffuse thickening from asbestos exposure, particularly if the disease is not symmetric. Features that suggest neoplasm are the presence of pleural nodularity or ring, parietal pleura thickening greater than 1 cm, or involvement of the mediastinal pleural surfaces (50).

The optimal management of patients with progressive pleural fibrosis due to asbestos exposure is unknown. Wright et al. (46) suggested that because these patients have an increased elastic recoil and a normal diffusing capacity when corrected for lung volume, they might benefit from decortication. Hillerdal, however, performed decortication on four patients and reported that only one of them improved subjectively (45). He attributed the lack of improvement to concomitant parenchymal fibrosis. Fielding et al. (54) subjected four patients with diffuse pleural thickening and opiate-resistant chest pain to thoracotomy and decortication; and reported that the results were disappointing.

ROUNDED ATELECTASIS

Rounded atelectasis refers to atelectasis of the peripheral lung resulting from pleural adhesions and fibrosis. Rounded atelectasis can mimic a pulmonary neoplasm because it presents as a peripheral mass. Rounded atelectasis consists of a peripheral part of the lung that has become atelectatic secondary to the pleural inflammation (55). Rounded atelectasis may occur anywhere in the chest, but by far the most common site is along the posterior surface of the lower lobe. Aerated lung is interposed between the mass and the diaphragm (55). It may be unilateral or bilateral. At thoracotomy, fibrous tissue can always be peeled off in several layers. After extensive dissection, the lung fully expands. The most probable explanation for rounded atelectasis is that an inflammatory reaction starts in the visceral pleura and leads to formation of fibrous tissue on the lung surface. This tissue consequently shrinks and causes atelectasis of the underlying lung (56).

Rounded atelectasis is usually due to asbestos exposure. Dernevik and Gatzinsky (56) reported pleural plaques in 29 of 37 cases (78%) of rounded atelectasis. Hillerdal and Ozesmi (57) reported that six of 60 patients (10%) with benign asbestos pleural effusion developed rounded atelectasis. Rounded atelectasis has also been reported in conjunction with tuberculosis, parapneumonic effusions, pulmonary embolization, and Dressler's syndrome (58). It is likely that any disease that produces localized inflammation of the visceral pleura can lead to rounded atelectasis.

The main importance of rounded atelectasis is that it must be differentiated from a malignant lung lesion. The rounded atelectasis itself does not produce symptoms. The roentgenologic picture is often suggestive of the diagnosis, whereas a CT scan is frequently diagnostic (Fig. 24.5). On the standard chest radiograph, rounded atelectasis appears as a spherical, sharply marginated mass abutting the pleura. Pleural thickening

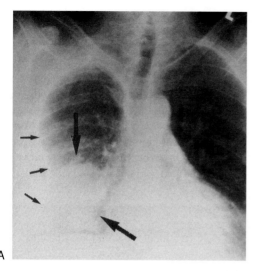

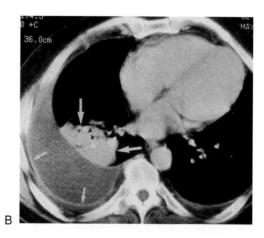

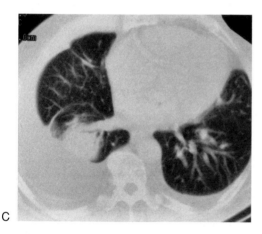

FIG. 24.5. Asbestos-related pleural disease and rounded atelectasis in a 62-year-old man with a 20-year history of asbestos exposure. **A:** PA chest radiograph shows a large right pleural effusion *(short arrows)* and a right lower lobe "mass" *(large arrows)*. **B:** CT scan with intravenous contrast demonstrates enhancement of the parietal pleura *(short arrows)*, indicating a chronic pleural effusion. The parenchyma "mass" *(long arrows)*, in contact with the visceral pleural surface, represents collapsed lung. The atelectatic lung has a rounded shape owing to fibrous adhesions and infolding of the visceral pleura. Air bronchograms are seen within the collapsed lung *(arrowhead)*. **C:** CT scan (lung windows) show the comet tail sign or the vacuum cleaner effect, both descriptions of how the vessels leading toward the atelectic lung diverge and arc around the undersurface of the atelectatic lung before merging with it.

is always present and frequently is thickest near the mass. The comet tail sign is produced by the crowding together of bronchi and blood vessels that extend from the lower border of the mass to the hilum (Fig. 24.5D). Although these features may be appreciated on standard radiographs, CT shows the characteristic features to better advantage, including the associated pleural thickening and peripheral location of the mass (59). Fine-needle biopsy can be performed easily because the lesion is pleural-based, but its utility is limited because malignancy cannot be excluded (58). Thoracotomy is definitive, but should rarely be necessary (24).

DIFFUSE BILATERAL PLEURAL THICKENING UNRELATED TO ASBESTOS

Although asbestos exposure accounts for most cases of diffuse bilateral pleural thickening, there are other causes. These include drugs, particularly bromocriptine (see Chapter 19); collagen vascular disease (see Chapter 18); and infectious diseases, which usually produce unilateral pleural thickening. Nevertheless, there are some cases for which no etiology is apparent. Buchanan et al. (60) described four patients with bilateral pleural effusions progressing to diffuse pleural thickening for which there was no evidence of an infective, embolic, or occupational cause. Histology showed that in all cases, both layers of the pleura were thickened by fibrous tissue and frequently the pleural space was obliterated. Interestingly, all four cases were HLA-B44 positive. Pleural decortication was successful in the three patients on whom this procedure was attempted (60). Pleural fibrosis can be familial. Azoulay et al. (61) reported three sisters with bilateral isolated apical pleural fibrosis that progressed to produce severe bilateral fibrosis (61). Two of the sisters died of respiratory failure, and the third received a lung transplant.

FIBROTHORAX

When pleural inflammation is intense, its resolution may be associated with the deposition of a thick layer of dense fibrous tissue on the visceral pleura. The patient is then said to have a fibrothorax. As a result of the marked pleural thickening, the hemithorax becomes contracted, and its mobility is reduced (62). As the fibrothorax progresses, the intercostal spaces may narrow, the size of the involved hemithorax may diminish, and the mediastinum may be displaced ipsilaterally. Radiologically, a peel of uniform thickness surrounds the lung. Calcification occurs frequently on the inner aspect of the peel (Fig. 24.3) and provides an indicator by which the thickness of the peel may be accurately measured (62). The three main causes of fibrothorax are hemothorax, tuberculosis, and bacterial lung infection (62), but pancreatitis (63), collagen vascular disease (64), and uremia (65) can lead to fibrothorax. In a few instances, no etiology is ever discovered (66).

Clinical Manifestations

Pulmonary function is severely compromised in fibrothorax. The degree of functional abnormality is much greater than one would expect from the degree of pleural disease (67). Pleural thickening in the costophrenic angle can cause profound alterations in the ventilation of and blood flow to the entire lung. Routine pulmonary func-

tion testing reveals mild-to-severe restrictive ventilatory dysfunction. Surprisingly, the blood flow is reduced more than the ventilation of the affected side (68). In a study of 127 patients (68), the mean oxygen uptake on the affected side was 19% of the total, whereas the mean ventilation was 33% of the total. This finding is in contrast to parenchymal diseases, in which the oxygen uptake and ventilation are reduced to the same degree (68). In severe disease, there is no ventilation or perfusion to the affected side (68).

Treatment

The only treatment available for fibrothorax is decortication, which involves removing the fibrous peel from the visceral pleura. The functional improvement following decortication has been variable (62, 67, 68). The most important clinical factor is the extent of the disease in the underlying lung (67, 68). The vital capacity may improve more than 50% following decortication if no underlying parenchymal disease is present, but the vital capacity may even decrease following decortication in patients with extensive parenchymal disease. Even in patients with longstanding fibrothorax, decortication can still lead to functional improvement. One case report noted a marked subjective improvement in a patient who had had a fibrothorax for 44 years (67).

Which patients should have decortication? Patients with recent hemothorax (see Chapter 22), recent empyema in which the infection is controlled (see Chapter 9), or recent tuberculous pleuritis (see Chapter 10) should not have a decortication because the pleural thickening frequently resolves by itself over several months. Therefore, decortication should be considered only if the pleural thickening has been stable or progressive over at least a 6-month period. If the pleural thickening has been present for several months and if the patient's way of life is compromised by exertional dyspnea, decortication should probably be performed unless previous chest radiographs demonstrated extensive parenchymal disease. Decortication is a major surgical procedure and should not be performed on patients debilitated by other diseases. In one series of

141 patients, the mortality rate with decortication was 3.5% (56).

INTRATHORACIC SPLENOSIS

Splenosis is defined as the autotransplantation of splenic tissue, usually after rupture of the spleen. Most commonly, it is discovered as innumerable purple nodules coating the mesentery, omentum, and peritoneal surfaces of the abdominal cavity. When the diaphragm and spleen are lacerated simultaneously, seeding of the pleural cavities can occur.

Intrathoracic splenosis can present with solitary or multiple pleural-based nodules (69). The presentation may be 15 years or more after the spleen was injured. A clue to the diagnosis is the absence of Howell-Jolly bodies, pitted erythrocytes, and siderocytes in the peripheral blood of asplenic individuals. Normally asplenic individuals have these abnormalities in their peripheral blood smear. However, if there is functional splenic tissue elsewhere, such as in the chest, these cells will be absent. Technetium-99m–labeled sulfur colloid radionucleotide scanning can identify residual splenic tissue. If the patient is asymptomatic, no therapy is indicated.

REFERENCES

1. Nishimura SL, Broaddus VC. Asbestos-induced pleural disease. *Clin Chest Med* 1998;19:311–329.
2. Hillerdal G. Pleural plaques in the general population. *Ann NY Acad Sci* 1991;643:430–437.
3. Bresnitz EA, Gilman MJ, Gracely EJ, et al. Asbestos-related radiographic abnormalities in elevator construction workers. *Am Rev Respir Dis* 1993;147:1341–1344.
4. Schwartz DA. New developments in asbestos-induced pleural disease. *Chest* 1991;99:191–198.
5. Karjalainen A, Karhunen PJ, Lalu K, et al. Pleural plaques and exposure to mineral fibres in a male urban necropsy population. *Occup Environ Med* 1994;51:456–460.
6. Epler GR, McLoud TC, Gaensler EA. Prevalence and incidence of benign asbestos pleural effusion in a working population. *JAMA* 1982;247:617–622.
7. Kilburn KH, Warshaw R, Thornton JC. Asbestos diseases and pulmonary symptoms and signs in shipyard workers and their families in Los Angeles. *Arch Intern Med* 1986;146:2213–2220.
8. Churg A, DePaoli L. Environmental pleural plaques in residents of a Quebec chrysotile mining town. *Chest* 1988;94:58–69.
9. Constantopoulos SH, Theodoracopoulos P, Dascalopoulos G, et al. Tremolite whitewashing and pleural calcifications. *Chest* 1987;92:709–712.
10. Kiviluoto R. Pleural calcification as a roentgenologic sign of non-occupational endemic anthophyllite-asbestosis. *Acta Radiol* 1960;194[Suppl]:1–67.
11. Hourihane DO'B, Lessof L, Richardson PC. Hyaline and calcified pleural plaques as an index of exposure to asbestos: a study of radiological and pathological features of 100 cases with a consideration of epidemiology. *Br Med J* 1966;1:1069–1074.
12. Hillerdal G, Lindgren A. Pleural plaques: correlation of autopsy findings to radiographic findings and occupational history. *Eur J Respir Dis* 1980;61:315–319.
13. Sargent EN, Jacobson G, Gordonson JS. Pleural plaques: a signpost of asbestos dust inhalation. *Semin Roentgenol* 1977;12:287–297.
14. Becklake MR. Asbestos-related diseases of the lung and other organs: their epidemiology and implications for clinical practice. *Am Rev Respir Dis* 1976;114:187–227.
15. Craighead JE, Mossman BT. The pathogenesis of asbestos-associated diseases. *N Engl J Med* 1982;306:1446–1455.
16. Roberts GH. The pathology of parietal pleural plaques. *J Clin Pathol* 1971;24:348–353.
17. Kishimoto T, Ono T, Okada K, et al. Relationship between number of asbestos bodies in autopsy lung and pleural plaques on chest x-ray film. *Chest* 1989;95:549–552.
18. Becklake MR, Cowie RL. Pneumoconioses. In: Murray JF, Nadel JA, eds. *Textbook of respiratory medicine.* Philadelphia: WB Saunders Company, 2000:1811–1851.
19. Churg A, Wright JL, Vedal S. Fiber burden and patterns of asbestos-related disease in chrysotile miners and millers. *Am Rev Respir Dis* 1993;148:25–31.
20. Gibbs GW. Etiology of pleural calcification: a study of Quebec chrysotile miners and millers. *Arch Environ Health* 1979;34:76–83.
21. Baris I, Simonato L, Artivinli M, et al. Epidemiological and environmental evidence of the health effects of exposure to erionite fibres: a four-year study in the Cappadocian region of Turkey. *Int J Cancer* 1987;39:10–17.
22. Casey KR, Shigeoka JW, Rom WN, et al. Zeolite exposure and associated pneumoconiosis. *Chest* 1985;87:837–840.
23. Huuskonen MS, Tossavainen A, Koskinen H, et al. Wollastonite exposure and lung fibrosis. *Environ Res* 1983;30:291–304.
24. Hillerdal G. Nonmalignant pleural disease related to asbestos exposure. *Clin Chest Med* 1985;6:141–152.
25. Hillerdal G. The pathogenesis of pleural plaques and pulmonary asbestosis: possibilities and impossibilities. *Eur J Respir Dis* 1980;61:129–138.
26. Viallat JR, Raybuad F, Passarel M, et al. Pleural migration of chrysotile fibers after intratracheal injection in rats. *Arch Environ Health* 1986;41:282–286.

27. Shore BL, Daughaday CC, Spilberg I. Benign asbestos pleurisy in the rabbit. *Am Rev Respir Dis* 1983;128: 481–485.

28. Sahn SA, Antony VB. Pathogenesis of pleural plaques: relationship of early cellular response and pathology. *Am Rev Respir Dis* 1984;130:884–887.

29. Kuwahara M, Kuwahara M, Verma K, et al. Asbestos exposure stimulates pleural mesothelial cells to secrete the fibroblast chemoattractant, fibronectin. *Am J Respir Cell Mol Biol* 1994;10:167–176.

30. Robledo R, Mossman B. Cellular and molecular mechanisms of asbestos-induced fibrosis. *J Cell Physiol* 1999;180:158–166.

31. Withers BF, Ducatman AM, Yang WN. Roentgenographic evidence for predominant left-sided location of unilateral pleural plaques. *Chest* 1989;95: 1262–1264.

32. Hu H, Beckett L, Kelsey K, et al. The left-sided predominance of asbestos-related pleural disease. *Am Rev Respir Dis* 1993;148:981–984.

33. Gallego JC. Absence of left-sided predominance in asbestos-related pleural plaques: a CT study. *Chest* 1998;113:1034–1036.

34. Gevenois PA, De Vuyst P, Dedeire S, et al. Conventional and high-resolution CT in asymptomatic asbestos-exposed workers. *Acta Radiol* 1994;35:226–229.

35. Sargent EN, Boswell WD Jr, Ralls PW, et al. Subpleural fat pads in patients exposed to asbestos: distinction from non-calcified pleural plaques. *Radiology* 1984;152: 273–277.

36. Friedman AC, Fiel SB, Fisher MS, et al. Asbestos-related pleural disease and asbestosis: a comparison of CT and chest radiography. *AJR Am J Roentgenol* 1988;150: 269–275.

37. Edelman DA. Asbestos exposure, pleural plaques and the risk of lung cancer. *Int Arch Occup Environ Health* 1988;60:389–393.

38. Weiss W. Asbestos-related pleural plaques and lung cancer. *Chest* 1993;103:1854–1859.

39. Hillerdal G. Pleural plaques and risk for bronchial carcinoma and mesothelioma. *Chest* 1994;105: 144–150.

40. Schwartz DA, Fuortes LJ, Galvin JR, et al. Asbestos-induced pleural fibrosis and impaired lung function. *Am Rev Respir Dis* 1990;141:321–326.

41. Schwartz A, Galvin JR, Yagla SJ, et al. Restrictive lung function and asbestos-induced pleural fibrosis. A quantitative approach. *J Clin Invest* 1993;91: 2685–2692.

42. Fridriksson HV, Hedenstrom H, Hillerdal G, et al. Increased lung stiffness in persons with pleural plaques. *Eur J Respir Dis* 1981;62:412–424.

43. Van Cleemput J, De Raeve H, Verschakelen JA, et al. Surface of pleural plaques quantitated by CT-scanning: no relation with cumulative asbestos exposure and no effect on lung function. *Am J Respir Crit Care Med* 2001 (*in press*).

44. Shih J-F, Wilson JS, Broderick A, et al. Asbestos-induced pleural fibrosis and impaired exercise physiology. *Chest* 1994;105:1370–1376.

45. Hillerdal G. Non-malignant asbestos pleural disease. *Thorax* 1981;36:669-675.

46. Wright PH, Hanson A, Keel L, et al. Respiratory function changes after asbestos pleurisy. *Thorax* 1980;35: 31–36.

47. Miller A, Teirstein AS, Selikoff I. Ventilatory failure due to asbestos pleurisy. *Am J Med* 1983;75:911– 919.

48. Shih J-F, Hunninghake GW, Goeken NE, et al. The relationship between HLA-A, B, DQ, and DR antigens and asbestos-induced lung disease. *Chest* 1993;104: 26–31.

49. Hillerdal G, Lee J, Blomkvist A, et al. Pleural disease during treatment with bromocriptine in patients previously exposed to asbestos. *Eur Respir J* 1997;10: 2711–2715.

50. Aberle DR, Balmes JR. Computed tomography of asbestos-related pulmonary parenchymal and pleural diseases. *Clin Chest Med* 1991;12:115–131.

51. Yates DH, Browne K, Stidolph PN, et al. Asbestos-related bilateral diffuse pleural thickening: natural history of radiographic and lung function abnormalities. *Am J Respir Crit Care Med* 1996;153: 301–306.

52. Picado C, Laporta D, Grassino A, et al. Mechanisms affecting exercise performance in subjects with asbestos-related pleural fibrosis. *Lung* 1987;165:45–57.

53. Leung AN, Muller NL, Miller RR. CT in differential diagnosis of diffuse pleural disease. *AJR Am J Roentgenol* 1990;154:487–492.

54. Fielding DI, McKeon JL, Oliver WA, et al. Pleurectomy for persistent pain in benign asbestos-related pleural disease. *Thorax* 1995;50:181–183.

55. Batra P, Brown K, Hayashi K, et al. Rounded atelectasis. *J Thorac Imaging* 1996;11:187–197.

56. Dernevik L, Gatzinsky P. Pathogenesis of shrinking pleuritis with atelectasis:"rounded atelectasis." *Eur J Respir Dis* 1987;71:244–249.

57. Hillerdal G, Ozesmi M. Benign asbestos pleural effusion: 73 exudates in 60 patients. *Eur J Respir Dis* 1987;71:113–121.

58. Szydlowski GW, Cohn HE, Steiner RM, et al. Rounded atelectasis: a pulmonary pseudotumor. *Ann Thorac Surg* 1992;53:817–821.

59. McLoud TC, Flower CD. Imaging the pleura: sonography, CT, and MR imaging. *AJR Am J Roentgnenol* 1991;156:1145–1153.

60. Buchanan DR, Johnston ID, Kerr IH, et al. Cryptogenic bilateral fibrosing pleuritis. *Br J Dis Chest* 1988;82: 186–193.

61. Azoulay E, Paugam B, Heymann MF, et al. Familial extensive idiopathic bilateral pleural fibrosis. *Eur Respir J* 1999;14:971–973.

62. Morton JR, Boushy SF, Guinn GA. Physiological evaluation of results of pulmonary decortication. *Ann Thorac Surg* 1970;9:321–326.

63. Shapiro DH, Anagnostopoulos CE, Dineen JP. Decortication and pleurectomy for the pleuropulmonary complications of pancreatitis. *Ann Thorac Surg* 1970;9: 76–80.

64. Brunk JR, Drash EC, Swineford O. Rheumatoid pleuritis successfully treated with decortication. Report of a case and review of the literature. *Am J Med Sci* 1966;251: 545–551.

65. Gilbert L, Bribot S, Franked H, et al. Fibrinous uremic pleuritis: a surgical entity. *Chest* 1975;67:53–56.

66. Lee-Chiong TL Jr, Hilbert J. Extensive idiopathic benign bilateral asynchronous pleural fibrosis. *Chest* 1996;109:564–565.

67. Hughes R, Jensik RJ, Faber LP, et al. Evaluation of unilateral decortication: a patient successfully treated 44 years after onset of tuberculosis. *Ann Thorac Surg* 1975;19:704–715.

68. Gaensler EA. Lung displacement: abdominal enlargement, pleural space disorders, deformities of the thoracic cage. In: Fenn WD, Rahn H, eds. *Handbook of physiology, section 3. Respiration*, volume II. Washington, D.C.: American Physiological Society, 1965:1623–1661.

69. Yousem SA. Thoracic splenosis. *Ann Thorac Surg* 1987;44:411–412.

Thoracentesis (Diagnostic and Therapeutic) and Pleural Biopsy

DIAGNOSTIC THORACENTESIS

Indications

A diagnostic thoracentesis should be performed on almost every patient with a pleural effusion of unknown origin. Empirically, I have found it difficult to obtain fluid with a diagnostic thoracentesis if the thickness of the fluid on the decubitus chest radiograph is less than 10 mm, and I usually do not attempt thoracentesis in such patients. If thoracentesis is attempted with small amounts of fluid, the proper location can be identified by using ultrasound (1).

Contraindications

The main contraindication to a diagnostic thoracentesis is a hemorrhagic diathesis. One should hesitate to perform a thoracentesis in a patient who is receiving anticoagulants, particularly thrombolytic agents. Depending on the urgency of the situation, however, diagnostic thoracentesis using a small (22-gauge) needle can be performed on almost any patient if one is careful. McVay et al. (2) demonstrated that there was no increased risk of bleeding if the prothrombin time or the partial thromboplastin time was not more than two times the normal value. Likewise, there was no increased risk of bleeding with low platelet counts (<25,000 per mm^3). Accordingly, these authors recommend that prophylactic blood product transfusions are not needed before thoracentesis in patients with mild coagulopathy and no clinical evidence of bleeding (2).

These authors did note an increased risk of bleeding if the creatinine level was elevated above 6 mg per dL (2), presumably due to decreased platelet function in the setting of uremia.

It appears that thoracentesis can be performed on patients who are undergoing mechanical ventilation. McCartney et al. (3) reported a series of 31 patients who underwent thoracentesis while they were receiving mechanical ventilation; 25 patients were receiving positive end-expiratory pressure (PEEP) between 5 and 20 cm H_2O. All thoracenteses were performed with patients in the lateral decubitus position. Only three of the patients (10%) developed a pneumothorax, and all were managed with a chest tube (3). In a second series, two of 32 patients (6%) developed a pneumothorax after undergoing a thoracentesis while on mechanical ventilation (4).

A thoracentesis should not be attempted through an area affected by a local cutaneous condition such as pyoderma or herpes zoster infection.

Positioning of Patient

For a diagnostic thoracentesis, and particularly for a therapeutic thoracentesis, the patient and the operator must be comfortable. I find that the patient is most comfortable when he or she sits on the side of the bed with his arms and head resting on one or more pillows on a bedside table (Fig. 25.1). A footstool is placed on the floor for the patient to have someplace to rest his feet. The bed is elevated so that the operator does not

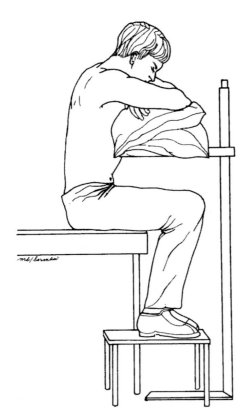

FIG. 25.1. Recommended position of the patient for diagnostic or therapeutic thoracentesis.

have to stoop over. The patient sits near the foot of the bed, with the side containing the fluid toward the foot of the bed. With the patient in this position, the operator does not have to reach across the entire bed, yet the foot of the bed can be covered with sterile drapes to provide a sterile area from which to work. The patient should be positioned with his back vertical so that the lowest part of his hemithorax is posterior. If the patient leans forward too far, the lowest part of the hemithorax may move anteriorly, and no fluid will remain posteriorly.

Some patients are too debilitated to assume a sitting position. The thoracentesis may then be performed with the patient lying on the side of the pleural effusion in the lateral decubitus position with his back near the edge of the operating table or bed. Alternately, the patient may sit in bed with the head of the bed maximally elevated. With

the patient in this position, the thoracentesis is performed in the midaxillary line.

Selection of Site

The site for the attempted thoracentesis should be selected with care. Most thoracenteses that fail to yield fluid are performed too low (5). A review of the chest radiographs indicates an approximate location. The physical examination of the patient's chest is most important in determining the site, however. When fluid is present between the lung and the chest wall, tactile fremitus is lost, and the light percussion note becomes dull. Accordingly, thoracentesis should be attempted one interspace below the spot where tactile fremitus is lost and the percussion note becomes dull. Thoracentesis should usually be performed posteriorly several inches from the spine, where the ribs are easily palpated. The exact location for the thoracentesis attempt should be just superior to a rib. The rationale for this location is that the arteries, veins, and nerves run just inferior to the ribs (Fig. 25.2), so that if the needle is just superior to a rib, the danger of damage to these structures is minimized.

Ultrasound has been proposed as being superior to chest roentgenography in identifying pleural fluid and choosing the optimal site for thoracentesis (6). One study (7), however, has demonstrated that it is not cost effective to obtain ultrasound routinely before thoracentesis. Kohan et al. (7) randomly allocated 205 patients to undergo or not undergo chest ultrasonography before thoracentesis. They reported that the incidence of dry attempts was significantly higher without ultrasound (33%) than with ultrasound (10%) in patients with small effusions, but there was no difference with large effusions. Moreover, the use of ultrasound did not lead to a lower rate of complications in patients with either small or large effusions (7). Based on this study, it is recommended that thoracentesis initially be attempted without ultrasound unless the amount of pleural fluid is very small. If no fluid is obtained after two or three attempts, then the fluid should be localized with ultrasound before additional attempts are made to obtain fluid.

It should be noted, however, that in a smaller study (8), the incidence of pneumothorax was much less if the thoracentesis was done with ultrasound guidance (8).

Thoracentesis Kits

The materials required to perform the diagnostic thoracentesis are listed in Table 25.1, and these kits should be assembled before the procedure is initiated. What is done more commonly, however, is to use a thoracentesis kit in which the materials have been preassembled. There are several thoracentesis kits available commercially, including the Pharmaseal distributed by Baxter, the Arrow-Clark Thoracentesis Kit distributed by Arrow, and the Argyle Turkel distributed by Kendall. The kit that is used most frequently is the Pharmaseal distributed by Baxter and this kit is unsatisfactory in my opinion. The primary needle for the aspiration is a 3-inch, 16-gauge needle. A needle this large should never be used for a diagnostic thoracentesis. If a therapeutic thoracentesis is going to be performed, it should not be done with a sharp needle because the sharp needle may lacerate the lung.

TABLE 25.1. *Materials needed for diagnostic thoracentesis*

Basic materials
  Lidocaine 1% or 2%
  Aqueous heparin, 1000 U/mL
  Atropine
  Antiseptic solution
  Alcohol swabs
  Sterile gloves
  Six 4 × 4-inch gauze pads
  Sterile drape with center hole
  Sterile drape (to cover bed)
  Adhesive tape
  Two 5- to 10-mL syringes
  One 50-mL syringe
  One No. 25 needle, $\frac{5}{8}$ inch long
  Two No. 20 to No. 22 needles, $1\frac{1}{2}$ inches long
  Band-Aids
Additional materials for therapeutic thoracentesis
  Two No. 14 needles and catheters
  One 3-way stopcock
  One sterile container for pleural fluid
  One 50-mL syringe (additional)
Additional materials for pleural biopsy
  Pleural biopsy needle
  Scalpel
  Formalin

One excellent thoracentesis kit is the Arrow-Clark Thoracentesis Kit manufactured by Arrow International, Reading, Pennsylvania (www.arrowintl.com, 800-233-3187). The basic thoracentesis apparatus in this kit is an 8 French gauge catheter over an 18-gauge needle with a 3-way stopcock and self-sealing valve. With this apparatus, one constantly aspirates as the catheter is advanced through the chest wall. Then, when a free flow of fluid is encountered, the catheter is advanced about 1 cm and the needle is withdrawn completely. One nice feature of this set is that there is a self-sealing valve so that air does not leak into the pleural space when the needle is withdrawn; however, the needle cannot be reinserted through the catheter. With this system, small amounts of fluid can be withdrawn by aspirating directly through the side port on the catheter. Another nice feature of this set is that one may easily withdraw large amounts of fluid either with a syringe or through vacuum bottles. If a syringe is used, aspiration is performed through a Y connector that has one-way valves so that no stopcocks need be turned with each aspiration. If vacuum bottles are used, there is vacuum bottle tubing included, which attaches directly to the sideport of the catheter. There is also a roller clamp to control the flow of fluid into the vacuum bottles. The cost of this thoracentesis kit is approximately $31.00.

Another excellent set is the Argyle Turkel Safety Thoracentesis Set manufactured by Kendall Company (St. Louis, MO, USA, www.kendallhq.com, 800-962-9888). This system incorporates a blunt, multiside fenestrated, spring-loaded inner cannula coaxially housed within a 16-gauge conventional sharp-beveled hollow needle. The advantage of this system is as the needle and blunt cannula penetrate the chest wall, the blunt cannula is forced into the shaft of the needle. Then when the tip of the needle encounters low resistance, such as an area of pleural effusion within the pleural space, the spring-loaded cannula automatically extends beyond the bevel, thus helping to protect the underlying tissue from further, inadvertent penetration. Another advantage of this system is an indicator in the needle housing that identifies the position of the blunt cannula; if resistance is being met such that the sharp end of the needle is exposed, then the indicator is red. In contrast, if no resistance is being met, then the indicator is green. Therefore, when the pleural space is entered, the indicator turns green. If a diagnostic thoracentesis is being performed, the pleural fluid can be withdrawn through the needle. If a therapeutic thoracentesis is being performed, the catheter assembly is advanced and then the needle assembly is withdrawn completely. There is a one-way valve such that there is no possibility of air leaking into the pleural space when the needle is withdrawn. There is a side port for fluid removal. The cost of these kits is approximately $24.00.

When comparing the two kits described earlier, the Argyle Turkel kit has the advantage of the spring-loaded inner cannula, which should decrease the incidence of lung laceration. The advantage of the Arrow-Clark system is the ease with which a therapeutic thoracentesis can be performed with either a syringe or with vacuum bottles.

Technique

The procedure should be carefully explained to the patient, and a signed consent form should be obtained. I do not routinely administer atropine to prevent vasovagal reactions as advocated by some (9), because I find such reactions to be uncommon. I do have atropine available, however, and I administer 1.0 mg subcutaneously or intramuscularly at the first sign of such a reaction. Similarly, I do not administer an analgesic, a sedative, or a tranquilizer routinely before the procedure unless the patient shows excessive anxiety. If there is excessive anxiety, I administer intravenous midazolam (Versed) just before the procedure.

Once the site for thoracentesis is identified, it is marked by exerting pressure using the end of a ballpoint pen with the tip retracted. This leaves a small indentation that will not be removed by subsequent cleansing of the area. Then the skin surrounding the site is cleansed thoroughly with an antiseptic solution over an area extending at least 4 inches in all directions from the proposed thoracentesis site. The sterile drape with the center hole is then taped to the patient's back, and another sterile drape is placed on the bed.

The next step is to obtain local anesthesia. It is necessary to anesthetize the skin, the periosteum of the rib, and the parietal pleura. The skin is anesthetized using a short 25-gauge needle by injecting enough lidocaine, about 0.5 mL, to raise a small wheal (Fig. 25.2A). The small needle is then replaced by a $1^{1}/_{2}$-inch long 22-gauge. This needle is inserted to the periosteum of the underlying rib and is moved up and over the rib with the frequent injection of small amounts (0.1 to 0.2 mL) of lidocaine (Fig. 25-2B). Once this needle is superior to the rib, it is slowly advanced toward the pleural space with aspiration, followed by the injection of 0.1 to 0.2 mL lidocaine every 1 to 2 mm (Fig. 25.2C). This frequent aspiration and the injection of lidocaine guarantee anesthesia of the parietal pleura. As soon as pleural fluid is aspirated through this needle into the syringe containing lidocaine, the needle should be withdrawn from the pleural space and reattached to a 50- to 60-mL syringe containing 1 mL heparin. Heparin is added to the syringe to prevent clotting of the pleural fluid as it is difficult to obtain differential white blood cell counts or pH determinations if the pleural fluid is clotted. The same needle is reintroduced along the same tract slowly with constant aspiration until pleural fluid is obtained. Aspiration is then continued until the syringe is filled. The needle is then withdrawn, and the procedure is finished. The commercially available kits can be used to perform a diagnostic thoracentesis. The special needles that come with these kits, however, have few advantages over a syringe and a needle for a diagnostic thoracentesis. They do have significant advantages for therapeutic thoracentesis, and they should be used in this situation.

At times, no pleural fluid is obtained when the $1^{1}/_{2}$-inch No. 22 needle is inserted all the way to its hub. In such a situation, the needle should be slowly withdrawn with constant aspiration. The rim of the pleural fluid is sometimes thin and may be missed as the needle is inserted. If no pleural fluid is obtained either as the needle is inserted or withdrawn, one of four possibilities exists: (a) the needle was too short; (b) placement of the needle was too far superior;

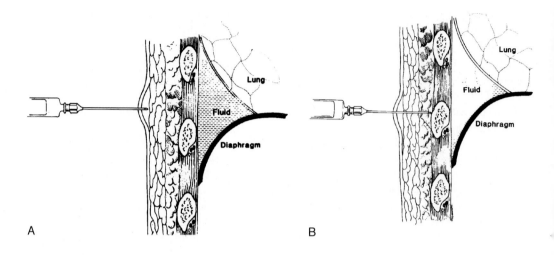

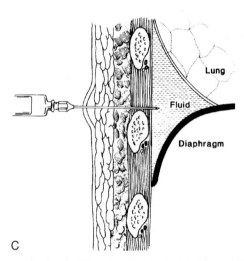

FIG. 25.2. Diagnostic thoracentesis. **A:** The skin is injected using a 25-gauge needle with a local anesthetic agent. **B:** The periosteum is injected with the local anesthetic. **C:** The pleural space is entered, and pleural fluid is obtained. **D:** The thoracentesis attempt is too high, and air bubbles are obtained. **E:** The thoracentesis attempt is too low, and neither bubbles nor fluid are obtained.

(c) placement of the needle was too far inferior; or (d) no pleural fluid is present. If the patient is markedly muscular or obese and if no air is obtained on the initial attempt, the $1\frac{1}{2}$-inch needle should be replaced with a longer needle such as a spinal needle, which is used for performing lumbar puncture, and the attempt should be repeated. If no fluid is aspirated, but air bubbles are obtained on the initial attempt with the local anes-

thetic, the lung parenchyma has been penetrated and the needle was inserted too far superiorly (Fig. 25.2D). Therefore, the procedure should be repeated one interspace inferiorly. Penetration of the lung with a small needle is not a catastrophe, and only occasionally does a pneumothorax result. If no fluid or air bubbles are obtained on the initial attempt, the needle was inserted too far inferiorly (Fig. 25.2E) and the procedure should

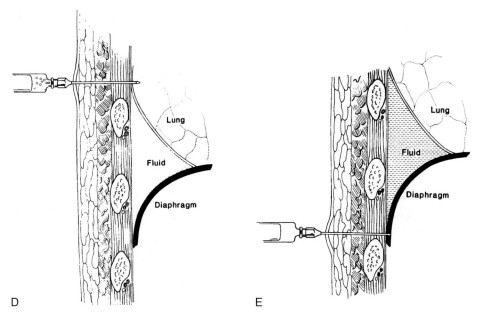

D   E

FIG. 25.2. *Continued.*

be repeated one interspace superiorly. Pleural fluid is almost never too thick to be aspirated through a No. 20 or a No. 22 needle. If no fluid is obtained after two or three attempts, ultrasound guidance of the thoracentesis is recommended.

Processing of Pleural Fluid

The main purpose of a diagnostic thoracentesis is to examine the pleural fluid. The recommended distribution of the pleural fluid to various laboratories is outlined in Table 25.2. For the cell count and differential, the fluid should be placed in EDTA-treated tubes (purple top tubes). If the fluid is placed in the tubes without anticoagulants that come with the thoracentesis trays, the cells are likely to clump or the fluid is likely to clot, giving inaccurate cell counts and differentials (10). For the determination of pleural fluid pH, the sample should be maintained anaerobically and the determination should be made with a blood gas machine (11), although it is not necessary to pack it in ice as long as

TABLE 25.2. *Laboratory distribution of pleural fluid obtained with diagnostic thoracentesis*

Laboratory	Amount (mL)	Test Ordered
Chemistry (Red top tube)	5	Protein Lactic acid dehydrogenase Glucose
Hematology (Purple top tube)	5	White blood cell count (WBC) Wright's stain Hematocrit (if pleural fluid is bloody)
Bacteriology	10	Aerobic and anaerobic cultures Gram's stain
Tuberculosis and mycology	5	Tuberculosis and fungal cultures Acid-fast stain
Cytology	5–25	Cytologic examination
Blood gas	5	pH
By blood gas machine		P_{CO_2}

pH determination is performed within an hour (12). Interpretation of the results of the various tests obtained in Table 25.2 is discussed in Chapters 4 and 5. If there is a good chance that the patient has a transudative pleural effusion, the most cost-effective approach is to measure only the lactate dehydrogenase (LDH) and protein in the pleural fluid. If these measurements demonstrate that the patient does not have a transudative pleural effusion (13), the remaining studies should be performed.

Complications

The most common complication of thoracentesis is pneumothorax. When three different series (7, 13, 14) involving 459 patients are combined, 51 of the patients (11%) developed a pneumothorax and chest tubes were necessary in 9 (2%). In a more recent report, the incidence of pneumothorax was 4% in a series of 506 thoracenteses and 2% received a chest tube (15). The incidence of pneumothorax following thoracentesis is reduced if experienced individuals such as pulmonary fellows or pulmonologists perform the procedure (16). The incidence of iatrogenic pneumothorax may also be lower if the procedure is performed under ultrasound guidance. Raptopoulos et al. reported that the incidence of pneumothorax was 18% for 154 thoracenteses performed with conventional techniques, whereas it was only 3% for 188 performed with ultrasound guidance (17). A second study with a comparable number of patients reported that the incidence of pneumothorax was similar whether or not the procedure was performed with ultrasound guidance (7). This difference in the incidence of complications in the first study is at least partially explained by the fact that the sonographers were more experienced in catheter placement (17).

It appears that the likelihood of the development of a pneumothorax may be higher in patients with chronic obstructive pulmonary (COPD) disease. Brandstetter et al. (18) performed thoracentesis in 106 patients, of whom 36 had COPD. The incidence of pneumothorax was significantly higher (41.7%) in those patients with COPD than in those without COPD (18.5%) (18). Nine of the 106 patients were treated with chest tubes and seven of them had COPD (18). The explanation of the very high incidence of pneumothorax in this series is not clear. In contrast, Raptopoulos et al. (17) were unable to find a relationship between the occurrence of a pneumothorax and the presence of underlying lung disease.

There are two different reasons that patients develop pneumothorax after a thoracentesis. First, air may flow from the atmosphere into the pleural space if the pleural space (with its negative pressure) communicates freely with the atmosphere. This most commonly happens when a syringe is removed from a needle or catheter and the air then flows from the atmosphere into the pleural space and produces a pneumothorax. This problem can be prevented if the special needles with one-way valves (such as the Arrow-Clark or Argyle Turkel) are used during thoracentesis. It can also be prevented if the patient hums (producing positive pleural pressure) while the needle is being changed. Second, the needle for thoracentesis may lacerate the lung and permit air to enter the pleural space from the alveoli. This can be prevented if catheters, rather than sharp needles, are used to perform therapeutic thoracenteses.

Should chest radiographs be obtained routinely after diagnostic thoracentesis? It appears that routine chest radiographs are not indicated. Aleman et al. (16) reported that only five of 488 patients without symptoms after thoracentesis developed a pneumothorax and that only one of these five patients required a chest tube. Gervais et al. (19) reported that the incidence of iatrogenic pneumothorax was approximately 1% in nonintubated patients undergoing ultrasound-guided thoracentesis and concluded that routine postprocedure chest radiographs are not indicated in spontaneously breathing patients who undergo thoracentesis. Doyle et al. (20) reviewed their experience with 174 thoracentesis and concluded that postprocedure chest radiographs were indicated only when a pneumothorax is suspected (20). In view of the above-mentioned series, I recommend postprocedure radiographs only when air is obtained during the thoracentesis, the patient develops symptoms, or when tactile fremitus is lost over the superior part of the aspirated hemithorax. The treatment of iatrogenic pneumothorax is discussed in Chapter 21.

Other common complications of thoracentesis are cough and chest pain (16). Cough most frequently complicates thoracentesis when it is performed for therapeutic reasons and usually occurs toward the end of the thoracentesis (16). Indeed if coughing occurs during a thoracentesis, it should serve as an indication to stop the procedure. The chest pain that complicates thoracentesis is of three types. First, the patient may experience sharp pain when the skin is anesthetized or when the parietal pleura is pierced. This pain should not be persistent if the parietal pleura is adequately anesthetized. Second, the patient may experience chest tightness or dull pain as fluid is removed during a therapeutic thoracentesis. This type of pain usually indicates that the patient's lung is not expanding rapidly and should serve as an indication to stop the procedure. Third, the patient may develop pleuritic chest pain after the procedure, which is usually due to the roughened pleural surfaces rubbing on each other after some of the fluid has been withdrawn. On auscultation, a pleural rub is often heard in these cases.

At times, a diagnostic thoracentesis provokes a vasovagal reflex characterized by bradycardia, a decreased stroke volume, and a resultant fall in cardiac output and blood pressure. This reaction is blocked by the intramuscular administration of 1 mg atropine. A similar syndrome may be provoked by various noxious, emotional, and physical stimuli such as apprehension, pain, or the sight of blood and is characterized by the sudden loss of peripheral vascular resistance without significant bradycardia. The patient develops hypotension, pallor, cold and clammy skin, and faintness. This syndrome is not blocked by atropine. The recommended treatment is termination of the procedure and the immediate placement of the patient in a reverse Trendelenberg position.

Another complication of thoracentesis is infection of the pleural space. Approximately 2% of all pleural infections are due to contamination of the pleural space at the time of thoracentesis. For this reason, sterile technique must be strictly followed during thoracentesis, and the skin must be thoroughly cleansed before the procedure is started. The treatment of pleural infections is discussed in Chapter 9.

Diagnostic thoracentesis can also produce a hemothorax if an intercostal artery is lacerated. This complication can usually be avoided if the thoracentesis is performed just superior to a rib, as previously described. In older patients, however, the intercostal arteries may be tortuous, and a hemothorax can result even with proper technique (21). The treatment of iatrogenic hemothorax is described in Chapter 22. Other rare complications of diagnostic thoracentesis include splenic or hepatic laceration, soft-tissue infection secondary to seeding of the needle tract with bacteria, seeding of the needle tract with tumor cells, and adverse reactions to the local anesthetic.

Another uncommon complication of which one should be aware is human immunodeficiency virus infection (HIV) infection with seroconversion. Oksenhendler et al. (22) reported an instance in which a nurse received a superficial self-inflicted needlestick injury to the finger while recapping a needle contaminated by the bloody pleural fluid of a patient with persistent generalized lymphadenopathy, pleural effusion, and seropositivity for HIV and hepatitis B surface antigen. Anicteric hepatitis developed 53 days later, and serum samples became HIV antibody positive by day 68. This case emphasizes the need for strict precautions regarding the handling of needles and body fluids from patients infected with HIV.

THERAPEUTIC THORACENTESIS

Indications

The three main indications for therapeutic thoracentesis are to remove the pleural fluid in patients with parapneumonic effusions or empyema, to relieve the symptom of dyspnea secondary to a pleural effusion, and to remove the pleural fluid so that the status of the lung underlying a pleural effusion can be evaluated. With the exception of patients with parapneumonic effusions or empyema (see Chapter 9), therapeutic thoracentesis provides symptomatic relief, but it is not the definitive therapy. Pleural fluid collects because the rate of pleural fluid formation has exceeded the rate of pleural fluid absorption. If nothing is done to change these two factors, then pleural fluid will reaccumulate after the therapeutic thoracentesis. The thoracentesis itself does not alter the basic condition that produced the pleural effusion. However, a therapeutic thoracentesis should always be performed in an acutely dyspneic patient with a large pleural effusion to alleviate the dyspnea.

Serial therapeutic thoracenteses can be performed in patients who are dyspneic from malignant pleural effusions with mediastinal shift toward the contralateral side in whom a pleurodesis cannot be successfully performed. It is recommended, however, that such patients have a pleuroperitoneal shunt placed. A therapeutic thoracentesis is also indicated in a patient with a malignant pleural effusion and dyspnea to determine whether the dyspnea can be relieved by the thoracentesis. This procedure should be performed before a chest tube is inserted and pleurodesis is attempted (see Chapter 7). The contraindications for therapeutic thoracentesis are the same as for diagnostic thoracentesis.

Technique

The positioning of the patient and the selection of the site for the thoracentesis are the same as for a diagnostic thoracentesis. The most important difference between a therapeutic and a diagnostic thoracentesis is that one must not use a sharp needle for the therapeutic thoracentesis. As the fluid is removed, the lung expands and can easily be lacerated if a sharp needle is present in the pleural space. Therefore, either a plastic catheter or a blunt pleural biopsy needle should be used for therapeutic thoracentesis. If a pleural biopsy is also indicated, the therapeutic thoracentesis can be performed through the pleural biopsy needle once the biopsy specimens have been obtained.

The additional materials required for the procedure are listed in Table 25.1. It is recommended that the Arrow-Clark or the Argyle Turkel thoracentesis kits be used for therapeutic thoracentesis. Directions for their use come with the kits. When these kits are used, it is important to make a large enough incision in the skin to allow easy passage for the needle with its overlying catheter.

If the incision is too small, the catheter may be damaged during the insertion. It is important to use a kit with a catheter over a needle, rather than one like the Pharmaseal that only has a sharp needle. The Arrow-Clark or the Argyle Turkel thoracentesis kits are recommended because they each contain the catheter and they each have a device that prevents air from entering the pleural space when the needle is withdrawn (see discussion of these kits earlier in this chapter).

If these kits are not available, the procedure can be performed with a plastic catheter (Intracath) as outlined in Fig. 25.3. When the fluid has been localized and identified by means of the lidocaine-filled syringe, as in diagnostic thoracentesis, a standard 16-gauge (Intracath) needle is attached to a plastic syringe. With gentle constant suction on the syringe, the needle is carefully and evenly advanced until pleural fluid is obtained. When the pleural fluid has been obtained, the syringe is disconnected from the needle, and the needle is temporarily occluded by a finger to prevent the development of a pneumothorax. Then, the 16-gauge (Intracath) catheter is inserted through the needle and is directed inferiorly toward the costodiaphragmatic recess. The catheter should not be advanced against resistance or its end may become traumatized and occluded. When the catheter has been advanced all the way to the hilt of the needle or when resistance is encountered, the needle is withdrawn carefully from the chest and the plastic catheter is left in the pleural space.

Immediately after withdrawing the needle, one should place the guard over the end of the needle so that the needle does not shear off the end of the catheter. The catheter should not be pulled back through the needle because the needle's sharp point may cut off a portion of the catheter. Once the needle is withdrawn from the pleural space, the catheter should be taped to the patient's skin so that it is not inadvertently removed from the pleural space.

The advantage of the plastic catheter system for therapeutic thoracentesis is that no sharp needle is present in the pleural space to lacerate the lung as it reexpands. Moreover, the patient can be repositioned with the catheter in place to allow more complete pleural fluid removal.

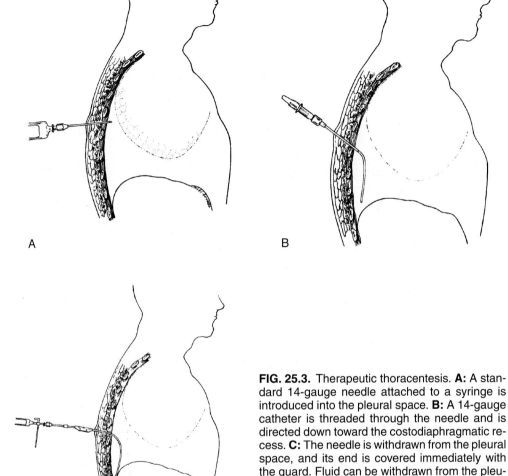

A

B

C

FIG. 25.3. Therapeutic thoracentesis. **A:** A standard 14-gauge needle attached to a syringe is introduced into the pleural space. **B:** A 14-gauge catheter is threaded through the needle and is directed down toward the costodiaphragmatic recess. **C:** The needle is withdrawn from the pleural space, and its end is covered immediately with the guard. Fluid can be withdrawn from the pleural space using the three-way stopcock and the syringe.

When the catheter has been positioned in the pleural space, the needle has been withdrawn, and the needle's end has been covered with the guard, a syringe with a three-way stopcock is attached to the end of the catheter, and the pleural fluid is withdrawn. Alternatively, the fluid can be drained by vacuum bottles. There are no studies comparing the side effects with syringe versus vacuum bottle drainage.

A chest radiograph should be obtained after a therapeutic thoracentesis to assess appearance of the lung in the absence of the fluid and to verify that no pneumothorax has occurred. If the

therapeutic thoracentesis was performed mainly for diagnostic purposes, it is sometimes useful to obtain bilateral decubitus radiographs after the procedure to delineate the amount of fluid remaining and to distinguish the remaining fluid from parenchymal infiltrates or masses. Similarly, it may be useful to inject 200 to 400 mL air into the pleural space at the end of the procedure before obtaining the radiographs. By means of this intentional iatrogenic pneumothorax, the thickness of the visceral and parietal pleura can be determined. If the therapeutic thoracentesis was performed strictly to relieve symptoms in a patient with a known diagnosis, a postprocedure chest radiograph is not indicated unless the patient has developed symptoms, air is obtained during the thoracentesis, or the tactile fremitus has disappeared over the superior aspect of the ipsilateral hemithorax.

How Much Pleural Fluid Can Be Withdrawn?

It is not clear how much fluid can be safely withdrawn during a therapeutic thoracentesis. Occasionally reexpansion pulmonary edema (see the following section) may develop following therapeutic thoracentesis. Because the reexpansion pulmonary edema is at times fatal, it is important to prevent it.

It has been hypothesized that the development of reexpansion pulmonary edema is related to the development of negative pleural pressure during therapeutic thoracentesis (23). We have demonstrated that large volumes of pleural fluid can be removed safely if the pleural pressure is monitored during thoracentesis and if thoracentesis is terminated when the pleural pressure falls below -20 cm H_2O (23). Pleural pressure can be monitored by a U-shaped manometer, as illustrated in Fig. 25.4. The change in the pleural pressure as fluid is withdrawn varies from patient to patient (Fig. 25.5). Frequently, neither the operator nor the patient is aware of the development of abnormally negative pleural pressure (23). In our series of 52 patients, 13 procedures (25%) were stopped because the patient's pleural pressures dropped below -20 cm H_2O. We have now removed more than 4,000 mL pleural fluid in a single thoracentesis from eight separate patients with no adverse consequences. Recently, Villena et al. (24) confirmed these observations in a series of 57 patients. They removed more than 1,500 mL from 29 patients with pleural pressure monitoring and had no instances of reexpansion pulmonary edema (24). In their 57 patients, the thoracentesis was stopped in 16 (28%) owing to excessively negative (<-20 cm H_2O) pleural pressure without any symptoms, in 29 patients (51%) owing to the development of symptoms (chest pain, cough, or chest tightness), in 10 patients (18%) because no more fluid could

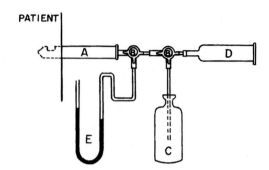

FIG. 25.4. Schematic diagram of apparatus used to measure pleural pressures and to aspirate pleural fluid. To measure the pleural pressure, the stopcock **(B)** adjacent to the Abram's needle **(A)** is turned so that the pleural space is in communication with the manometer **(E)**. It is important in measuring the pressure not to let fluid enter the plastic catheter between the tube and the manometer. Bottle **(C)**; 60-mL syringe **(D)**. (From Light RW, Jenkinson SG, Minh V, et al. Observations on pleural pressures as fluid is withdrawn during thoracentesis. *Am Rev Respir Dis* 1980;121:799–804, with permission.)

be obtained, and in two patients (5%) because the physician considered that too much fluid had been evacuated.

In view of the above-mentioned problems, it is recommended that the volume of a therapeutic

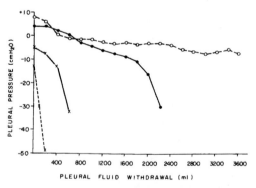

FIG. 25.5. Changes in pleural pressure as fluid is withdrawn during therapeutic thoracentesis in two patients with malignant pleural disease (*circles*) and in two patients with trapped lung (*x's*). Note how rapidly the pleural pressures fall in the patients with trapped lung. (From Light RW, Jenkinson SG, Minh V, et al. Observations on pleural pressures as fluid is withdrawn during thoracentesis. *Am Rev Respir Dis* 1980;121: 799–804, with permission.)

thoracentesis be limited to 1,000 mL unless pleural pressures are monitored. If the patient develops pernicious coughing, chest tightness, or chest pain, the procedure should be stopped before 1,000 mL of fluid are withdrawn. If pleural pressures are monitored, the procedure can be safely continued as long as the pleural pressure is above -20 cm H_2O and the patient does not have any symptoms.

Complications

Therapeutic thoracentesis is associated with the same complications as diagnostic thoracentesis, including vasovagal reaction, pneumothorax, pleural infection, and hemothorax. In addition, reexpansion pulmonary edema and hypovolemia may complicate therapeutic thoracentesis, and, as mentioned earlier, these complications may be related to the development of abnormally negative pleural pressures. Pneumothorax is more common with therapeutic than with diagnostic thoracentesis for two reasons. First, if a sharp needle is used for therapeutic thoracentesis, the lung is likely to be lacerated as it reexpands, leading to a bronchopleural fistula and a pneumothorax. Second, because the pleural pressure at times becomes quite negative during a therapeutic thoracentesis, air is more likely to enter the pleural space through faulty technique or even through the thoracentesis tract.

The treatment of iatrogenic pneumothorax is discussed in Chapter 21. A special situation exists in some patients with malignant pleural effusion who undergo therapeutic thoracentesis. In the series of Boland et al. (25), therapeutic thoracentesis was performed on 512 patients with malignant pleural effusion over a 3-year period. Pneumothoraces were documented in 40 patients (8%), and 29 were treated with tube thoracostomy. However, the pneumothorax in 17 of the 29 (59%) persisted despite the application of suction and the insertion of larger (28 to 36 F) chest tubes. After the drainage catheters were removed, the effusion completely reaccumulated in all patients. This study demonstrates that a small subgroup of patients with malignant pleural effusions who undergo therapeutic thoracentesis develop asymptomatic hydropneumothoraces due to poor lung compliance. If a chest tube is inserted in these patients, the lung will not reexpand and there will be no evidence of a bronchopleural fistula. In such a situation, the chest tube should be removed as soon as the situation is recognized.

REEXPANSION PULMONARY EDEMA

Reexpansion pulmonary edema is characterized by the development of unilateral pulmonary edema in a lung that has been rapidly reinflated following a variable period of collapse secondary to a pleural effusion or pneumothorax (26). The unilateral pulmonary edema is associated with a variable degree of hypoxia and hypotension, sometimes requiring intubation and mechanical ventilation, and occasionally leading to death (27, 28).

Pathophysiologic Features

The exact mechanisms responsible for reexpansion pulmonary edema are not known. In the experimental animal, reexpansion pulmonary edema occurs only if the lung has been collapsed for several days and if negative pressure is applied to the pleural space. Miller et al. (29) studied monkeys in which a pneumothorax had been present for 1 hour or 3 days. These researchers found that reexpansion pulmonary edema occurred only when the pneumothorax had been present for 3 days and the lung was reexpanded with -10 mm Hg pleural pressure. No pulmonary edema developed if the lung was reexpanded by underwater-seal drainage after 3 days of collapse or if negative pressure was used in a lung that had been collapsed for only 1 hour.

In a study of rabbits, Pavlin and Cheney found that reexpansion pulmonary edema was much more extensive in lungs that had been collapsed for 7 days than in those that had been collapsed for 3 days (30). Reexpansion with -20 mm Hg pleural pressure led to no more edema than did reexpansion with positive airway pressure, but reexpansion with -40 mm Hg or -100 mm Hg increased the amount of edema. In some of these animals, contralateral pulmonary edema also developed, but to a lesser extent than in the ipsilateral lung (30). Some cases of reexpansion pulmonary edema in humans, however, have occurred when no negative pressure was applied to the pleural space (31, 32). Almost all cases of reexpansion pulmonary edema occur when the pneumothorax or pleural effusion has been present for at least 3 days.

Reexpansion pulmonary edema appears to be due to increased permeability of the pulmonary vasculature. In both humans (33) and rabbits (34), the edema fluid has a high protein content, suggesting that it is leakiness of the capillaries rather than an increased hydrostatic pressure difference that leads to the edema. Pavlin et al. (35) have hypothesized that the mechanical stresses applied to the lung during reexpansion damage the capillaries and lead to the development of pulmonary edema. There is no evidence that the collapsed lung has increased permeability before reinflation (35).

An alternate hypothesis that has become popular is that reexpansion pulmonary edema is due to a reperfusion injury (36). With atelectasis, hypoxia of the atelectatic lung may be severe because oxygen delivery to the lung is reduced by absent ventilation and hypoperfusion. Then when the hypoxic areas are reperfused, oxygen-free radical formation is promoted and lung injury can result. If the lung is only partially collapsed, the reexpansion edema sometimes only occurs in the part of the lung that has been atelectic (37). Mechanical stress is probably not the sole factor responsible for reexpansion pulmonary edema, because the edema is associated with neutrophil influx into the lung in both animals (38) and humans (39), and the edema fluid contains interleukin-8 and leukotriene B_4. Neutrophils are not responsible for the reexpansion edema, however, because neutrophil depletion in the animal model does not prevent its occurrence (38). The reperfusion injury hypothesis is supported by the observation that the administration of an increased FI_2 (40%) for the duration of the pneumothorax prevents edema when lungs are reexpanded (40). The supplemental oxygen eliminates the systemic hypoxemia while the lung is collapsed. Additional support for this hypothesis is provided by the observation that the administration of antioxidants before reexpansion minimizes both the permeability edema and the degree of inflammation in rabbits (41).

Clinical Manifestations

Patients who develop reexpansion pulmonary edema typically develop pernicious coughing or chest tightness during or immediately following thoracentesis or chest tube placement. The cough sometimes is productive of copious amounts of frothy pink sputum. Other symptoms include dyspnea, tachypnea, tachycardia, fever, hypotension, nausea, vomiting, and cyanosis. The symptoms progress for 24 to 48 hours, and the chest radiograph reveals pulmonary edema throughout the ipsilateral lung. Pulmonary edema may also develop in the contralateral lung (31). If the patient does not die within the first 48 hours, recovery is usually complete. The seriousness of the syndrome is emphasized by reports that it has been responsible for the death of healthy, young people. In one review of the subject (31), the outcome was fatal in 11 of 53 reported cases (20%). The overall mortality rate is probably much less than 20% because fatal cases are more likely to be reported than are nonfatal cases.

The incidence of reexpansion pulmonary edema is not known, but it is thought to be uncommon. Until 1988, a total of only 53 cases had been reported (41). With therapeutic thoracentesis, the incidence is very low. Moyers et al. (42) reported that none of 251 patients undergoing thoracentesis developed reexpansion pulmonary edema. In this series, no pleural pressure monitoring was performed and 25 patients had more than 1,500 mL pleural fluid withdrawn. Milanez de Campos et al. (43) reported that reexpansion pulmonary edema occurred in 2% of 500 patients who underwent thoracoscopy and talc insufflation for treatment of recurrent pleural effusion. In the Veterans Administration (VA) cooperative study on spontaneous pneumothorax there were no cases of reexpansion pulmonary edema among the 229 study subjects despite the use of suction in over 80% of the cases (44). In another study of 320 patients treated with tube thoracostomy for spontaneous pneumothorax, the incidence of reexpansion pulmonary edema was 1% (45).

Prevention

The possibility of reexpansion pulmonary edema should be considered in patients with large pleural effusions or pneumothoraces of more than a few days' duration who are undergoing tube thoracostomy or thoracentesis. When tube thoracostomy is performed for spontaneous pneumothorax, the tubes should be connected to an underwater-seal drainage apparatus rather than to a negative pressure apparatus in view of the animal studies of Miller et al. (29) and Pavlin and Cheney (30). If underwater-seal drainage does not effect reexpansion of the underlying lung within 24 to 48 hours, then negative pressure can be applied to the pleural space.

The amount of pleural fluid withdrawn during thoracentesis should be limited to 1,000 mL unless pleural pressures are monitored, as discussed earlier. In addition, if the patient develops chest tightness or pernicious coughing at any time during a therapeutic thoracentesis, the procedure should be stopped.

Treatment

The treatment of reexpansion pulmonary edema is primarily supportive with intravenous fluids, oxygen, and morphine. Diuresis may be detrimental and should be avoided (45). Suggested escalating levels of treatment include no treatment for an abnormality on radiography alone; nasal supplemental oxygen for mild hypoxemia; intubation, mechanical ventilation, and positive end expiratory pressure (PEEP) for severe hypoxemia; and volume replacement and inotopic agents for hypotension with low cardiac output (26).

NEEDLE BIOPSY OF THE PLEURA

Indications

With a needle biopsy of the pleura, a small piece of the parietal pleura is obtained for microscopic or microbiologic evaluation. The main diagnoses established with a needle biopsy of the pleura are tuberculous pleuritis and malignancy of the pleura. A pleural biopsy is now used less than in the past because the diagnosis of tuberculous pleuritis can be made by measuring the adenosine deaminase (ADA) or interferon-gamma level in the pleural fluid, and the diagnosis of pleural malignancy is usually established by pleural fluid cytology or thoracoscopy (46).

A needle biopsy of the pleura is currently recommended when tuberculous pleuritis is suspected and the pleural fluid ADA or interferon-gamma levels are not definitive. A needle biopsy of the pleura is also recommended when malignancy is suspected but the pleural fluid cytology is negative and thoracoscopy is not readily available.

Contraindications

The main contraindication to a pleural biopsy is a bleeding diathesis. A pleural biopsy should not be performed in patients who are taking anticoagulants or whose bleeding parameters are prolonged. If the platelet count is below 50,000 per mm^3, platelet transfusion should be given before the procedure is attempted. If the patient has borderline respiratory failure, one should hesitate to perform a pleural biopsy because the production of a pneumothorax could precipitate respiratory failure.

Another contraindication to needle biopsies is the presence of an empyema. In one series, subcutaneous abscesses developed at the biopsy site in two of five patients with empyema in whom a pleural biopsy was attempted (47). Other contraindications include an uncooperative patient and local cutaneous lesions such as pyoderma or herpes zoster infection.

Technique

The materials necessary for pleural biopsy are listed in Table 25.1. Most frequently, one uses a thoracentesis kit plus the pleural biopsy needle. When there is a moderate or larger pleural effusion, the biopsy is usually done with no imaging. If the effusion is small or loculated, then either ultrasound or CT can accurately identify the location of the fluid. Ultrasound is the preferred technique for guiding biopsy because it offers the advantage of a real-time approach to the biopsy and has the added advantages of the absence of ionizing radiation, portability, ready availability, and low expense. Because the patient can be imaged in the erect position, the depth of the fluid is maximized, thus minimizing complications (48).

The patient is positioned, and the site is selected as for diagnostic thoracentesis (described earlier in this chapter). The skin is cleaned, and the local anesthetic is administered as for diagnostic thoracentesis. Liberal amounts of lidocaine should be injected once the rib is passed to ensure adequate anesthesia of the parietal pleura. In general, if no fluid is obtained with the local anesthetic, the biopsy should not be attempted. When pleural fluid has been obtained with the lidocaine syringe and needle, a pleural biopsy can be performed with an Abram's or a Cope needle.

A biopsy is sometimes attempted without free pleural fluid. If there is no fluid, the procedure should be performed with ultrasonic or CT guidance (48).

Abram's Needle

The Abram's needle (Fig. 25.6) consists of three parts: a large outer trocar, an inner cutting cannula, and an inner solid stylet. The end of the outer trocar is blunt so that the instrument will not lacerate the lung, but the bluntness of the instrument requires one to make a small scalpel incision in the anesthetized skin and subcutaneous tissue to permit insertion of the biopsy needle without undue force. This incision should be made along the lines of cleavage to minimize postoperative scarring. The inner cutting cannula (Fig. 25.6B) fits tightly in the outer trocar (Fig. 25.6A) and can be locked in one of two positions: (a) a closed position, in which the inner cannula obstructs the notch on the outer trocar to make the needle airtight, and (b) an open position, in which the inner cannula is slightly withdrawn so that the notch on the outer trocar is not occluded. An indicator knob in the hexagonal grip of the

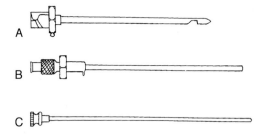

FIG. 25.6. Abram's pleural biopsy needle. **A:** Large outer trocar. **B:** Inner cutting cannula. **C:** Stylet.

larger outer trocar indicates the position of the notch in the distal end of the trocar.

To insert the Abram's pleural biopsy needle, the stylet is placed in the inner cannula, which, in turn, is placed in the outer trocar. The inner cannula (Fig. 25.6B) is twisted clockwise to close the distal notch of the outer trocar. The needle is pushed into the pleural space by exerting firm pressure on the stylet. Because the needle has a large diameter and is blunt, a substantial amount of pressure is needed. Usually, a pop is heard as the needle enters the pleural space. The inability to pass the needle into the pleural space is usually due to an insufficiently large skin incision. At times, the ribs are too close together to allow the needle to pass. In such situations, rotation of the patient's arm and shoulder over his or her head frequently separates the ribs sufficiently.

Once the tip of the needle is thought to be in the pleural space, the inner stylet (Fig. 25.6C) is removed, and with the inner cannula in the closed position, a syringe is attached to the connection on the inner cannula. Then, the inner cannula is rotated counterclockwise in the outer trocar so that the distal notch is locked open (Fig. 25.7A). At this time, pleural fluid may be aspirated for diagnostic studies. When the desired fluid has been obtained, the inner cannula of the needle is rotated clockwise to occlude the distal notch so that the syringe can be changed without creating a pneumothorax. A 10- to 20-mL syringe is then attached to the needle, and the inner cannula is rotated to open the distal notch. The entire needle is then rotated so that the knob on the outer trocar is inferior. This is important so that the blood vessels and nerves that lie immediately below the rib will not be biopsied. The biopsy needle is then slowly withdrawn with constant aspiration until it hooks onto the pleura (Fig. 25.7B). When the needle hooks, one can be sure that parietal pleura is in the notch of the needle if pleural fluid can still be aspirated through the syringe. When the needle is hooked on the pleura, the outer trocar is held firmly with one hand while the inner cannula is rotated into the closed position with the other hand to cut off a small piece of parietal pleura (Fig. 25.7C). Usually, mild resistance is met immediately before the needle is completely closed, and this resistance is due to

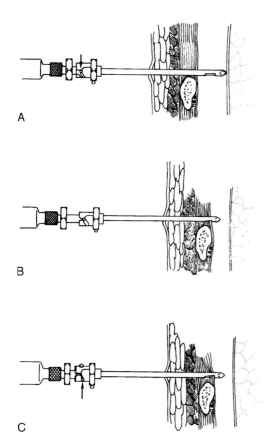

A

B

C

FIG. 25.7. A: Abram's needle in pleural space with notch open so that fluid can be aspirated. **B:** Abram's needle snagging the parietal pleura. **C:** The biopsy is obtained when the inner cutting cannula closes the notch in the outer trocar and shears off parietal pleura and anything else that remains in the notch. The arrows point to the pin on the inner cannula that locks into the outer trocar in either the open or closed position.

the inner cannula's severing the entrapped pleura for the biopsy specimen.

Once the initial biopsy specimen is obtained, the needle can either be withdrawn from the pleural space in the closed position or reinserted into the pleural space. If the needle is withdrawn from the chest, the pleural biopsy specimen is found in the tip of the needle and can be closely examined, but the needle then has to be reinserted. Reinsertions of the needle are through the same tract, however, and are easier than the original insertion. If the needle is reinserted into the pleural space without a complete withdrawal, the tissue

specimen can be aspirated through the syringe. The biopsy procedure can be repeated without removing the biopsy needle. The difficulty in not withdrawing the needle is that the biopsy specimen sometimes becomes lodged in the syringe or is confused with a pleural fluid clot. I prefer to remove the pleural biopsy needle after obtaining each biopsy specimen. Whenever the Abram's pleural biopsy needle is withdrawn from the pleural space, the biopsy tract should be occluded with a finger immediately after the needle is withdrawn to decrease the likelihood of a pneumothorax.

At least four separate biopsy specimens should be obtained. Three of the four should be placed in formalin and taken to the pathology laboratory, and the fourth should be placed in a saline-containing sterile tube and sent to the tuberculosis laboratory to be ground up and cultured for mycobacterium and fungus. If electron microscopy is indicated, for example, for suspected mesothelioma, an additional pleural biopsy should be placed in glutaraldehyde. Once the biopsy specimens are obtained, a therapeutic thoracentesis can be performed through the Abram's needle. The pleural fluid should be removed only after obtaining the biopsy specimens because the pleural fluid separates the parietal and visceral pleura, and increases the safety of the procedure.

When the Abram's needle is withdrawn for the last time, the biopsy site should be massaged for a short time before placement of the bandage to eradicate the needle tract. Then a small adhesive bandage should be placed over the biopsy incision in a crosswise fashion to act as a butterfly-type dressing. Occasionally, pleural fluid exits or air enters through the biopsy tract after the procedure, particularly in patients who are debilitated and thin with poor tissue turgor. If this should happen, the biopsy site should be closed with a purse-string suture. Chest radiographs should be obtained on all patients after pleural biopsies.

Raja Needle

The Raja needle is very similar in design to the Abram's needle except that it has a self-opening stainless steel biopsy flap mounted on the inner tube (49, 50). When the Raja needle is withdrawn from the pleural space, the biopsy flap catches the parietal pleura. In the hands of the inventor, the Raja needle provides larger biopsy specimens in the experimental situation (49). In addition, the developer has reported that there is a significantly higher diagnostic yield with the Raja needle compared with the Abram's needle (50). Until these findings are confirmed by investigators without a personal interest in the Raja needle, the Raja needle is not recommended.

Cope Needle

The Cope needle (Fig. 25.8) consists of four separate parts: (a) a large outer cannula with a square but sharp end; (b) a hollow, blunt-tipped, hooked biopsy trocar; (c) a hollow-beveled trocar, and (d) a solid thin obturator or stylet. To insert the outer cannula (Fig. 25-8A) into the pleural space, the stylet (Fig. 25.8D) is inserted into the hollow-beveled trocar (Fig. 25.8C), which, in turn, is placed in the large outer cannula. Then, this apparatus is inserted through the small skin incision into the pleural space. The stylet and the hollow-beveled trocar must then be removed from the outer cannula and replaced by the hollow, blunt-tipped, hooked biopsy trocar (Fig. 25.8B). This maneuver is performed at the end of a normal expiration while the patient is holding his breath, by removing the hollow-beveled trocar and the stylet, and by placing the operator's thumb over the end of the outer cannula to prevent a pneu-

mothorax. A syringe may be attached to the outer cannula to obtain fluid for diagnostic studies at this time. Then, with the patient again holding his breath, the hooked biopsy trocar, to which a 10- to 20-mL syringe has been attached, is inserted through the large outer cannula into the pleural space. If a syringe is not attached to the hooked biopsy trocar, it should be occluded with a stopcock or the operator's thumb.

The right-angled projection on the proximal end of the hooked biopsy trocar indicates the direction of the distal biopsy hook. To obtain a biopsy, the apparatus is withdrawn with the hook directed inferiorly so as not to ensnare any nerves, veins, or arteries until the hooked biopsy trocar engages the parietal pleura (Fig. 25.9A). Then, with one hand, the engaged hook is held steady with a continual outward pulling motion, while the other hand advances the large outer cannula toward the pleural space using a rotary motion to sever the engaged piece of pleura (Fig. 25.9B). Then, the hooked biopsy trocar containing the tissue specimen is removed while the patient holds his breath, and the hooked trocar is replaced with the beveled trocar and obturator before the procedure is repeated for an additional biopsy specimen. Once the required biopsy specimens have been obtained, a therapeutic thoracentesis may be performed by attaching a large syringe and a three-way stopcock to the outer cannula.

The biopsy site and the biopsy specimens are handled identically with both Abram's and Cope pleural biopsy needles.

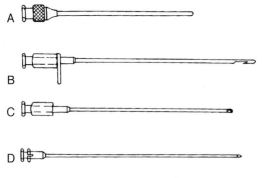

FIG. 25.8. Cope pleural biopsy needle. **A:** Outer cannula. **B:** Hollow, blunt-tipped, hooked biopsy trocar. **C:** Hollow-beveled trocar. **D:** Obturator or stylet.

Abram's versus Cope Needles

The rate of success in obtaining a pleural biopsy specimen depends more on the skill of the operator than on the choice of instruments (51). Morrone et al. (52) obtained pleural biopsies simultaneously with the Abram's and Cope needles, and they reported that the diagnostic yields were virtually identical. The Abram's needle provided slightly larger specimens and was slightly superior in detecting mesothelial cells. The Cope needle provided larger specimens of intercostal muscle. The Abram's needle is generally preferred over the Cope needle, however, because

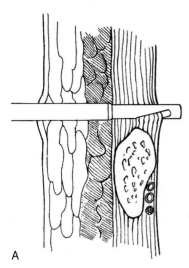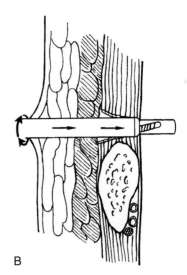

A   B

FIG. 25.9. A: The parietal pleura is hooked with the hollow, blunt-tipped biopsy trocar. **B:** The biopsy specimen is obtained by advancing the outer cannula with a rotary motion (*arrows*) to sever the engaged piece of pleura.

it is easier to use, it is a closed system and hence the likelihood of a pneumothorax is decreased, it provides a larger biopsy specimen, and it is safer for concomitant therapeutic thoracentesis because the end of the outer cannula is blunt.

Complications

Pleural biopsy has the same complications as diagnostic thoracentesis. One might expect pneumothorax to be more common with pleural biopsy than with thoracentesis for two reasons. First, the atmosphere has much more opportunity to be in communication with the pleural space with the biopsy, particularly when the Cope needle is used. Second, when the biopsy specimen is obtained, the visceral pleura may be inadvertently incised, leaving a small bronchopleural fistula that can lead to a large pneumothorax. The incidence of pneumothorax and the requirement for tube thoracostomy are comparable after thoracentesis and pleural biopsy, however (53). This is probably because more experienced individuals usually perform the pleural biopsy.

The second major complication of pleural biopsy is bleeding. If an intercostal artery or vein is inadvertently biopsied, a hemothorax can result

(47, 54). There is one case report of an arteriovenous fistula from an intercostal artery to an intercostal vein developing after pleural biopsy (55). The fistula subsequently ruptured causing a hemothorax. The pleural biopsy needle can also be mistakenly inserted into the liver, spleen, or kidney. Even though hepatic or kidney tissue may be demonstrated in the biopsy specimen, the patient usually suffers no significant adverse effects. Penetration of the spleen frequently requires splenectomy (56), however, and one should therefore be careful not to perform pleural biopsy or thoracentesis too far inferiorly on the left side.

REFERENCES

1. Adams FV, Galati V. M-mode ultrasonic localization of pleural effusion. *JAMA* 1978;239:1761–1764.
2. McVay PA, Toy PT. Lack of increased bleeding after paracentesis and thoracentesis in patients with mild coagulation abnormalities. *Transfusion* 1991;31:164–171.
3. McCartney JP, Adams JW, Hazard PB. Safety of thoracentesis in mechanically ventilated patients. *Chest* 1993;103:1920–1921.
4. Godwin JE, Sahn SA. Thoracentesis: a safe procedure in mechanically ventilated patients. *Ann Intern Med* 1990;113:800–802.
5. Weingardt JP, Guico RR, Nemcek AA Jr, et al. Ultrasound findings following failed, clinically directed thoracenteses. *J Clin Ultrasound* 1994;22:419–426.

6. Lipscomb DJ, Flower CDR, Hadfield JW. Ultrasound of the pleura: an assessment of its clinical value. *Clin Radiol* 1981;32:289–290.

7. Kohan JM, Poe RH, Israel RH, et al. Value of chest ultrasonography versus decubitus roentgenography for thoracentesis. *Am Rev Respir Dis* 1986;133:1124–1126.

8. Grogan DR, Irwin RS, Channick R, et al. Complications associated with thoracentesis. A prospective, randomized study comparing three different methods. *Arch Intern Med* 1990;150:873–877.

9. Rhodes ML. Thoracentesis. In: Jay SJ, Stonehill RB, eds. *Manual of pulmonary procedures*. Philadelphia: WB Saunders, 1980:1–11.

10. Ayo DS, Lee YC, Conner B, et al. Pleural fluid white blood cell count variation using different sample containers and methods at 4 and 24 hours after collection. *Chest* 1999;116:357S.

11. Cheng D-S, Rodriguez RM, Rogers J, et al. Comparison of pleural fluid pH values obtained using blood gas machine, pH meter, and pH indicator strip. *Chest* 1998;114:1368–1372.

12. Sarodia BD, Goldstein LS, Laskowski DM, et al. Does pleural fluid pH change significantly at room temperature during the first hour following thoracentesis? *Chest* 2000;117:1043–1048.

13. Seneff MG, Corwin RW, Gold LH, et al. Complications associated with thoracocentesis. *Chest* 1986;90:97–100.

14. Collins TR, Sahn SA. Thoracocentesis: clinical value, complications, technical problems, and patient experience. *Chest* 1987;91:817–822.

15. Bartter T, Mayo PD, Pratter MR, et al. Lower risk and higher yield for thoracentesis when performed by experienced operators. *Chest* 1993;103:1873–1876.

16. Aleman C, Alegre J, Armadans L, et al. The value of chest roentgenography in the diagnosis of pneumothorax after thoracentesis. *Am J Med* 1999;107:340–343.

17. Raptopoulos V, Davis LM, Lee G, et al. Factors affecting the development of pneumothorax associated with thoracentesis. *AJR Am J Roentgenol* 1991;156:917–920.

18. Brandstetter RD, Karetzky M, Rastogi R, et al. Pneumothorax after thoracentesis in chronic obstructive pulmonary disease. *Heart Lung* 1994;23:67–70.

19. Gervais DA, Petersein A, Lee MJ, et al. US-guided thoracentesis: requirement for postprocedure chest radiography in patients who receive mechanical ventilation versus patients who breathe spontaneously. *Radiology* 1997;204:503–506.

20. Doyle JJ, Hnatiuk OW, Torrington KG, et al. Necessity of routine chest roentgenography after thoracentesis. *Ann Intern Med* 1996;124:816–820.

21. Carney M, Ravin CE. Intercostal artery laceration during thoracentesis. Increased risk in elderly patients. *Chest* 1979;75:520–521.

22. Oksenhendler E, Harzic M, Le Roux JM, et al. HIV infection with seroconversion after a superficial needlestick injury to the finger. *N Engl J Med* 1986;315:582.

23. Light RW, Jenkinson SG, Minh V, et al. Observations on pleural pressures as fluid is withdrawn during thoracentesis. *Am Rev Respir Dis* 1980;121:799–804.

24. Villena V, Lopez-Encuentra A, Pozo F, et al. Measurement of pleural pressure during therapeutic thoracentesis. *Am J Respir Crit Care Med* 2000;162:1534–1538.

25. Boland GW, Gazelle GS, Girard MJ, et al. Asymptomatic hydropneumothorax after therapeutic thoracentesis for malignant pleural effusions. *AJR Am J Roentgenol* 1998;170:943–946.

26. Tarver RD, Broderick LS, Conces DJ Jr. Reexpansion pulmonary edema. *J Thorac Imaging* 1996;11:198–208.

27. Trapnell DH, Thurston JGB. Unilateral pulmonary edema after pleural aspiration. *Lancet* 1970;1:1367–1369.

28. Peatfield RC, Edwards PR, Johnson NM. Two unexpected deaths from pneumothorax. *Lancet* 1979;1:356–358.

29. Miller WC, Toon R, Palat H, et al. Experimental pulmonary edema following re-expansion of pneumothorax. *Am Rev Respir Dis* 1973;108:664–666.

30. Pavlin J, Cheney FW Jr. Unilateral pulmonary edema in rabbits after re-expansion of collapsed lung. *J Appl Physiol* 1979;46:31–35.

31. Mahfood S, Hix WR, Aaron Bl, et al. Re-expansion pulmonary edema. *Ann Thorac Surg* 1988;45:340–345.

32. Olcott EW. Fatal reexpansion pulmonary edema following pleural catheter placement. *J Vasc Interv Radiol* 1994;5:176–178.

33. Waqaruddin M, Bernstein A. Re-expansion pulmonary edema. *Thorax* 1975;30:54–60.

34. Sprung CL, Loewenherz JW, Baier H, et al. Evidence for increased permeability in re-expansion pulmonary edema. *Am J Med* 1981;71:497–500.

35. Pavlin DJ, Nessly ML, Cheney FW. Increased pulmonary vascular permeability as a cause of re-expansion edema in rabbits. *Am Rev Respir Dis* 1981;124:422–427.

36. Pavlin DJ. Lung re-expansion: for better or worse. *Chest* 1986;89:2–3.

37. Woodring JH. Focal reexpansion pulmonary edema after drainage of large pleural effusions: clinical evidence suggesting hypoxic injury to the lung as the cause of edema. *South Med J* 1997;90:1176–1182.

38. Jackson RM, Veal CF, Alexander CB, et al. Neutrophils in reexpansion pulmonary edema. *J Appl Physiol* 1988;65:228–234.

39. Nakamura H, Ishizaka A, Sawafuji M, et al. Elevated levels of interleukin-8 and leukotriene B_4 in pulmonary edema fluid of a patient with reexpansion pulmonary edema. *Am J Respir Crit Care Med* 1994;149:1037–1040.

40. Pavlin DJ, Nessly ML, Cheney FW. Hemodynamic effects of rapidly evacuating prolonged pneumothorax in rabbits. *J Appl Physiol* 1987;62:477–484.

41. Jackson RM, Veal CF, Alexander CB, et al. Re-expansion pulmonary edema: a potential role for free radicals in its pathogenesis. *Am Rev Respir Dis* 1988;137:1165–1171.

42. Moyers JP, Starnes DL, Bienvenu GL, et al. Thoracentesis performed by radiologist using ultrasound guidance is safe regardless of the amount of fluid withdrawn. *Chest* 1998;114:368S.

43. Milanez de Campos JR, Vargas FS, Werebe EC, et al. Thoracoscopy talc poudrage: 15 years experience. *Chest* 2001 (*in press*).

44. Light RW, O'Hara VS, Moritz TE, et al. Intrapleural tetracycline for the prevention of recurrent spontaneous pneumothorax. *JAMA* 1990;264:2224–2230.

45. Rozenman J, Yellin A, Simansky DA, et al. Re-expansion pulmonary oedema following spontaneous pneumothorax. *Respir Med* 1996;90:235–238.

46. Light RW. Closed needle biopsy of the pleura is a valuable diagnostic procedure. Con closed needle biopsy. *J Bronchol* 1998;5:332–336.

47. Levine H, Cugell DW. Blunt-end needle biopsy of pleura and rib. *Arch Intern Med* 1971;109:516–525.

48. Screaton NJ, Flower CD. Percutaneous needle biopsy of the pleura. *Radiol Clin North Am* 2000;38:293–301.

49. Ogirala RG, Agarwal V, Aldrich TK. Raja pleural biopsy needle. A comparison with the Abrams needle in experimental pleural effusion. *Am Rev Respir Dis* 1989;139:984–987.

50. Ogirala RG, Agarwal V, Vizioli LD, et al. Comparison of the Raja and the Abrams pleural biopsy needles in patients with pleural effusion. *Am Rev Respir Dis* 1993;147:1291–1294.

51. Walsh LJ, Macfarlane JT, Manhire AR, et al. Audit of pleural biopsies: an argument for a pleural biopsy service. *Respir Med* 1994;88:503–505.

52. Morrone N, Algranti E, Barreto E. Pleural biopsy with Cope and Abram's needles. *Chest* 1987;92:1050–1052.

53. Poe RH, Israel RH, Utell MJ, et al. Sensitivity, specificity, and predictive values of closed pleural biopsy. *Arch Intern Med* 1984;144:325–328.

54. Ali J, Summer WR. Hemothorax and hyperkalemia after pleural biopsy in a 43-year-old woman on hemodialysis. *Chest* 1994;106:1235–1236.

55. Lai JH, Yan HC, Kao SJ, et al. Intercostal arteriovenous fistula due to pleural biopsy. *Thorax* 1990;45:976–978.

56. Mearns AJ. Iatrogenic rupture of the spleen. *Br Med J* 1973;1:395–396.

26
Chest Tubes

Chest tubes are frequently used in the practice of pulmonary medicine. Indeed, in 1995, it was estimated that 1,330,000 chest tubes were placed (1). However, it has been my impression that many medical personnel do not understand how the drainage system for chest tubes functions and how to troubleshoot problems with chest tubes. In this chapter, the various methods of inserting chest tubes are discussed, followed by a more in-depth discussion of the different drainage systems used with chest tubes, plus recommendations for troubleshooting related problems. The indications for chest tube insertion with pneumothorax, hemothorax, empyema, and malignant pleural effusion are discussed in the respective chapters on these entities.

CHEST TUBE INSERTION

In general, chest tubes are inserted into the pleural space by three methods: tube thoracostomy with a guidewire and dilators, tube thoracostomy with a trocar, and operative tube thoracostomy. If the chest tube is inserted to drain blood, pus, or another fluid from the pleural space, the patient should be seated when the tube is inserted to ensure that the diaphragm is in the most dependent position and the fluid is collected in the lower part of the chest. When a chest tube is placed for a pneumothorax, the patient should be recumbent if an anterior chest tube is placed, and should be in the decubitus position if an axillary tube is placed.

Guidewire Tube Thoracostomy

This is probably the easiest way to insert a chest tube. In many hospitals, chest tubes are inserted by a radiologist, who uses this technique with either ultrasound or computed tomography (CT) guidance (2). Commercial kits are available for guidewire tube thoracostomy. This procedure uses the Seldinger technique with guidewires and dilators (3). In general, after the skin, periosteum, and parietal pleura are anesthetized, as is done for pleural biopsy (Chapter 25), an incision is made in the skin that is ample to permit passage of the desired size chest tube (Fig. 26.1A). Then a 18-gauge needle attached to a syringe is introduced into the pleural space. Fluid or air is aspirated to confirm the intrapleural position (Fig. 26.1B). The syringe is removed, and the "J" wire is threaded through the needle in the desired direction into the pleural space. The needle is then removed, and more local anesthetic is injected into the intercostal muscles surrounding the wire (Fig. 26.1C). The smallest dilator is inserted, and with a rotating movement, it is advanced into the pleural space over the guidewire (Fig. 26.1D). The wire should always project out beyond the end of the dilator or inserter. The first dilator is removed, leaving the wire in place. Then the next size dilator is advanced over the guidewire into the pleural space and removed. Finally, the chest tube containing the inserter is threaded over the guidewire (Fig 26.1E). The tube should pass readily, following the path made by the dilators and guided by the wire (3). It is important to make certain that all of the side holes in the tube are in the pleural space.

Once the tube is in place, the inserter and the guidewire are withdrawn (Fig. 26.1F). The tube is then clamped until it is attached to the chest drainage system. The tube is anchored in place by means of a long suture through the skin and

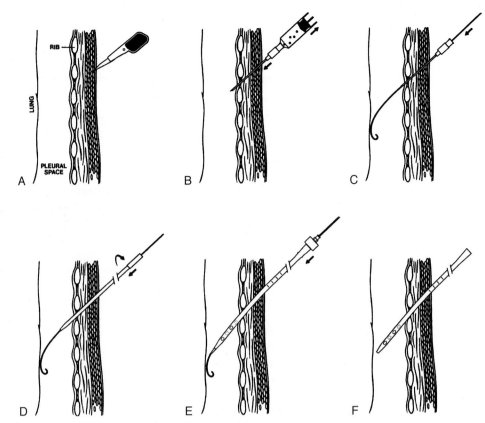

FIG. 26.1. Guidewire tube thoracostomy. **A:** Making a small skin incision slightly larger than the diameter of the chest tube. **B:** Introduction of 18-gauge needle into the pleural space. **C:** Insertion of wire with "J" end into the pleural space. **D:** With guidewire in place, the tract is enlarged by advancing progressively larger dilators over the wire guide. Introduction of the dilators is facilitated by rotating and advancing the dilators in the same plane of the wire guide. **E:** Introduction of the chest tube inserter/chest tube assembly over the guidewire. **F:** The guidewire and the chest tube inserter have been removed, leaving the chest tube positioned within the pleural space.

around the tube. The incision is sutured without tension to avoid necrosis of the skin next to the tube. The operative area is cleaned and is covered with plain 4 × 4 gauze pads. The gauze is then covered with tape, and additional fixation of the tube is obtained by the tape.

There are many different types of chest tubes that can be inserted with the above-mentioned technique. Kits are made so that chest tubes from 8.0 to 36.0 F can be inserted. The kits with the smaller chest tubes (less than 12.0 F) have no dilators. Some catheters have different characteristics. For example with the Wayne Pneumothorax Set (Cook Critical Care), a 14.0 F size catheter is inserted over a 19-gauge needle; the catheter

with this set is curved at the end like a pig's tail, and hence the name pigtail catheter. The Thal-Quick Chest Tube Sets come with chest tube sizes from 8.0 F to 36.0 F (Cook Critical Care, 800-457-4500, www.cookgroup.com).

Trocar Tube Thoracostomy

This method is similar to the guidewire tube thoracostomy, except that there is no guidewire or dilators. In general, it is not recommended (1). This method initially requires a 2 to 4 cm incision parallel to the superior border of the rib through the skin and subcutaneous tissues after local anesthesia is obtained. The trocar can

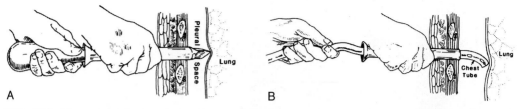

FIG. 26.2. Trocar tube thoracostomy. **A:** Insertion of trocar into the pleural space. Note the position of the hands, the position of the trocar relative to the ribs, and the cephalad position of the flat edge of the trocar. **B:** Insertion of chest tube through the trocar.

then be inserted between the ribs into the pleural cavity, with the flat edge of the stylet tip cephalad to prevent damage to the intercostal vessels (Fig. 26.2A). Because significant force is often required to insert the trocar, the hand not applying the force should be placed next to the patient's chest wall to control the depth of penetration. Once the trocar is in the pleural space, the stylet is removed. When the stylet is removed, the operator should immediately cover the trocar with the thumb to prevent a pneumothorax. Then, when the operator's thumb is removed, the chest tube, with its distal end clamped, is quickly inserted into the pleural space (Fig. 26.2B). The trocar is removed by sliding it back over the tube. When the trocar has been removed from the chest, the chest tube is clamped between the trocar and the chest wall so that the clamp on the distal end of the chest tube can be removed. This maneuver allows the trocar to be withdrawn from around the tube. The chest tube must remain clamped until it is attached to an underwater seal to prevent air from entering the pleural space.

An alternate trocar method uses a chest tube with a trocar positioned inside the tube. The procedure with this apparatus is similar to that already detailed. Once the pleural cavity is entered, the inner trocar is gradually removed from the chest tube. When the proximal end of the trocar clears the chest wall, a clamp is placed between the trocar and the chest wall until the trocar can be completely withdrawn and the tube attached to a water-seal drainage system.

Operative Tube Thoracostomy

With this method, an incision is made in the chest wall, and then after blunt dissection with a hemo-stat, the operator places his finger into the pleural space, to break adhesions between the lung and chest wall, and to ascertain the position of the chest tube. It is a more extensive procedure than guidewire tube thoracostomy or trocar tube thoracostomy, but it is probably safer. The most serious complications of tube thoracostomy are insertion of the tube ectopically, namely, into the lung, stomach, spleen, liver, or heart. These complications are more likely when a trocar chest tube is used. With the operative method, digital exploration of the insertion site delineates whether the tract leads into the pleural space and whether any tissue or organ is adherent to the parietal pleura at the planned site of tube insertion (4).

It is important to emphasize that operative tube thoracotomy can be very painful. Therefore, it is recommended that patients be given a narcotic or an anxiolytic medication 10 to 15 minutes before the procedure and that liberal doses of the local anesthetic be used (5). To perform an operative tube thoracostomy, a 3 to 4 cm incision is made in the skin parallel to the chosen intercostal space. The incision should be made down to the fascia overlying the intercostal muscle. This fascia is then incised throughout the length of the incision, with care taken not to cut the muscle. Once the fascia has been incised, the muscle fibers are spread with a blunt-tipped hemostat until the intercostal interspace is identified. Then, an incision is made in the intercostal fascia just above the superior border of the inferior rib over which the tube will pass. The parietal pleura is then penetrated by pushing a blunt-tipped hemostat through it. The hole in the parietal pleura is then enlarged by means of the operator's index finger (Fig. 26.3A). At this time, the operator should

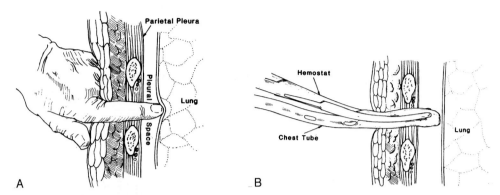

FIG. 26.3. Operative tube thoracostomy. **A:** The physician's index finger is used to enlarge the opening and to explore the pleural space. **B:** Placement of chest tube intrapleurally using a large hemostat.

palpate the adjacent pleural space to detect any adhesions. Then, the chest tube with its distal end clamped is inserted into the pleural space. A hemostat is used to guide the tube into the pleural space as the operator's finger is withdrawn (Fig. 26.3B). The last hole in the chest tube should be at least 2 cm inside the pleural space. The tube is sutured in place, and the incision is cleaned as in guidewire tube thoracostomy.

Verification of Chest Tube Placement

After the chest tube has been inserted and connected to a drainage system, a chest radiograph should be obtained to verify the correctness of its position. Ideally, both a posteroanterior (PA) and a lateral view should be obtained, because certain ectopic locations may not be apparent on the PA view alone (6). One advantage of performing the procedure under CT guidance is that position of the tube and the completeness of the drainage can be immediately assessed with repeat scans. If there are undrained locules of fluid, additional chest tubes can be inserted (2). Interestingly, the chest tubes frequently end up in the fissures, even with operative tube thoracostomy. Curtin et al. (7) reviewed the PA and lateral chest radiographs in 50 patients who had 66 chest tubes placed in the emergency room for trauma. They reported that 38 of the 66 chest tubes (58%) were within a fissure. There was no evidence, however, that the presence of the tube within the fissure decreased its functional effectiveness (7). It is pos-

sible that some of the chest tubes were not in the fissures originally but became positioned in the fissures after the fluid was drained.

PLEURAL DRAINAGE SYSTEMS

Chest tubes are inserted into the pleural space to evacuate air or fluid. Because the pleural pressure is usually negative, at least during part of the respiratory cycle, various methods have been developed to prevent air from entering the pleural space when the pleural pressure is negative but to permit air or fluid, or both, to drain from the pleural space continuously. When managing patients with chest tubes, one must understand how these various drainage systems operate. In the past, the bottle system (described later) was used for pleural drainage. Commercially manufactured collection systems have subsequently replaced the bottle system. Nevertheless, the bottle system is described in detail because all the commercially manufactured systems are based on the same principles as is the bottle system.

One-Way (Heimlich) Valve

This drainage system is by far the simplest. The chest tube is attached to a one-way flutter valve assembly, which is constructed so that the flexible tubing is occluded whenever the pressure inside the tubing is less than atmospheric pressure and is patent whenever the pressure inside the tubing is above atmospheric pressure. Therefore,

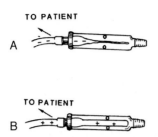

FIG. 26.4. Flutter valve. A: When the pleural pressure, and hence the intratube pressure, is negative (inspiration), the flexible tube is occluded because the pressure outside the tube is greater than the pressure inside the tube. B: When the pleural pressure is positive (expiration), the flexible tube is held open by the positive pressure, allowing the egress of air from the pleural space.

when the pleural pressure, and hence the pressure in the tube, are negative (Fig. 26.4A), the flutter valve is closed and no air enters the pleural space. When the pleural pressure becomes positive (Fig. 26.4B), however, the tube is patent and air or fluid can egress from the pleural space. This drainage system is only useful when the chest tube is placed for pneumothorax because with it, there is no good manner by which fluid, blood, or pus can be collected. The main advantages of the flutter valve are its simplicity and the freedom of the patient from bulky drainage apparatus. The flutter valve is effective, however. In one study of patients with postoperative air leaks, it was shown that the pleural pressure was more negative when the flutter valve was used than when underwater seal was used (8). When using the flutter valve, it is important to attach it with the correct orientation. Cases have been reported in which tension pneumothorax developed because the flutter valve was attached backwards (9).

One-Bottle Collection System

This system consists of one bottle that serves as both a collection container and a water seal (Fig. 26.5). The chest tube is connected to a rigid straw inserted through a stopper into a sterile bottle. Enough sterile saline solution is instilled into the bottle so that the tip of the rigid straw is about 2 cm below the surface of the saline solution. The

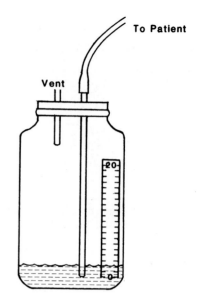

FIG. 26.5. One-bottle collection system. See text for details.

bottle's stopper must have a vent to prevent pressure from building up when air or fluid coming from the pleural space enters the bottle. The bottle usually is provided with a cap on the vent, and it is crucial to remove this cap before the system is connected to the patient.

This system works as follows. When the pleural pressure is positive, the pressure in the rigid straw becomes positive, and if the pressure inside the rigid straw is greater than the depth to which the straw is inserted into the saline solution, air (or liquid) will enter the bottle and will be vented to the atmosphere (or collect in the bottle). If the pleural pressure is negative, fluid will be drawn from the bottle into the rigid straw and no extra air will enter the system of the pleural space and the rigid straw. This system is called a water seal because the water in the bottle seals the pleural space from air or fluid from outside the body. Obviously, if the straw is above the fluid level in the bottle, the system will not operate and a large pneumothorax will develop.

This one-bottle system works well for uncomplicated pneumothorax. If substantial amounts of fluid are draining from the patient's pleural space, however, the level of fluid will rise in the one-bottle system, and therefore, the pressure will have to be higher and higher in the rigid straw to

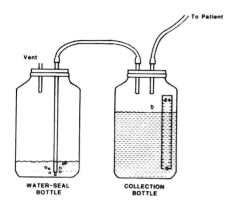

FIG. 26.6. Two-bottle collection system. See text for details.

allow additional air or fluid to exit from the pleural space. Another disadvantage of this system is that if the bottle is inadvertently placed above the level of the patient's chest, fluid can run back into the pleural cavity.

Two-Bottle Collection System

This system (Fig. 26.6) is preferred to the one-bottle collection system when substantial amounts of liquid are draining from the pleural space. With this system, the bottle adjacent to the patient acts as a collection bottle for the drainage, and the second bottle provides the water seal and the air vent. Therefore, the degree of water seal

does not increase as the drainage accumulates. The water seal bottle functions identically in both one- and two-bottle systems.

Suction and Three-Bottle Collection Systems

At times, it is desirable to apply negative pressure to the pleural space to facilitate reexpansion of the underlying lung or to expedite the removal of air or fluid from the pleural space. Suction at a fixed level, usually -15 to -20 cm H_2O, can be applied to the vent on a one- or two-bottle collection system with an Emerson pump. In many facilities, however, suction is provided by wall suction or other pumps in which the level of suction is not easily controlled. Because uncontrolled high levels of suction are considered dangerous, it is necessary to have some means of controlling the amount of suction.

Controlled amounts of suction can be readily applied to the system if a third bottle, the suction-control bottle, is added to the system, as illustrated in Fig. 26.7. A vent on the suction-control bottle is connected to a vent on the water-seal bottle. The suction-control bottle has a rigid straw similar to that of the water-seal bottle. The suction is connected to a second vent on the suction-control bottle. When suction is applied to the suction-control bottle, air enters this bottle

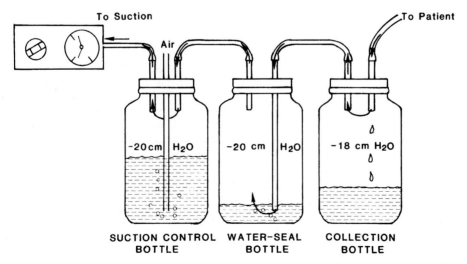

FIG. 26.7. Three-bottle collection system. The arrows describe the pathway for air to leave the pleural space. See text for details.

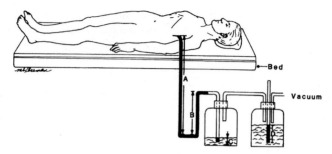

FIG. 26.8. The presence of liquid in the tube can affect the amount of negative pressure applied to the pleural space. The actual negative pressure in the chest = A − B − C + D.

through its rigid straw if the pressure in the bottle is more negative than the depth to which the straw is submerged. Therefore, the amount of negative pressure in the system is equal to the depth to which the rigid straw in the suction-control bottle is submerged below the surface as long as bubbles are entering the suction-control bottle through its rigid straw. In the example in Fig. 26.7, air enters the suction-control bottle from the atmosphere while its rigid straw is submerged 20 cm H_2O. Therefore, the pressure in the suction-control bottle is −20 cm H_2O. The same pressure exists in the water-seal bottle because these two bottles are in direct communication. The pressure in the drainage collection bottle is less negative than that in the other bottles, however, on account of the intervening water seal. In this case, the depth of the water seal is 2 cm, so the pressure in the drainage collection bottle and the pleural space (if no liquid is present in the chest tube) is −18 cm H_2O.

The amount of negative pressure in the system can be changed by adjusting the position of the rigid straw in the suction-control bottle or by changing the depth of the water in the suction control bottle. Bubbles must come continuously from the bottom of the suction-control straw if one is to have the expected degree of negative pressure. The bubbling does not need to be vigorous, just continuous; vigorous bubbling only creates more noise and hastens evaporation of the solution in the control bottle.

INTRINSIC NEGATIVE PRESSURE IN CHEST TUBES

The presence of liquid in the chest tubes can markedly influence the negative pressure that is applied to the pleural space, as illustrated in Fig. 26.8. The liquid in the tube that runs from the patient to the floor produces the effects of a siphon (10, 11). If the distance from the patient's chest to the top of the collection apparatus is 50 cm and the tube is filled with liquid, there will be a negative pressure of 50 cm H_2O in the pleural space if no suction is applied. The actual negative pressure applied to the pleural space from the entire system is the net vertical distance that the liquid occupies in the tube (A − B) minus the level of fluid in the waterseal (C) plus the negative pressure applied through the suction (D). Of course, if there is no liquid in the tube, the actual applied pressure will be the suction pressure minus the depth of the water seal. In the clinical situation, the presence of fluid in a dependent loop will result in an increased pressure at the connection between the chest tube and the drainage system and will result in a decrease in the hourly drainage (12).

COMMERCIALLY AVAILABLE DRAINAGE SYSTEMS

As can be appreciated from Fig. 26.7, three-bottle systems are unhandy to set up and are cumbersome to move if the patient needs to be transported. Therefore, a number of more compact and convenient chest-drainage units are commercially available. The main disadvantage of these units is that they are more expensive than the older systems. The average cost is about $75. The most popular system is a one-piece disposable, molded-plastic unit called the Pleur-Evac. Other available systems include the Atrium Total Recovery Water-Seal Chest Drains, Sentinel Seal, the Aquaseal, and the Thoraseal. An acceptable drainage system should have the following characteristics: (a) the water seal should be easily visualized, so one can determine whether the chest tube is patent and whether a bronchopleural fistula is present; (b) the tube should be functional when no suction is applied; (c) the volume of the collection chamber should be adequate and the markings should be such that the drainage is easily quantitated; and (d) there should be a pop-off valve to provide a safety factor if pressure builds up in the system. If the patient has a large amount of blood in their pleural space, consideration should be given to using a unit with autotransfusion capabilities such as the Atrium Blood Recovery Water Seal Chest Drain or the Davo Thora-Klex Chest Drainage System with Autotransfusion.

Pleur-Evac Unit

The Pleur-Evac system is a disposable, molded-plastic unit with three chambers duplicating the classic three-bottle system (Fig. 26.9). The chamber to the right is equivalent to the drainage collection bottle, whereas the middle chamber is equivalent to the water-seal bottle, and the chamber on the left is equivalent to the suction-control bottle. The height of water in the suction-control chamber minus the height of water in the water-seal compartment again determines the amount of pressure applied to the pleural space when suction is being applied. A valve located in the water-seal portion of the Pleur-Evac unit also vents air whenever the pressure in the system is greater than +2 cm H_2O.

The advantages of the Pleur-Evac unit are that it is simple to use, the amount of drainage can be easily measured, and the amount of negative pressure can be easily controlled. If the suction rate is turned up too high, the fluid will evaporate from the suction-control chamber and the system will be exceedingly noisy. If no suction is applied and the suction port is vented to room air, the system functions as a two-bottle collection system. When the patient is not receiving suction, the patency of the chest tube can be assessed by

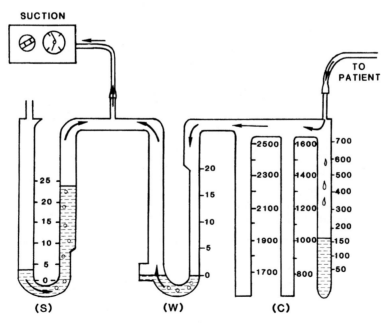

FIG. 26.9. Pleur-evac collection system, which is analogous to a three-bottle collection system. The area labeled C is the calibrated collection system; W is the water-seal chamber; S is the suction-control chamber. Arrows demonstrate the pathway for air to leave the pleural space. If the suction vent is left open to atmospheric pressure, the Pleur-evac system functions as a two-bottle collection system. When suction is applied, atmospheric air enters through S and leaves through the suction apparatus.

observing oscillations in the water-seal chamber with respiratory movements. In addition, if the patient is not receiving suction, the pressure in the chest tube can be calculated as the difference in the level of water in the two arms of the water-seal chamber after taking into consideration the amount of fluid in the tubes.

Other Chest Drainage System

Most of the other commercially available units are similar in design to the Pleur-Evac unit. Auto-transfusion can be performed with the Atrium Blood Recovery Water Seal Chest Drain or the Davo Thora-Klex Chest Drainage System with Autotransfusion. The Thora-Klex Chest Drainage System is unique in that it does not require water for either the water seal or the suction control. For the water seal, this system uses a one-way valve rather than a water seal and there is a relatively large chamber in which air leaks can be observed. The suction can be set between 0 and 40 cm H_2O with a suction control knob. The advantage of this system is that one need not worry about it tipping over since it contains no water.

INJECTION OF MATERIALS THROUGH CHEST TUBES

There are circumstances in which one would like to inject various materials through the chest tubes. For example, one might want to inject urokinase or streptokinase through the chest tube in a patient with a complicated parapneumonic effusion or one might want to inject talc in a slurry or a tetracycline derivative through the chest tube in a patient with a malignant pleural effusion. This is usually done by taking the chest tube apart and injecting the material through a Toomey syringe. This procedure is less than ideal because the sterility of the system is compromised if the tubes are disconnected, and there is always the possibility of a pneumothorax if the tubes are not clamped properly.

There is a commercially available adapter called a Thal-Quick Chest Tube Adapter (Cook Critical Care, 800-457-4500, www.cookgroup. com) that will fit in any chest tube. This unit

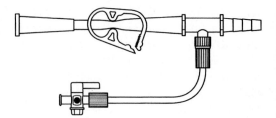

FIG. 26.10. Thal-Quick Chest Tube Adapter. This adapter provides an easy means by which materials can be injected into the pleural space through chest tubes. See text for details.

(Fig. 26.10) consists of two adapters separated by flexible tubing with a clamp. On the proximal end there is a sideport with a short segment of connecting tubing to which is attached a three-way stopcock. When one wishes to inject anything through the chest tube, the tube is clamped and the material is injected via the three-way stopcock. This system is recommended when a sclerosing agent is injected for pleurodesis or when a fibrinolytic agent is injected to break down loculi.

CARE OF A CHEST TUBE

The following three questions should be answered each time the condition of a patient with a chest tube is evaluated:

1. Is there bubbling through the water-seal bottle or the water-seal chamber on the disposable unit?
2. Is the tube functioning?
3. What is the amount and type of drainage from the tube?

Bubbling through Water-Seal Chamber

If air bubbles are escaping through the water seal, it means that air is entering the chest tube between the pleural space and the water seal. If the patient is receiving water-seal drainage without suction, the presence of bubbling in the water seal usually indicates a persistent air leak from the lung into the pleural space. If no air bubbles are seen on the initial inspection of the water seal, the patient should be asked to cough, and the water seal should be observed for bubbling. The coughing maneuver increases the patient's pleural pressure and should demonstrate small air leaks into the pleural space.

If the patient is receiving suction, disconnection or partial disconnection anywhere between the water seal and the patient will lead to bubbling through the water seal. For example, if the cap on the collection bottle in Fig. 26.7 is not airtight, air will be pulled into the collection bottle by the negative pressure and will exit through the water-seal bottle producing bubbling. Leaks in the system may be detected by clamping the chest tube at the point where it exits from the chest. If bubbling through the water seal persists, the drainage system itself is responsible for the leak, and the system should be examined thoroughly for leaks. If the bubbling stops when the chest tube is clamped, then the air is coming from the pleural space.

The presence of bubbling through the water seal does not necessarily indicate a communication between the lung and the pleural space. If the chest tube is not inserted far enough into the pleural space, one or more of the holes in the chest tube may lie outside the pleural space. Obviously, in such a situation, air enters the chest tube directly from the atmosphere. The possibility is evaluated by inspecting the chest tube. At times, particularly in debilitated patients with poor tissue turgor, the negative pleural pressure will cause air to enter the pleural space around the chest tube at the insertion site. At times it may be difficult to tell whether the air is leaking around the chest tube or whether it is due to a bronchopleural fistula. One may make this differentiation by measuring the level of Pco_2 in the air coming from the chest tube. The air from the chest tube is collected in a syringe and analyzed with the regular blood gas analyzer. Usually, a simple modification must be made on the analyzer so that it can analyze gas rather than liquid. If the air came from the lung via a bronchopleural fistula, then the Pco_2 should be greater than 20 mm Hg. Alternatively, if the air leaked around the chest tube, it will not have participated in gas exchange in the lung, and the Pco_2 should be less than 10 mm Hg. In such patients, additional sutures should be placed to make the chest tube insertion site airtight.

Bubbling through the water-seal chamber should not be confused with bubbling through the suction-control chamber. If suction is working properly, bubbling through the suction-control chamber or the suction-control bottle will always be present. When suction is being applied, the suction control chamber should be checked to make certain that there is a continuous stream of small bubbles and that the liquid is at the desired height.

Is the Chest Tube Functioning?

Each time the condition of a patient with a chest tube is evaluated, the functional status of the chest tube itself should be evaluated. If the patient is not receiving suction, one should observe the level of the liquid in the water seal. If the chest tube is patent and in the pleural space, the level of the liquid should move higher on inspiration in the limb of the water seal proximal to the patient, indicating a more negative pleural pressure. Of course, if the patient is receiving mechanical ventilation, the level of liquid in the proximal limb will go down on inspiration because the pleural pressure becomes more positive. When no fluctuations are observed synchronous with respiratory movements, the patient should be asked to make a maximal inspiratory effort, and if still no movement is observed, the chest tube is not functioning.

When the patient is receiving suction, it may be more difficult to ascertain chest tube function. If large bubbles of air are entering the suction-control chamber, the level of liquid in the water-seal chamber will fluctuate, depending on the number and size of bubbles in the chamber. These fluctuations should not be mistaken for evidence that the tube is functional. When the patient is receiving suction, the negative pressure in the suction-control chamber should be transmitted to the pleural space continuously to keep the pleural pressure constant. Therefore, to detect changes in pleural pressures with respiration, the suction must be temporarily discontinued. When suction is discontinued, the volume of air and liquid between the water seal and the pleural space should not change, and therefore, the level of liquid in the water-seal chamber should rise to be equivalent to the suction previously applied. This initial rise occurs whether or not the chest tube is patent. After this initial rise, the level of the fluid in the water-seal should be observed for fluctuations with the respiratory cycle to verify patency of the chest tube.

If a chest tube is not functioning, its functional status should be restored, or it should be removed. Chest tubes can become obstructed with tissue around the holes or by clots within the tube. The simplest method for restoring patency is to flush the tube with 50 mL of saline. This frequently clears the tube by pushing the clot out of the tube or by pushing the tissue away from the holes in the tube. The patency of a chest tube obstructed by clots in the extrathoracic portion of the tube can frequently be restored by "stripping" the tube. The usual technique is to grip and stabilize the tubing adjacent to the chest with the thumb and index finger of one hand and then to slide the other hand toward the drainage unit to compress a section of the tubing. Then, the first hand is repositioned adjacent to the second hand, and the procedure is repeated until the entire length of the tubing is cleared. A special chest tube roller is sometimes used. Stripping may relieve the obstruction in the tube. An alternate strategy is to instill the fibrinolytic enzyme streptokinase into the chest tube. The utility of streptokinase in clearing obstructed peritoneal catheters has been documented. The instillation of 250,000 IU streptokinase successfully relieved the obstruction in 13 of 19 episodes of catheter failure (13).

Chest tubes that are no longer patent and are no longer draining fluid should be removed because they serve as conduits for bacterial infection of the pleural space. Chest tubes frequently become colonized with bacteria, and when the tube becomes obstructed with a clot, the clot may contain bacteria. At times, a chest tube does not fluctuate but continues to drain fluid. In such a situation, the chest tube need not be removed.

Amount and Type of Drainage

The amount and the character of the drainage from the chest tube should be recorded for each 24-hour period. The amount of drainage is most easily quantitated by marking the level of the liquid in the collection chamber each day. This record-keeping is important because many therapeutic decisions are based on the quantity of the drainage. The character of the drainage is best described by quantitating the percentage of solid drainage material. This quantitation is easily done by marking the level of the sediment in the collection chamber each day. If the increase in volume of the entire collection system is known and if the increase in volume of the solid sediment is known, it is simple to calculate what percentage of the daily drainage is solid.

COMPLICATIONS OF TUBE THORACOSTOMY

There are numerous complications of tube thoracostomy. One of the most common complications is misplacement of the chest tube. The incidence of this complication has varied markedly. In one recent study, the incidence of malpositioned chest tubes was 26% with the emergency insertion of 77 tubes (14). In contrast, the incidence of chest tube malposition was only 1% in one series of 447 patients in whom the chest tubes were inserted through blunt dissection (15). A PA and lateral chest radiograph should always be obtained after a chest tube is inserted. It should be noted, however, that frequently the malposition is not diagnosed by these routine films. Accordingly, if a patient has an air or fluid collection that is not being drained adequately, a chest CT scan should be obtained to assess the position of the chest tube (and the presence of loculi). In one series, malpositioned chest tubes were diagnosed only by CT scan in 13 of 20 (65%) patients (14).

Many life-threatening complications occur when the tube is first inserted and include insertion of the chest tube into the lung, stomach, spleen, liver, or heart (4). These complications occur very rarely and are more likely when a trocar chest tube is used or when the tube is inserted without digital exploration of the insertion site. There is one case report in which a patient developed reversible cardiogenic shock owing to chest tube compression of the right ventricle (16). There is another report of two patients who developed tension pneumothoraces because the flutter valves were hooked up backward to the chest tube (9).

Pleural infection is another complication of tube thoracostomy. The administration of antibiotics to patients who have chest tubes for thoracic trauma may decrease the prevalence of empyema. Brunner et al. (17) randomly allocated 90 such patients to receive cefazolin or nothing immediately before and then every 6 hours until tube removal. They reported that there were six empyemas and three cases of pneumonia in the control group but only one case of pneumonia and no empyema in the antibiotic group (17). Two subsequent studies, which also evaluated trauma patients, reported similar results (18, 19). In view of these three studies, prophylactic antibiotics are recommended for all trauma patients who receive a chest tube. The antibiotic chosen should have activity against *Staphylococcus aureus* because this is the organism that causes the most infections (19). The utility of prophylactic antibiotics in other situations such as in postoperative patients, patients with spontaneous pneumothorax and patients with malignant effusions undergoing pleurodesis, is yet to be evaluated.

The insertion of a chest tube creates inflammation in the pleural space. Carvalho et al. (20) studied the pleural fluid characteristics of sheep with an experimental pleural effusion and an Argyle 32-Fr tube in the pleural space. The white blood cell count in the pleural effusion increased from 125 to over 6,000 per mm^3 within 6 hours. In this model, the pleural fluid protein level increased from 0 to 3.7 g per dL by 48 hours, and the pleural fluid lactate dehydrogenase increased from 44 IU per L to 638 IU per L by 24 hours. There is one report of three patients (all with quadriplegia) who developed lung entrapment as a result of prolonged chest tube drainage. They could only be weaned from the ventilator after a decortication was performed (21).

AUTOTRANSFUSION

Autotransfusion involves the collection, filtration, and reinfusion of the patient's shed blood for repletion of intravascular volume and the diminution of transfusion requirements. Postoperative patients with chest tubes and patients with hemothorax should be considered as candidates for autotransfusion. Several autotransfusion systems are commercially available. Atrium Medical Corporation manufactures a system capable of continuous infusion.

CHEST TUBE REMOVAL

The indications for the discontinuation of the tube thoracostomy for various conditions are discussed in the respective chapters on these conditions. In general, chest tubes for pneumothorax are removed when the lung has reexpanded and no air leaks are present. Chest tubes for hemothorax and empyema are removed when pleural drainage of blood or pus, respectively, has ceased.

Before chest tube removal is attempted, the procedure should be explained to the patient. In addition, petrolatum-impregnated gauze and an occlusive bandage should be prepared for use in a sterile field. Then, the dressing covering the thoracostomy site is removed, and the suture restraining the chest tube is cut. Petrolatum-impregnated gauze is placed around the tube on the patient's chest wall so that it can be moved to cover the wound when the tube is removed. It is important that the pleural pressure be positive when the chest tube is removed so that air will not enter the pleural space. This can be accomplished by having the patient hum or perform a Valsalva maneuver. The chest tube is quickly pulled out of the chest, and the wound is covered immediately with the gauze. The wound usually closes sufficiently without using sutures. The procedure is completed by placing an occlusive dressing over the gauze.

REFERENCES

1. Munnell ER. Thoracic drainage. *Ann Thorac Surg* 1997;63:1497–1502.
2. Moulton JS. Image-guided management of complicated pleural fluid collections. *Radiol Clin North Am* 2000;38:345–474.
3. Thal AP, Quick KL. A guided chest tube for safe thoracostomy. *Surg Gynecol Obstet* 1988;167:517.
4. Symbas PN. Chest drainage tubes. *Surg Clin North Am* 1989;69:41–46.
5. Luketich JD, Kiss M, Hershey J, et al. Chest tube insertion: a prospective evaluation of pain management. *Clin J Pain* 1998;14:152–154.

6. Gilbert TB, McGrath BJ, Soberman M. Chest tubes: indications, placement, management and complications. *J Intensive Care Med* 1993;8:73–86.

7. Curtin JJ, Goodman LR, Quebbeman EJ, et al. Thoracostomy tubes after acute chest injury: relationship between location in a pleural fissure and function. *AJR Am J Roentgenol* 1994;163:1339–1942.

8. Waller DA, Edwards JG, Rajesh PB. A physiological comparison of flutter valve drainage bags and underwater seal systems for postoperative air leaks. *Thorax* 1999;54:442–443.

9. Mainini SE, Johnson FE. Tension pneumothorax complicating small-caliber chest tube insertion. *Chest* 1990; 97:759–760.

10. Enerson DM, McIntyre J. A comparative study of the physiology and physics of pleural drainage systems. *J Thorac Cardiovasc Surg* 1966;52:40–46.

11. Kam AC, O'Brien M, Kam PC. Pleural drainage systems. *Anaesthesia* 1993;48:154–161.

12. Schmelz JO, Johnson D, Norton JM, et al. Effects of position of chest drainage tube on volume drained and pressure. *Am J Crit Care* 1999;8:319–323.

13. Wiegmann TB, Stuewe B, Duncan KA, et al. Effective use of streptokinase for peritoneal catheter failure. *Am J Kidney Dis* 1985;6:119–123.

14. Baldt MM, Bankier AA, Germann PS, et al. Complications after emergency tube thoracostomy: assessment with CT. *Radiology* 1995;195:539–543.

15. Millikan JS, Moore EE, Steiner E, et al. Complications of tube thoracostomy for acute trauma. *Am J Surg* 1980;140:738–741.

16. Kollef MH, Dothager DW. Reversible cardiogenic shock due to chest tube compression of the right ventricle. *Chest* 1991;99:976–980.

17. Brunner RG, Vinsant GO, Alexander RH, et al. The role of antibiotic therapy in the prevention of empyema in patients with an isolated chest injury (ISS 9-10): a prospective study. *J Trauma* 1990;30:1148–1153.

18. Nichols RL, Smith JW, Muzik AC, et al. Preventive antibiotic usage in traumatic thoracic injuries requiring closed tube thoracostomy. *Chest* 1994;106: 1493–1498.

19. Gonzalez RP, Holevar MR. Role of prophylactic antibiotics for tube thoracostomy in chest trauma. *Am Surg* 1998;64:617–620.

20. Carvalho P, Kirk W, Butler J, et al. Effects of tube thoracostomy on pleural fluid characteristics in sheep. *J Appl Physiol* 1993;74:2782–2787.

21. Peterson WP, Whiteneck GG, Gerhart KA. Chest tubes, lung entrapment, and failure to wean from the ventilator. Report of three patients with quadriplegia. *Chest* 1994;105:1292–1294.

27

Thoracoscopy

Although thoracoscopy has been a part of thoracic surgical practice for many years, the advent of video-assisted techniques has greatly expanded the indications and the uses of this procedure. Where previously thoracoscopy was performed mainly for diagnostic purposes, video-assisted thoracic surgery (VATS) now has assumed a major role in the therapy of chest pathology. Indeed, in some institutions it is now the most commonly used operative approach in the general thoracic surgical practices (1). The primary advantage of VATS is that it produces less morbidity and mortality, and shorter hospitalization times than does thoracotomy. At present, VATS is used for many surgical procedures in the chest other than those related to pleural disease including pulmonary nodule removal, lobectomy, lung biopsy, exploration of the mediastinum, myotomy for achalasia, sympathectomy, and pericardial window creation. In this chapter, we discuss only those procedures that deal with pleural disease.

It is important to understand that there are two different techniques for thoracoscopy—VATS and medical thoracoscopy. VATS is performed in an operating room under general anesthesia with the patient selectively intubated to allow for single lung ventilation. Multiple puncture sites are made in the chest wall through which the thoracoscope and surgical instruments are introduced. Medical thoracoscopy differs from VATS in that the patient may not be intubated and usually breathes spontaneously (2). The procedure is usually performed with conscious sedation and local anesthesia. Medical thoracoscopy primarily serves as a diagnostic tool rather than for intervention. Medical thoracoscopy is usually performed by pulmonologists, whereas VATS is performed by thoracic surgeons (2). The primary advantages of medical thoracoscopy are that it can be performed in an endoscopy suite, it does not involve general anesthesia, and it is less expensive than VATS (2). For diagnostic purposes, either VATS or medical thoracoscopy is appropriate and the choice of procedure depends primarily on its availability at one's institution.

HISTORY

Thoracoscopy was developed by Jacobaeus in the early 1900s because a method was needed to break down adhesions in patients with pulmonary tuberculosis so that an artificial pneumothorax could be produced (3). Thoracoscopy was used extensively for this purpose up until 1945, at which time streptomycin was introduced for the treatment of tuberculosis (4). In one report, the results in 1,000 patients in whom thoracoscopy was used to breakdown adhesions were detailed (5). Jacobaeus also published an early report on the use of thoracoscopy to localize and diagnose benign and malignant lesions of the pleura and pulmonary parenchyma (6).

After 1950, thoracoscopy was rarely performed in the United States, although some physicians in Europe continued to perform the procedure. During this period, thoracoscopy was used primarily to assist in diagnosing pleural effusions, although pleurodesis was sometimes attempted with talc (7, 8) or silver nitrate (9, 10). A number of instruments were employed including rigid bronchoscopes, mediastinoscopes, flexible bronchoscopes, and specialized rigid fiberoptic thoracoscopes (11). Two books published in the past 15 years provide state-of-the-art discussions on thoracoscopy before the advent of VATS, which has become available mainly since 1990 (12, 13).

The recent revival of thoracoscopy was made possible by the tremendous advances in endoscopic technology (14). The development of the charged coupling device, a silicon chip that is light sensitive, led to the sufficient miniaturization of a video camera. When attached to a fiberoptic telescope, the video camera produces a well-defined, magnified image on a video monitor that allows the operating surgeon to work with an assistant. Previously, the surgeon had to hold the thoracoscope, and only he could look into it while working, which did not allow for the aid of an assistant and, thus, limited the complexity of the procedures undertaken (11).

PROCEDURE

There are two fundamental techniques by which medical thoracoscopy is performed, namely, single puncture and double puncture (15). Both techniques require a xenon light source, which satisfies the requirements for high-quality visual exploration and video documentation. For the single puncture technique, a rigid thoracoscope with a working channel of 3 to 5 mm is used. With the single puncture technique various instruments such as the biopsy forceps, needle biopsy, and suction catheter are used through the working channel, which also accommodates electrocautery. For the double puncture technique, a rigid thoracoscope is also used. A second smaller trocar is used, which accommodates biopsy forceps, brushes, needles, and laser fibers. The single puncture technique is the easiest method to learn and is commonly used by the chest physician (15).

Most VATS procedures are performed under general anesthesia because with general anesthesia, endoscopic surgical manipulation can be accomplished safely and expeditiously (1). It is imperative that the anesthesia personnel be experienced in open thoracic procedures. In addition, they must be well versed with the principles of selective one-lung ventilation. Ventilation for the patient is provided through the contralateral lung. It is most convenient to work with two video

monitors, one on each side, so that both the operator and the assistant may have an unobstructed view.

The patient is placed on the operating table, and the chest is prepared and draped as for a thoracotomy. After general anesthesia is induced, the thoracoscope is inserted and the ipsilateral lung is collapsed for unimpaired visibility of the intrathoracic structures. At this time, the thoracic cavity is systematically examined. After the initial thoracoscopic exploration of the pleural cavity is concluded, further intercostal access for VATS instrumentation is achieved under direct thoracoscopic vision. Usually, three incisions are made to create a triangular configuration, an arrangement that facilitates instrument placement and allows one to work in coordination with an assistant. The incisions are placed along a line of the proposed thoracotomy incision so that if a thoracotomy is required, the incisions simply are joined. At the completion of the VATS procedure, a single chest tube is placed into the pleural space.

Instrumentation for VATS is slowly improving. Initially, instruments designed for laparoscopy were used but were less than ideal, particularly for grasping lung parenchyma, which has a tendency to tear. The most significant advance in instrumentation was the development of an endoscopic linear stapler, which simultaneously cuts while laying down parallel rows of staples that are both hemostatic and aerostatic (Endo:GIA, U.S. Surgical Corp., Norwalk, CT, USA).

CONTRAINDICATIONS TO THORACOSCOPY

The two primary contraindications to thoracoscopy are the inability to tolerate one lung ventilation and pleural adhesions of sufficient density to preclude entry into the chest (11). Of course the patient must be able to tolerate general anesthesia and must not have bleeding abnormalities that would preclude other surgical procedures.

INDICATIONS AND RESULTS

Undiagnosed Pleural Effusion

On occasion, the etiology of a pleural effusion remains uncertain after the initial diagnostic workup, which includes a diagnostic thoracentesis with pleural fluid cytology, a pleural fluid marker for tuberculosis and an evaluation for pulmonary embolus. Such patients are possible candidates for thoracoscopy to establish the etiology of the pleural effusion.

Thoracoscopy is an efficient way to establish the diagnosis of malignancy. In the early 1990s, two separate studies, each with 102 patients, were published that reported diagnostic yields of 93% (16) and 80% (17). However, when these two studies are examined in detail, one finds that the only diagnosis that was definitely established is malignancy. When the above-mentioned two studies are combined, the diagnosis of malignancy was established in 99 of the 117 patients (85%) with malignancy, including 51 of 56 (91%) with mesothelioma. In a more recent study from Denmark, thoracoscopy established the diagnosis in 89 of 101 patients (88%) with malignancy (18). Thoracoscopy can also establish the diagnosis of tuberculosis (18–20).

Where is the rightful place of thoracoscopy in the management of the patient with an undiagnosed pleural effusion? Thoracoscopic procedures should be used only when the less invasive methods of diagnosis such as pleural aspiration for cytologic, bacteriologic, and chemical examinations have not yielded a diagnosis. In one series of 620 patients with pleural effusions, only 48 (8%) remained without a diagnosis and were subjected to thoracoscopy (21). In these 48 patients, a diagnosis of malignancy was established in 24 (50%), and in an additional 16 patients, the diagnosis of benign disease was established when the thoracoscopic and clinical findings were considered jointly. In the remaining eight patients (16%), no diagnosis was established at thoracoscopy, but six of the patients were subsequently diagnosed as having malignancy (21).

Thoracoscopy is recommended for the patient with an undiagnosed pleural effusion in whom the diagnosis of malignancy is suspected, and in whom at least one pleural fluid cytology and one pleural fluid marker for tuberculosis (adenosine deaminase, interferon-gamma, or polymerase chain reaction [PCR]) have been negative. When one performs thoracoscopy for diagnostic purposes, it is important to be prepared to perform a procedure to create a pleurodesis at the time of surgery. Our preferred method is pleural abrasion. Although talc insufflation was recommended in the previous edition of this book, concerns about respiratory failure occurring after talc administration (see Chapter 7) have led to this different recommendation. It should also be noted that the performance of thoracoscopy without any attempt to create a pleurodesis will result in a pleurodesis in over 50% of patients with malignant pleural effusions (22, 23).

Malignant Pleural Effusion

If a patient has a known malignancy, should thoracoscopy be performed to effect a pleurodesis? It appears that the success rates are comparable for pleurodesis with thoracoscopy and with tube thoracostomy. In a recent study, Heffner et al. (24) reported that the failure rate was 18% in 231 patients subjected to thoracoscopy, whereas it was 19.6% in 188 patients in which pleurodesis was attempted through a chest tube. Yim et al. (25) randomized 55 patients to pleurodesis with thoracoscopy and talc insufflation or pleurodesis with tube thoracostomy and talc slurry, and found that there was no significant differences in the results with the two treatment methods (25). Therefore, it does not seem reasonable to subject a patient to general anesthesia and the extra expense of thoracoscopy when he or she could be managed just as effectively with tube thoracostomy and a tetracycline derivative intrapleurally.

If a patient has a malignant pleural effusion that is loculated, it is possible that the loculations can be broken down and the pleural space cleared with thoracoscopy.

Parapneumonic Pleural Effusion

Thoracoscopy should be considered for the patient with a parapneumonic effusion that is not drained with either a therapeutic thoracentesis or tube thoracostomy. At the time of thoracoscopy, the loculi in the pleural space can be disrupted, the pleural space can be completely drained, and the chest tube can be optimally placed. In addition, the pleural surfaces can be inspected to determine the necessity for further intervention such as decortication. A chest computed tomography (CT) scan should be obtained before thoracoscopy to provide anatomic information about the size and extent of the empyema cavity and the thickness of the peel over the visceral pleura.

Incompletely drained parapneumonic effusions are treated very effectively with thoracoscopy. When four recent series (26–29) are combined, thoracoscopy was the definitive procedure in 178 of 232 patients (77%). The overall mortality was 3%. The median time for chest tube drainage after the procedure ranged from 3.3 to 7.1 days, and the median hospital stay after thoracoscopy ranged from 5.3 to 12.3 days.

When faced with a patient with a complicated parapneumonic effusion that is not completely drained, there are basically four alternatives: (a) insert additional chest tubes, (b) instill fibrinolytics intrapleurally, (c) perform thoracoscopy, or (d) perform decortication. The insertion of additional chest tubes is not recommended because it usually is ineffective. Fibrinolytics intrapleurally have been recommended by some and are a viable alternative (see Chapter 9). If fibrinolytics are used and drainage is incomplete after 3 to 5 days, thoracoscopy should be performed (30). Some have recommended not using the fibrinolytics and proceeding directly to thoracoscopy. Wait et al. (31) randomized 20 patients with parapneumonic effusions and either a loculated pleural effusion or a pleural fluid pH of less than 7.20 to receive either streptokinase via tube thoracostomy or thoracoscopy. They reported that thoracoscopy was the definitive procedure in 10 of 11 patients (91%), whereas streptokinase was definitive in only 4 of 9 (44%). They concluded that a primary treatment strategy of VATS was associated with a higher efficacy, shorter hospitalization, and less cost than a treatment strategy of intrapleural fibrinolytics (31). Thoracotomy is reserved for those cases in which thoracoscopy fails or in which thoracoscopy is indicated but is unavailable.

Thoracoscopy also appears to be useful in patients with postpneumonectomy empyemas. Hollaus et al. (32) reported that debridement of the pleura with thoracoscopy in five patients with postpneumonectomy empyema without bronchopleural fistula, facilitated control of the pleural infection (32).

Pneumothorax

Thoracoscopy is effective in the treatment of spontaneous pneumothorax and the prevention of recurrent pneumothorax. With thoracoscopy, there are two primary objectives: (a) to treat the bullous disease responsible for the pneumothorax and (b) to create a pleurodesis. The most common means by which the bullae are treated at the present time is with an endoscopic stapling device. The primary disadvantage of the endo-stapler is cost, which is about $1,000 per procedure (33). Previously, the bullae were treated with electrocoagulation, which was associated with a higher recurrence rate (34). An alternative method of dealing with the apical bullae is to ligate the bullae with a Roeder loop (35). However, Inderbitzi et al. (35) reported a relatively high recurrence rate after use of the loop and recommend that it be abandoned in favor of wedge resection with the endo-stapler. The best way to induce a pleurodesis appears to be with pleural abrasion. It is comparable in effectiveness to talc insufflation and does not carry the risk of inducing acute respiratory failure. It is also comparable in effectiveness to partial parietal pleurectomy but is easier to perform.

The effectiveness of VATS in conjunction with endo-stapling has been demonstrated in several large series, which were recently reported. Cardillo et al. (36) used VATS to treat 432 patients with primary spontaneous pneumothorax between 1992 and 1998. They used subtotal pleurectomy to induce a pleurodesis in some patients and talc insufflation in others. In 2.3% of their 432 patients, conversion to an open procedure was necessary, usually because of extensive adhesions. The recurrence rate was 4.4%, with a mean follow-up of 38 months (36). Yim and Liu (37) treated 483 patients with primary spontaneous pneumothorax creating a pleurodesis with mechanical abrasion. In this series, the mean postoperative stay was only 3 days and the recurrence rate was only 1.74%, with a mean follow-up of 20 months (37). Thoracoscopy is also effective for treating secondary spontaneous pneumothorax (38, 39).

Which patients with spontaneous pneumothorax should be subjected to thoracoscopy? In some centers, all patients with spontaneous pneumothorax are subjected to thoracoscopy to evaluate the status of the underlying lung (40). This approach seems overly aggressive because approximately 50% of patients with their initial pneumothorax will never have a recurrence without any treatment. Patients with primary pneumothorax in whom aspiration therapy has failed or who have a recurrent pneumothorax are best managed with thoracoscopy. The reason for this recommendation is that the hospital stays are comparable with thoracoscopy and tube thoracostomy, but the recurrence rates are much less after thoracoscopy. Because the recurrence of a pneumothorax is more life threatening in patients with secondary spontaneous pneumothorax, it is recommended that thoracoscopy be performed in most patients with secondary spontaneous pneumothorax after they are initially managed with tube thoracostomy (see Chapter 21).

Hemothorax

Thoracoscopy may replace thoracotomy in some patients with traumatic hemothorax who otherwise would have been subjected to thoracotomy. Thoracotomy rather than thoracoscopy should be performed if there is exsanguinating hemorrhage through the chest tubes (41). Villavicencio et al. (42) reviewed the literature and reported that VATS was effective in controlling the bleeding in 33 of 40 (82%) of the patients on whom it was attempted. Thoracoscopy was effective in controlling the bleeding when it arose from intercostal vessels or from lung lacerations.

If more that 30% of the hemithorax is occupied by clotted blood after tube thoracostomy, removal of the blood is usually recommended. Traditionally, the clotted blood has been removed through a thoracotomy. However, thoracoscopy now appears to be the optimal method for the removal of this clotted blood (42, 43). Carrillo and Richardson (43) reviewed 25 patients with retained thoracic collections who underwent 26

VATS procedures for this problem. They reported that the procedure was successful in 19 of the 25 patients. If the procedure was performed less than 7 days after the initial injury, it was more likely to be successful.

Chylothorax

One of the options for the treatment of a chylothorax is ligation of the thoracic duct. It is possible to ligate the thoracic duct through thoracoscopy. Although thoracoscopy has not been widely employed for the control of chylothorax, there are anecdotal reports documenting its successful use (44–46). Kent and Pinson (44) successfully ligated the thoracic duct in one patient who developed a chylothorax after a radical neck dissection. Shirai et al. (45) performed thoracoscopy on a patient who developed a chylothorax postoperatively. They could identify the site of leakage, and the leakage stopped with the application of fibrin glue. Zoetmulder et al. (46) reported on a 51-year-old patient who developed a chylothorax 4 years after treatment of a soft-tissue sarcoma. At thoracoscopy, the thoracic duct leak could be identified and oversewn. The patient had no recurrence of her pleural effusion. It remains to be seen whether the endoscopic closure of chylous leaks is more successful or better tolerated than current open techniques (47).

COMPLICATIONS OF THORACOSCOPY

Thoracoscopy has a relatively low rate of complications. Data collected on 1,820 patients from the VATS Study Group Registry revealed that the overall mortality was 2%. Prolonged air leak was the most frequent complication and occurred in 3.2%; significant bleeding resulting in transfusion occurred in only 1%. Pneumonia and empyema occurred in 1.1% and 0.6%, respectively (48). Thoracoscopy is tolerated relatively well by the patient with chronic obstructive pulmonary disease. In the above-mentioned study, there were 59 patients who had an FEV_1 below 1 L who underwent thoracoscopy. There was one death (1.7%), and the average postprocedure hospital stay was only 5.4 days (48). Jancovici et al. (49)

reviewed 937 VATS procedures at four surgical institutions from June 1991 through May 1995. In this series approximately half the procedures were performed for pleural problems. They reported that the in-hospital mortality rate was 0.5%, and death occurred principally in patients operated on for malignant pleural effusions. In their series, the overall incidence of postoperative complications was 10.9%; the most common complications were prolonged air leak (6.7%) and pleural effusion (0.7%). There have also been at least 21 instances of tumor seeding of VATS incisions reported by the VATS study group (50). The complications of medical thoracoscopy are even less than those of VATS (15). The mortality rate is less than 0.5%, and most deaths are thought to be unrelated to the procedure (15).

REFERENCES

1. Landreneau RJ, Mack MJ, Hazelrigg SR, et al. The role of thoracoscopy in the management of intrathoracic neoplastic processes. *Semin Thorac Cardiovas Surg* 1993;5:219–228.
2. Loddenkemper R. Thoracoscopy—state of the art. *Eur Respir J* 1998;11:213–221.
3. Jacobaeus HC. Ueber die Môglichkeit die Zystoskopie bei untersuchung serôser hôhlungen anzuwenden. *München Med Wochenschr* 1910;57:2090–2092.
4. Braimbridge MV. The history of thoracoscopic surgery. *Ann Thorac Surg* 1993;56:510–614.
5. Day JC, Chapman PT, O'Brien EJ. Closed intrapleural pneumonolysis: an analysis of 1000 consecutive operations. *J Thorac Surg* 1948;17:537–554.
6. Jacobaeus HC. The practical importance of thoracoscopy in surgery of the chest. *Surg Gynecol Obstet* 1922;34:289–296.
7. Adler RH, Rappole BW. Recurrent malignant pleural effusions and talc powder aerosol treatment. *Surgery* 1967;62:1000–1006.
8. Weissberg D, Ben-Zeev I. Talc pleurodesis. Experience with 360 patients. *J Thorac Cardiovasc Surg* 1993;106:689–695.
9. Andersen I, Poulsen T. Surgical treatment of spontaneous pneumothorax. *Acta Chir Scand* 1959;118:105–112.
10. Wied U, Andersen K, Schultz A, et al. Silver nitrate pleurodesis in spontaneous pneumothorax. *Scand J Thorac Cardiovasc Surg* 1981;15:305–307.
11. Kaiser LR. Video-assisted thoracic surgery. Current state of the art. *Ann Surg* 1994;220:720–734.
12. Brandt H-J, Loddenkemper R, Mai J. *Atlas of diagnostic thoracoscopy.* New York: Thieme Inc., 1985.
13. Boutin C, Viallat JR, Aelony Y. *Practical thoracoscopy.* Berlin: Springer-Verlag, 1991.
14. Loddenkemper R, Boutin C. Thoracoscopy: present diagnostic and therapeutic indications. *Eur Respir J* 1993;6:1544–1555.
15. Mathur PN, Astoul P, Boutin C. Medical thoracoscopy. Technical details. *Clin Chest Med* 1995;16:479–486.
16. Hucker J, Bhatnagar NK, al-Jilaihawi AN, et al. Thoracoscopy in the diagnosis and management of recurrent pleural effusions. *Ann Thorac Surg* 1991;52:1145–1147.
17. Menzies R, Charbonneau M. Thoracoscopy for the diagnosis of pleural disease. *Ann Intern Med* 1991;114:271–276.
18. Hansen M, Faurschou P, Clementsen P. Medical thoracoscopy, results and complications in 146 patients: a retrospective study. *Respir Med* 1998;92:228–232.
19. de Groot M, Walther G. Thoracoscopy in undiagnosed pleural effusions. *S Afr Med J* 1998;88:706–711.
20. Emad A, Rezaian GR. Diagnostic value of closed percutaneous pleural biopsy vs pleuroscopy in suspected malignant pleural effusion or tuberculous pleurisy in a region with a high incidence of tuberculosis: a comparative, age-dependent study. *Respir Med* 1998;92:488–492.
21. Kendall SW, Bryan AJ, Large SR, et al. Pleural effusions: is thoracoscopy a reliable investigation? A retrospective review. *Respir Med* 1992;86:437–440.
22. Groth G, Gatzemeier U, Haubingen K, et al. Intrapleural palliative treatment of MPEs with mitoxantrone versus placebo (pleural tube alone). *Ann Oncol* 1991;2:213–215.
23. Sorensen PG, Svendsen TL, Enk B. Treatment of MPE with drainage, with and without instillation of talc. *Eur J Respir Dis* 1984;65:131–135.
24. Heffner JE, Nietert PJ, Barbieri C. Pleural fluid pH as a predictor of pleurodesis failure: analysis of primary data. *Chest* 2000;117:87–95.
25. Yim AP, Chan AT, Lee TW, et al. Thoracoscopic talc insufflation versus talc slurry for symptomatic malignant pleural effusion. *Ann Thorac Surg* 1996;62:1655–1658.
26. Landreneau RJ, Keenan RJ, Hazelrigg SR, et al. Thoracoscopy for empyema and hemothorax. *Chest* 1995;109:18–24.
27. Cassina PC, Hauser M, Hillejan L, et al. Video-assisted thoracoscopy in the treatment of pleural empyema: stage-based management and outcome. *J Thorac Cardiovasc Surg* 1999;117:234–238.
28. Lawrence DR, Ohri SK, Moxon RE, et al. Thoracoscopic debridement of empyema thoracis. *Ann Thorac Surg* 1997;64:1448–1450.
29. Striffeler H, Gugger M, Im Hof V, et al. Video-assisted thoracoscopic surgery for fibrinopurulent pleural empyema in 67 patients. *Ann Thorac Surg* 1998;65:319–323.
30. Silen ML, Naunheim KS. Thoracoscopic approach to the management of empyema thoracis. Indications and results. *Chest Surg Clin N Am* 1996;6:491–499.
31. Wait MA, Sharma S, Hohn J, et al. A randomized trial of empyema therapy. *Chest* 1997;111:1548–1551.
32. Hollaus PH, Lax F, Wurnig PN, et al. Videothoracoscopic treatment of postpneumonectomy empyema. *J Thorac Cardiovasc Surg* 1999;117:397–398.
33. Hazelrigg SR, Landreneau RJ, Mack M, et al. Thoracoscopic stapled resection for spontaneous pneumothorax. *J Thorac Cardiovasc Surg* 1993;105:389–393.
34. Takeno Y. Thoracoscopic treatment of spontaneous pneumothorax. *Ann Thorac Surg* 1993;56:688–690.
35. Inderbitzi RGC, Leiser A, Furrer M, et al. Three years' experience in video-assisted thoracic surgery (VATS) for spontaneous pneumothorax. *J Thorac Cardiovasc Surg* 1994;107:1410–1415.

36. Cardillo G, Facciolo F, Giunti R, et al. Videothoraco-scopic treatment of primary spontaneous pneumothorax: a 6-year experience. *Ann Thorac Surg* 2000;69:357–361.

37. Yim AP, Liu HP. Video assisted thoracoscopic manage-ment of primary spontaneous pneumothorax. *Surg Laparosc Endosc* 1997;7:236–240.

38. Wait MA. AIDS-related pneumothorax. *Ann Thorac Surg* 1997;64:290–291.

39. Waller DA. Video-assisted thoracoscopic surgery for spontaneous pneumothorax—a 7-year learning experi-ence. *Ann R Coll Surg Engl* 1999;81:387–392.

40. Janssen JP, van Mourik J, Cuesta Valentin M, et al. Treat-ment of patients with spontaneous pneumothorax during videothoracoscopy. *Eur Respir J* 1994;7:1281–1284.

41. Smith RS, Fry WR, Tsoi EK, et al. Preliminary report on videothoracoscopy in the evaluation and treatment of thoracic injury. *Am J Surg* 1993;166:690–693.

42. Villavicencio RT, Aucar JA, Wall MJ Jr. Analysis of tho-racoscopy in trauma. *Surg Endosc* 1999;13:3–9.

43. Carrillo EH, Richardson JD. Thoracoscopy in the man-agement of hemothorax and retained blood after trauma. *Curr Opin Pulm Med* 1998;4:243–246.

44. Kent RB 3d, Pinson TW. Thoracoscopic ligation of the thoracic duct. *Surg Endosc* 1993;7:52–53.

45. Shirai T, Amano J, Takabe K. Thoracoscopic diagnosis and treatment of chylothorax after pneumonectomy. *Ann Thorac Surg* 1991;52:306–307.

46. Zoetmulder F, Rutgers E, Baas P. Thoracoscopic ligation of a thoracic duct leakage. *Chest* 1994;106:1233–1234.

47. Ferguson MK. Thoracoscopy for empyema, bron-chopleural fistula, and chylothorax. *Ann Thorac Surg* 1993;56:644–645.

48. Hazelrigg SR, Nunchuck SK, LoCicero J, and the Video Assisted Thoracic Surgery Study Group. Video assisted thoracic surgery study group data. *Ann Thorac Surg* 1993;56:1039–1044.

49. Jancovici R, Lang-Lazdunski L, Pons F, et al. Complica-tions of video-assisted thoracic surgery: a five-year ex-perience. *Ann Thorac Surg* 1996;61:533–537.

50. Downey RJ, McCormack P, LoCicero J 3rd. Dis-semination of malignant tumors after video-assisted thoracic surgery: a report of twenty-one cases. The Video-Assisted Thoracic Surgery Study Group. *J Tho-rac Cardiovasc Surg* 1996;111:954–960.

Subject Index

Note: Page numbers in *italics* indicate figures; page numbers followed by t indicate tables.